Microbial Cell Factories

Microbial Cell Factories

Edited by
Deepansh Sharma
Baljeet Singh Saharan

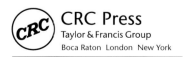

CRC Press
Taylor & Francis Group
Boca Raton London New York

CRC Press is an imprint of the
Taylor & Francis Group, an **informa** business

CRC Press
Taylor & Francis Group
6000 Broken Sound Parkway NW, Suite 300
Boca Raton, FL 33487-2742

First issued in paperback 2020

© 2018 by Taylor & Francis Group, LLC
CRC Press is an imprint of Taylor & Francis Group, an Informa business

No claim to original U.S. Government works

ISBN 13: 978-0-367-65730-7 (pbk)
ISBN 13: 978-1-138-06138-5 (hbk)

Library of Congress Cataloging-in-Publication Data

Names: Sharma, Deepansh, editor. | Saharan, Baljeet Singh, editor.
Title: Microbial cell factories / Deepansh Sharma and Baljeet Singh Saharan, editors.
Other titles: Microbial cell factories (Boca Raton, Fla.)
Description: Boca Raton : Taylor & Francis, CRC Press, 2018. | Includes bibliographical references.
Identifiers: LCCN 2017050618 | ISBN 9781138061385 (hardback : alk. paper)
Subjects: LCSH: Microbial biotechnology. | Industrial microbiology. | Cells, Cultured--Industrial applications.
Classification: LCC TP248.27.M53 M533 2018 | DDC 660.6/2--dc23
LC record available at https://lccn.loc.gov/2017050618

Visit the Taylor & Francis Web site at
http://www.taylorandfrancis.com

and the CRC Press Web site at
http://www.crcpress.com

Contents

v

Preface

Microbial Cell Factories consists of 19 chapters from diverse research groups. Each group exemplifies the development of, research in, and future prospects of microbial cell factories.

Microorganisms, also called microbial cell factories, are now in great demand due to their role as sustainable and healthy food additives; a realistic alternative for agricultural and environmental remedies; and minimization of greenhouse gas emissions by accumulating ethanol as a next-generation energy alternative. The idea of editing a book on *Microbial Cell Factories* came to me after we started working with various microbial strains for food, environmental, and industrial applications. During a vigorous discussion with my Ph.D. supervisor, we came up with the idea of editing a book that would compile the various aspects of microbial cells for environmental, medical, food, and recent industrial applications. We listed some of the major areas of applications of microorganisms to start the first draft of the book and contacted all those who are experts in the area of microbial cell factories. Through their treasured contributions, the expert and encouraging commitments from my dear colleagues and global experts made our hope of completing this book an actuality. Their work and contributions are appreciated and cherished. This compilation of work about various aspects of the microbial world and future advances in the field promises to be an exceptional addition to the captivating field of microbial research. I hope it meets the expectations of the scholars in academia and industry.

We wish to acknowledge the contributing writers of this book for the extraordinary eminence of their work, willingness to accommodate suggestions, and devoting their time to writing chapter-length papers.

We acknowledge Chuck Crumly and Jennifer Blaise for their support in the editing process, and CRC Press/Taylor & Francis Group for publishing this text.

Dr. Deepansh Sharma

Dr. Baljeet Singh Saharan

Editors

Dr. Deepansh Sharma is presently working as assistant professor at the Amity Institute of Microbial Technology, Amity University, Rajasthan, India. He joined the world of academia in 2015 at Lovely Professional University, Phagwara, India, after receiving his doctoral degree in microbiology with a specialization in biosurfactant research. He is M. Phil (Microbiology) from CCS University, Meerut, and M.Sc. (Microbiology) from Gurukula Kangri University, Haridwar, India, with ICAR-ASRB-NET. He has over eight years of research and teaching experience. He has successfully completed several recent food fermentation industrial consultancy projects. Dr. Sharma is a recipient of the DAAD (Germany) short-term fellowship for doctoral studies in Karlsruhe Institute of Technology, Karlsruhe, Germany.

Dr. Sharma has published over 25 research papers and reviews in national and international journals and consortium proceedings along with 5 book chapters on various aspects of the microbial world. He is author of *Biosurfactants of Lactic Acid Bacteria* and *Biosurfactants in Food* (2016) published by Springer International Publishing. His research interests include biosurfactants, bacteriocins, and microbial food additives.

Dr. Baljeet Singh Saharan is presently working as assistant professor in the Department of Microbiology at Kurukshetra University, Kurukshetra, India. He joined the faculty in 2006 after receiving his postdoctoral and doctoral degrees in microbiology. He is MSc (Microbiology) from CCS HAU Hisar and UGC-CSIR-NET and ICAR-ASRB-NET qualified. He has over 16 years of teaching and research experience. He has successfully completed three major research projects financed by the University Grant Commission (UGC), Department of Science and Technology (DST), and Haryana State Council for Science and Technology (HSCST). Dr. Saharan is a recipient of the DAAD (Germany) and Raman (the United States) fellowships for postdoctoral studies in UFZ Leipzig Germany, and Department of Plant Pathology, United States Department of Agriculture, Washington State University, Pullman, Washington, United States, during 2003–2004 and 2013–2014, respectively. He has visited the Helmholtz Centre for Environmental Research—UFZ, Leipzig; Karlsruhe Institute of Technology (KIT), Karlsruhe (Germany); University of Bath, United Kingdom; Natural History Museum, London; University of Zurich, Switzerland; Washington State University, Pullman, Washington, United States; and several other institutions as an honorary guest, distinguished scientist, and adjunct faculty member.

Dr. Baljeet Singh Saharan has published more than 53 research papers and reviews in national and international journals and consortium proceedings. He is co-author of *Biosurfactants of Lactic Acid Bacteria* (2016) published by Springer International Publishing.

He has visited more than 10 countries, including Germany, the United Kingdom, the United States, Switzerland, the Czech Republic, and France, to conduct and/or attend conferences and workshops and to complete scientific assignments. He chaired the November 2015 session during the international conference in London organized by WASET. He is a member of the UG and PG Board of Studies in the Department of Microbiology at Kurukshetra University, Kurukshetra, India. He has supervised over 15 doctoral students pursuing their degrees. His research interests include biosurfactants, bacteriocins, plant-growth-promoting rhizobacteria, and bioremediation.

Contributors

Dipesh Aggarwal
Lady Irwin College
University of Delhi
New Delhi, India

Nahid Akhtar
Department of Molecular Biology and
    Genetics
School of Bioengineering and
    Biosciences
Lovely Professional University
Phagwara, India

Santosh Anand
National Dairy Research Institute
Karnal, India

Mattia Pia Arena
Dipartimento di Scienze degli Alimenti
Facoltà di Agraria
Università degli Studi di Foggia
Foggia, Italy

Ibrahim M. Banat
School of Biomedical Sciences
University of Ulster
Coleraine, North Ireland, United
    Kingdom

Chinnappan Baskar
THDC Institute of Hydropower
    Engineering and Technology Tehri
Uttarakhand Technical University
Dehradun, India

Arun Beniwal
Dairy Microbiology Division
National Dairy Research Institute
Karnal, India

Kaushik Bhattacharjee
Microbiology Laboratory
Department of Biotechnology and
    Bioinformatics
North-Eastern Hill University
Shillong, India

Vittorio Capozzi
Dipartimento di Scienze degli Alimenti
Facoltà di Agraria
Università degli Studi di Foggia
Foggia, Italy

Arun Chauhan
Department of Zoology
School of Bioengineering and
    Biosciences
Lovely Professional University
Phagwara, India

Anila Fariq
Microbiology & Biotechnology
    Research Lab
Department of Environmental Sciences
Fatima Jinnah Women University
Rawalpindi, Pakistan

Daniela Fiocco
Dipartimento di Medicina Clinica e
    Sperimentale
Polo Biomedico E. Altomare
Università degli Studi di Foggia
Foggia, Italy

Rajesh Gopaul
Microbial Biosensors and Food Safety
    Laboratory
Dairy Microbiology Division
ICAR-National Dairy Research Institute
Karnal, India

S. R. Joshi
Microbiology Laboratory
Department of Biotechnology and
    Bioinformatics
North-Eastern Hill University
Shillong, India

Shailly Kapil
Whey Fermentation and Bio-Active
    Peptide Laboratory
Dairy Microbiology Division
National Dairy Research Institute
Karnal, India

Robinka Khajuria
School of Bioengineering and
    Biosciences
Lovely Professional University
Phagwara, India

Ajay Kumar
Department of Bioengineering and
    Biosciences
Lovely Professional University
Phagwara, India

Gaurav Kumar
Department of Microbiology
School of Bioengineering and
    Biosciences
Lovely Professional University
Phagwara, India

Naresh Kumar
Microbial Biosensors and Food Safety
    Laboratory
Dairy Microbiology Division
ICAR-National Dairy Research
    Institute
Karnal, India

Navneet Kumar
Department of Biochemistry
School of Bioengineering and
    Biosciences
Lovely Professional University
Phagwara, India

Sanjeev Kumar
Department of Genetics and Plant
    Breeding
School of Agriculture
Lovely Professional University
Phagwara, India

Vineet Kumar
Department of Environmental
    Microbiology
School for Environmental Sciences
Babasaheb Bhimrao Ambedkar
    University
Lucknow, India

Shriya Mehta
Functional Fermented Foods and
    Bioactive Peptides Lab
Dairy Microbiology Division
National Dairy Research Institute
Karnal, India

Jagrani Minj
Functional Fermented Foods and
    Bioactive Peptides Lab
Dairy Microbiology Division
National Dairy Research Institute
Karnal, India

Shayanti Minj
Functional Fermented Foods and
    Bioactive Peptides Lab
Dairy Microbiology Division
National Dairy Research Institute
Karnal, India

Monika
Department of Microbiology
School of Bioengineering and
    Biosciences
Lovely Professional University
Phagwara, India

H. V. Raghu
Microbial Biosensors and Food Safety
    Laboratory
Dairy Microbiology Division
ICAR-National Dairy Research Institute
Karnal, India

Pasquale Russo
Dipartimento di Scienze degli Alimenti
Facoltà di Agraria
Università degli Studi di Foggia
Foggia, Italy

Priyanka Saini
Dairy Microbiology Division
National Dairy Research Institute
Karnal, India

Surekha K. Satpute
Department of Microbiology
Institute of Bioinformatics &
    Biotechnology
Savitribai Phule Pune University
Pune, India

Amarish Kumar Sharma
Department of Bioengineering and
    Biosciences
Lovely Professional University
Phagwara, India

Anjana Rana Sharma
Department of Bioengineering and
    Biosciences
Lovely Professional University
Phagwara, India

Deepansh Sharma
Lovely Professional University
Phagwada, India

Pradip Kumar Sharma
Microbial Biosensors and Food Safety
    Laboratory
Dairy Microbiology Division
ICAR-National Dairy Research
    Institute
Karnal, India

Joginder Singh
Department of Bioengineering and
    Biosciences
Lovely Professional University
Phagwara, India

Kumar Siddharth Singh
Lovely Professional University
Phagwara, India

Rahul Singh
Department of Zoology
School of Bioengineering and
    Biosciences
Lovely Professional University
Phagwara, India

Shalini Singh
School of Bioengineering and
    Biosciences
Lovely Professional University
Phagwara, India

Giuseppe Spano
Dipartimento di Scienze degli
    Alimenti
Facoltà di Agraria
Università degli Studi di Foggia
Foggia, Italy

Nimisha Tehri
Microbial Biosensors and Food Safety
   Laboratory
Dairy Microbiology Division
ICAR-National Dairy Research
   Institute
Karnal, India

Shilpa Vij
Dairy Microbiology Division
National Dairy Research Institute
Karnal, India

Pratibha Vyas
Microbiology Domain
School of Bioengineering and
   Biosciences
Lovely Professional University
Phagwara, India

Shivani Yadav
Department of Genetics and Plant
   Breeding
School of Agriculture
Lovely Professional University
Phagwara, India

Azra Yasmin
Microbiology & Biotechnology
   Research Lab
Department of Environmental
   Sciences
Fatima Jinnah Women University
Rawalpindi, Pakistan

Smita S. Zinjarde
Institute of Bioinformatics &
   Biotechnology
Savitribai Phule Pune University
Pune, India

1 Recent Updates on Biosurfactants in the Food Industry

Surekha K. Satpute, Smita S. Zinjarde, and Ibrahim M. Banat

CONTENTS

INTRODUCTION

Surfactants and emulsifiers have gained a large market share during the past few decades that seems to be growing with a compound annual growth rate estimate of 6% (Markets and Markets, 2016). Along with synthetic surfactant, biosurfactants (BSs) and bioemulsifiers (BEs) are also beginning to create their own commercial demand with a compound annual growth rate forecast of 8%–9% (Markets and Markets, 2016). In industry terms, it is crucial to accentuate that the use of renewable substrates tender immense competition with other markets (Satpute et al., 2017). Nature offers us several different BSs/BEs from diverse origins having varied structural and functional diversity. Saponin obtained from soap nuts (*Sapindus mukorosi*) (Ghagi et al., 2011), cereals (soya, wheat, and oats), lecithin from egg yolk and other proteins, casein, gelatin, wax, cholesterol, and so on are some representative examples. Among the different plant-based surfactants, lecithin has been a widely explored, natural,

1

low-molecular-weight BS used for industrial purposes (Dickinson, 1993). The type II alveolar cells in our own lungs produce a phospholipoprotein-based surfactant to facilitate breathing and gaseous exchange. Infants lacking the ability to produce surfactant suffer from respiratory distress syndrome (Xu et al., 2011). In addition to plant- and animal-produced BSs/BEs, microorganisms represent some of the most suitable candidates for production of diverse forms of surface-active compounds.

When we consider the microbial-originated BSs/BEs, the available global literature reflects great diversity with respect to structure, composition, and properties. This wide diversity among BSs/BEs therefore offers huge applications not only in the food industry (Kralova and Sjöblom, 2009; Mnif and Ghribi, 2016; Sharma et al., 2016) but also in bioremediation (Satpute et al., 2005; Sáenz-Marta et al., 2015), agriculture (Sachdev and Cameotra, 2013), medicine (Rodrigues et al., 2006; Santos et al., 2016), and cosmetics and pharmaceuticals (Fracchia et al., 2010). In addition to the naturally available BSs/BEs, humanmade synthetic surfactants, namely, sodium dodecyl sulfate (SDS), aerosol-OT (AOT), cetytrimethyl bromide (CTAB), Triton derivatives, Sorbitan esters (also known as Spans, Tween, etc.), have been exploited extensively for various commercial applications. However, considering their toxic, nonbiodegradable nature they are not eco-friendly in nature), synthetic surfactants are not the preferred choice for biological-based applications and/or green sustainability (Kourkoutas and Banat, 2004; Campos et al., 2013).

BSs/BEs have been utilized in a variety of food formulations, preparations, and dressings as food additives. BSs like rhamnolipids (RHLs), surfactin, and sophorolipids (SLs) have been exploited in various food preparations. Presently, BS-based products are frequently seen in the market. For example, JBRR products coming from Jeneil Biosurfactant Co. US sell RHLs in different aqueous solutions of different purity levels as biofungicide. The RHL products have been proved with great potential for numerous uses. Understanding the promising implication of RHL, the United States Environmental Protection Agency (USEPA) has permitted the broad use of RHL in or on all food merchandises. RHL is anticipated to avoid and regulate zoosporic, pathogenic fungi found on horticultural and agricultural harvests (Nitschke and Costa SGVAO, 2007; ZONIX Biofungicide, 2012). The literature also depicts the frequent use of lactic acid bacterial–originated BS/BE from the genus *Lactobacillus* genus due to their benefits in the food industry. This chapter deals with different properties of BSs/BEs, for example, their antimicrobial, antibiofilm, antiadhesive, and nonfouling features, which are finding special services and application for the food industry. A brief description of actual and potential uses of different BSs/BEs in various sectors of the food industry and inclusion in different food formulations available in the market are detailed. Discussion on utilization of certain food and food wastes for BS production is also included.

DIVERSE BIOLOGICAL–FUNCTIONAL ALLIED PROPERTIES OF BIOSURFACTANTS/BIOEMULSIFIERS

The amphiphilic (hydrophilic and hydrophobic) nature of BSs/BEs confers unique properties, such as the ability to reduce surface and interfacial tension. Other interesting properties such as aggregation, cleansing, emulsification, foaming, wetting,

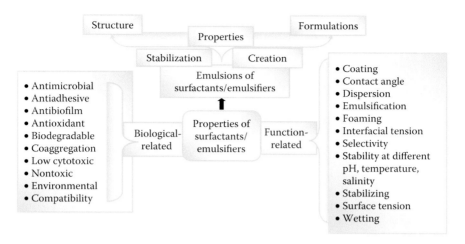

FIGURE 1.1 Representation of various biological and functional properties of biosurfactant (BS)/bioemulsifiers (BE) to be considered for potential applications.

phase separation, surface activity, and reduction in oil viscosity permit their exploitation in various industries. The diversity of their microbial origin—for example fungi (Zinjarde and Pant, 2002; Rufino et al., 2014), bacteria (Satpute et al., 2016), and actinomycetes (Zambry et al., 2017)—gives BSs/BEs wide structural, compositional, and functional properties. Figure 1.1 shows the main characteristics most BSs/BEs may have to be considered *surfactant* or *emulsifier*. However, it is not suggested that all the properties mentioned in Figure 1.1 are shared by all surfactant- or emulsifier-type compounds. Their basic structural organization is the main reason for their differences. The molecules with such diverse properties provide a broad range of applications and are therefore motivating researchers worldwide.

ROLE OF ADDITIVES IN FOOD PREPARATIONS/ DRESSINGS/FORMULATIONS

The use of flavoring and preserving substances in food has been a routine practice for maintaining good quality of foods since ancient times. Good flavor, rich nutrition, safety, and appealing appearance were always minimum criteria to be fulfilled in food products. In addition, cost and affordability are always main concerns for food. Many additives/ingredients are in use by the food industries, and customers today have become quite demanding in their current food requirements and constituents. We have become much more conscious of food products with regard to safety and originality. Some additives like pentosanases, hydrocolloids, and enzymes (amylases, lipases, hemicellulases, etc.) are used intensively to improve the texture and consistency of food. Other additional benefits from additives include enhancing freshness and increasing shelf life (Mnif et al., 2012). Here are some important points that should be considered during formulating any preparations in the food industry:

1. *Maintaining freshness*: We are aware of the hazardous effect of food-borne diseases; botulism is one of those life-threatening toxins of microbial origin. The use of antioxidants as preservatives is quite common for preventing oxidation of oils and fats in food and thus delaying or reducing the development of bad flavor.

2. *Safety maintenance*: Food products are subject to spoilage caused by the presence of various microorganisms like bacteria, yeast, fungi, molds, and actinomycetes. Air is an important source and facilitator of microbial growth in food products. Therefore, retaining the desired quality of the food is quite challenging, and making food safe is a major concern for all food products used for human and animal consumption.

3. *Improvement and maintenance of nutritional value*: Most food products contain several minerals, vitamins, fibers, sugars, fats, and proteins that ultimately affects their utilization and nutritive value. Under certain circumstances, additional nutritional components may have to be added to enrich the nutritional value of the food products; however, retaining the quality and taste of food is highly critical in performing such alterations.

4. *Enhancing the texture and appearance*: The addition of naturally available spices and sweeteners often improves the taste of various food products, and coloring agents are generally included to improve the appearance and appeal to consumers. In addition to spices and sweeteners, emulsifiers, stabilizers, and thickeners are used to achieve the desired homogeneity, rheological behavior, appearance, texture, acidity, and alkalinity of food (Kourkoutas and Banat, 2004).

USE OF SURFACTANTS/EMULSIFIERS IN THE FOOD INDUSTRY

Emulsifier and surfactant compounds are not new to the food industry and have been routinely used in the formulation of numerous food products over the centuries. Dairy producers, producers of fermented foods, bakeries, and breweries regularly use synthetic and natural emulsifiers and surfactants. In most dairy-based products like milk, curd, cheese, and cream, food-grade surfactants/emulsifiers are always permissible. Other products like salad, dressings, mayonnaise, deserts, and so on are often supplemented with such compounds to improve their flavor, appearance, and storage rather than as nutritional aids. Other properties that are conferred by BSs are stabilization of flavor oils and property improvement in bakery and dairy formulations (Kosaric, 2001; Kosaric and Sukan, 2014). Monoglycerides, for examples, are currently utilized as emulsifiers for numerous food products; synthetic surfactants like sorbitan esters and their ethoxylate derivatives have been added to many food products (Hasenhuettl, 2008; Tadros, 2013, 2016).

Understanding the various properties of surfactants/emulsifiers is essential to exploit them for wider industrial applications. Low-molecular-weight compounds like monoglycerides, lecithins, glycolipids, and fatty alcohols effectively reduce surface and also interfacial tension. High-molecular-weight compounds mostly composed of protein, polysaccharide-type molecules facilitate stabilization of emulsions (Satpute et al., 2010a,b). Under these circumstances, electrostatic interactions promote effective penetrating power. Different kinds of foods represent colloidal systems consisting of various forms of aggregations made up of particles and drops, thus giving the appearance of "gels." Surfactant and polymer molecules aggregate due to a number of interactions, including van der Waals forces and repulsive forces. The mechanisms are absolutely suitable for foods with oil and fat content. Reduction in surface tension aids formation of emulsions between immiscible phases and improves the texture.

Similar mechanisms are also seen in the formation of foam in liquid systems having surface-active molecules (Campos et al., 2013). A food formulation determines various phases among particles (Kralova and Sjöblom, 2009). Basically three major types of emulsions are important in a variety of foods, as shown in Figure 1.2.

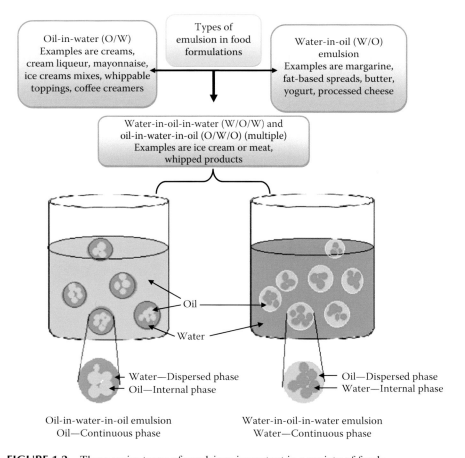

FIGURE 1.2 Three major types of emulsions important in a variety of foods.

This precise structural organization of surfactant molecules empowers surface active agents and emulsifiers to quintessence at the oil/water (O/W) interphase, leading to an increase in the thermodynamic stability of an unstable system (Berton-Carabin et al., 2014). Emulsifiers get their emulsifying abilities from their amphiphilic nature, making it feasible to mold with starchy and proteins fractions of food products. BSs/BEs competently emulsify and homogenize the partially digested fatty fractions. The emulsifier becomes associated with protein fractions of food ingredients, leading to their aggregations (Mnif et al., 2012). Mannoprotein-producing *Saccharomyces cerevisiae* facilitates the stabilization of O/W emulsions for products like ice creams and mayonnaise (Cameron et al., 1988; Moreira et al., 2016). More complex duplex and multiple emulsions, such as water in oil in water (W/O/W) and oil in water in oil (O/W/O), are also achievable (Figure 1.2).

The purpose of adding BSs/BEs is mainly to alter or retain certain chemical (pH, temperature, and taste), biological (safe for consumption), and physical (constancy and appearance) features unique to food products that undergo several procedures like preparation, processing, manufacturing, storage, packaging, handling, and transport. Extensive use of carboxymethyl cellulose and glyceryl monostearate is a regular practice. The emulsification properties of BSs/BEs chiefly used as thickening, stabilizing, and gelling agents cannot be ignored when considering them for food applications. These products dramatically affect the texture and consistency of foods. At the same time, other interesting parameters, including phase dispersion and aroma solubilization, are also influenced by the emulsification phenomena and characteristics of emulsifiers. The main objective of emulsion stabilization is achieved by the aggregation of the fat globules by the emulsifier and the stabilizing aerated systems. Thus, two heterogenous systems are homogenized, and the SFT reduces energy between the two phases, preventing particles coalescence (Berton-Carabin et al., 2014).

Cream, margarine, mayonnaise, butter, chocolate, and salad dressing require extensive use of emulsifiers (Nitschke and Costa SGVAO, 2007). The best example is RHL in the preparation of frozen pastries and cream filling for Danish pastries by adding in sufficient amount. L-Rhamnose is already used as a high-quality flavor compound (Van Haesendonck and Vanzeveren, 2002). In addition to bakery products, RHL also helps in improving the properties of dairy products like butter cream and frozen products (Van Haesendonck and Vanzeveren, 2004). BE from *Candida utilis* is used in salad dressings and is proving to be highly useful for innovative texture modifications. BEs (e.g., liposan) with good emulsification properties can be used successfully to emulsify commercial edible oils (Shepherd et al., 1995). Most BEs, particularly those of high molecular weight, exhibit superior stabilizing behavior compared to carboxymethlyl cellulose and Arabic acid. Excellent alterations are displayed due to the addition of BSs/BEs in food (Marchant and Banat, 2012). BEs isolated from *Enterobacter cloaceae* works as a viscosity enhancer, which allows their use in low-pH-acid-containing products like ascorbic acid and citric acid (Iyer et al., 2006). Even though several reports discuss BS/BE production, a small number of BSs/BEs have been studied specifically for food products at commercial scale.

DIMINUTION OF ADHESION AND ERADICATION
OF BIOFILM FORMERS FROM FOOD PRODUCTS
WITH THE AID OF BIOSURFACTANTS/BIOEMULSIFIERS

The applications of microbial surfactants is well established in a range of food formulations, dressings, and food processing. In addition to surface-active properties, their antiadhesive, antimicrobial, and antibiofilm properties make BSs extra special molecules. Table 1.1 summarizes different BSs that exhibit potential activities against pathogens. It is important to highlight that BSs/BEs represent a new generation of food additives as well as antiadhesive agents. The noteworthy application of BSs/BEs in food formulations are as agglomeration of fat molecules, which ultimately extends the shelf life of food. Other properties like rheological behavior and the texture of dough are also improved in oil- and fat-based food dressings and formulations (Guerra-Santos et al., 1984). Well-explored glycolipid type BSs, namely RHL and sophorolipids (SLs), have enriched salad dressings and sweet/confectionary preparations (Guerra-Santos et al., 1986). In the case of meat products, BSs proficiently emulsify the partially digested fatty molecules. Another interesting role played by BSs/BEs for food products is impeding the growth of harmful microbial biofilms. Thus, microbial colonization has been successfully prevented and/or removed through application of various kinds of BSs/BEs. The production of microbial biofilms through secretion of extracellular polysaccharides (EPSs) leads to severe spoilage of food (Sharma and Malik, 2012). Therefore, defensive procedures are important to reduce the adherence and establishment of pathogens in and on food surfaces. The role of microbial-originated surfactants in biofilm disruption and/or prevention has become an important topic related to food and pharmaceutical applications.

Preconditioning of inanimate surfaces with popular BSs like surfactin and RHL successfully prevents the adhesion of food-spoiling and pathogenic bacteria. Both types of BSs effectively disrupt preformed biofilms (Gomes et al., 2012). RHL and surfactin have been proved to inhibit the adhesion of *Listeria monocytogenes* on polystyrene surfaces. The effective role of surfactin in reducing the adhesion of *L. monocytogenes* on stainless steel and polypropylene is well accepted (Nitschke et al., 2009). Polystyrene is used extensively in various food industries, and its surfaces are frequently exposed to food; hence, development of biofilm on such surfaces raises the risk of food contamination. Like polystyrene, metallic surfaces have been tested to prevent microbial colonization of pathogens. Meylheuc et al. (2006) tested two types of BSs, namely, Pf (*P. fluorescens*) and Lh (*L. helveticus*) against biofilms formed by *L. monocytogenes* on stainless steel surfaces. Such experimental design supports antiadhesive biological coating abilities of BSs on different surfaces. Research contributed by Zeraik and Nitschke (2010) describes the effects of surfactin and RHL against attachment of *Staphylococcus aureus*, *Micrococcus luteus*, and *L. monocytogenes* on polystyrene surfaces. Even after surface-conditioning tests, including high-temperature treatment, surfactin displays an antiadhesive activity and therefore is suitable as an antiadhesive agent to protect various surfaces from pathogens. De Araujo et al. (2011) investigated the adhesion profiles of biofilm-forming strains and reported that both BSs effectively reduce

TABLE 1.1
Summary for Biosurfactants/Bioemulsifiers Exhibiting Potential Activity against Pathogens

Biosurfactant/ Bioemulsifier	Potential Activity	Used Against	References
Rhamnolipid	• Increasing shelf life of fruit	Inhibiting bacteria, molds, fungi growth	Dilarri et al. (2016)
Rhamnolipid	• Antimicrobial activity	Inhibiting the growth of gram positive and gram negative bacteria and yeasts	Al-Asady et al. (2016)
Glycolipid from marine actinobacterium *Brachybacterium paraconglomeratum*	• Antibacterial activities	*S. aureus, B. subtilis, C. albicans, K. pneumonia, Mi. luteus, S. epidermidis, E. faecalis, P. aeruginosa, E. coli, P. mirabilis*	Kiran et al. (2014)
Glycolipid *Streptomyces*	• Antimicrobial activities	*B. megaterium, B. cereus, S. aureus, E. faecalis, Salmonella shigella, S. dysenteriae, S. boydii, C. albicans, A. niger*	Haba et al. (2014)
Surfactin and rhamnolipid	• Removing biofilms, • Modifying surface properties	*S. aureus, L. monocytogenes, S. Enteritidis*	Gomes and Nitschke (2012)
Rhamnolipid	• Antimicrobial activity	*C. albicans* and *S. aureus*	Manivasagan et al. (2014)
Rhamnolipid	• Antifungal activity	*Botrytis* sp. *Rhizoctonia* sp. *Pythium* sp. *Phytophtora* sp., *Plasmopara* sp.	Vatsa et al. (2010)
Rhamnolipids	• Inhibits spore germination and mycelial growth protection of vines	*Botrytis cinerea*	Varnier et al. (2009)
Bacillus licheniformis VS16	• Antibacterial activities • Inhibiting biofilm formation • Removal of cadmium (Cd) from vegetables	*Brevibacterium casei, Nocardiopsis, Vibrio alginolyticus*	Giri et al. (2017)

the attachment of biofilm formers. In fact, RHL strongly impedes the adherence of *L. monocytogenes*. This work demonstrated the usefulness and effectiveness of this approach in controlling the growth of bacterial populations formed during biofilm formation.

Food, fermentation, medical, and environmental industries are all concerned with the attachment of bacteria to surfaces and consequent biofilm formation. The occurrence of biofilm in food-processing areas can lead to food spoilage and the transmission of dreaded diseases, resulting in health concerns and greater risks.

Salmonella enteritidis and *Staphylococcus aureus* are known as prominent food-borne pathogens. Various platforms and surfaces, like plastics, glass, stainless steel, and rubber, are generally affected by the growth of biofilm-forming microorganisms. The economic losses resulting from such circumstances are very high for the food industry (Simões et al., 2010).

Like medical industries, various food industries are severely affected due to colonization of pathogenic organisms. Since food is directly consumed by humans, it has serious health implications. Food materials are rich with carbon, nitrogen, vitamins, and minerals, and a wide variety of microorganisms can easily grow in and on food surfaces. It is highly impossible to eradicate well-established microbial biofilms. This is the way microbial biofilms prove to be one of the foremost sources of food contamination (Zhang et al., 2008). Researchers have concentrated on tackling this challenging situation through use of lactic acid bacteria (LABs) or probiotic microorganisms and their BSs/BEs to fight against microbial growth on inert surfaces (Sharma et al., 2015; Satpute et al., 2016). LAB-derived BSs/BEs have been cherished as antimicrobial, antiadhesive, antibiofilm agents to eliminate the colonization of dangerous organisms. This issue is discussed in more detail in the next section.

The use of BSs/BEs on any surface alters the hydrophobicity of the surface and in turn interferes with adhesion of microbial mats. Recent research illustrates the active role of LAB-derived BS for antibiofilm properties (Sharma and Saharan, 2014, 2016; Sharma et al., 2015). BSs obtained from microbes of dairy origin are found to be useful in removal of established biofilms through changes in the morphology of developed microbial mats. A xylolipid-type BS produced by *Lactococcus lactis* exhibits remarkable antibacterial activity against several clinical pathogens. The organism *L. lactis* was isolated from a fermented dairy preparation by Saravanakumari and Mani (2010). Thus, such nontoxic BSs are completely safe for human and animal health. The BSs obtained from LABs appear to be very effective against multidrug-resistant microorganisms (Falagas and Makris, 2009). The unique properties of BSs/BEs thus offer exceptional antimicrobial, antiadhesive, emulsifying, and antibiofilm characteristics. Thus, BSs/BEs create possibilities for further improvisation in the food products in more positive ways.

USE OF LACTIC ACID BACTERIA FOR BIOSURFACTANT/BIOEMULSIFIER PRODUCTION

LABs are a noteworthy group of organisms that contribute toward natural microbiota of human's genitourinary and gastrointestinal tracts. Thus, they play a key role in maintaining homeostasis within those habitats by preventing colonization by pathogenic microorganisms. LABs are represented as probiotic agents, suggesting that the consumption of live microbial preparations in sufficient quantity confers innumerable health benefits to the consumer. LABs successfully impede the growth of pathogens through production of various antibacterial compounds, including bacteriocins, lactic acid, and hydrogen peroxide. In addition to all those molecules, LABs also secrete cell-bound or cell-associated BSs/BEs (Satpute et al., 2016). The food-based industries have comprehensively explored lactic acid–producing strains of *Lactobacilli*, among several other metabolites. The global literature depicts BS-producing LABs as useful strains to be exploited commercially in various formulations (Sharma and Saharan, 2014; Sharma et al., 2015).

Streptococcus thermophilus releases BS that detaches previously existing adhered cells and makes an antiadhesive coating on a substratum. In addition, BSs have the capacity to be adsorbed by heat exchanger plates in pasteurizers and impede aggregation of microorganisms. Thermoresistant microorganisms are known to form heavy deposits in different sections of pasteurizer plants, which lead the development of fouling. The growth of thermoresistant microbes ultimately affects the quality, texture, and appearance of dairy products. It also depletes nutritional value. The fouling deposits are also responsible for the diminished efficiency of heat transfer in pasteurizing plants. Therefore, it is essential to control fouling in heat-exchanger pasteurizing systems (Busscher et al., 1996). *S. thermophilus is* one of the well-identified, fouling-forming thermoresistant bacteria. Heavy biofilm formation is observed more often in pasteurized milk than in raw milk (which may contain some inhibitory compounds). As the growth of *S. thermophilus* continues, the well-established cells are progressively detached, giving the appearance of a clean surface. Newly cultured organisms cannot adhere to the surface. This might be happening due to production of BS by adhering *S. thermophilus*, which does not allow the organisms to deposit and develop the colonization. In fact, *S. thermophilus* cells are well known for their own detachment, through release and further adsorption of BSs (Busscher et al., 1990).

Among LABs, several species of *Lactobacillus* are used in combination with *Streptococcus* for forming a range of dairy-based products. Due to their acid and flavor production capabilities, they are the preferred bacteria among LAB. *Lactobacilli* species have been explored thoroughly for production of BS. Generally, *L. acidophilus*, *L. brevis*, *L. plantarum*, *L ruteri*, *L. rhamnosus*, *L. acidophilus*, *L. pentosus*, *L. fermentum*, and *L. casei* are known for BS/BE production. Although *Lactobacilli* species have been known for some time for BS production, complete characterization of their BSs appears to be challenging as they basically appear to be a multicomponent mixture containing various percentages of protein and polysaccharides. Therefore, it has been tedious to predict the complete structure of BSs produced by *Lactobacillus* spp. BSs produced by *lactobacilli* especially reduce the adherence abilities of pathogens on surfaces and thus prevent their proliferation and biofilm formation (Satpute et al., 2016b). Due to the presence of antimicrobial activities, BSs interfere with the adhesion mechanisms of pathogens to urogenital and intestinal tract epithelial cells. As a result, BSs derived from *Lactobacillus* spp. can function as antibiofilm agents. About 46 articles have reported on production of BSs from *Lactobacilli* spp., and they can be broadly classified as cell-free, and cell-associated or cell-bound. Among all 46 reports, 40 came from cell-associated BS type, and merely half of those reports discussed their detailed composition. A survery of the literature survey reveals that glycolipidic, proteinaceous, gycoproteins, or glycolipopeptides-type BSs are produced from several *Lactobacilli* spp. Most BSs are of the proteinaceous type and are therefore generally termed as surlactin. Most of the cell-associated and cell-bound BS types are specially known for their antibiofilm and antiadhesive properties (Rodrigues et al., 2006; Walencka et al., 2008). We are frequently responsive with harmless nature of the genus *Lactobacillus*; however, certain strains may prove to be pathogenic under certain circumstances.

It is important to highlight that the protein and polysaccharide components of BSs obtained from *Lactobacilli* spp. are altered because of changes in the composition of the fermentation medium, pH, temperature and time of incubation, inoculum volume, as well as the growth phase of bacteria (Fouad et al., 2010). Yeast extract is responsible for the growth of bacteria used in the fermentation process; at the same time, peptone is essential for synthesis of BS. Gudiña et al. (2011) showed that the use of peptone and meat extract can result in a large amount of BS production in comparison with De-Man, Rogosa, and Sharpe medium, which is used regularly used for cultivation, production, and purification of BS from *Lactobacilli* spp. (De Man et al., 1960). The addition of manganese and magnesium has been proved to support bacterial growth and production of surlactin-, protein-rich BS (Fracchia et al., 2010). In addition to growth supplements, environmental parameters like pH and temperature also establish the type and activity of BS (Gudiña et al., 2010).

ROLE OF FOOD AND FOOD WASTE IN PRODUCTION OF BIOSURFACTANTS/BIOEMULSIFIERS

The routine use of various cheap and renewable waste substrates from dairies, distilleries, agriculture, animal fat processing, the food processing industry, oil processing mills, and the fruit processing industry represents rich sources for several oils, sugars, minerals, and vitamins. In spite of this, the lower yield of BS at commercial scale is a major concern. High monetary inputs are indispensable in order to drive large-scale fermentation processes. To some extent, use of renewable substrates has provided some relief against the cost-related issues (Banat et al., 2014).

Among different dairy-based products, cheese whey seems to be very popular alternative substrates. Maximum work documents the use of cheese whey for BS production at industrial scale. Rodrigues and Teixeira (2008) reported *L. pentosus* CECT-4023 as a strong BS-producing strain on whey cheese. Gudiña et al. (2015) demonstrated BS production from different *Lactobacillus* strains on conventional MRS medium, which is well known for growth and production of BS from lactic acid bacteria. Glycoprotein-type BS produced by *L. agilis* reduces SFT up to 42.5 mN/m, with an emulsification activity (E24) of 60% with the utilization of cheese whey as a culture medium. BS production by *L. agilis* was enhanced from 84 to 960 mg/L. BS does exhibit substantial antiadhesive activity against *S. aureus*. Some BSs also possess antimicrobial activity against bacterial pathogens like *S. aureus*, *S. agalactiae*, and *P. aeruginosa*. Such studies are applicable for inhibition of the adherence of pathogens on biomedical devices. The abundant availability of agricultural residues has drawn the attention of several researchers for use in BS production processes. However, agriculture residues frequently need prior treatments, including acid hydrolysis and thermal treatment, before their actual use in fermentation industries. These steps provide predigested substrates, which can be utilized efficiently by organisms considered in the different fermentation processes.

Surfactin production from *Bacillus* spp. is widespread; newer substrates have been tested by several investigators. Portilla-Rivera et al. (2007a,b, 2008) and Paradelo et al. (2009) reported the use of agriculture-based digested substrates for growing this bacterial system efficiently and found them suitable for the same. *L. pentosus* grows and produces BSs on grape marc hydrolysates and is efficient in the reduction of water repellence of hydrophobic material, which is superior in comparison to synthetic surfactants. In addition, sugars from vineyard pruning waste have been tested for large-scale production of BS from *Lactobacillus* spp. Such production would reduce environmental impacts from the disposal of waste material (Moldes et al., 2013).

BIOSURFACTANT-/BIOEMULSIFIER-BASED FOOD FORMULATIONS AND OTHER APPLICATIONS

Diverse emulsifiers have been previously tested to improve the texture of crumbs, bread volume, and dough rheological proprieties. Edible-grade emulsifiers provide strength and softness to crumbs. BS is continuously utilized by bread makers. Thus, emulsifiers greatly affect the functional properties of wheat bread. BS obtained from *B. subtilis* SPB1 improves the quality and shelf life of bread (Mnif et al., 2012). The authors have claimed that results are quite interesting with respect to improvement in shape and also superior specific volume and voided fraction of loaves in comparison to soya lecithin, a well-known commercial surfactant. The BE SPB1 noticeably improves the texture profiles of bread when a concentration of 0.075% (w/w) is applied. In addition, it also leads to decreased chewiness and firmness along with adhesion values. The BE SPB1 increases cohesion for bread compared with soya lecithin. The emulsifier results in a strong protein network and enhances the gas retention ability of dough during fermentation, thereby increasing the volume of bread. Hydrophilic emulsifiers encourage the formation of lamellar liquid-crystalline phases in water. Van Haesendonck and Vanzeveren (2002) have filed a patent on the use of RHL to enhance dough or batter stability and the dough texture of bakery products. RHL also has a positive effect on properties of butter cream, fresh or frozen sweet, decoration cream, and so on. The composition of a liquid, powder, or emulsion having RHL works synergistically to lengthen the emulsion stability of the dough or batter. Lactic acid esters of monoglycerides, diglycerides, and glycerides of fatty acids can be substituted by RHL for various dairy and nondairy products.

BSs are now used for synthesis and/or capping agents for green nanoparticles (NPs) (Kiran et al., 2010a,b; Kumar et al., 2010). The appearance of such reports encourages more research in this area. *P. aeruginosa* produces RHL-mediated silver NPs (Kumar et al., 2010). Such preparations are facilitated in a water-in-oil microemulsion system (Xie et al., 2006). Another *P. aeruginosa* strain, namely, NaBH 4, demonstrates the synthesis of RHL reverse micelles. A review of the global literature reveals that maximum work is reported on RHL-mediated NP synthesis. NiO NP has been synthesized by using a microemulsion system in heptane (Palanisamy et al., 2009). Rods of ZnS nanoparticles are formulated by using the capping agents (Narayanan et al., 2010). Other microbial systems, like *Brevibacterium casei,* have been used for glycolipid-based formulations in combination with Ag NP. Like RHL, surfactin can stabilize gold and silver NPs (Reddy et al., 2009) and cadmium sulfide NPs (Singh et al., 2011). Other types of BS, like mannosylerythritol lipids (MELs), exhibit self-assembling capacities and are therefore suitable candidates for diverse properties (Kitamoto et al., 2009). Thus, BSs represent a "green" alternative for synthesis as well as stabilization of metal NPs, and they have proved to be effective for various applications.

REMOVAL OF HEAVY METALS FROM FOOD BY USING BIOSURFACTANTS

The presence of heavy metals in food products is extremely hazardous when health-related issues are concerned. The variety of plant, its growth phase, the soil condition, and the presence of heavy metals in the surrounding environment are the parameters in determining the uptake of heavy metals. Therefore, it is essential to keep track of their presence and accumulation in and on food surfaces to prevent damage that could be caused by these heavy metals. To date, efforts have been directed toward treating wastewater plants near food industries. Newer technologies are definitely trying to tackle the heavy metal contamination issues. Nevertheless, no guaranteed solutions have been proposed to eradicate the heavy metal contamination of foods. The available methodologies are ineffective and expensive (Hidayati et al., 2014).

Ionic surfactants bind to heavy metals via ion exchange phenomena and are precipitated. Thus, the metals are removed in the form of aggregates (Wang and Mulligan, 2004); see Figure 1.3. An amalgamation procedure using foam technology and BS also seems to be interesting. The capacity of RHL in the formation of microemulsion results in efficient removal of heavy metals in comparison with plain distilled water and/or surfactant solution (Mulligan and Wang, 2006). Based on the literature, it can be proposed that heavy metals form complexes with BSs on food surfaces similar to the soil surface, and they finally are separated from food and remain in the surrounding solution. BSs predominantly of anionic type i.e. (RHL) can efficiently remove positively charged metals because of surface activity between BS and metal (Xu et al., 2011).

Work carried out by Anjum et al. (2016) is significant because it reports successful removal of cadmium (Cd) (up to 70%) from various vegetables like potato, radish, garlic, and onion by using surfactin isolated from *Bacillus* sp. MTCC 5877. The BSs are capable of removing heavy metals from contaminated food material. In addition, BSs have the capacity to reduce biofilm formation and therefore can prevent the adherence of microbes from various surfaces. Another recent work published by Giri et al. (2017) demonstrated that BS derived from *B. licheniformis* VS16 is capable of removing Cd from carrot, ginger, radish, and potato; it can also inhibit biofilms of various pathogenic organisms. BSs find definite applications in food industry at the commercial level. Thus, surface-active molecules definitely assist in cleaning the environmental pollutants.

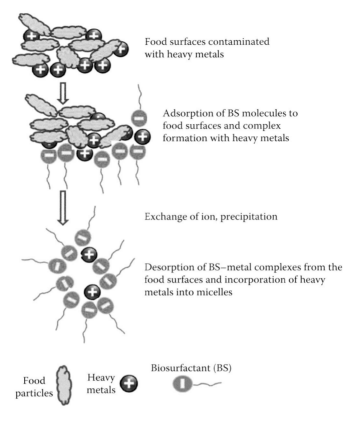

FIGURE 1.3 Mechanism of heavy metal removal by biosurfactant from food surfaces. Note: The different properties of BS like hydrophobicity, molecular size, solubility, flexibility, and surface charge do impart during interaction all above interactions with heavy metals.

ROLE OF BIOSURFACTANTS IN FOOD-PROCESSING SANITATION

Well-known facts about food spoilage caused by microorganisms compel explorations for new techniques to tackle the food spoilage challenges. Fruits, vegetables, and other food products should retain their nutritional value and safety until they are consumed. The use of chlorine compounds, organic acids, trisodium phosphate, iodine solutions, and ammonia compounds are common in overcoming food spoilage (Hricova et al., 2008). On the other hand, these conventional techniques have many drawbacks. They often fall short in maintaining the integrity of products with respect to taste, color, and appearance. Therefore, the search for new methodologies becomes indispensable to eliminate microbes in food (Dilarri et al., 2016). Considerable studies about reducing the food susceptibility against microbial contamination have been done.

Many microbial systems can survive in a variety of surrounding environments, and BS production by microbial cells can endure in foods (Mellor et al., 2011). These authors suggested that bacterial count can increase in the stored food in the presence of BS. Their work gave the evidence of increase in the total bacterial count of *P. fluorescens* on chicken that is stored aerobically up to 3 days. BS affects the bioavailability of nutrients for the bacteria, making them aggressive about sustaining and improving the decomposition of food materials. It should be noted that the exact physiological role of BS is not known completely (Jirku et al., 2015). One of the reports from Lima et al. (2013) suggested that a food-borne pathogen, namely, *S. enteritidis*, possesses a natural tendency to adhere to the surfaces of lettuce leaves. Recent studies demonstrated by Rossi et al. (2016) revealed that *S. enteritidis* SE86 c produce BS that affects its adherence to lettuce leaves and confers resistance to sanitizers. The studies used scanning electron microscopy (SEM) to indicate the formation of lumps by organisms, and BS produced by this bacterium favors invasion of stomata. The studies are remarkable in understanding how BS affects the adherence capacity and therefore enhances the organism's resistance against sanitizers.

A germicidal composition having SDS and sophorolipid (US 6262038) was developed by Pierce and Heilman (2001) for sanitization of fruits and vegetables. The composition is extremely suitable for 100% killing of dangerous pathogens like *E. coli*, *Salmonella*, and *Shigella*. Foliage of agricultural plants are also cleaned with the help of BE in combination with acids and alkyl sulfonates. In addition to the food surfaces, containers like milk tanks are also covered by biofilm formed by *B. cereus* where surfactin, a well-known BS produced by *Bacillus* spp., facilitates their survival (Shaheen et al., 2010). We need to understand the possible function of BSs produced by microorganisms while in contact with food surfaces. BSs do not necessarily have a role in enhancing the adherence of organisms to the surfaces. Differing reports suggest that the BS produced by *P. aeruginosa* NBIMCC 1390 increasing the cell hydrophobicity, leading to alterations in the cell surfaces (Sotirova and Vasileva-Tonkova, 2009).

RHL has been evaluated for fruit washing and sanitation purposes. The studies included tap water, electrolyzed water, and RHL solution for examination of impeding effect on microbial growth. RHL is very efficient for preventing the growth of microorganisms and also for increasing the shelf life of fruit. Hence, RHL fruit sanitation is one of the most recommended methods (Dilarri et al., 2016). RHL inhibits various bacteria as well as fungi (Murray et al., 2006). RHL-type BS, although important in improving the food textures, is not practical because of human safety concerns. In spite of all this, glycolipid BSs have achieved a significant place in food-processing technologies (Mnif and Ghribi, 2016).

FUTURE PROSPECTS

BSs/BEs are metabolites with a broad spectrum of functional/biological properties for use in various food industries. Accurate utilization of BSs/BEs requires knowledge about toxicity prior to their applications to the food industry. Pioneering applications of BSs/BEs in food manufacturing and processing are providing encouragement for researchers studying these surface-active molecules. Although there is ample knowledge on diverse functional and biological properties of BSs/BEs, the food-related applications are few. We need to study probable roles and interactions exhibited by organisms when they are in contact with variety of food surfaces. Novel strategies used in the medical and pharmaceutical fields can be extended to the food industries. The problems for BS/BE production engineering are the large-scale production, structural characterization, and cost. Further work in these proposed areas may facilitate commercial exploitation of BSs/BEs.

CONCLUSIONS

Different biological and functional properties of BSs/BEs address their uses as active components in various food formulations and preparations. Some newer approaches can be tried to broaden their applications in food industries. The ever-increasing demand for the use of BSs/BEs is prompting researchers to investigate newer microbial cell systems with innovative structural and functional diversity. One of the recent approaches—amalgamation of BS with NPs—finds valuable applications for designing newer food formulations. Metal NPs can be used in different food formulations and in the packaging of food. Applications of BSs/BEs in the food industries can be achieved with innovative modifications, which was impossible with conventional emulsifiers. The ambitious objectives of designing innovative BS/BE-based formulations can be achieved with the aid of recent advanced technologies.

REFERENCES

Anjum F. et al., 2016. Biosurfactant production through *Bacillus* sp. MTCC 5877 and its multifarious applications in food industry, *Bioresource Technology* 213: 262.

Banat I. M. et al., 2014. Cost effective technologies and renewable substrates for biosurfactants' production, *Frontiers in Microbiology* 5: 697.

Berton-Carabin C. C., Hélène Ropers M.-H., and Geno C. 2014. Lipid oxidation in oil-in-water emulsions: Involvement of the interfacial layer, *Comprehensive Reviews in Food Science and Food Safety* 13: 945.

Busscher H. J., van der Kuijl-Booij M., and van der Mei H. C., 1996. Biosurfactants from thermophilic dairy streptococci and their potential role in the fouling control of heat exchanger plates, *Journal of Industrial Microbiology* 16: 21.

Busscher H. J. et al., 1990. Deposition of *Leuconostoc mesenteroides* and *Streptococcus thermophilus* to solid substrata in a parallel plate flow cell, *Biofouling* 2: 55.

Cameron D. R., Cooper D. G., and Neufeld R. J., 1988. The mannoprotein of *Saccharomyces cereuisiae* is an effective bioemulsifier, *Applied and Environmental Microbiology* 54: 1420.

Campos J. M. et al., 2013. Microbial biosurfactants as additives for food industries, *Biotechnology Progress* 29: 1097.

De Araujo L. V. et al., 2011. Rhamnolipid and surfactin inhibit Listeria monocytogenes adhesion, *Food Research International* 44: 481.

De Man J. C., Rogosa M., and Sharpe M. E., 1960. A medium for cultivation of Lactobacilli, *Journal of Applied Bacteriology* 23: 130.

Dickinson E., 1993. Towards more natural emulsifiers, *Trends Food Science Technology* 4: 330.

Dilarri G. et al., 2016. Electrolytic treatment and biosurfactants applied to the conservation of Eugenia uniflora fruit, *Food Science Technology* (*Campinas*) 36: 456.

Falagas M. E. and Makris G. C., 2009. Probiotic bacteria and biosurfactants for nosocomial infection control: A hypothesis, *Journal of Hospital Infection* 71: 301.

Fouad H. K., Hanaqa H. H., and Munira C. H. I., 2010. Purification and characterization of surlactin produced by *Lactobacillus acidophilus*, *IRAQI Academic Sciences Journal* 8: 34.

Fracchia L. et al., 2010. A Lactobacillus-derived biosurfactant inhibits biofilm formation of human pathogenic *Candida albicans* biofilm producers, in current research, *Technology and Education Topics in Applied Microbiology and Microbial Biotechnology*, FORMATEX, Spain Microbiology Book Series, No. 2: 827.

Ghagi R. et al., 2011. Study of functional properties of *Sapindus mukorossi* as a potential bio-surfactant, *Indian Journal of Science and Technology* 4: 231.

Giri S. S., Sen S. S., Jun J. W., Sukumaran V., and Park S. C., 2017. Role of *Bacillus licheniformis* VS16-derived biosurfactant in mediating immune responses in carp rohu and its application to the food industry, *Frontiers in Microbiology* 8: 514.

Gomes M. Z do V. and Nitschke M., 2012. Evaluation of rhamnolipid and surfactin to reduce the adhesion and remove biofilms of individual and mixed cultures of food pathogenic bacteria, *Food Control* 25: 441.

Gudiña E. J, Teixeira J. A, and Rodrigues L. R., 2010. Isolation and functional characterization of a biosurfactant produced by *Lactobacillus paracasei*, *Colloids and Surfaces B* 76: 298.

Gudiña E. J, Teixeira J. A, and Rodrigues, L. R., 2011. Biosurfactant-producing lactobacilli: Screening, production profiles, and effect of medium composition, *Applied and Environmental Soil Science* 2011: 1.

Gudiña E. J. et al., 2015. Antimicrobial and anti-adhesive activities of cell-bound biosurfactant from *Lactobacillus agilis* CCUG31450, *RSC Advances* 5: 909.

Guerra-Santos L., Käppeli O., and Fiechter A., 1984. *Pseudomonas aeruginosa* biosurfactant production in continuous culture with glucose as carbon source, *Applied and Environmental Microbiology* 48: 301.

Guerra-Santos L. H., Käppeli O., and Fiechter A., 1986. Dependence of *Pseudomonas aeruginosa* continuous culture biosurfactant production on nutritional and environmental factors, *Applied Microbiology and Biotechnology* 24: 44.

Haba E. et al., 2014. Rhamnolipids as emulsifying agents for essential oil formulations: Antimicrobial effect against *Candida albicans* and methicillin-resistant *Staphylococcus aureus*, *International Journal Pharmacy* 476: 134.

Hasenhuettl G. L., 2008. Synthesis and commercial preparation of food emulsifiers, in *Food Emulsifier and Their Applications*, Chapter 2, Hasenhuettl G. L. and Hartel, R. W. (Eds.), New York: Springer Science.

Hidayati N. Surtiningsih T., and Ni'matuzahroh., 2014. Removal of heavy metals Pb, Zn and Cu from sludge waste of paper industries using biosurfactant, *Journal of Bioremediation and Biodegradation* 5: 255. doi:10.4172/2155-6199.1000255.

Hricova D., Stephan R., and Zweifel C., 2008. Electrolyzed water and its application in the food industry, *Journal of Food Protection*, 71: 1934.

Iyer A., Mody K., and Jha B., 2006. Emulsifying properties of a marine exopolysaccharide, *Enzyme Microbial Technology*, 38: 220.

Jirku V.et al., 2015. Multicomponent biosurfactants: A green toolbox, extension, *Biotechnology Advances* 33: 1272.

Kiran G. S., Sabu A., and Selvin J., 2010a. Synthesis of silver nanoparticles by glycolipid biosurfactant produced from marine *Brevibacterium casei* MSA 19, *Journal of Biotechnology* 148: 221.

Kiran G. S.et al., 2010b. Optimization and characterization of a new lipopeptide biosurfactant produced by marine *Brevibacterium aureum* MSA13 in solid state culture, *Bioresource Technology* 101: 2389.

Kiran G. S. et al., 2014. Production of glycolipid biosurfactant from sponge-associated marine actinobacterium *Brachybacterium paraconglomeratum* MSA21, *Journal of Surfactant and Detergent* 17: 531.

Kitamoto D. et al., 2009. Self-assembling properties of glycolipid biosurfactants and their potential applications, *Current Opinion in Colloid and Interface Science* 14: 315.

Kosaric N., 2001. Biosurfactants and their applications for soil bioremediation, *Food Technology Biotechnology* 39: 295.

Kosaric N. and Sukan F. V., 2014. *Biosurfactants: Production and Utilization—Processes, Technologies and Economics*, Boca Raton, FL: CRC Press, p. 389.

Kourkoutas Y. and Banat I. M., 2004. Biosurfactant production and application, in *The Concise Encyclopedia of Bioresour Technology*, Pandey A. P. (Ed.), Philadelphia, PA: Haworth Reference Press, p. 505.

Kralova I. and Sjöblom J., 2009. Surfactants used in food industry: A review, *Journal of Dispersion Science and Technology* 30: 1363.

Kumar C. G. et al., 2010. Synthesis of biosurfactant-based silver nanoparticles with purified rhamnolipids isolated from *Pseudomonas aeruginosa* BS-161R, *Journal of Microbiology and Biotechnology*, 20: 1061.

Lima, P. M. et al., 2013. Interaction between natural microbiota and physicochemical characteristics of lettuce surfaces can influence the attachment of *Salmonella* Enteritidis, *Food Control* 30: 157–161.

Manivasagan P. et al., 2014. Optimization, production and characterization of glycolipid biosurfactant from the actinobacterium, *Streptomuces* sp. MAB36, *Bioprocess Biosystem Engineering* 37: 783.

Marchant R. and Banat I. M., 2012. Biosurfactants: A sustainable replacement for chemical surfactants?, *Biotechnol Letter* 34: 1597.

Mellor G. E., Bentley J. A., and Dykes G. A., 2011. Evidence for a role of biosurfactants produced by *Pseudomonas fluorescens* in the spoilage of fresh aerobically stored chicken meat, *Food Microbiology* 28: 1101.

Meylheuc T. et al., 2006. Adsorption on stainless steel surfaces of biosurfactants produced by gram-negative and gram-positive bacteria: Consequence on the bioadhesive behavior of *Listeria monocytogenes*, *Colloids and Surfaces B: Biointerfaces* 52: 128.

Mnif I. and Ghribi D. 2016. Glycolipid biosurfactants: Main properties and potential applications in agriculture and food industry, *Journal of Science Food Agriculture* 96: 4310.

Mnif I. et al., 2012. Improvement of bread dough quality by *Bacillus subtilis* SPB1 biosurfactant addition: Optimized extraction using response surface methodology, *Journal of the Science of Food and Agriculture* 21: 3055.

Moldes A. B. et al., 2013. Partial characterization of biosurfactant from *Lactobacillus pentosus* and comparison with sodium dodecyl sulphate for the bioremediation of hydrocarbon contaminated soil, *BioMed Research International* 2013: 1.

Moreira T. C. et al., 2016. Stabilization mechanisms of oil-in-water emulsions by *Saccharomyces cerevisiae*, *Colloids Surf B Biointerfaces* 143: 399.

Mulligan C. N. and Wang S., 2006. Remediation of a heavy metal-contaminated soil by a rhamnolipid foam, *Engineering Geology* 85: 75.

Murray P. R., Rosenthal K. S., and Pfaller M. A., 2006. *Microbiologia Médica*, Rio de Janeiro, Brazil: Elsevier.

Narayanan J. et al., 2010. Synthesis, stabilization and characterization of rhamnolipid-capped ZnS nanoparticles in aqueous medium, *IET Nanotechnology* 4: 29.

Nitschke M. and Costa SGVAO, 2007. Biosurfactants in food industry, *Trends Food Science Technology* 18: 252.

Nitschke M. et al., 2009. Surfactin reduces the adhesion of food-borne pathogenic bacteria to solid surfaces, *Letters in Applied Microbiology* 49: 241.

Palanisamy P. and Raichur A. M., 2009. Synthesis of spherical NiO nanoparticles through a novel biosurfactant mediated emulsion technique, *Materials Science and Engineering* 29: 199.

Paradelo R. et al., 2009. Reduction of water repellence of hydrophobic plant substrates using biosurfactant produced from hydrolyzed grape marc, *Journal of Agricultural and Food Chemistry* 10: 4895.

Pierce D. and Heilman T. J., 2001. Germicidal composition, US6262038 B1 US 09/284,687.

Portilla-Rivera O. M. et al., 2007a. Biosurfactants from grape marc: Stability study, *Journal of Biotechnology*, 131: S136.

Portilla-Rivera O. M. et al., 2007b. Lactic acid and biosurfactants production from hydrolyzed distilled grape marc, *Process Biochemistry* 42: 1010.

Portilla-Rivera O. M. et al., 2008. Stability and emulsifying capacity of biosurfactants obtained from lignocellulosic sources using *Lactobacillus pentosus*, *Journal of Agricultural and Food Chemistry* 56: 8074.

Reddy A. S. et al., 2009. Synthesis of gold nanoparticles via an environmentally benign route using a biosurfactant, *Journal of Nanoscience and Nanotechnology* 9: 6693.

Rodrigues L. R. and Teixeira J. A., 2008. Biosurfactants production from cheese whey, in *Advances in Cheese Whey Utilization*, Cerdan M. E., Gonzalez-Siso M. I., and Becerra M. (Eds.), Kerala, India: Transworld Research Network, p. 81.

Rodrigues L. et al., 2006. Biosurfactants: Potential applications in medicine, *Journal of Antimicrobial Chemotherapy* 57: 609.

Rossi E. M. et al., 2016. Biosurfactant produced by *Salmonella Enteritidis* SE86 can increase adherence and resistance to sanitizers on lettuce leaves (*Lactuca sativa* L., *cichoraceae*). *Frontiers in Microbiology* 7: 9.

Rufino R. D., de Luna J. M., de Campos Takaki G. M., and Sarubbo L. A., 2014. Characterization and properties of the biosurfactant produced by *Candida lipolytica* UCP 0988, *Electronic Journal of Biotechnology* 17: 34.

Sachdev D. P. and Cameotra S. S., 2013. Biosurfactants in agriculture, *Applied Microbiology Biotechnology* 97: 1005.

Sáenz-Marta C. I. et al., 2015. Biosurfactants as useful tools in bioremediation, in *Advances in Bioremediation of Waste Water and Polluted Soil*, Shiomi N. (Ed.), Rijeka, Croatia: In Tech.

Santos D. K. et al., 2016. Biosurfactants: Multifunctional biomolecules of the 21st century. *International Journal of Molecular Sciences* 17: 1.

Saravanakumari P. and Mani K., 2010. Structural characterization of a novel xylolipid biosurfactant from *Lactococcus lactis* and analysis of antibacterial activity against multidrug resistant pathogens, *Bioresource Technology* 101: 8851.

Satpute S. K., Dhakephalkar P. K., and Chopade B. A., 2005. Biosurfactants and bioemulsifiers in hydrocarbon biodegradation and spilled oil bioremediation, Indo-Italian brain storming workshop on technology transfer for industrial applications of novel methods and materials for environmental problem, pp. 1–18.

Satpute S. K., Płaza G. A., and Banpurkar A. G., 2017. Biosurfactants' production from renewable natural resources: Example of innovative and smart technology in circular bioeconomy, *Management Systems in Production Engineering* 1: 46.

Satpute S. K. et al., 2010a. Biosurfactants, bioemulsifiers and exopolysaccharides from marine microorganisms, *Biotechnology Advances* 28: 436.

Satpute S. K. et al., 2010b. Methods for investigating biosurfactants and bioemulsifiers: A review, *Critical Reviews in Biotechnology* 30: 127.

Satpute S. K. et al., 2016a. Biosurfactant/s from Lactobacilli species: Properties, challenges and potential biomedical applications, *Journal of Basic Microbiology* 56: 1140.

Satpute S. K. et al., 2016b. Multiple roles of biosurfactants in biofilms, *Current Pharmaceutical Design* 22: 429.

Shaheen R. et al., 2010. Persistence strategies of *Bacillus cereus* spores isolated from dairy silo tanks, *Food Microbiology* 27: 347.

Sharma D. and Malik A., 2012. Incidence and prevalence of antimicrobial resistant Vibrio cholera from dairy farms, *African Journal of Microbiology Research* 6: 5331.

Sharma D. and Saharan B. S., 2014. Simultaneous production of biosurfactants and bacteriocins by probiotic *Lactobacillus casei* MRTL3, *International Journal of Microbiology*: 698713.

Sharma D. and Saharan B. S., 2016. Functional characterization of biomedical potential of biosurfactant produced by *Lactobacillus helveticus*, *Biotechnology Reports* 11: 27.

Sharma D., Saharan B. S., and Shailly K. (Eds.), 2016. Biosurfactants of lactic acid bacteria, in *Springer Briefs in Microbiology*, New York: Springer–Verlag.

Sharma D. et al., 2014. Production and structural characterization of *Lactobacillus helveticus* derived biosurfactant, *The Scientific World Journal*.

Sharma D. et al., 2015. Isolation and functional characterization of novel biosurfactant produced by *Enterococcus faecium*, *Springer Plus* 4: 1.

Shepherd R., Rockey J., Shutherland I. W., and Roller S., 1995. Novel bioemulsifiers from microorganisms for use in foods, *Journal of Biotechnology* 40: 207.

Simões L. C., Simões M., and Vieira M. J., 2010. Adhesion and biofilm formation on polystyrene by drinking water-isolated bacteria, *Antonie Van Leeuwenhoek* 98: 317.

Singh B. R. et al., 2011. Synthesis of stable cadmium sulfide nanoparticles using surfactin produced by *Bacillus amyloliquifaciens* strain KSU-109, *Colloids and Surfaces B: Biointerfaces* 85: 207.

Surfactants market by type, applications and geography—Global forecasts to 2021, 2016. www.marketsandmarkets.com.

Tadros T. F., 2016. *Emulsions: Formation, Stability, Industrial Applications*, Berlin, Germany: Walter de Gruyter GmbH and Co.

Van Haesendonck I. and Vanzeveren E. C. A., 2002. Rhamnolipids in bakery products, Pub. No.: US 2006/0233935 A1.

Van Haesendonck I. and Vanzeveren E. C. A., 2004. Rhamnolipids in bakery products, International application patent (PCT).

Varnier A. L. et al., 2009. Bacterial rhamnolipids are novel MAMPs conferring resistance to *Botrytis cinerea* in grapevine, *Plant, Cell and Environment* 32: 178.

Walencka E. et al., 2008. The influence of *Lactobacillus acidophilus* derived surfactants on staphylococcal adhesion and biofilm formation, *Folia Microbiology* 53: 61.

Wang, S. and Mulligan, C. N., 2004. An evaluation of surfactant foam technology in remediation of contaminated soil, *Chemosphere* 57: 1079.

Xie Y., Ye R., and Liu H., 2006. Synthesis of silver nanoparticles in reverse micelles stabilized by natural biosurfactant, *Colloids and Surfaces A: Physicochemical and Engineering Aspects* 2: 175.

Xu Q. et al., 2011. Biosurfactants for microbubble preparation and application, *International Journal of Molecular Sciences* 12: 462.

Zambry N. S., Ayoib A., Md Noh N. A., and Yahya A. R. M., 2017. Production and partial characterization of biosurfactant produced by *Streptomyces* sp. R1, *Bioprocess and Biosystem Engineering*. doi:10.1007/s00449-017-1764-4.

Zeraik A. E. and Nitschke M. 2010. Biosurfactants as agents to reduce adhesion of pathogenic bacteria to polystyrene surfaces: Effect of temperature and hydrophobicity, *Current Microbiology* 61: 554.

Zhang T. et al., 2008. Antifungal compounds from *Bacillus subtilis* BFS06 inhibiting the growth of *Aspergillus flavus*, *World Journal of Microbiology and Biotechnology* 24: 783.

Zinjarde S. S. and Pant A., 2002. Emulsifier from a tropical marine yeast, *Yarrowia lipolytica* NCIM 3589, *Journal of Basic Microbiology* 42: 67.

ZONIX™ Biofungicide., 2012. EPA Reg. No. 72431-1 Label amendment (FAST TRACK) to modify active ingredient statement and add dilution Ratios MASTER LABEL—Version (15), p. 17. https://www3.epa.gov/pesticides/chem_search/ppls/072431-00001-20121016.pdf.

2 Exopolysaccharides Produced by Lactic Acid Bacteria and Their Role in the Food Industry

Mattia Pia Arena, Pasquale Russo,
Giuseppe Spano, Vittorio Capozzi,
and Daniela Fiocco

CONTENTS

INTRODUCTION

Bacteria can produce a wide range of biopolymers (mainly polyesters, polyamides, inorganic polyanhydrides, and polysaccharides), with significant and heterogeneous physiological functions in prokaryotes (Rehm, 2010). Several of these compounds find application in the industrial and medical field, often offering—because of their biocompatibility and biodegradability—sustainable solutions from the economic, environmental, and social point of view (Rehm, 2010; Ates, 2015).

Among biopolymers, microbial polysaccharides (PSs) are varied in terms of chemical structure and biological function. Regarding their biological function, we can distinguish (1) intracellular storage PS, such as starch; (2) exopolysaccharides (EPSs) (e.g., xanthan); and (3) capsular PS (CPSs) (e.g., K30) (Ates, 2015; Schmid and

Sieber, 2015). Both EPSs and CPSs are secreted, but CPSs are covalently bound to the bacterial cell wall, while EPSs are released and present no specific chemical association with the cell envelope (Schmid and Sieber, 2015). With a focus on the industrial and medical applications, it is crucial to underline that the exploitation of EPSs is simpler because they do not require any effort to be extracted or harvested from the cell (Schmid and Sieber, 2015). This fact justifies the considerable interest EPSs have been receiving and explains why we focus, in this chapter, on this specific class of bacterial polysaccharides. Considering chemical composition and structure, EPSs comprise homo(exo)polysaccharides (HoPSs) and hetero(exo)polysaccharides (HePSs), if composed by the repetition of the same monosaccharide unit (e.g., glucose) or of repeating units comprising multiple monosaccharides, respectively (Schmid and Sieber, 2015). As a function of the kind of linkage (and of the position of the linked carbon involved in the bond among sugars), HoPSs can be mainly classified as α-D-glucans (e.g., α-(1,6)), β-D-glucans (e.g., β-(1,3)) and fructans (Ates, 2015). Additionally, HePSs exist as branched sugars/sugar derivatives (sugars substituted with various chemical aglycones such as phosphate, acetyl, and glycerol) (Kleerebezem et al., 1999; Zannini et al., 2016). Normally, the biosynthesis of EPSs takes place in the cytoplasm with a subsequent secretion outside the cell, while only for some cells is the biosynthetic enzyme secreted directly to the outside of the cells and HoPS are synthetized extracellularly (Freitas et al., 2011). The biosynthetic routes encompass substrate uptake, central metabolite pathways, and polysaccharide synthesis, with general intracellular pathways such as the Wzx/Wzy dependent pathway, the ABC transporter dependent pathway, the synthase dependent pathway, and the extracellular synthesis catalyzed by single sucrase protein (Freitas et al., 2011; Ates, 2015).

In nature, bacterial EPSs have prominent structural and functional roles in phenomena such as (1) cellular adhesion to solid surfaces, (2) protection from abiotic and biotic stresses, (3) development and maintenance of microbial biofilms, (4) cell-to-cell interactions, (5) water retention, (6) sink for excess energy and nutrient source, (7) organic compound and inorganic ion sorption, (8) binding of enzymes, and (9) passive bacterial motility (Nwodo et al., 2012; Ates, 2015; Pérez-Mendoza and Sanjuàn, 2016; Zannini et al., 2016; Hölscher and Kovács, 2017). Microbial EPSs, such as xanthan from *Xanthomonas campestris*, gellan from *Sphingomonas elodea*, and dextran from *Leuconostoc* subsp. are renewable polymers currently used to design hydrocolloids employed in medical and industrial applications, with specific uses in the pharmaceutical and food sectors (Ahmad et al., 2015). In this regard, it is interesting to underline that few microbial EPSs are already commercialized (e.g., alginate, dextran, gellan gum, and xanthan) and, in some cases, their use is considered compliant with the United States and European Union (food and drug) regulatory frameworks (e.g., gellan was approved by the U.S. Food and Drug Administration as a food stabilizer and thickener; xanthan was approved as food additive in Europe as E415) (United States Pharmacopeia [USP]—National Formulary [NF], 2012; European Pharmacopeia [EP], 2014; Ahmad et al., 2015; Kielak et al., 2017).

Lactic acid bacteria (LABs) comprise a heterogeneous group of Gram-positive, catalase-negative cocci and bacilli, all sharing the ability to catabolize fermentable sugars, resulting in the production of lactic acid. Several LABs live in association with host species: they colonize the surfaces of plants and animals, including the gut mucosa of mammals and humans, where some commensal strains are thought to play probiotic functions (Douillard and de Vos, 2014). Considering their use, LABs are generally nonpathogenic and safe for human and animal applications (with few exceptions of species/strains belonging to the genera *Streptococcus*, *Lactococcus*, *Enterococcus* and *Carnobacterium*). As a matter of fact, they usually possess the so-called Generally Recognized as Safe (GRAS) and Qualified Presumption of Safety (QPS)-status recognized, respectively, by the U.S. Food and Drug Administration and European Food Safety Authority (Russo et al., 2017). This historical safe use is well testified by the applications of LAB in the food sector as protechnological microbes, protective cultures, aroma enhancers, detoxificant agents, biofortifiers, and probiotics (Bove et al., 2012a; Capozzi et al., 2012a,b; Coelho et al., 2014; Benozzi et al., 2015; Berbegal et al., 2016; Russo et al., 2017). On the other hand, their safety also explains the continuous interest in innovative applications of LABs in the medical and industrial sectors (e.g., biocontrol, vaccine delivery, and cell factories) (Arena et al., 2016; Brown et al., 2017; Szatraj et al., 2017).

The increasing interest in microbial EPSs–based sustainable solutions for the medical and industrial sector and the evergreen attention to the exploitation of LABs because of their general safe status justify the growing scientific appeal of EPSs from LABs (e.g., Ryan et al., 2015; Caggianiello et al., 2016; Leroy and De Vuyst, 2016; Salazar et al., 2016; Zannini et al., 2016). Considering LAB HoPS, the α-D-glucans structure is generally more represented than the β-D-glucans one (Ryan et al., 2015). Among LAB α-D-glucans, we can recognize dextran (producer organisms: species/strains belonging to the genera *Lactobacillus*, *Leuconostoc*, *Streptococcus*, and *Weisella cibaria*), mutan (producer organisms: strains belonging to the species *Lactobacillus reuteri*, *Streptococcus mutans, Streptococcus downei*, and *Streptococcus sobrinus*), alternan (*Leuconostoc mesenteroides*), and reuteran (*L. reuteri*) (Zannini et al., 2016). β-D-glucans are mainly produced by strains belonging to the species *Pediococcus damnosus*, *Pediococcus parvulus*, and *Lactobacillus diolivorans* (Zannini et al., 2016). Additionally, we have to consider that levan (producer organisms: strains belonging to the species *L. reuteri*, *Lactobacillus sanfranciscensis*, *Lc. mesenteroides*, *S. sobrinus*, and *Streptococcus salivarius*) and inulin-like EPSs (*L. reuteri*, *Leuconostoc citreum*, and *S. mutans*) belong to the class of fructans (Zannini et al., 2016). However, the majority of EPSs released by LABs are HePSs, composed of three to eight repeating units, each made up of two or more monosaccharides (usually rhamnose, fructose, galactose, or glucose), with, in some cases, modifications such as phosphorylations, pyruvylations, and acetylations, resulting in a wide assortment of structures (Ryan et al., 2015).

In LABs, the genes coding for enzymes involved in EPS biosynthesis belong to definite clusters annotated as *eps* or *cps*, with a prevalent genomic location in species such as *S. thermophilus* or *Lactobacillus plantarum*, while often located on plasmids in LABs such as *Lactococcus lactis* and *P. damnsosus* (Caggianiello et al., 2016). Among the general intracellular pathways, the Wzx/Wzy dependent pathway and the ABC transporter dependent pathway have been found active in LABs (Caggianiello et al., 2016). HoPS synthesis is quite a simple process, with the major energy expense on the biosynthesis of the extracellular enzymes responsible for the process

(Ryan et al., 2015). The synthesis of LAB HePSs, in terms of amount and type, is a function of growth phases and of fermentation conditions (De Vuyst and Degeest, 1999). Moreover, the capacity to synthesize EPSs is often a strain-specific feature. Because of the previously encompassed, specific roles of LABs in human life, other than the general structural and functional roles reported for bacterial EPSs, LAB-associated EPSs have been found to be implicated in peculiar biological functions, such as adhesion to human cells and immunomodulation of the host (Yasuda et al., 2008; Lebeer et al., 2011; Polak-Berecka et al., 2013; Ghadimi et al., 2014; Lee et al., 2016).

In this chapter we will discuss some of the different use of EPS-producing bacteria in the food industry, with a particular focus on technological or probiotic features.

THE IMPACT OF EXOPOLYSACCHARIDES ON SOME TECHNOLOGICAL ASPECTS OF FOOD AND FOOD MANUFACTURING

Food and beverage industries are increasingly leaning toward a limited use of chemical additives and excessive treatments, preferring natural compounds and mild technologies, due to growing consumer demand for natural food products (Dickson-Spillmann et al., 2011). The use of LAB starter cultures to ferment raw material produce end products with specific technofunctional traits with mild bioprocessing technology (Di Cagno et al., 2013; Paramithiotis, 2017). More specifically, the use of EPS-producing starter cultures might ameliorate the texture and the stability of several food matrices, such as milk-based products, vegetables, and starchy foods.

The first polysaccharide produced by LABs to be applied in the food industry was probably dextran, from *L. mesenteroides* (Monsan et al., 2001). Dextran, whose backbone chain consists of α-1$\rightarrow$6 glycosidic linkages branched through α-1$\rightarrow$2, α-1$\rightarrow$3, and α-1$\rightarrow$4 side ramifications, was used in thickening and gelation of the syrups from sugar cane and beet (Patel and Prajapat, 2013). Besides improving viscosity and moisture retention, avoiding sugar crystallization, and promoting food gelling and mouth feel, dextran protects the starter cultures from adverse food processing and storing conditions (Kim et al., 2000). In 2001, the commercialization of a *Lc. mesenteroides* dextran preparation was approved by the European Commission as a food ingredient in bakery applications (up to a level of 5%) in order to improve the softness, crumb texture, and loaf volume (Byrne, 2001). Also well known is kefiran, the polysaccharide responsible for the slimy texture of the alcoholic fermented milk called Kefir, which is traditionally manufactured in Eastern Europe. Kefiran is produced by homofermentative and heterofermentative LABs, yeasts, and acetic acid bacteria and acts as a natural thickening agent (Duboc and Mollet, 2001; Shah and Prajapati, 2013). *Lactobacillus kefiranofaciens* subsp. *kefiranofaciens* is the most important bacterium with the ability to produce large amounts of kefiran, which includes an equal proportion of glucose and galactose monomers and has been applied to improve viscoelastic properties of acid milk gels (Micheli et al., 1999). Alternan, a polymer with a backbone structure of alternating α-1$\rightarrow$6 and α-1$\rightarrow$3-D-glucosidic linkages, is naturally produced by *Lc. mesenteroides* strains and is commercially exploited as a low-viscosity bulking agent and carrier in the food industry; alternan-derived oligosaccharides, obtained by the microbial extracellular enzyme alternanase, are used as low-glycemic sweeteners (Leathers et al., 2003, 2010). Reuteran, which owes its name to the EPS-producing *L. reuteri*, is characterized by α-1→4 and α-1→6 glycosidic bonds in the backbone chain and is involved in the thickening of fermented dairy products and in enhancing the shelf life of baked goods (Meng et al., 2004; Arendt et al., 2007).

Several LABs are able to synthesize β-glucans, a group of polysaccharides exhibiting a principal chain of (1,3)-linked β-glucopyranosyl units. β-glucans have been applied in yogurt manufacturing and confer value-added microbiological and physicochemical properties to the end product (Kılıç and Akpınar, 2013). Fructans, synthesized by the genera *Streptococcus, Leuconostoc*, and *Lactobacillus*, are EPSs consisting of chains of fructosyl units linked by β-2→1 or β-2→6 linkages, called inulin or levan, respectively (Seibel and Buchholz, 2010). Levan, produced by *S. salivarius, S. mutans, Lc. mesenteroides, L. sanfranciscensis*, and *L. reuteri*, can stabilize, emulsify, and intensify flavors and fragrances in various food matrices, and can retain water (Korakli et al., 2003). Inulin, mainly produced by *Lactobacillus johnsonii, S. mutans, Lc. citreum*, and *L. reuteri* strains, is said to be a prebiotic; it can also be used as a natural agent to improve organoleptic quality and to achieve a better-balanced nutritional composition, as well as a texturizer, emulsion stabilizer, and partial replacement for fat (Franck, 2002).

The ability to produce EPSs by LABs during the process of food fermentation has been found to improve several technological aspects of the fermented end products (Ravyts et al., 2011; Leroy and De Vuyst, 2016). In the dairy industry, the inoculation of EPS-producing strains of *Bifidobacterium longum* and *Bifidobacterium infantis* in yogurt led to a better end product in terms of lower syneresis, greater storage modulus and firmness, and a more appreciable microstructure of yogurt due to the interaction between EPS and milk proteins (Prasanna et al., 2013). The textural and rheological improvements of yogurt, due to the production of EPS by *Lactobacillus mucosae* strain, resulted in a greater acceptance of EPS-enriched yogurt by consumers (London et al., 2015). Moreover, the *in situ* production of EPS by a strain of *S. thermophilus* during the manufacture of ayran, which is a traditional Turkish yogurt drink, led to improved viscosity, probably because of the interactions of EPS with the milk protein network (Yilmaz et al., 2015). EPS-producing *L. rhamnosus,* isolated from Chinese sauerkrauts, could increase the water-holding capacity and viscosity of yogurt samples and can also reduce milk solids (Yang et al., 2010).

EPS-producing strains were also found to positively affect tome sensory attributes, for example, taste, moisture, intensity of flavor, and chewability of low-fat Caciotta-type cheeses inoculated with *S. thermophilus* (Di Cagno et al., 2014) and Cheddar cheese inoculated with *W. cibaria* and *Lactobacillus reuteri* strains (Lynch et al., 2014). An interaction between EPS molecules and milk proteins during the production of fresh cheese inoculated with EPS-producing strain of *Lc. lactis* subsp. *cremoris* has been indicated as the main reason for the reduction of rough particles, which correlated to a decreased in-mouth creaminess (Hahn et al., 2014). The technological use of EPS has been also proposed for the production of Mexican manchego-type cheese fermented by ropy strains of *S. thermophiles*, which were appreciated for their capability to improve water and fat retention and thus cheese yield. The ability to raise the moisture value has been correlated with the production of EPS, which bound water molecules within the protein matrix of the cheese (Lluis-Arroyo et al., 2014).

In recent years, the use of natural biothickening microbes, which can produce *in situ* compounds such as EPS that are useful for ameliorating the quality of end products, has been also exploited in countries where the lack of commercial starter cultures prompted work on isolating in investigating LAB indigenous to the food matrix. In India, several studies have aimed at screening the autochthonous microflora of fermented milks prepared in rural and urban areas in order to identify EPS-producing strains (Behare et al., 2009a,b). A strain of *L. fermentum*, isolated from one of the most consumed fermented types of milk in India (dahi, which is traditionally made without inoculation of starter cultures), was shown to produce EPSs during the fermentation that determined lower whey separation, higher viscosity, and high adhesiveness and stickiness values (Behare et al., 2013).

In addition to milk-based products, the technological use of EPSs is gaining attention in nondairy food matrices. Dextran, levan, and β-glucan, which are the EPSs mainly produced by selected strains of *Lactobacillus*, *Leuconostoc*, and *Weissella*, are able to modify the texture of liquid carrot to improve the thick texture and possibly replace the hydrocolloid additives (Juvonen et al., 2015). Moreover, EPS-producing LABs were shown to extend the shelf life and enhance the structure of sourdough breads and cereal-based drinks (Katina et al., 2009; Waldherr and Vogel, 2009). Furthermore, the viscoelastic property and the volume of bread could be increased by including EPS-synthesizing LAB cultures, such as strains of *Lactobacillus delbueckii* and *Lactobacillus helveticus*, while bread staling was reduced (Tamani et al., 2013). The application of EPS in gluten-free bread prepared with buckwheat, quinoa, sorghum, and teff flours led to excellent results, specifically the rheology, bread quality, and sensory properties of these increasingly demanded healthy products (Wolter et al., 2014).

The growing interest in a healthy and natural diet, for example, lactose free, low alcoholic, nonalcoholic drinks, includes also functional beverages. In this regard, EPS-producing strains of *Weisiella cibaria* can potentiate the rheological profile of sucrose-supplemented barley-malt-derived wort, due to the EPS (dextran) and oligosaccharides (glucooligosaccharides) produced during the fermentation process (Zannini et al., 2013). The addition of sucrose to raw material is a relevant technological step that correlates with the ability of cereal-associated LABs to produce EPSs starting just from sucrose, through the activity of glucansucrase or glycansucrases (Tieking and Ganzle, 2005; Korakli and Vogel, 2006). Moreover, EPSs can be synthetized also from maltose, or other acceptor carbohydrates, by glycansucrases (Ganzle et al., 2009). Among fermented beverages, soymilk drinks, fermented by selected EPS-producing *L. plantarum* and *L. rhamnosus* cultures, gain higher bacteria viability, water-holding capacity, viscosity values, and an overall improved texture due to EPS-protein mesh-like structure (Li et al., 2014). EPS-producing LABs also attract the attention of gluten-free food manufacturing because of the possibility of obtaining an acceptable network matrix comparable to gluten-based counterparts. Such a food matrix can bind water, thus improving shelf life and representing a natural alternative to hydrocolloids for application in cereal food production, such as bread (Lynch et al., 2017).

Overall, the impact of EPS on food technological characteristics depends on both the food matrix microstructure and the specific EPS structure, that is, capsular or free, homopolysaccharides or heteropolysaccharides (Gentès et al., 2013; Mende et al., 2013). Thus, depending on food manufacturing and the requisites of the end product, it is necessary to select the appropriate EPS-producing strains and to optimize their application (Ruas-Madiedo and de los Reyes-Gavilán, 2005). Indeed, EPS-producing starter cultures, selected according to the high production of EPS *in vitro*, do not always exhibit an adequate performance during food manufacturing for a variety of reasons and processing conditions that may influence EPS yield (e.g., bacterial growth rate, carbon and nitrogenous sources, pH, temperature, presence of metals) and to the chemical characteristics of the synthesized EPS (e.g., structure, polymerization degree, side chains, biodegradability, hydrophobicity, or hydrophilicity) (More et al., 2014; Şanli et al., 2014).

HEALTH-PROMOTING EFFECTS OF EXOPOLYSACCHARIDES FROM LABs AND THEIR POTENTIAL USE AS INGREDIENTS OF FUNCTIONAL FOOD

Beyond the physiological functions that EPSs have for the producing cells, there is a growing interest in their interactions with a host and consequently their possible impact on human health. Indeed, LAB EPSs are endowed with a broad range of biological activities (Table 2.1), which probably underlie many of the health-promoting properties ascribed to EPS-producing probiotic species. Because of such features, LAB EPSs could be used to develop and formulate food additives, therapeutic

TABLE 2.1

Some of the Biological Properties Ascribed to EPSs from LABs

EPS Source	Observed Effect	Experimental Procedure	References
		Immunomodulation	
L. kefiranofaciens; kefiran	Increased number of IgA+ cells in small and large intestine lamina propria	*In vivo* (mice)-oral administration	Vinderola et al. (2006)
L. casei Shirota	Lower production of TNF-α, interleukin-12 (IL-12), IL-10, and IL-6 (anti-inflammatory effect)	*In vitro* (mice spleen cell and macrophages)	Yasuda et al. (2008)
P. parvulus 2.6; purified (and recombinant) β-glucans	Activation of human macrophages/cytokine induction with anti-inflammatory effect	*In vitro* (human macrophages)	Notararigo et al. (2014)
L. plantarum N14	Modulation of pro-inflammatory cytokines; anti-inflammatory effect	*In vitro* (pig intestinal epithelial cells)	Murofushi et al. (2015)

(Continued)

TABLE 2.1 (*Continued*)
Some of the Biological Properties Ascribed to EPSs from LABs

EPS Source	Observed Effect	Experimental Procedure	References
L. plantarum	Modulation of nitric oxide and cytokines in intestinal fluid and serum; phenotypic maturation of dendritic cells	*In vivo* (mice)-administration by gavage; *in vitro*	Tang et al. (2015)
L. mesenteroides NTM048 (vegetable isolate)	Increased IgA content in fecal samples and plasma	*In vitro* and *in vivo* (mice)-dietary supplementation	Matsuzaki et al. (2014)
L. paraplantarum BGCG11	Modulated cytokine production in human PBMC; increase IL-10/IL-12 (pro-Th2-Treg) and IL-1β/IL-12 (pro-Th17 response) ratios	*In vitro* (human PBMC)	Nikolic et al. (2012)
L. delbrueckii TUA4408L	Downregulate inflammatory cytokines; reduce activation MAPK and NF-κB pathways after enterotoxigenic *Escherichia coli* (ETEC) stimulation	*In vitro* (pig intestinal epithelial cells)	Wachi et al. (2014)
L. rhamnosus RW-9595M	Increase IL-10 production; lower levels of pro-inflammatory TNF-α, IL-6, and IL-12	*In vitro* (mice macrophages)	Bleau et al. (2010)
Hypocholesterolemic Activity			
L. lactis subsp. *cremoris* SBT 0495 (fermented milk)	Reduce serum cholesterol level	*In vivo* (rats)-dietary intake of fermented milk	Nakajima et al. (1992)
β-glucan-producing recombinant *L. paracasei* (NFBC) (expressing the Gtf gene from *P. parvulus* 2.6) and naturally EPS-producing *L. mucosae* (DPC) 6426	Reduce serum cholesterol level and modulated enteric microbiota	*In vivo* (apoE-deficient mice)-dietary administration	London et al. (2014)

(Continued)

TABLE 2.1 (*Continued*)
Some of the Biological Properties Ascribed to EPSs from LABs

EPS Source	Observed Effect	Experimental Procedure	References
L. kefiranofaciens (kefiran)	Reduce blood cholesterol level and decrease blood pressure Reduce the size of atherosclerotic lesions (i.e., anti-atherogenic effect); lower cholesterol content in liver	*In vivo* (spontaneously hypertensive stroke-prone rats; hypercholesterolemic rabbits)-dietary intake	Maeda et al. (2004); Uchida et al. (2010)
β-glucan producing *P. damnosus* 2.6 (fermented oat-based product)	Decrease serum cholesterol concentration	*In vivo* (human volunteers)-dietary administration	Mårtensson et al. (2005)
Gastrointestinal Mucosa and Physiology			
S. thermophilus CRL 1190 (fermented milk)	Gastro-protective effect: prevention and relief of (ASA-induced) gastritis	*In vivo* (mice)-dietary administration	Rodríguez et al. (2009, 2010)
S. thermophilus CRL 1190 (purified EPS from fermented milk)	Stimulate human gastric epithelial cell proliferation	*In vitro*	Marcial et al. (2013)
Probiotic lactobacilli (i.e., *L. delbrueckii* subsp. *bulgaricus* B3 and A13)	Attenuate inflammation scores in experimental colitis	*In vivo* (rats)-intra-stomach administration	Şengül et al. (2006)
Protection from Pathogens			
L. rhamnosus GG	Abrogate cytotoxic effects of bacterial toxins	*In vitro* (Caco-2 cells; erythrocytes)	Ruas-Madiedo and De Los Reyes-Gavilán (2010)
L. reuteri (reuteran)	Antiadhesive properties against enterotoxigenic *Escherichia coli* (ETEC); protect weanling piglets from ETEC colonization	*In vitro; ex vivo* (pig intestinal segments); *in vivo* (piglets)-dietary intake	Wang et al. (2010); Chen et al. (2014); Yang et al. (2015)
L. acidophilus A4	Reduce biofilm formation by ETEC	*In vitro*	Kim et al. (2009)

(*Continued*)

TABLE 2.1 (*Continued*)
Some of the Biological Properties Ascribed to EPSs from LABs

EPS Source	Observed Effect	Experimental Procedure	References
L. kefiranofaciens (kefiran)	Antagonize cytopathic effects of *Bacillus cereus* B10502 Antimicrobial effect and healing activity on skin lesion	*In vitro* *In vitro* and *in vivo* (rats)	Medrano et al. (2008, 2009); Rodrigues et al. (2005)
L. plantarum YW32	Inhibit biofilms formation by pathogenic bacteria	*In vitro*	Wang et al. (2015)
Anti-oxidative, Anti-tumour, and Anti-toxic			
L. casei Zhang	Modulate oxidative stress-associated enzymatic activities (including malondialdehyde [MDA], superoxide dismutase [SOD] and glutathione peroxidase [GSH-Px]) levels in serum and liver	*In vivo*–oral administration to hyperlipidemic rats	Zhang et al. (2010)
L. plantarum strains	Resistance to hydrogen peroxide and hydroxyl radical; DPPH scavenging; increase SOD activity in serum, increase GSH-Px activity and total antioxidant capacity in liver; decrease MDA level in liver	*In vitro*; *in vivo*-oral administration to senescent mice	Li et al. (2012); Wang et al. (2015)
P. acidilactici M6; *L. plantarum* LP6; *L. helveticus* MB2-1; *L. plantarum* C88; *L. paracasei* NTU 101 and *L. plantarum* NTU 102; *L. rhamnosus* E/N	Anti-oxidant ability; radical scavenging properties	*In vitro*	Song et al. (2013); Li et al. (2013, 2014); Zhang et al. (2013); Liu et al. (2011a); Polak-Berecka et al. (2013)
L. acidophilus 606	Inhibit cancer cell proliferation, antioxidant activity Antitumorigenic against colon cancer cells; induce autophagy	*In vitro* (various of cell lines); *in vitro* (HT-29 cells)	Choi et al. (2006); Kim et al. (2010)

(Continued)

TABLE 2.1 (*Continued*)
Some of the Biological Properties Ascribed to EPSs from LABs

EPS Source	Observed Effect	Experimental Procedure	References
L. plantarum strains	Antiproliferative activity	*In vitro* (HT-29 cells)	Wang et al. (2014, 2015)
L. casei 01	Antiproliferative activity; reduce cytotoxicity of genotoxic agent	*In vitro* (HT-29 cells; intestine 407 cells)	Liu et al. (2011b)
L. plantarum 301102; *L. casei 01*	Bind and inactivate mutagens	*In vitro*	Tsuda et al. (2008); Liu et al. (2011b)
L. plantarum (isolate from Chinese Paocai)	Lead adsorption	*In vitro*	Feng et al. (2012)

adjuncts, drugs, dietary supplements, and functional food (i.e., food that provides specific benefits beyond its basic nutritional function [German et al., 1999]) that could be helpful in the prevention and/or treatment of human and animal diseases.

Despite their potential, however, there are still major limitations to the applications of EPSs at the industrial level. First, most of the bioactivities attributed to LAB EPSs are based on *in vitro* or preliminary studies. Therefore, additional research is necessary to test their efficacy *in vivo*, as well as to understand their mechanism of action, before planning any application in the field of functional food and drugs. Another important consideration is that the EPS structure-function relationship is remarkably tight and, at the same time, LAB EPSs are extremely variable when one considers their chemical composition and structure (e.g., differences in bond types, chemical substitutions, branching, and molecular mass). Thus, EPSs of different origin act differently, and their biological properties vary in a species- or strain-dependent fashion. Last but not the least, the commercial exploitation of LAB EPSs as purified chemicals appears infeasible because of the high production costs arising from their generally low yield, especially in comparison to other polymers of microbial origin (Salazar et al., 2016). Conversely, the use of the whole EPS-producing strains, particularly LABs with food grade and/or probiotic status, seems more feasible and would result in a better *in situ* production, within the product itself, being it either a mere vehicle, a fermented food, or a specific symbiotic preparation.

Immunomodulation by Exopolysaccharides

As extracellular bacterial components, EPSs are involved in interactions with the environment, including protection from harsh conditions and niche colonization. In commensal LABs inhabiting the gut, EPSs are key microbe-associated molecular patterns (MAMPs) that promote the interplay with host cells, especially in terms of eliciting an immune response. Indeed, the genetic repertoire enabling EPS biosynthesis is extremely widespread among intestine-adapted LABs, hence corroborating a role for such surface components in microbe–host relationships, specifically those that improve survival chances in the gut. In this regard, under an ecological perspective, Sims et al. (2011) suggested that, after adopting a commensal relationship with vertebrate hosts, LAB EPSs would have acquired novel roles, including immunomodulation. This would enhance colonization of the host, for instance, by regulating gut mucosal immune homeostasis to induce an immunological tolerance toward the commensal. The relevance of EPS in immune interactions with host was emphasized also by recent studies finding how composition and properties of EPSs from intestinal commensal species, including lactobacilli (Górska et al., 2016) and bifidobacteria (Ferrario et al., 2016), may be consistently modulated by host gut conditions (i.e., inflammation state and age, respectively).

The physical-chemical features of bacterial EPSs appear closely related to their immunomodulatory ability. Indeed, based on analysis of the available literature, it was proposed that low molecular weight and/or negatively charged (i.e., typically containing phosphate groups) EPSs would act as mild immune stimulators, while neutral and large EPSs would have immunosuppressive properties (Hidalgo-Cantabrana et al., 2012). Several studies report the ability of LAB EPSs to elicit immune responses, especially in relation to the intestinal mucosa. Anti-inflammatory and immunosuppressive properties have been demonstrated for EPSs from LABs, including *Lactobacillus casei, Lc. lactis, P. parvulus, L. plantarum, L. rhamnosus, Lactobacillus paraplantarum, L. kefiranofaciens* (Vinderola et al., 2006; Yasuda et al., 2008; Bleau et al., 2010; Nikolic et al., 2012; Notararigo et al., 2014; Wachi et al., 2014; Murofushi et al., 2015; Tang et al., 2015). Overall, such studies describe the ability of EPSs to interact with different types of immune cells (including intestinal epithelial cells, which are considered major components of the gastrointestinal immune system) and modulate the production of specific cytokines.

Oral administration of kefiran, that is, the main EPS produced by *L. kefiranofaciens,* a species commonly found among kefir microbiota, led to increased secretion of immunoglobin A (IgA) in the small and large intestine (Vinderola et al., 2006). IgA-inducing activities were ascribed also to EPS from a vegetal isolate of *Leuconostoc mesenteroides* (Matsuzaki et al., 2014). As IgA plays an important role as the first line of defense in the host, the authors suggest a protective role for EPS on the intestinal mucosa. Purified EPS from *L. rhamonosus* RW-9595M could inhibit the production of TNF, IL-6, and IL-12, while stimulating the secretion of the anti-inflammatory cytokine IL-10 in murine macrophages, thus pointing to their anti-inflammatory potential (Bleau et al., 2010). Wild type *L. casei* Shirota, which produces high-molecular-weight (HMW) EPS, attenuated cytokine production and immune reaction in murine spleen cells and macrophages, compared to the EPS-KO mutant strain, which was unable to synthesize EPS (Yasuda et al., 2008). According to the authors, HMW EPS of *L. casei* Shirota would act as a suppressor for its own immunologic activity. A similar conclusion was drawn by studying *L. paraplantarum* BGCG11 EPS-producing (parental) strain and its non-ropy derivatives, in relation to the cytokine pattern induced in human peripheral blood mononuclear cells (Nikolic et al., 2012): the former induced a cytokine ratio suggestive of Th2-Treg and Th17 response (i.e., suppressive and immunoregulatory functions), while the latter induced a pro-Th1 (pro-inflammatory) response. Purified β-glucans from *P. parvulus* 2.6

activated human macrophages and had anti-inflammatory effects (Notararigo et al., 2014). Both *L. delbrueckii* TUA4408L EPS and acidic EPS from *L. plantarum* N14 attenuated enterotoxigenic *Escherichia coli* (ETEC)-induced inflammatory response in porcine intestinal epithelial, and the modulation of pro-inflammatory cytokine was mediated by specific members of the Toll-like receptor family (Wachi et al., 2014; Murofushi et al., 2015). Based on *in vivo* and *in vitro* assays, Tang et al. (2015) suggested that purified EPS from *L. plantarum* induced variations of the cytokine level in mice intestinal fluid and promoted the maturation of dendritic cells.

Although more investigations are required to understand the mechanisms underlying the immunomodulative effect of EPSs from (probiotic) LABs, many of the above studies suggest that they are good candidates for developing functional food that protects against immune-related disorders, particularly those entailing intestinal inflammatory damage.

METABOLIC EFFECTS: HYPOCHOLESTEROLEMIC ACTIVITY

The saccharides included in dietary fibers, especially those of plant origin, reduce the risk of cardiovascular diseases and are known to have a positive influence on constipation, hyperlipidemias, diabetes, obesity, and diverticular disease (German et al., 1999). One of their main features is their acknowledged hypocholesterolemic property. For instance, the dietary assumption of oat β-glucan fibers is associated with the reduction of blood cholesterol level, and both the U.S. Food and Drug Administration (FDA) and the European Food Safety Authority (EFSA) have approved health claims for that (EFSA, 2010; FDA, 2010).

A few studies have investigated the hypoglycemic and hypocholesterolemic effects of bacterial EPS and hint that dietary interventions based on EPS-producing probiotic strains may represent a valuable opportunity for managing lipid metabolism (Maeda et al., 2004; London et al., 2014). It was suggested that the cholesterol-lowering ability of LAB EPSs could be due, at least in part, to their thickening property and their ability to absorb cholesterol, thus hampering its assimilation by intestinal cells (Nakajima et al., 1992; Tok and Aslim, 2010). In a human study, the administration of an oat-based product, co-fermented with a β-glucan EPS-producing *Pediococcus* strain, significantly reduced serum cholesterol concentrations (Mårtensson et al., 2005). In lipid-fed apolipoprotein E (apoE)-deficient mice, the dietary intake of EPS-producing probiotic lactobacilli resulted in lower serum levels of cholesterol and triglycerides, underpinning an improvement in the lipid metabolism; moreover, such a diet modulated the composition of the gut microbiota (London et al., 2014). Kefiran, from *L. kefiranofaciens*, has been ascribed hypotensive and hypocholesterolemic effects (Maeda et al., 2004), and its administration was found to prevent atherosclerosis in hypercholesterolemic rabbits (Uchida et al., 2010).

EFFECTS ON GUT MUCOSA AND PHYSIOLOGY

Several studies provide the rationale for the therapeutic use of LAB EPSs in the prevention or treatment of gastrointestinal disorders. For instance, the EPS produced by *S. thermophilus* CRL1190 (in the form of *S. thermophilus*-fermented milk) could both prevent the development and alleviate the symptoms of gastritis in mice (Rodríguez et al., 2009, 2010). Besides, its dietary intake was shown to preserve and/or increase the thickness of the mucus gel layer in murine gastric mucosa, thus contributing to strengthen this important defense barrier (Rodríguez et al., 2010). Notably, a similar effect was previously observed upon administration of *L. rhamnosus* GG, an EPS-producing probiotic strain (Lam et al., 2007). Interestingly, the antigastritis and anti-inflammatory actions were achieved only when EPSs were suspended in milk but not in water; therefore, the authors suggested that interactions between microbial EPSs and milk proteins could underlie the observed gastroprotective effect (Rodríguez et al., 2009). Molecular size and polymer composition seem relevant for the therapeutic effect of EPSs on the gastric function, although with different results according to studies. For instance, Nagaoka et al. (1994) noticed that *Lactobacilli* and *Streptococci* EPSs with higher rhamnose content were more effective in healing gastric ulcers in rats, while Rodríguez et al. (2009) found that, independently on composition, only HMW EPS could exert a consistent prevention of gastritis. In following *in vitro* studies, purified EPSs, isolated from milk fermented by *S. thermophilus* CRL1190, were chemically characterized and shown to stimulate regeneration and innate defense mechanisms in human gastric and mouth epithelial cells (Marcial et al., 2013). As indicated by the authors, the signals promoting such an effect could arise from the ability of EPSs to adhere on the cell surface and to be partially taken up via endosomal transport.

The EPSs produced by probiotic LABs have a promising therapeutic role also for dysfunctions at the intestinal level, such as those leading to food allergy reactions or chronic inflammation. In this regard, EPS-producing probiotic lactobacilli significantly attenuated experimental colitis in rats, with an EPS dose-dependent effect (Şengül et al., 2006), thus providing a natural alternative in the treatment of inflammatory bowel diseases.

PROTECTION AGAINST PATHOGENS

Another promising application of LAB EPSs relates to their ability to antagonize microbial pathogens, especially those acting in the intestine. The livestock industry is constantly looking for alternatives to antibiotic treatments, with the aim to reduce infections and ensure animal and consumers' health. The potential of bacterial EPS has been investigated also in this field. Reuteran and levan, EPSs synthesized by *L. reuteri* (i.e., a LAB that occurs in the swine commensal microbiota and is also used industrially as a starter culture in cereal fermentations), protected piglet intestinal mucosa from enterotoxigenic *E. coli* (ETEC) infection (Chen et al., 2014). Furthermore, administration of a reuteran-containing diet consistently reduced the level of ETEC colonization in weaning piglets (Yang et al., 2015), thus proposing an EPS-enriched functional feed as a possible method for controlling ETEC infections. EPS from *L. reuteri* and from *Lactobacillus acidophilus* A4 were ascribed antiadhesive and antibiofilm properties against ETEC (Kim et al., 2009; Wang et al., 2010).

The fermented dairy product kefir and its main EPS component kefiran, produced by *L. kefiranofaciens*, showed antimicrobial activity against various microbial pathogens and exerted a cicatrizing effect on wounded skin (Rodrigues et al., 2005). Kefiran also protected human enterocytes from the structural damages induced by a pathogenic *Bacillus cereus* strain (Medrano et al., 2008, 2009), which was probably due to its ability to interact with both bacterial and eukaryotic cells, thus antagonizing the interactions necessary for the pathogen biological effects.

The study by Ruas-Madiedo et al. (2010) revealed another mechanism possibly underlying the antagonism of probiotics against pathogens. The EPS produced by probiotic strains of bifidobacteria and lactobacilli were able to counteract *in vitro* the cytotoxic effect of bacterial toxins. According to the authors, bacterial EPSs could act either by blocking the toxin receptors on the animal cell or by capturing the toxin, thus avoiding its interaction with the infected animal cells. Even in such cases, some physical–chemical characteristics of EPSs, including molecular mass and radius of gyration, were directly related to the observed antitoxin effect (Ruas-Madiedo et al., 2010).

Antioxidant and Antitumor Properties

Accumulation of reactive oxygen species and oxidative stress can mine the structural integrity and functionality of cellular components, which is associated with the onset of inflammatory disorders, degenerative disease, and cancer. Synthetic antioxidants are commonly used drugs to treat effectively oxidative stress-associated pathologies; however, concerns about their safety prompt an ongoing search for natural, less toxic alternatives. Food-grade antioxidative agents are also helpful for food preservation, and so they are in constant demand by the food industry.

Some studies have focused on the antioxidant and free radical scavenging abilities of LAB EPSs. Şengül et al. (2006) attributed to the EPS produced by *Lactobacillus bulgaricus* B3 the capacity to alleviate acetic acid–induced experimental colitis *in vivo*, ascribing such effect to their antioxidant and metal ion-chelating abilities. Likewise, some recent *in vivo* studies demonstrated that the dietary administration of *L. casei* and *L. plantarum* strains could alleviate oxidative stress and ameliorate antioxidant indexes, suggesting that such capacity was associated with the production of EPS (Zhang et al., 2010; Li et al., 2012; Zhang et al., 2013). Several subsequent reports have described how purified EPSs from diverse LAB species are able to chelate ferrous ions, inhibit lipid peroxidation, provide reducing power, and/or act as radical scavengers *in vitro* (Liu et al., 2011a; Li et al., 2013; Polak-Berecka et al., 2013; Song et al., 2013; Zhang et al., 2013; Li et al., 2014; Wang et al., 2015).

According to some preliminary *in vitro* studies, EPS could provide promising natural adjuncts also for the prevention and treatment of cancer. The soluble polysaccharide fraction isolated from *L. acidophilus* 606 heat-killed cells was found to inhibit cancer cell proliferation, while being much less cytotoxic to normal cells (Choi et al., 2006). The observed inhibitory effect was tentatively attributed to the induction of apoptosis. Later, Kim et al. (2010) found that purified cell-bound EPS from that same *L. acidophilus* strain promoted autophagic death of tumor cells. Consistently, antiproliferative activities on human colon cancer cells have also been reported for EPSs isolated from *L. casei 01* (Liu et al., 2011b) and *L. plantarum* strains (Wang et al., 2014, 2015).

INACTIVATION OF TOXIC COMPOUNDS

The capacity of LAB EPSs to interact with toxic compounds has also been investigated by a few *in vitro* studies, though this beneficial property deserves further attention for its intriguing applications, not only in the area of food and pharmaceuticals but also in view of bioremediation interventions. EPS from *L. plantarum* 301102 were shown to bind and inactivate mutagens (Tsuda et al., 2008). Similarly, EPS from *L. casei 01* protected intestinal cells against the cytotoxicity of a genotoxic compound (Liu et al., 2011b). Additionally, EPS from a *L. plantarum* strain, isolated from Chinese traditional fermented foods, acted as a biosorbent of lead, hence suggesting its practical application for the removal of heavy metals from environmental samples or for excretion of lead from human body (Feng et al., 2012).

THE PREBIOTIC POTENTIAL OF LAB EXOPOLYSACCHARIDES

The dietary assumption of probiotics, prebiotics and/or their synergistic combination (i.e., synbiotics) represents an intriguing nutritional strategy for modulating the composition of the enteric microbial communities, with the aim to improve human health. Prebiotics are healthful, nondigestible food ingredients that selectively stimulate growth and/or activities of beneficial members of the gut microbiota, consequently enhancing their health benefits to the host (Gibson and Roberfroid, 1995; Roberfroid et al., 2010). Well-known prebiotics comprise nondigestible oligosaccharides, mainly of plant origin, such as inulins, fructo-oligosaccharides (FOSs), and galactooligosaccharides (GOSs) (Charalampopoulos and Rastall, 2012). Such carbohydrates withstand the host gastrointestinal (GI) digestion, thus reaching (undigested) the colon, where they can be fermented by health-promoting commensal microbes, that is, typically bifidobacteria and lactobacilli.

Recently, LAB EPSs have also been evaluated as potential prebiotics (reviewed by Salazar et al., 2016). According to their proposed physiological role, EPSs are not meant to be used as growth substrate by the producing bacteria, yet those synthesized by intestinal LABs might act as a carbon-source for the gut microbiota, through metabolic cross-interactions among its members. In line with this, some LAB EPSs were shown to be biodegraded by human fecal microbes (Ruijssenaars et al., 2000), and EPSs produced by LABs isolated from the digestive tract of marine fishes resisted to simulated GI conditions, showing a strong bifidogenic effect (Hongpattarakere et al., 2012). Bifidogenic effects have been proven *in vitro* for EPSs isolated from sourdough *L. sanfranciscensis* (Dal Bello et al., 2001; Korakli et al., 2002), probiotic *L. rhamnosus* E/N (Polak-Berecka et al., 2013), and *L. plantarum* DM5 (Das et al., 2014). While EPS from *L. rhamnosus* RW-9595M were not metabolized by infant fecal microbiota and lacked any prebiotic effect (Cinquin et al., 2006), EPS from *P. parvulus* 2.6 were suggested to be used as a carbon source by some probiotic strains *in vitro* (Russo et al., 2012), and an oat-based product, fermented with the same EPS-producing *P. parvulus* strain, exhibited a bifidogenic effect in humans (Mårtensson et al., 2005). However, administration of those purified EPSs to mice did not result in any prebiotic effect, whereas assumption of live EPS-producing bacteria antagonized *Enterobacteriaceae* without disturbing the homeostasis of the gut microbiota (Lindström et al., 2013).

From this early set of studies, it is apparent that LAB EPSs of different origins and with diversified chemical structures are prone to varying degrees to biodegradability by members of the enteric microbiota. Moreover, their prebiotic potential needs to be assayed *in vivo* (Roberfroid et al., 2010), where the endogenous microbiota provides a large pool of hydrolytic enzymes that can break down potential prebiotics. It is also evident that, given the complexity of gut ecosystems and the differences between animal models and even among individuals, the evaluation of a prebiotic activity is a challenging task. Not surprisingly, the abovementioned studies provide only fragmentary indications about whether LAB EPSs comply with three main requisites of prebiotics: that is, (1) be resistant to hydrolytic action of the host digestive tract, (2) provide fermentable substrates to beneficial gut microbes, and (3) benefit the host by selective modulation of the enteric microbiota. However, if we broaden the concept of prebiotic, we can assume that a prebiotic compound is not only a mere carbon source (Figure 2.1). Hence, LAB EPSs could enhance the activity of endogenous and/or dietary assumed probiotics by other means, not necessarily involving their use as fermentable substrates. Indeed, several experimental observations indicate that EPSs can improve the overall performance of probiotics because they influence important characteristics, including their ability to survive

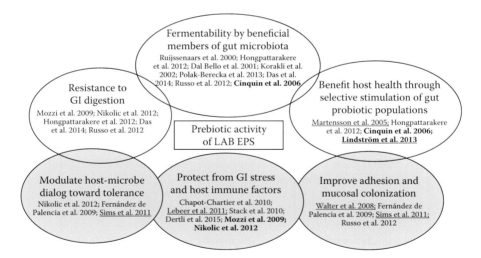

FIGURE 2.1 *Characteristics of prebiotics.* Stringent requisites of prebiotic substrates and, according to a broader concept, other beneficial activities (gray-shaded circles) that can promote the performance of probiotics, resulting in benefits for the host. Indicated are the references that support or contrast (in dark) such properties for EPSs from LABs. References based on *in vivo* experiments are underlined. GI, gastrointestinal.

in the digestive tract, their immunomodulatory properties, and their adhesion to the intestinal mucosa. For instance, EPSs physically shielded LAB cells from host immune factors (Chapot-Chartier et al., 2010; Lebeer et al., 2011); moreover, they modulate the cross talk between bacteria and host, hence inducing an immune reaction that favors the persistence of the EPS-producing LAB strain (see also above) (Fernández de Palencia et al., 2009; Sims et al., 2011; Nikolic et al., 2012). Likewise, in bifidobacteria, EPSs were assigned a beneficial role in modulating various aspects of the interaction with the host, including the ability of commensal species to remain immunologically silent (Fanning et al., 2012a). In a few cases, LAB EPSs also were found to enhance the resistance to the harsh physical–chemical stress typically encountered along the GI tract (Stack et al., 2010; Dertli et al., 2015). In spite of contrasting evidence on the role of EPSs in LAB adhesion, sometimes EPSs were reported to act as positive mediators because the production and/or exogenous addition of LAB EPSs could potentiate probiotic adherence to human intestinal cells *in vitro* (Fernández de Palencia et al., 2009; Russo et al., 2012) and intestinal colonization *in vivo* (Walter et al., 2008). Their antiadhesive properties against pathogenic bacteria (Wang et al., 2010; Chen et al., 2014) might give a competitive advantage to the EPS-producing cells. In addition, EPSs promote the formation of biofilms (i.e., probably the preferential growth mode of gut commensal microbes), which enables a stable gut colonization (Walter et al., 2008) and were recently shown to boost some desirable effects of probiotics (Rieu et al., 2014; Aoudia et al., 2016). Besides, the increased viscosity of EPS-containing matrices, when used as vehicle to deliver dietary probiotics, might increase the length of their stay in the GI tract, thus prolonging their beneficial effects (German et al., 1999).

Overall, considering both the experimental findings and the high frequency of EPS-producing strains among LABs and bifidobacteria isolated from the intestine (Ruas-Madiedo et al., 2007), EPSs are very likely to enhance the fitness of probiotics to the gut niche (Fanning et al., 2012a,b). Therefore, the inclusion of LAB EPSs in functional food products and/or the direct administration of EPS-producing beneficial LABs should be considered as a way to enhance the efficacy of probiotics.

In summary, EPS-producing LABs, particularly probiotic strains hold promising applications in the functional food area; however, in order to realize such opportunity, *in vivo* investigations, especially human interventions proving their (prebiotic) functionality, need to be performed.

CONCLUSION

Considering the future uses of LAB EPSs as a possible driver of innovation in the food industry, there are important trends that deserve attention. First, the potential of data obtained by application of next-generation sequencing approaches is remarkable in order to elucidate the EPSs biosynthesis genetic determinants in LABs (including both plasmidia and genomic gene clusters) (e.g., Lamontanara et al., 2015; Li et al., 2015; Bai et al., 2016; Malik et al., 2016; Pérez-Ramos et al., 2016; Puertas et al., 2016; Gangoiti et al., 2017). Indeed, comparative genomics analysis could provide further insights for the industrial exploitation of LAB EPSs. This could also be accomplished from a systems biology perspective (Ates, 2015). Furthermore, the genome sequence data are extremely helpful to better assess the safety of EPS-producing LABs (Salvetti et al., 2016).

On the other hand, there is increasing evidence indicating a relevant role of EPSs in the stress response of LABs (e.g., Mozzi et al., 2009; Wu et al., 2014; Caggianiello et al., 2016). An ameliorated stress response in LABs is of considerable industrial importance for the preservation and survival of the microbial food cultures (MFCs) (i.e., starter cultures, protective cultures and probiotics) (Bourdichon et al., 2012) when exposed to the stresses associated with (1) MFC preparation, (2) MFC storage, (3) food matrices, and (4) the orogastrointestinal human tract (van de Guchte et al., 2002; Capozzi et al., 2009, 2010; Bove et al., 2012b; Bove et al., 2013).

More generally, this chapter focused on biopolymers that could be released by the producing bacteria directly *in situ*, thus avoiding several phases in this type of production, such as synthesis, separation, production, delivery of the alternative additives/functional molecules. As already demonstrated for some biofortifications (e.g., riboflavin in bread; Capozzi et al., 2011), the in situ EPSs enrichment by food-grade LAB cultures would represent a sustainable solution to achieve similar technological and better functional properties when compared with the use of traditional additives.

REFERENCES

Ahmad, N. H., Mustafa, S., and Y. B. C. Man. 2015, Microbial polysaccharides and their modification approaches: A review. *International Journal of Food Properties* 18:332–347. doi:10.1080/10942912.2012.693561.

Aoudia, N., Rieu, A., Briandet, R., Deschamps, J., Chluba, J., et al. 2016. Biofilms of *Lactobacillus plantarum* and *Lactobacillus fermentum*: Effect on stress responses, antagonistic effects on pathogen growth and immunomodulatory properties. *Food Microbiology* 53:51–59.

Arena, M. P., Silvain, A., Normanno, G., Grieco, F., Drider, D., et al. 2016. Use of *Lactobacillus plantarum* strains as a bio-control strategy against food-borne pathogenic microorganisms. *Frontiers in Microbiology* 7:464. doi:10.3389/fmicb.2016.00464.

Arendt, E. K., and E. Zannini. 2013. 12—Quinoa in *Cereal Grains for the Food and Beverage Industries*, (Eds.) E.K. Arendt and E. Zannini, Cambridge, UK: Woodhead Publishing, pp. 409–438.

Ates, O. 2015. Systems biology of microbial exopolysaccharides production. *Frontiers in Bioengineering and Biotechnology* 3:200. doi:10.3389/fbioe.2015.00200.

Bai, Y., Sun, E., Shi, Y., Jiang, Y., Chen, Y., et al. 2016. Complete genome sequence of *Streptococcus thermophilus* MN-BM-A01, a strain with high exopolysaccharides production. *Journal of Biotechnology* 224:45–46. doi:10.1016/j.jbiotec.2016.03.003.

Behare, P. V., Singh, R., Nagpal, R., Kumar, M., Tomar, S. K., and J. B. Prajapati. 2009b. Comparative effect of exopolysaccharides produced in situ or added as bioingredients on dahi properties. *Milchwissenschaft* 64:396–400.

Behare, P. V., Singh, R., Nagpal, R., and K. H. Rao. 2013. Exopolysaccharides producing *Lactobacillus fermentum* strain for enhancing rheological and sensory attributes of low-fat dahi. *Journal of Food Science and Technology* 50:1228–1232.

Behare, P., Singh, R., and R. P. Singh. 2009a. Exopolysaccharide-producing mesophilic lactic cultures for preparation of fat-free Dahi–an Indian fermented milk. *Journal of Dairy Research* 76:90–97.

Benozzi, E., Romano, A., Capozzi, V., Makhoul, S., Cappellin, L., et al. 2015. Monitoring of lactic fermentation driven by different starter cultures via direct injection mass spectrometric analysis of flavour-related volatile compounds. *Food Research International* 76:682–688. doi:10.1016/j.foodres.2015.07.043.

Berbegal, C., Peña, N., Russo, P., Grieco, F., Pardo, I., et al. 2016. Technological properties of *Lactobacillus plantarum* strains isolated from grape must fermentation. *Food Microbiology* 57:187–194. doi:10.1016/j.fm.2016.03.002.

Bleau, C., Monges, A., Rashidan, K., Laverdure, J. P., Lacroix, M., et al. 2010. Intermediate chains of exopolysaccharides from *Lactobacillus rhamnosus* RW-9595M increase IL-10 production by macrophages. *Journal of Applied Microbiology* 108:666–675.

Bourdichon, F., Casaregola, S., Farrokh, C., Frisvad, J. C., Gerds, M. L., et al. 2012. Food fermentations: Microorganisms with technological beneficial use. *International Journal of Food Microbiology* 154:87–97. doi:10.1016/j.ijfoodmicro.2011.12.030.

Bove, P., Fiocco, D., Gallone, A., Perrotta, C., Grieco, F., et al. 2012b. Abiotic stress responses in lactic acid bacteria (pp. 355–403). Chapter in *Stress Response of Foodborne Microorganisms*, (Ed.) Hin-chung Wong. https://www.novapublishers.com/catalog/product_info.php?products_id=34460 (accessed May 4, 2017).

Bove, P., Gallone, A., Russo, P., Capozzi, V., Albenzio, M., et al. 2012a. Probiotic features of *Lactobacillus plantarum* mutant strains. *Applied Microbiology and Biotechnology* 96:431–441. doi:10.1007/s00253-012-4031-2.

Bove, P., Russo, P., Capozzi, V., Gallone, A., Spano, G., and D. Fiocco. 2013. *Lactobacillus plantarum* passage through an oro-gastro-intestinal tract simulator: Carrier matrix effect and transcriptional analysis of genes associated to stress and probiosis. *Microbiological Research* 168:351–359. doi:10.1016/j.micres.2013.01.004.

Brown, L., Pingitore, E. V., Mozzi, F., Saavedra, L., Villegas, J. M., and E. M. Hebert. 2017. Lactic acid bacteria as cell factories for the generation of bioactive peptides. *Protein and Peptide Letters* 24:146–155. doi:10.2174/0929866524666161123111333.

Byrne D. 2001. Commission decision of January 30, 2001 on authorising the placing on the market of a dextran preparation produced by *Leuconostoc mesenteroides* as a novel food ingredient in bakery products under Regulation (EC) No. 258/97 of the European Parliament and of the Council Official. *Journal European Commission* L44.

Caggianiello, G., Kleerebezem, M., and G. *Spano*. 2016. Exopolysaccharides produced by lactic acid bacteria: From health-promoting benefits to stress tolerance mechanisms. *Applied Microbiology and Biotechnology* 100:3877–3886. doi:10.1007/s00253-016-7471-2.

Capozzi, V., Fiocco, D., Amodio, M. L., Gallone, A., and G. Spano. 2009. Bacterial stressors in minimally processed food. *International Journal of Molecular Science* 10:3076–3105. doi:10.3390/ijms10073076.

Capozzi, V., Fiocco, D., and G. Spano. 2011a. Responses of lactic acid bacteria to cold stress, in E. Tsakalidou and K. Papadimitriou (Eds.), *Stress Responses of Lactic Acid Bacteria, Food Microbiology and Food Safety*. New York: Springer, pp. 91–110.

Capozzi, V., Menga, V., Digesù, A. M., De Vita, P., van Sinderen, D., et al. 2011b. Biotechnological production of vitamin B2-enriched bread and pasta. *Journal of Agriculture and Food Chemistry* 59:8013–8020. doi:10.1021/jf201519h.

Capozzi, V., Russo, P., Fragasso, M., De Vita, P., Fiocco, D., et al. 2012a. Biotechnology and pasta-making: Lactic acid bacteria as a new driver of innovation. *Frontiers in Microbiology* 3:94. doi:10.3389/fmicb.2012.00094.

Capozzi, V., Russo, P., Ladero, V., Fernández, M., Fiocco, D., et al. 2012b. Biogenic amines degradation by *Lactobacillus plantarum*: Toward a potential application in wine. *Frontiers in Microbiology* 3:122. doi:10.3389/fmicb.2012.00122.

Chapot-Chartier, M. P., Vinogradov, E., Sadovskaya, I., Andre, G., Mistou, M. Y., et al. 2010. Cell surface of *Lactococcus lactis* is covered by a protective polysaccharide pellicle. *Journal of Biological Chemistry* 285(14):10464–10471. doi:10.1074/jbc. M109.082958.

Charalampopoulos, D., and R. A. Rastall. 2012. Prebiotics in foods. *Current Opinion in Biotechnology* 23:187–191.

Chen, X. Y., Woodward, A., Zijlstra, R. T., and M. G. Gänzle. 2014. Exopolysaccharides synthesized by *Lactobacillus reuteri* protect against enterotoxigenic *Escherichia coli* in piglets. *Applied and Environmental Microbiol*ogy 80:5752–5760. doi:10.1128/ AEM.01782-14.

Choi, S. S., Kim, Y., Han, K. S., You, S., Oh, S., et al. 2006. Effects of *Lactobacillus* strains on cancer cell proliferation and oxidative stress in vitro. *Letters in Applied Microbiology* 42:452–458.

Cinquin, C., Le Blay, G., Fliss, I., and C. Lacroix. 2006. Comparative effects of exopolysaccharides from lactic acid bacteria and fructo-oligosaccharides on infant gut microbiota tested in an in vitro colonic model with immobilized cells. *FEMS Microbiology and Ecology* 57:226–238.

Coelho, M. C., Silva, C. C. G., Ribeiro, S. C., Dapkevicius, M. L. N. E., and H. J. D. Rosa. 2014. Control of Listeria monocytogenes in fresh cheese using protective lactic acid bacteria. *International Journal of Food Microbiology* 191:53–59. doi:10.1016/j. ijfoodmicro.2014.08.029.

Dal Bello, F., Walter, J., Hertel, C., and W. P. Hammes. 2001. In vitro study of prebiotic properties of levan-type exopolysaccharides from lactobacilli and non-digestible carbohydrates using denaturing gradient gel electrophoresis. *System Applied Microbiology* 24:232–237.

Das, D., Baruah, R., and A. Goyal. 2014. A food additive with prebiotic properties of an α-D-glucan from *Lactobacillus plantarum* DM5. *International Journal of Biological Macromolecules* 69:20–26.

Dertli, E., Mayer, M. J., and A. Narbad. 2015. Impact of the exopolysaccharide layer on biofilms, adhesion and resistance to stress in *Lactobacillus johnsonii* FI9785. *BMC Microbiology* 15:8–12.

Di Cagno, R., Coda, R., De Angelis, M., and M. Gobbetti. 2013. Exploitation of vegetables and fruits through lactic acid fermentation. *Food Microbiology* 33:1–10.

Di Cagno, R., De Pasquale, I., De Angelis, M., Buchin, S., Rizzello, C. G., et al. 2014. Use of microparticulated whey protein concentrate, exopolysaccharide-producing *Streptococcus thermophilus*, and adjunct cultures for making low-fat Italian Caciotta-type cheese. *Journal of Dairy Science* 97:72–84.

Dickson-Spillmann, M., Siegrist, M., and C. Keller. 2011. Attitudes toward chemicals are associated with preference for natural food. *Food Quality and Preference* 22:149–156.

Douillard, F. P., and W. M., de Vos. 2014. Functional genomics of lactic acid bacteria: From food to health. *Microbial Cell Factory* 13:S8.

Duboc, P., and B. Mollet. 2001. Applications of exopolysaccharides in the dairy industry. *International Dairy Journal* 11:759–768.

EFSA—Panel on Dietetic Products, Nutrition and Allergies. 2010. Scientific Opinion on the substantiation of a health claim related to oat beta glucan and lowering blood cholesterol and reduced risk of (coronary) heart disease pursuant to Article 14 of Regulation (EC) No 1924/2006. *EFSA Journal* 8(12):1885. doi:10.2903/j. efsa.2010.1885.

European Pharmacopeia [EP]. 2014. *1506, 0999, 1000, 1001 (dextran), 1277 (xanthan), 0625 (sodium alginate), 1472 (sodium hyaluronate), 2603 (pullulan)*, 8th ed., Pharmacopeia Commission-European Directorate for the Quality of Medicines and Healthcare of the Council of Europe, Strasbourg, France.

Fanning, S., Hall, L. J., Cronin, M., Zomer, A., MacSharry, J., et al. 2012a. Bifidobacterial surface-exopolysaccharide facilitates commensal-host interaction through immune modulation and pathogen protection. *Proceedings of the National Academy of Sciences U S A* 109:2108–2113. doi:10.1073/pnas.1115621109.

Fanning, S., Hall, L. J., and D., van Sinderen. 2012b. *Bifidobacterium* breve UCC2003 surface exopolysaccharide production is a beneficial trait mediating commensal-host interaction through immune modulation and pathogen protection. *Gut Microbes* 3:420–425.

FDA. 2010. A rule by the Food and Drug Administration. Food labelling: Health claims: Oat and coronary heart disease. *Federal Register* 62:15.

Feng, M., Chen, L. I. C., Nurgul, R., and M. Dong. 2012. Isolation and identification of an exopolysaccharide-producing lactic acid bacterium strain from Chinese Paocai and biosorption of Pb(II) by its exopolysaccharide. *Journal of Food Science* 77:111–117.

Fernández de Palencia, P., Werning, M. L., Sierra-Filardi, E., Dueñas, M. T., Irastorza, A., et al. 2009. Probiotic properties of the 2-substituted (1,3)-β-D-glucan-producing bacterium *Pediococcus parvulus* 2.6. *Applied and Environmental Microbiology* 75:4887–4891.

Ferrario, C., Milani, C., Mancabelli, L., Lugli, G. A., Duranti, S., et al. 2016. Modulation of the eps-ome transcription of bifidobacteria through simulation of human intestinal environment. *FEMS Microbiology Ecology* 92(4):fiw056. doi:10.1093/femsec/fiw056.

Franck A., 2002. Technological functionality of inulin and oligofructose. *British Journal of Nutrition* S2:S287–S291.

Freitas, F., Alves, V. D., and M. A. M. Reis. 2011. Advances in bacterial exopolysaccharides: From production to biotechnological applications. *Trends Biotechnolology* 29:388–398. doi:10.1016/j.tibtech.2011.03.008.

Galle, S. and E. K. Arendt. 2014. Exopolysaccharides from sourdough lactic acid bacteria. *Critical Reviews in Food Science and Nutrition* 54:891–901. doi:10.1080/10408398.2011.617474.

Gangoiti, J., Meng, X., Bueren, A. L. van, and L. Dijkhuizen. 2017. Draft genome sequence of *Lactobacillus reuteri* 121, a source of α-glucan and β-fructan exopolysaccharides. *Genome Announcements* 5:e01691-16. doi:10.1128/genomeA.01691-16.

Ganzle, M. G., Zhang, C. G., Monang, B. S., Lee, V., and C. Schwab. 2009. Novel metabolites from cereal-associated lactobacilli—Novel functionalities for cereal products? *Food Microbiology* 26:712–719.

Gentès, M. C., St-Gelais, D., and S. L. Turgeon. 2013. Exopolysaccharide-milk protein interactions in a dairy model system simulating yoghurt conditions. *Dairy Science and Technology* 93:255–271.

German, B., Schiffrin, E., Reniero, R., Mollet, B., Pfeifer, A., and J. R. Neeser. 1999. The development of functional foods: Lessons from the gut. *Trend Biotechnol*ogy 17:492–499.

Gibson, G. R., and M. B. Roberfroid. 1995. Dietary modulation of the human colonic microbiota: Introducing the concept of prebiotics. *Journal of Nutrition* 125:1401–1412.

Górska, S., Sandstrőm, C., Wojas-Turek, J., Rossowska, J., Pajtasz-Piasecka, E., et al. 2016. Structural and immunomodulatory differences among lactobacilli exopolysaccharides isolated from intestines of mice with experimentally induced inflammatory bowel disease. *Scientific Reports* 6.

Hahn, C., Müller, E., Wille, S., Weiss, J., Atamer, Z., et al. 2014. Control of microgel particle growth in fresh cheese (concentrated fermented milk) with an exopolysaccharide-producing starter culture. *International Dairy Journal* 36:46–54.

Hidalgo-Cantabrana, C., López, P., Gueimonde, M., Clara, G., Suárez, A., et al. 2012. Immune modulation capability of exopolysaccharides synthesised by lactic acid bacteria and bifidobacteria. *Probiotics and Antimicrobial Proteins* 4:227–237.

Hölscher, T. and Á. T. Kovács. 2017. Sliding on the surface: Bacterial spreading without an active motor. *Environmental Microbiology* doi:10.1111/1462-2920.13741.

Hongpattarakere, T., Cherntong, N., Wichienchot, S., Kolida, S., and R. A. Rastall. 2012. In vitro prebiotic evaluation of exopolysaccharides produced by marine isolated lactic acid bacteria. *Carbohydate Polymers* 87:846–852.

Juvonen, R., Honkapää, K., Maina, N. H., Shi, Q., Viljanen, K., et al. 2015. The impact of fermentation with exopolysaccharide producing lactic acid bacteria on rheological, chemical and sensory properties of pureed carrots (Daucus carota L.). *International Journal of Food Microbiology*, 207:109–118.

Katina, K., Maina, N. H., Juvonen, R., Flander, L., Johansson, L., et al. 2009. In situ production and analysis of *Weissella confusa* dextran in wheat sourdough. *Food Microbiology* 26:734–743.

Kielak, A. M., Castellane, T. C. L., Campanharo, J. C., Colnago, L. A., Costa, O. Y. A., et al. 2017. Characterization of novel Acidobacteria exopolysaccharides with potential industrial and ecological applications. *Science Report* 7: doi:10.1038/srep41193.

Kılıç, G. B., and D. Akpınar. 2013. The effects of different levels of β-glucan on yoghurt manufactured with Lactobacillus plantarum strains as adjunct culture. *Journal of Food, Agriculture and Environment* 11:281–287.

Kim, D. S., Thomas, S., and H. S. Fogler. 2000. Effects of pH and trace minerals on long-term starvation of *Leuconostoc mesenteroides*. *Applied Environmental Microbiology* 66:976–981.

Kim, Y., Oh, S., and S. H. Kim. 2009. Released exopolysaccharide (r-EPS) produced from probiotic bacteria reduce biofilm formation of enterohemorrhagic *Escherichia coli* O157:H7. *Biochememical and Biophysical Research Communications* 379:324–329.

Kim, Y., Oh, S., Yun, H. S., and S. H. Kim. 2010. Cell-bound exopolysaccharide from probiotic bacteria induces autophagic cell death of tumour cells. *Letters Applied Microbiology* 51:123–130.

Kleerebezem, M., van Kranenburg, R., Tuinier, R., Boels, I. C., Zoon, P., et al. 1999. Exopolysaccharides produced by *Lactococcus lactis*: From genetic engineering to improved rheological properties? *Antonie Van Leeuwenhoek* 76:357–365.

Korakli, M., Gänzle, M. G., and R. F. Vogel. 2002. Metabolism by bifidobacteria and lactic acid bacteria of polysaccharides from wheat and rye, and exopolysaccharides produced by *Lactobacillus sanfranciscensis*. *Journal of Applied Microbiology* 92:958–965.

Korakli, M., Pavlovic, M., Ganzle, M. G., and R. F. Vogel. 2003. Exopolysaccharide and kestose production by *Lactobacillus sanfranciscensis* LTH2590. *Applied Environmental Microbiology* 69:2073–2079.

Korakli, M., and R. F. Vogel. 2006. Structure/function relationship of homopolysaccharide producing glycansucrases and therapeutic potential of their synthesised glycans. *Applied Microbiology and Biotechnology* 71:790–803.

Lam, E. K., Tai, E. K., Koo, M. W., Wong, H. P., Wu, W. K., et al. 2007. Enhancement of gastric mucosal integrity by *Lactobacillus rhamnosus* GG. *Life Sciences* 80:2128–2136.

Lamontanara, A., Caggianiello, G., Orrù, L., Capozzi, V., Michelotti, V., et al. 2015. Draft genome sequence of *Lactobacillus plantarum* Lp90 isolated from wine. *Genome Announcements* 3: doi:10.1128/genomeA.00097-15.

Leathers, T. D., Nunnally, M. S., Ahlgren, J. A., and G. L. Cote. 2003. Characterization of a novel modified alternan. *Carbohydrates Polymers* 54:107–113.

Leathers, T. D., Nunnally, M. S., and G. L. Côté. 2010. Optimization of process conditions for enzymatic modification of alternan using dextranase from *Chaetomium erraticum*. *Carbohydrates Polymers* 81:732–736.

Lebeer, S., Claes, I. J., Verhoeven, T. L., Vanderleyden, J., and S. C. De Keersmaecker. 2011. Exopolysaccharides of *Lactobacillus rhamnosus* GG form a protective shield against innate immune factors in the intestine. *Microbial Biotechnology* 4:368–374.

Lee, I.-C., Caggianiello, G., van Swam, I. I., Taverne, N., Meijerink, M., et al. 2016. Strain-specific features of extracellular polysaccharides and their impact on *Lactobacillus plantarum*-host interactions. *Applied Environmental Microbiology* 82:3959–3970. doi:10.1128/AEM.00306-16.

Leroy, F., and L. De Vuyst. 2016. Advances in production and simplified methods for recovery and quantification of exopolysaccharides for applications in food and health. *Journal of Dairy Science* 99:3229–3238.

Li, C., Li, W., Chen, X., Feng, M., Rui, X., et al. 2014a. Microbiological, physicochemical and rheological properties of fermented soymilk produced with exopolysaccharide (EPS) producing lactic acid bacteria strains. *LWT-Food Science and Technology* 57:477–485.

Li, J.-Y., Jin, M.-M., Meng, J., Gao, S.-M., and R. R. Lu. 2013. Exopolysaccharide from *Lactobacillus plantarum* LP6: Antioxidation and the effect on oxidative stress. *Carbohydrate Polymers* 98:1147–1152.

Li, S., Zhao, Y., Zhang, L., Zhang, X., Huang, L., et al. 2012. Antioxidant activity of *Lactobacillus plantarum* strains isolated from traditional Chinese fermented foods. *Food Chemistry* 135:1914–1919.

Li, W., Ji, J., Chen, X., Jiang, M., Rui, X. et al. 2014b. Structural elucidation and antioxidant activities of exopolysaccharides from *Lactobacillus helveticus* MB2-1. *Carbohydrate Polymers* 102:351–359.

Li, W., Xia, X., Chen, X., Rui, X., Jiang, M., et al. 2015. Complete genome sequence of *Lactobacillus helveticus* MB2-1, a probiotic bacterium producing exopolysaccharides. *Journal of Biotechnolology* 209:14–15. doi:10.1016/j.jbiotec.2015.05.021.

Lindström, C., Xu, J., Oste, R., Holst, O., and G. Molin. 2013. Oral administration of live exopolysaccharide-producing *Pediococcus parvulus*, but not purified exopolysaccharide, suppressed Enterobacteriaceae without affecting bacterial diversity in ceca of mice. *Applied Environmental Microbiology* 79:5030–5037. doi:10.1128/AEM.01456-13. *Epub* 2013 Jun 14.

Liu, C.-F., Tseng, K.-C., Chiang, S.-S., Lee, B.-H., Hsu, W.-H., et al. 2011a. Immunomodulatory and antioxidant potential of *Lactobacillus* exopolysaccharides. *Journal of Science of Food Agriculture* 91:2284–2291.

Liu, C.-T., Chu, F.-J., Chou, C. C. and R. C. Yu. 2011b. Antiproliferative and anticytotoxic effects of cell fractions and exopolysaccharides from *Lactobacillus casei* 01. *Mutation Research* 721:157–162.

Lluis-Arroyo, D., Flores-Nájera, A., Cruz-Guerrero, A., Gallardo-Escamilla, F., Lobato-Calleros, C., et al. 2014. Effect of an exopolysaccharide-producing strain of *Streptococcus thermophilus* on the yield and texture of Mexican Manchego-type cheese. *International Journal of Food Properties* 17:1680–1693.

London, L. E., Chaurin, V., Auty, M. A., Fenelon, M. A., Fitzgerald, G. F., et al. 2015. Use of *Lactobacillus mucosae* DPC 6426, an exopolysaccharide-producing strain, positively influences the techno-functional properties of yoghurt. *International Dairy Journal* 40:33–38.

London, L. E., Kumar, A. H., Wall, R., Casey, P. G., O'Sullivan, O., et al. 2014. Exopolysaccharide-producing probiotic Lactobacilli reduce serum cholesterol and modify enteric microbiota in ApoE-deficient mice. *Journal of Nutrition* 144:1956–1962.

Lynch, K. M., Coffey, A., and E. K. Arendt. 2017. Exopolysaccharide producing lactic acid bacteria: Their techno-functional role and potential application in gluten-free bread products. *Food Research International*.

Lynch, K. M., McSweeney, P. L., Arendt, E. K., Uniacke-Lowe, T., Galle, S., et al. 2014. Isolation and characterisation of exopolysaccharide-producing *Weissella* and *Lactobacillus* and their application as adjunct cultures in Cheddar cheese. *International Dairy Journal* 34:125–134.

Maeda, H., Zhu, X., Suzuki, S., Suzuki, K., and S. Kitamura. 2004. Structural characterization and biological activities of an exopolysaccharide kefiran produced by *Lactobacillus kefiranofaciens* WT-2B(T). *Journal of Agriculture and Food Chemistry* 52:5533–2238.

Malik, A., Sumayyah, S., Yeh, C.-W., and N. C. K. Heng. 2016. Identification and sequence analysis of pWcMBF8-1, a bacteriocin-encoding plasmid from the lactic acid bacterium *Weissella confusa. FEMS Microbiological Letters* 363. doi:10.1093/femsle/fnw059.

Marcial, G., Messing, J., Menchicchi, B., Goycoolea, F. M., Faller, G., et al. 2013. Effects of polysaccharide isolated from *Streptococcus thermophilus* CRL1190 on human gastric epithelial cells. *International Journal of Biological Macromolecules* 62:217–224. doi:10.1016/j.ijbiomac.2013.08.011.

Mårtensson, O., Biörklund, M., Lambo, A. M., Dueñas-Chasco, M., Irastorza, A., et al. 2005. Fermented, ropy, oat-based products reduce cholesterol levels and stimulate the bifidobacteria flora in humans. *Nutrition Research* 25:429–442.

Matsuzaki, C., Kamishima, K., Matsumoto, K., Koga, H., Katayama, T., et al. 2014. Immunomodulating activity of exopolysaccharide-producing *Leuconostoc mesenteroides* strain NTM048 from green peas. *Journal of Applied Microbiology* 116:980–989.

Medrano, M., Hamet, M. F., Abraham, A. G., and P. F. Pérez. 2009. Kefiran protects Caco-2 cells from cytopathic effects induced by *Bacillus cereus* infection. *Antonie van Leeuwenhoek* 96:505–513.

Medrano, M., Pérez, P. F., and A. G. Abraham. 2008. Kefiran antagonizes cytopathic effects of Bacillus cereus extracellular factors. *International Journal of Food Microbiology* 122:1–7.

Mende, S., Peter, M., Bartels, K., Rohm, H., and D. Jaros. 2013. Addition of purified exopolysaccharide isolates from *S. thermophilus* to milk and their impact on the rheology of acid gels. *Food Hydrocolloids* 32:178–185.

Meng, X., Dobruchowska, J. M., Gerwig, G. J., Kamerling, J. P., and L. Dijkhuizen. 2004. Synthesis of oligo- and polysaccharides by *Lactobacillus reuteri* 121 reuteransucrase at high concentrations of sucrose. *Carbohydrate Research* 414:85–92.

Micheli, L., Uccelletti, D., Palleschi, C., and V. Crescenzi. 1999. Isolation and characterisation of a ropy *Lactobacillus* strain producing the exopolysaccharide kefiran. *Applied Microbiology and Biotechnology* 53:69–74.

Monsan, P., Bozonnet, S., Albenne, C., Joucla, G., Willemot, R. M., et al. 2001. Homopolysaccharides from lactic acid bacteria. *International Dairy Journal* 11:675–685.

More, T. T., Yadav, J. S. S., Yan, S., Tyagi, R. D., and R. Y. Surampalli. 2014. Extracellular polymeric substances of bacteria and their potential environmental applications. *Journal of Environmental Management* 144:1–25.

Mozzi, F., Gerbino, E., Font de Valdez, G., and M. I. Torino. 2009. Functionality of exopolysaccharides produced by lactic acid bacteria in an in vitro gastric system. *Journal of Applied Microbiology* 107:56–64. doi:10.1111/j.1365-2672.2009.04182.x.

Murofushi, Y., Villena, J., Morie, K., Kanmani, P., Tohno, M., et al. 2015. The toll-like receptor family protein RP105/MD1 complex is involved in the immunoregulatory effect of exopolysaccharides from *Lactobacillus plantarum* N14. *Molecular Immunology* 64:73–75.

Nagaoka, M., Hashimoto, S., Watanabe, T., Yokokura, T., and Y. Moro. 1994. Anti-ulcer effects of lactic acid bacteria and their cell wall polysaccharides. *Biological and Pharmaceutical Bulletin* 17:1012–1017.

Nakajima, H., Suzuki, Y., Kaizu, H., and T. Hirota. 1992. Cholesterol lowering activity of ropy fermented milk. *Journal of Food Science* 57:1327–1329.

Nikolic, M., López, P., Strahinic, I., Suárez, A., Kojic, M., et al. 2012. Characterisation of the exopolysaccharide (EPS)-producing *Lactobacillus paraplantarum* BGCG11 and its non-EPS-producing derivative strains as potential probiotics. *International Journal of Food Microbiology* 158:155–162.

Notararigo, S., de las Casas-Engel, M., de Palencia, P. F., Corbí, A. L., and P. López. 2014. Immunomodulation of human macrophages and myeloid cells by 2-substituted (1–3)-β-d-glucan from *P. parvulus* 2.6. *Carbohydrate Polymers* 112:109–113.

Nwodo, U. U., Green, E., and A. I. Okoh. 2012. Bacterial exopolysaccharides: Functionality and prospects. *International Journal of Molecular Science* 13:14002–14015. doi:10.3390/ijms131114002.

Paramithiotis, S. (Ed.). 2017. *Lactic Acid Fermentation of Fruits and Vegetables*. Boca Raton, FL: CRC Press.

Patel, A., and J. B. Prajapat. 2013. Food and health applications of exopolysaccharides produced by lactic acid bacteria. *Advances in Dairy Research* 2003:1–8.

Pérez-Mendoza, D., and J. Sanjuán. 2016. Exploiting the commons: Cyclic diguanylate regulation of bacterial exopolysaccharide production. *Current Opinion in Microbiology* 30:36–43. doi:10.1016/j.mib.2015.12.004.

Pérez-Ramos, A., Mohedano, M. L., Puertas, A., Lamontanara, A., Orru, L., et al. 2016. Draft genome sequence of *pediococcus parvulus* 2.6, a Probiotic β-Glucan Producer Strain. *Genome Announcements* 4. doi:10.1128/genomeA.01381-16.

Polak-Berecka, M., Wasko, A., Szwajgier, D., and A. Chomaz. 2013. Bifidogenic and antioxidant activity of exopolysaccharides produced by *Lactobacillus rhamnosus* E/N cultivated on different carbon sources. *Polish Journal of Microbiology* 62:181–189.

Prasanna, P. H. P., Grandison, A. S., and D. Charalampopoulos. 2013. Microbiological, chemical and rheological properties of low-fat set yoghurt produced with exopolysaccharide (EPS) producing Bifidobacterium strains. *Food Research International* 51:15–22.

Puertas, A. I., Capozzi, V., Llamas, M. G., López, P., Lamontanara, A., et al. 2016. Draft genome sequence of *Lactobacillus collinoides* CUPV237, an exopolysaccharide and riboflavin producer isolated from cider. *Genome Announcements* 4. doi:10.1128/genomeA.00506-16.

Ravyts, F., De Vuyst, L. U. C., and F. Leroy. 2011. The effect of heteropolysaccharide-producing strains of *Streptococcus thermophilus* on the texture and organoleptic properties of low-fat yoghurt. *International Journal of Dairy Technology* 64:536–543.

Rehm, B. H. A. 2010. Bacterial polymers: Biosynthesis, modifications and applications. *Nature Reviews Microbiology* 8:578–592. doi:10.1038/nrmicro2354.

Rieu, A., Aoudia, N., Jego, G., Chluba, J., Yousfi, N., Briandet, R., Deschamps, J., Gasquet, B., Monedero, V., Garrido, C., and J. Guzzo. 2014. The biofilm mode of life boosts the anti-inflammatory properties of *Lactobacillus*. *Cellular Microbiology* 16:1836–1853.

Roberfroid, M., Gibson, G. R., Hoyles, L., McCartney, A. L., Rastall, R., et al. 2010. Prebiotic effects: Metabolic and health benefits. *British Journal of Nutrition* 104:S1–S63.

Rodrigues, K. L., Gaudino-Caputo, L. R., Tavares-Carvalho, J. C., Evangelista, J., and J. M. Schneedorf. 2005. Antimicrobial and healing activity of kefir and kefiran extract. *International Journal of Antimicrobial Agents* 25:404–408.

Rodríguez, C., Medici, M., Mozzi, F., and G. Font de Valdez. 2010. Therapeutic effect of *Streptococcus thermophilus* CRL 1190-fermented milk on chronic gastritis. *World Journal of Gastroenterology* 16:1622–1630.

Rodríguez, C., Medici, M., Rodríguez, A. V., Mozzi, F., and G. Font de Valdez. 2009. Prevention of chronic gastritis by fermented milks made with exopolysaccharide-producing *Streptococcus thermophilus* strains. *Journal of Dairy Science* 92:2423–2434. doi:10.3168/jds.2008-1724.

Ruas-Madiedo, P., and C. G. De Los Reyes-Gavilán. 2005. Invited review: Methods for the screening, isolation, and characterization of exopolysaccharides produced by lactic acid bacteria. *Journal of Dairy Science* 88:843–856.

Ruas-Madiedo, P., Medrano, M., Salazar, N., De Los Reyes-Gavilán, C. G., Pérez, P. F., et al. 2010. Exopolysaccharides produced by *Lactobacillus* and *Bifidobacterium* strains abrogate in vitro the cytotoxic effect of bacterial toxins on eukaryotic cells. *Journal of Applied Microbiology* 109:2079–2086. doi:10.1111/j.1365-2672.2010.04839.

Ruas-Madiedo, P., Moreno, J. A., Salazar, N., Delgado, S., Mayo, B., et al. 2007. Screening of exopolysaccharide-producing Lactobacillus and Bifidobacterium strains isolated from the human intestinal microbiota. *Applied and Environmental Microbiology* 73:4385–4388.

Ruijssenaars, H. J., Stingele, F., and S. Hartmans. 2000. Biodegradibility of food-associated extracellular polysaccharides. *Current Microbiology* 40:194–199.

Russo, P., Arena, M. P., Fiocco, D., Capozzi, V., Drider, D., et al. 2017. *Lactobacillus plantarum* with broad antifungal activity: A promising approach to increase safety and shelf-life of cereal-based products. *International Journal of Food Microbiol*ogy 247:48–54. doi:10.1016/j.ijfoodmicro.2016.04.027.

Russo, P., López, P., Capozzi, V., De Palencia, P. F., Dueñas, M. T., et al. 2012. Beta-glucans improve growth, viability and colonization of probiotic microorganisms. *International Journal of Molecular Sciences* 13:6026–6039.

Ryan, P. M., Ross, R. P., Fitzgerald, G. F., Caplice, N. M., and C. Stanton. 2015. Sugar-coated: Exopolysaccharide producing lactic acid bacteria for food and human health applications. *Food and Function* 6:679–693. doi:10.1039/c4fo00529e.

Salazar, N., Gueimonde, M., de Los Reyes-Gavilán, C. G., and P. Ruas-Madiedo. 2016. Exopolysaccharides produced by lactic acid bacteria and *Bifidobacteria* as fermentable substrates by the intestinal microbiota. *Critical Reviews in Food Science and Nutrition.* 56:1440–1453. doi:10.1080/10408398.2013.770728.

Salvetti, E., Orrù, L., Capozzi, V., Martina, A., Lamontanara, A., et al. 2016. Integrate genome-based assessment of safety for probiotic strains: *Bacillus coagulans* GBI-30, 6086 as a case study. *Applied Microbiology and Biotechnology* 100:4595–4605. doi:10.1007/s00253-016-7416-9.

Şanlı, T., Şenel, E., Sezgin, E., and M. Benli. 2014. The effects of using transglutaminase, exopolysaccharide-producing starter culture and milk powder on the physicochemical, sensory and texture properties of low-fat set yoghurt. *International Journal of Dairy Technology* 67:237–245.

Schmid, J. and V. Sieber. 2015. Enzymatic transformations involved in the biosynthesis of microbial exo-polysaccharides based on the assembly of repeat units. *ChemBioChem* 16:1141–1147. doi:10.1002/cbic.201500035.

Schmid, J., Sieber, V., and B. Rehm. 2015. Bacterial exopolysaccharides: Biosynthesis pathways and engineering strategies. *Frontiers in Microbiology* 6:496. doi:10.3389/fmicb.2015.00496.

Seibel, J., and K. Buchholz. 2010. Tools in oligosaccharide synthesis current research and application. *Advances in Carbohydrate Chemistry and Biochemistry* 63:101–138.

Şengül, N., Aslím, B., Uçar, G., Yücel, N., Işık, S., et al. 2006. Effects of exopolysaccharide-producing probiotic strains on experimental colitis in rats. *Diseases of the Colon and Rectum* 49:250–258.

Shah, N., and J. B. Prajapati. 2013. Effect of carbon dioxide on sensory attributes, physico-chemical parameters and viability of Probiotic *L. helveticus* MTCC 5463 in fermented milk. *Journal of Food Science and Technology* 51:3886–3893.

Sheppard, D. C., and P. L. Howell. 2016. Biofilm exopolysaccharides of pathogenic fungi: Lessons from bacteria. *Journal of Biological Chem*istry 291:12529–12537. doi:10.1074/jbc. R116.720995.

Sims, I. M., Frese, S. A., Walter, J., Loach, D., Wilson, M., et al. 2011. Structure and functions of exopolysaccharide produced by gut commensal Lactobacillus reuteri 100–123. *The ISME Journal* 5:1115–1124.

Song, Y. R., Jeong, D. Y., Cha, Y. S., and S. H. Baik. 2013. Exopolysaccharide produced by *Pediococcus acidilactici* M76 isolated from the Korean traditional rice wine, makgeolli. *Journal of Microbiology and Biotechnology* 23:681–688.

Stack, H. M., Kearney, N., Stanton, C., Fitzgerald, G. F., and R. P. Ross. 2010. Association of beta-glucan endogenous production with increased stress tolerance of intestinal lactobacilli. *Applied and Environmental Microbiology* 76:500–507. doi:10.1128/AEM.01524-09.

Szatraj, K., Szczepankowska, A. K., and M. Chmielewska-Jeznach. 2017. Lactic acid bacteria—Promising vaccine vectors: Possibilities, limitations, doubts. *Journal of Applied Microbiology* doi:10.1111/jam.13446.

Tamani, R. J., Goh, K .K. T., and C. S. Brennan. 2013. Physico-chemical properties of sourdough bread production using selected lactobacilli starter cultures. *Journal of Food Quality* 36:245–252.

Tang, Y., Dong, W., Wan, K., Zhang, L., Li, C., et al. 2015. Exopolysaccharide produced by *Lactobacillus plantarum* induces maturation of dendritic cells in BALB/c mice. *PloS one* 10:e0143743.

Tieking, M., and M. G. Ganzle. 2005. Exopolysaccharides from cereal-associated lactobacilli. *Trends Food Science Technology* 16:79–84.

Tok, E., and B. Aslim. 2010. Cholesterol removal by some lactic acid bacteria that can be used as probiotics. *Microbiology and Immunology* 54:257–264.

Tsuda, H., Hara, K., and T. Miyamoto. 2008. Binding of mutagens to exopolysaccharide produced by *Lactobacillus plantarum* mutant strain 301102S. *Journal of Dairy Science* 91:2960–2966.

Uchida, M., Ishii, I., Inoue, C., Akisato, Y., Watanabe, K., et al. 2010. Kefiran reduces atherosclerosis in rabbits fed a high cholesterol diet. *Journal of Atherosclerosis and Thrombosis* 17:980–988.

United States Pharmacopeia [USP] 35th Edn—National Formulary [NF] 30th Edn. 2012. (dextran), 2017 (xanthan), 1950 (sodium alginate), 1328 (gellan), 1938 (pullulan). Rockville, MD: United States Pharmacopeial Convention, pp. 2851–2853.

van de Guchte, M., Serror, P., Chervaux, C., Smokvina, T., Ehrlich, S. D., et al. 2002. Stress responses in lactic acid bacteria. *Antonie Van Leeuwenhoek* 82:187–216.

Varsha, K. K., and K. M. Nampoothiri. 2016. Appraisal of lactic acid bacteria as protective cultures. *Food Control* 69:61–64. doi:10.1016/j.foodcont.2016.04.032.

Vinderola, G., Perdigon, G., Duarte, J., Fanrworth, E., and C. Matar. 2006. Effects of the oral administration of the exopolysaccharide produced by *Lactobacillus kefiranofaciens* on the gut mucosal immunity. *Cytokine* 36:254–260.

Wachi, S., Kanmani, P., Tomosada, Y., Kobayashi, H., Yuri, T., et al. 2014. *Lactobacillus delbrueckii* TUA4408L and its extracellular polysaccharides attenuate enterotoxigenic *Escherichia coli*-induced inflammatory response in porcine intestinal epitheliocytes via Toll-like receptor-2 and 4. *Molecular Nutrition and Food Research* 58:2080–2093.

Waldherr, F. W., and R. F. Vogel. 2009. Commercial exploitation of homo-exopolysaccharides in nondairy food systems, in M. Ullrich (Ed.), *Bacterial Polysaccharides: Current Innovations and Future Trends*. Norfolk, VA: Caister Academic Press, pp. 313–329.

Walter, J., Schwab, C., Loach, D. M., Ganzle, M. G., and G. W. Tannock. 2008. Glucosyltransferase A (GtfA) and inulosucrase (Inu) of *Lactobacillus reuteri* TMW1.106 contribute to cell aggregation, *in vitro* biofilm formation, and colonization of the mouse gastrointestinal tract. *Microbiology* 154:72–80.

Wang, J., Zhao, X., Yang, Y., Zhao, A., and Z. Yang. 2015. Characterization and bioactivities of an exopolysaccharide produced by *L. plantarum* YW32. *International Journal of Biological Macromolecules* 74:119–126. doi:10.1016/j.ijbiomac.2014.12.006.

Wang, K., Li, W., Rui, X., Chen, X., Jiang, M., et al. 2014. Characterization of a novel exopolysaccharide with antitumor activity from *Lactobacillus plantarum* 70810. *International Journal of Biological Macromolecules* 63:133–139. doi:10.1016/j.ijbiomac.2013.10.036.

Wang, Y., Gänzle, M. G., and C. Schwab. 2010. Exopolysaccharide synthesized by *Lactobacillus reuteri* decreases the ability of enterotoxigenic *Escherichia coli* to bind to porcine erythrocytes. *Applied and Environmental Microbiology* 76:4863–4866. doi:10.1128/AEM.03137-09.

Welman, A. D., and I. S. Maddox. 2003. Exopolysaccharides from lactic acid bacteria: Perspectives and challenges. *Trends in Biotechnology* 21:269–274. doi:10.1016/S0167-7799(03)00107-0.

Wolter, A., Hager, A. S., Zannini, E., Czerny, M., and E. K. Arendt. 2014. Influence of dextran-producing *Weissella cibaria* on baking properties and sensory profile of gluten-free and wheat breads. *International Journal of Food Microbiology* 172:83–91.

Wu, Q., Tun, H. M., Leung, F. C.-C., and N. P. Shah. 2014. Genomic insights into high exopolysaccharide-producing dairy starter bacterium *Streptococcus thermophilus* ASCC 1275. *Science Reports* 4. doi:10.1038/srep04974.

Yang, Y., Galle, S., Le, M. H., Zijlstra, R. T., and M. G. Gänzle. 2015. Feed fermentation with reuteran- and levan-producing *Lactobacillus reuteri* reduces colonization of weanling pigs by enterotoxigenic *Escherichia coli*. *Applied and Environmental Microbiology* 81:5743–5752. doi:10.1128/AEM.01525-15.

Yang, Z., Li, S., Zhang, X., Zeng, X., Li, D., et al. 2010. Capsular and slime-polysaccharide production by *Lactobacillus rhamnosus* JAAS8 isolated from Chinese sauerkraut: Potential application in fermented milk products. *Journal of Bioscience and Bioengineering* 110:53–57.

Yasuda, E., Serata, M., and T. Sako. 2008. Suppressive effect on activation of macrophages by *Lactobacillus casei* strain Shirota genes determining the synthesis of cell wall-associated polysaccharides. *Applied and Environmental Microbiology* 74:4746–4755.

Yilmaz, M. T., Dertli, E., Toker, O. S., Tatlisu, N. B., Sagdic, O., et al. 2015. Effect of in situ exopolysaccharide production on physicochemical, rheological, sensory, and microstructural properties of the yogurt drink ayran: An optimization study based on fermentation kinetics. *Journal of Dairy Science* 98:1604–1624.

Zannini, E., Mauch, A., Galle, S., Gänzle, M., Coffey, A., et al. 2013. Barley malt wort fermentation by exopolysaccharide-forming *Weissella cibaria* MG1 for the production of a novel beverage. *Journal of Applied Microbiology* 115:1379–1387.

Zannini, E., Waters, D. M., Coffey, A., and E. K. Arendt. 2016. Production, properties, and industrial food application of lactic acid bacteria-derived exopolysaccharides. *Applied Microbiology and Biotechnology* 100:1121–1135. doi:10.1007/s00253-015-7172-2.

Zhang, L., Liu, C., Li, D., Zhao, Y., Zhang, X., et al. 2013. Antioxidant activity of an exopolysaccharide isolated from *Lactobacillus plantarum* C88. *International Journal of Biological Macromolecules* 54:270–275.

Zhang, Y., Du, R., Wang, L., and H. Zhang. 2010. The antioxidative effects of probiotic *Lactobacillus casei* Zhang on the hyperlipidemic rats. *European Food Research and Technology* 231:151–215.

3 Lithic Bacteria
A Lesser-Known Group in the Biomining Arena

Kaushik Bhattacharjee and S. R. Joshi

CONTENTS

INTRODUCTION

With increasing population and globalizing of the world economy, the demand for mineral and energy resources has been increasing. But high-grade ore reserves are deteriorating, and efficient techniques for the conversion of this raw material to renewable resources is also lacking (Acharya, 1990; Schippers et al., 2014). Since traditional techniques such as pryometallurgy and chemical processing are becoming obsolete, efficient recovery, recycling, and processing of mineral and energy resources are of significant importance today (Schippers et al., 2014).

Microorganisms are a notable addition to new development in this field (Acharya, 1990). Biomining refers to the use of microorganisms to facilitate the extraction and recovery of metals from metal containing ores and concentrates (Rawlings and Johnson, 2007). The substantial growth in scale and application of biomining started in the 1960s with the recovery of copper from ores in basically engineered rock "dumps" (Rawlings and Johnson, 2007). Biomining is becoming increasingly important among available mining technologies (Acharya, 1990). It has a clear advantage over hydrometallurgical or chemical procedures, with wider biotechnological applications (Schippers et al., 2014). Conventional techniques used in the mining industry for recovery of metals from low- and lean-grade ores are very expensive due to high energy and capital inputs, and they pollute the environment. In this regard, biomining offers an economic alternative for the mining industry (Alting and Chaerun, 2010), and it is environmentally friendly because it generates a minimal amount of pollutants. It has the added benefit of mining low-grade ore and/or mine tailings.

Metals play an integral role in the life process of microorganisms, but increasing concentrations of metals lead to damage of DNA structure and cell membranes, disruption in cellular functions, and alterations in enzyme specificity. Rock composed of minerals is the niche of lithobiontic bacterial community (Orell et al., 2013). Generally, microorganisms growing in such mineral-rich environments are, in most cases, remarkably tolerant of a wide range of metal ions due to the presence of robust metal resistance mechanisms (Rawlings et al., 2003; Orell et al., 2013). Hence, there is growing interest in discovering how microbes participate in biomining.

LITHIC BACTERIA

WHAT ARE LITHIC BACTERIA?

The earth is thought to be approximately 4.6 eons old (Jacobsen, 2003). Primitive life probably appeared 0.5–0.7 eons after formation of the planet, and the earliest forms of cellular life were reported as prokaryotes. The surface of the earth comprises the lithosphere, hydrosphere, and atmosphere, which are habitable by microbes to a greater or lesser extent (Ehrlich and Newman, 2009). One of the components of lithosphere of the Earth is rock. Geologically, a rock refers to a massive and solid matter that is the combination of one or more minerals. Geologists classify rocks into three major groups (igneous, sedimentary, and metamorphic) based on their mode of formation (Ehlers and Blatt, 1997; Best, 2003). Sedimentary rocks form 66% of the earth's crust; igneous and metamorphic rocks form the remaining 34% (Ehlers and Blatt, 1997).

Igneous rocks may arise from magma that cools either underground or on earth's surface. Sedimentary rocks (e.g., limestone, shale, and sandstone) are formed from the accumulation and compaction of sediment mainly derived from the breakdown of other rocks or cementation of the accumulated inorganic sediment (Figure 3.1). Metamorphic rocks are formed from igneous or sedimentary rocks that have been changed by temperature, pressure, or chemical reactions. Microorganisms that live in rock are termed as lithobiontic microorganisms (Golubic et al., 1981). Rocks appear to be similar superficially, although each habitat may host different microclimatic conditions due to various properties of rock, including porosity, translucence, and thickness (Cockell et al., 2005).

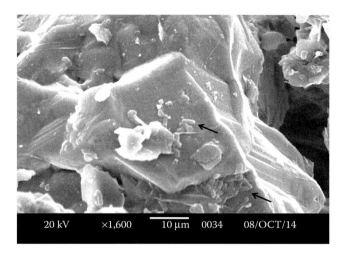

FIGURE 3.1 Scanning electron micrograph (SEM) of endolithic bacteria in greywacke sandstone from Mawsynram Village (Meghalaya, India), showing lithic bacterial colonization (arrow).

TYPES OF LITHIC BACTERIA

Lithobiontic bacterial colonization can be on the rock surface (epiliths), at the rock–soil interface (hypoliths), and inside the rocks (endoliths) (Friedmann, 1971; Broady, 1981; Stivaletta and Barbieri, 2009). Epilithic bacterial colonization mainly depends on ambient moisture content. Such colonization is rare in deserts due to rapid desiccation and intense solar radiation on rock surfaces (Wynn-Williams, 2000; Cockell et al., 2008). Epilithic bacteria display adaptations to ultraviolet (UV) light and to xeric and other stress conditions due to their exposure to the harsh epilithic environment (Cockell et al., 2008; Omelon, 2016).

However, the interior of lithic niche, that is, the endolithic environment, can retain moisture in the substrata, thus protecting the bacterial colonizations from direct exposure to UV light and temperature fluctuations (Wynn-Williams, 2000; Bhatnagar and Bhatnagar, 2005; Cockell et al., 2008). Endolithic habitats provide microorganisms with a stable substrate and protection from intense solar radiation, temperature fluctuations, wind, and desiccation (DiRuggiero et al., 2013). The endolithic bacteria are present in various types of rock, including sandstone (Bell 1993), limestone (Gerrath et al., 2000), gypsum (Hughes and Lawley, 2003; Stivaletta et al., 2010; Rhind et al., 2014), dolomite (Sigler et al., 2003; Horath and Bachofen, 2009), carbonates (Hoppert et al., 2004), ignimbrite (Wierzchos et al., 2013), and granite (Li et al., 2013).

According to different studies on lithic environments, the endolithic bacteria can be further subdivided into cryptoendolithic, chasmoendolithic, and euendolithic (Golubic et al., 1981). Chasmoendoliths reside in existing cracks or fissures of rocks. They are sometimes perceived as a transition between the epilithic habitats to the endolithic habitats. In some cases where cracks are not distinctive, they may appear as cryptoendoliths (Nienow and Friedmann, 1993). Chasmoendoliths are found mainly in desert condition (DiRuggiero et al., 2013). Euendoliths are rock-boring microorganisms that pierce actively into the interior of rocks (Friedmann et al., 1967; Golubic et al., 1981). They are found mostly in calcite, dolomite, and marble (Garcia-Pichel, 2006). Euendoliths play a major role in numerous geologic phenomena, including the bioerosion of limestones and other biogenic carbonates, and microbial cementation of carbonates, stromatolites, and microbialites (Hillgartner et al., 2001; Garcia-Pichel 2006). Cryptoendoliths are found in preexisting fissures, structural cavities, and pore spaces produced and vacated by euendoliths (Golubic et al., 1981). They can colonize the interstitial spaces of porous rocks and rather translucent rocks (Nienow and Friedmann, 1993), and were first reported by Friedmann et al. (1967) in the hot Negev desert. Since then, crypto-endolithic bacteria have been found in Antarctic sandstone (Hirsch et al., 2004), varnish on rocks (Kuhlman et al., 2008), and volcanic ignimbrite rocks (Wierzchos et al., 2013). They generally develop in areas where the microclimate prevents epithilic microbial growth (Bell, 1993; see Figure 3.2).

Hypolithic microbial communities are co-occurring phototrophic and heterotrophic consortia found on the undersides of translucent and opaque rocks that make contact with the underlying soil (Nienow and Friedmann, 1993; Cockell and Stokes, 2004;

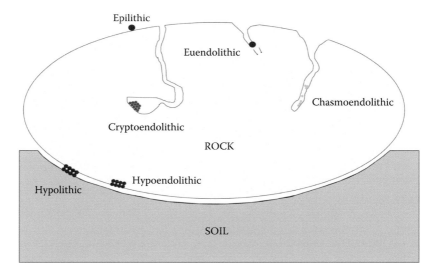

FIGURE 3.2 The possible lithobiontic habitats of microorganisms: epilithic (rock surface), hypolithic (rock underside in contact with the soil), endolithic (inside the rock, not in contact with the soil, and further divided into cryptoendolithic, chasmoendolithic, euendolithic, and hypoendolithic).

Wierzchos et al., 2011; Vitek et al., 2013; Warren-Rhodes et al., 2013) (Figure 3.1). Generally, the translucent and opaque rocks (quartz, granite, limestone, and gypsum) are suitable habitats for hypolithic microbial communities. They allow transmission of sufficient light at a depth where moisture availability, UV irradiance, and substrate stability are sufficiently minimized, and thus they support photosynthesis and the development of hypolithic microbial communities (Cary et al., 2010; Wong et al., 2010; Cowan et al., 2011; Warren-Rhodes et al., 2013). Researchers mention another lithic habitat, that is, hypoendolithic, where pore spaces are not in contact with the soil but occur on the underside of the rock and make contact with the underlying soil (Wierzchos et al., 2011).

CHARACTERIZATION OF LITHIC BACTERIA

Researchers have reported different methods with various media compositions suitable for isolating lithobiontic bacterial communities. However, the method for isolating bacterial communities from epilithic, endolithic, and hypolithic sources differs significantly depending on where they colonize.

For the isolation of epilithic microbial communities, Mitchell and Gu (2000) described the swab technique. Epilithic microbial communities can also be recovered by the printing-off method, where the microbial surface is rubbed directly on the medium (Staley, 1968). Eckhardt (1979) used an agar impression technique to investigate microbes on the surfaces of rock (Etienne and Dupont, 2002). For the isolation of endolithic microbial community, the rocks have to be sterilized to get rid of epilithones and other dirt particles, and then the core must be crushed, as described by Weirich and Schweisfurth (1985). After crushing, the rock powder has to be suspended in 100 mL of 0.2% Na-pyrophosphate solution and mixed for 15 min on a reciprocal shaker, followed by plating the dilution on media plate (Hirsch et al., 1995).

Epilithic microorganisms are counted by measuring the numbers of organisms per unit area of rock surface (Taylor-George et al., 1983). Endolithic microorganisms are counted by measuring the colony forming unit per gram of powdered rock. Since the hypolithic bacterial community exists at the interface between rock and underlying soil, the combined methods of soil dilution and epilithic microbial community can be used for the isolation of hypolithic bacterial community.

It is generally accepted that the success of the cultivation-based technique is primarily based on a suitable culture medium to isolate them (Bhattacharjee and Joshi, 2016). It is an axiom of microbiology that most culture media are selective for subsets of the total bacterial community; therefore, a variety of culture media is required to maximize the recovery of diverse microorganisms from different niches (Stevens, 1995).

To isolate the lithic bacteria, researchers have experimented with various media compositions (Table 3.1). Each of the media has different components that can influence the growth of lithic bacterial community specific to a niche. The source and concentration of nutrients of a medium, accompanied by the environmental factors, are known to have a profound effect on the isolation of microbes.

TABLE 3.1

Some of the Bacteriological Media Used for Isolation of Lithic Bacteria

Rock	Type	Media	References
Stone samples	Ep	Trypticase soy agar, Na and Mg supp. with 15% NaCl	Ettenauer et al. (2014)
	Ep	Trypticase soy agar, Na and Mg supp.	Ettenauer et al. (2014)
	Ep	Nutrient agar diluted 1:100	Ettenauer et al. (2014)
	Ep	Nutrient agar with 3% NaCl	Ettenauer et al. (2014)
Stone samples, bio-deteriorated monument	Ep	DSMZ media 372	Ettenauer et al. (2014)
Stone samples	Ep	DSMZ media 1018	Ettenauer et al. (2014)
Gravel particles	Ep	Solid mineral medium	Radwan et al. (2010)
Volcanic rocks	Ep	CDM agar	Campos et al. (2011)
Rock particles of cave	Ep	Peptone–yeast extract-brain heart infusion medium	Groth et al. (1999)
	Ep	Casein mineral medium	Groth et al. (1999)
	Ep	Bactotryptic soy agar	Groth et al. (1999)
	Ep	Starch–casein agar	Groth et al. (1999)
	Ep	Glycerol–asparagine agar (ISP 5)	Groth et al. (1999)
	Ep	Cycloheximide agar	Groth et al. (1999)
	Ep	Humic acid agar	Groth et al. (1999)
	Ep	Malt–yeast extract agar	Groth et al. (1999)
	Ep	Tap water agar	Groth et al. (1999)
Dolomite and limestone	En	Tryptone–soy agar	Fike et al. (2002)
Granite samples	En	LB medium or SSM	Fajardo-Cavazos and Nicholson (2006)
Red sandstone	En	Marine agar	Tanaka et al. (2003)
	En	BY medium; pH 7.4	Tanaka et al. (2003)
Siliceous rocks	En	Solid mineral media	Gaylarde et al. (2012)
Antarctic sandstone	En	PYGVagar	Hirsch et al. (2004)
	En	PYGV-8x, with peptone, yeast extract, and glucose	Hirsch et al. (2004)
Ancient stone	En	Starch–casein agar	Abdulla et al. (2008)
	En	Arginine glycerol salt medium	Abdulla et al. (2008)
	En	Starch nitrate medium	Abdulla et al. (2008)
	En	M3 medium	Abdulla et al. (2008)

(Continued)

TABLE 3.1 (*Continued*)
Some of the Bacteriological Media Used for Isolation of Lithic Bacteria

Rock	Type	Media	References
Granitic rock	En	Starch–casein agar	Abdulla (2009)
	En	Starch–casein agar with 20% rock extract	Abdulla (2009)
	En	Potato dextrose agar	Abdulla (2009)
	En	CYC agar	Abdulla (2009)
	En	MGA medium	Abdulla (2009)
	En	Arginine glycerol salts agar	Abdulla (2009)
Quartz pebble, lateritic sandstone, friable sandstone, basalt, decomposed granite, granitic pebble, quartzite, and phyllite	En	LM10	Bhattacharjee and Joshi (2016)

Note: supp: Supplemented; Ep: Epithilic; En: Endolithic

For characterization of epilithic, endolithic, and hypolithic bacterial community, a combination of biochemical, physiological, chemosystematics, and molecular biological methods are useful to obtain information about the bacterial community composition, and its ecological and physiological function (Vandamme et al., 1996). Of the various molecular biology techniques used to characterize cultivable bacterial community structures in diverse environments, 16Sr RNA gene analysis is the most useful (Cottrell and Kirchman, 2000) (Figure 3.3).

BIOMINING

Biomining is the generic term for describing when microorganisms are used for processing of metal-containing ores and concentrates (Johnson et al., 2013). It is an alternative to traditional physical–chemical methods of mineral processing (Rawlings and Johnson, 2007). Microbes interact with metals and metalloids for their own benefit or sometimes for their detriment (Ehrlich, 1997). Microorganisms involved in mineral processing have been around for almost 3.5 billion years (Brierley, 1984; Birgitta et al., 2004). Bacteria can interact with metals through chemotaxis, quorum sensing, adhesion, and biofilm formation. These are considered key phenomena for understanding the process of biomining. Bacteria have the ability to bind metal ions at the cell surface or to transport them into the cell for various intracellular functions (Ehrlich, 1997). This mechanism is being used to recover metals such as gold, copper, nickel, cobalt, zinc, iron, and uranium (Siddiqui et al., 2009). "Bioleaching" and "bio-oxidation" are two different processes of biomining (Pollmann et al., 2016). Bioleaching is referred as a simple and potent technology in biomining (Alting and Chaerun, 2010).

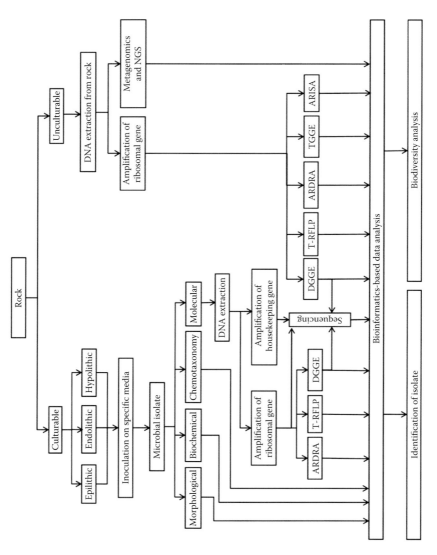

FIGURE 3.3 Flow diagram depicting the characterization and diversity analysis of lithic bacteria.

It is the biological conversion of an insoluble metal compound into a water-soluble form by means of microorganisms (Orell et al., 2013). Bio-oxidation is also caused by microorganisms; the valuable metal remains in the solid phase, but it becomes enriched (Pollmann et al., 2016).

Bioleaching is the biological and economical method for the recovery of metals, especially from low-grade ores (Rohwerder et al., 2003). Previously, bioleaching was focused on sulfidic ores; today, however, nonsulfidic (phosphates, oxides, carbonates, silicates) and complex ores are also targeted (Pollmann et al., 2016). During bioleaching of sulfidic ores, sulfuric acid and ferric iron are produced as by-products, and they contribute to the degradation of mineral. During the process, acid is produced; thus, acidophilic (pH 1.5–2.0) and chemolithoautotrophic bacteria (*Acidithiobacillus* sp., *Ferrimicrobium* sp., and *Leptospirillum* sp.) are normally used for bioleaching of sulfidic ores (Pollmann et al., 2016). Thiosulfate and polysulfide are the two different mechanisms that control the dissolution of metal sulfides. In the thiosulfate pathway, metal sulfides (pyrite, molybdenite, and tungstenite) are attacked by Fe^{3+}, which reduces to Fe^{2+}. As a result, the metal sulfide releases M^{2+} (metal cations) and thiosulfate. This thiosulfate is oxidized via tetrathionate and other polythionates, and finally to sulfate. From the requirement of an electron extraction reaction, iron-oxidizing bacteria such as *Acidithiobacillus ferrooxidans* and *Leptospirillum ferrooxidans* can catalyze the recycling of Fe^{3+} in acidic solutions (Rohwerder et al., 2003).

In the polysulfide pathway, metal sulfides (sphalerite, galena, arsenopyrite, chalcopyrite, and hauerite) are attacked both by Fe^{3+} and protons. During the reaction, bonds between metal and sulfur moiety are broken, and hydrogen sulfide (H_2S) is liberated, and it can spontaneously dimerize to free disulfide (H_2S_2); it is further oxidized via higher polysulfides and polysulfide radicals to elemental sulfur. The sulfur compounds are oxidized abiotically or biotically by sulfur-oxidizing bacteria such as *At. ferrooxidans* and *At. Thiooxidans* (Rohwerder et al., 2003).

For bioleaching of nonsulfidic ores, heterotrophic bacteria are used (Jain and Sharma, 2004). In this process, for growth and as a source of energy, the heterotrophic bacteria require an organic carbon source because they cannot gain energy from those ores. During this consumption, bacteria produce organic acids, extracellular polymeric substances (EPS), or siderophores that may interact with mineral surfaces and can solubilize the metals (Pollmann et al., 2016). Methods of leaching vary, from in situ dump leaching and heap leaching, with circulation, percolation, and irrigation of the leaching medium, to various tank or reactor leaching (Rawlings and Silver, 1995).

Microorganisms also play an important role in bioleaching of rare earth elements (REEs) by producing organic acids. Earlier, several researchers reported that chemolithoautotrophic bacteria such as *A. ferrooxidans* can degrade highly resistant zircon mineral by producing gluconic acids (Pollmann et al., 2016) and that heterotrophic bacteria such as *Acetobacter* sp., *Pseudomonas aeruginosa* can perform bioleaching of REEs from Egyptian monazite and monazite-bearing ores (Hassanien et al., 2014; Shin et al., 2015; Pollmann et al., 2016).

Bio-oxidation is the microbial process where the valuable metal remains in the solid phase. This process is used commercially for refractory sulfidic gold ores such as arsenopyrite before cyanide leaching (Rawlings et al., 2003). During the process, iron, arsenic, and sulfur are removed from gold deposits and render the gold accessible to cyanide and oxygen (Rawlings 2005). The advantage of bio-oxidation compared to roasting is that it is less expensive and it is safer for the environment, but it is a more time-consuming process than roasting (Grund et al., 2008). Munoz et al. (2006) and Escobar et al. (2000) have also tested this process for the pretreatment of copper minerals such as enargite. However, in contrast to the bio-oxidation of arsenopyrite, a minor amount of enargite oxidation was observed (Corkhill et al., 2008).

MICROBES IN BIOMINING AND THEIR CHARACTERISTICS

A variety of acidophilic, autotrophic, heterotrophic, and chemolithotrophic iron- and sulfur-oxidizing bacteria can oxidize minerals or mineral concentrates such as copper, gold, and uranium to recover metals. Autotrophic microorganisms associated with biomining are found to be strictly chemolithotrophic and acidophilic. They utilize inorganic carbon as a carbon source and gain energy by oxidation of reduced sulfur compounds such as pyrites. During the process, they produce nitric or sulfuric acid, which can react with minerals, leading to partial or complete dissolution or alteration in the mineralogy of the matrix (Sukla et al., 2014). *Pseudomonas arsenitoxidans* is the first obligate autotroph that was found to utilize arsenic as its sole energy source (Sukla et al., 2014). *Acidithiobacillus ferrooxidans, A. thiooxidans, A. caldus, Leptospirillum ferrooxidans, L. ferriphilum,* and *S. thermosulfidooxidans* are some of the other autotrophic microorganisms involved in bio-oxidation and bioleaching (Nagpal et al., 1993; Leduc and Ferroni, 1994; Clark and Norris, 1996; Suzuki, 2001; Rawlings, 2002).

Heterotrophic microorganisms utilize organic carbon as a carbon and energy source for their growth. The process produces organic acids, which leads to the partial or complete dissolution or alteration of the mineral surface. They can also solubilize the metals through different mechanisms, including production of exopolysaccharides, amino acids, or siderophores (Sukla et al., 2014; Roy and Roy, 2015). They are also beneficial for biomining of nonsulfide minerals. For example, *Bacillus circulans* was reported for use in the removal of heavy metals such as Cu, Ni, Pb, and Co by membrane-bound reductase enzyme (Roy and Roy, 2015).

Most bacteria capable of biomining have several common physiological characteristics. They are resistant to a range of metal ions, can fix CO_2 and N_2 from the air, can grow within the pH range from 1.5 to 2.0 and are able to use ferrous iron or reduced inorganic sulfur sources (or both) as electron donors (Rawlings, 2002) (Table 3.2).

TABLE 3.2
Bacterial Strains Reported to be Involved in Biomining

Microorganisms	Energy Pathway	Biomining Mechanism	References
Acidithiobacillus ferrooxidans	Obligate chemoautolithotroph	Desulfurization	Acharya et al. (2001)
Acidithiobacillus ferrooxidans	Obligate chemoautolithotroph	Fe oxidizing	Clark and Norris (1996)
Acidithiobacillus ferrooxidans	Obligate chemoautolithotroph	S oxidizing	Siddiqui et al. (2009)
Acidithiobacillus ferrooxidans	Obligate chemoautolithotroph	EPS production	Michel et al. (2009)
Acidithiobacillus ferrooxidans	Obligate chemoautolithotroph	Cu leaching	Pradhan et al. (2008)
Acidithiobacillus ferrooxidans	Obligate chemoautolithotroph	Arsenic leaching	Makita et al. (2004)
Acidithiobacillus ferrooxidans	Obligate chemoautolithotroph	Bioleaching	Martinez et al. (2015)
Acidithiobacillus ferrooxidans	Obligate chemoautolithotroph	Bioleaching of zinc	Bayat et al. (2009)
Acidithiobacillus ferrooxidans	Obligate chemoautolithotroph	Bioleaching of iron	Bayat et al. (2009)
Acidithiobacillus thiooxidans	Chemolithotroph	S oxidizing	Siddiqui et al. (2009)
Acidithiobacillus thiooxidans	Chemolithotroph	Bioleaching	Martinez et al. (2015)
Acidithiobacillus caldus	Chemolithotroph	S oxidizing	Siddiqui et al. (2009)
Acidithiobacillus caldus	Chemolithotroph	Bioleaching of chalcopyrite and bornite	Zhao et al. (2015)
Leptospirillum ferrooxidans	Autotroph	Fe oxidizing	Siddiqui et al. (2009)
Leptospirillum ferrooxidans	Autotroph	EPS production	Michel et al. (2009)
Leptospirillum ferriphilum	Obligate chemoautolithotroph	Fe oxidizing	Siddiqui et al. (2009)
Leptospirillum ferriphilum	Obligate chemoautolithotroph	Bioleaching of chalcopyrite and bornite	Zhao et al. (2015)
Sulfobacillus thermosulfidooxidans	Autotroph, mixotroph	Fe oxidizing	Dopson and Lindstrom (1999)
Acidithiobacillus caldus and *Sulfobacillus thermosulfidooxidans*		Arsenopyrite leaching	Dopson and Lindstrom (1999)

(*Continued*)

TABLE 3.2 (*Continued*)
Bacterial Strains Reported to be Involved in Biomining

Microorganisms	Energy Pathway	Biomining Mechanism	References
Acidithiobacillus thiooxidans	Chemolithotroph	Bioleaching, toxic metal sulfides to less toxic sulfates	Roy and Roy (2015)
Bacillus	Heterotroph	Mn bioleaching	Roy and Roy (2015)
Micrococcus	Heterotroph	Mn bioleaching	Roy and Roy (2015)
Pseudomonas	Heterotroph	Mn bioleaching	Roy and Roy (2015)
Achromobacter	Heterotroph	Mn bioleaching	Roy and Roy (2015)
Enterobacter	Heterotroph	Mn bioleaching	Roy and Roy (2015)
Bacillus circulans	Heterotroph	Cu, Ni, Pb, and Co leaching	Roy and Roy (2015)
Brevibacterium casei	Heterotroph	Mn bioleaching	Das et al. (2003)
Acidomonas methanolica (Acetobacter methanolicus)	Methanol was the sole source of carbon and energy	Leach by producing gluconate	Brandl et al. (2016)
Acidimicrobium ferrooxidans	Autotroph	Leach by producing gluconate	Brandl et al. (2016)
Acidiphilium angustum	Heterotroph	Leach by producing gluconate	Brandl et al. (2016)
Acidiphilium cryptum	Heterotroph	Leach by producing organic acid	Brandl et al. (2016)
Acidiphilium symbioticum	Heterotroph	Leach by producing organic acid	Brandl et al. (2016)
Acidobacterium capsulatum	Chemoorganotrophic	Leach by producing organic acid	Brandl et al. (2016)
Acidocella sp.	Heterotroph	Leach by producing organic acid	Brandl et al. (2016)
Acidomonas methanolica	Methanol was the sole source of carbon and energy	Leach by producing organic acid	Brandl et al. (2016)
Arthrobacter sp.	Heterotroph	Leach by producing organic acid	Brandl et al. (2016)
Microbacterium (Aureobacterium) liquefaciens	Heterotroph	Leach by producing organic acid	Brandl et al. (2016)
Bacillus sp.	Heterotroph	Leach by producing organic acid	Brandl et al. (2016)
Bacillus coagulans	Heterotroph	Leach by producing organic acid	Brandl et al. (2016)
Bacillus licheniformis	Heterotroph	Leach by producing organic acid	Brandl et al. (2016)
Bacillus megaterium	Heterotroph	Leach by producing citrate	Brandl et al. (2016)

(*Continued*)

TABLE 3.2 (*Continued*)
Bacterial Strains Reported to be Involved in Biomining

Microorganisms	Energy Pathway	Biomining Mechanism	References
Bacillus polymyxa	Heterotroph	Leach by producing citrate	Brandl et al. (2016)
Pantoea (Enterobacter) agglomerans	Heterotroph	Ferric iron	Brandl et al. (2016)
Enterobacter cloacae	Heterotroph	Ferric iron	Brandl et al. (2016)
Lactobacillus acidophilus	Heterotroph	Ferric iron	Brandl et al. (2016)
Propionibacterium acnes	Heterotroph	Ferric iron	Brandl et al. (2016)
Pseudomonas cepacia	Heterotroph	Ferric iron	Brandl et al. (2016)
Pseudomonas putida	Heterotroph	Leach by producing citrate and gluconate	Brandl et al. (2016)
Serratia ficaria	Chemoheterotrophic	Leach by producing citrate and gluconate	Brandl et al. (2016)
Staphylococcus lactis	Heterotroph	ferric iron	Brandl et al. (2016)
Pantoea (Enterobacter) agglomerans	Heterotroph	Solubilize manganese from ores	Baglin et al. (1992)
Enterobacter cloacae	Heterotroph	Solubilize manganese from ores	Baglin et al. (1992)
Achromobacter sp.	Heterotroph	Solubilize manganese from ores	Baglin et al. (1992)
Bacillus sp.	Heterotroph	Solubilize manganese from ores	Baglin et al. (1992)
Enterobacter sp.	Heterotroph	Solubilize manganese from ores	Baglin et al. (1992)
Bacillus cereus	Heterotroph	Leaching of copper	Farbiszewska-Kiczma et al. (2004)
Bacillus cereus	Heterotroph	Leaching of nickel	Farbiszewska-Kiczma et al. (2004)
Bacillus cereus	Heterotroph	Leaching of zinc	Farbiszewska-Kiczma et al. (2004)
Acinetobacter sp.	Heterotroph	Mn-oxidizing bacterium	Su et al. (2016)
Acidiphilium cryptum	Heterotroph	Bioleaching	Martinez et al. (2015)
Alicyclobacillus acidocaldarius	Heterotroph	Bioleaching	Martinez et al. (2015)

(*Continued*)

TABLE 3.2 (*Continued*)
Bacterial Strains Reported to be Involved in Biomining

Microorganisms	Energy Pathway	Biomining Mechanism	References
Anoxybacillus flavithermus	Chemolithoautotroph	Bioleaching	Martinez et al. (2015)
Acidiphilium multivorum	Heterotroph	Bioleaching	Martinez et al. (2015)
Sulfobacillus acidophilus	Autotroph, mixotroph	Bioleaching	Martinez et al. (2015)
Anoxybacillus kamchatkensis	Heterotroph	Bioleaching	Martinez et al. (2015)
Alicyclobacillus contaminans	Heterotroph	Bioleaching	Martinez et al. (2015)
Alicyclobacillus herbarius	Heterotroph	Bioleaching	Martinez et al. (2015)
Alicyclobacillus pomorum	Heterotroph	Bioleaching	Martinez et al. (2015)
Anoxybacillus gonensis	Heterotroph	Bioleaching	Martinez et al. (2015)
Anoxybacillus tepidamans	Heterotroph	Bioleaching	Martinez et al. (2015)
Thiobacillus prosperus	Obligate chemolithotroph	Bioleaching	Martinez et al. (2015)
Pseudomonas aeruginosa	Heterotroph	Bioleaching of copper oxide	Shabani et al. (2013)
Bacillus cereus	Heterotroph	Bioleaching of kaolin and quartz sands	Styriakova et al. (2003)
Thiobacillus denitrificans	Chemolithotroph, Lithotroph	Fe oxidizing, Sulfur oxidizing	Beller et al. (2006)
Sulphurihydrogenibium sp.	Chemolithoautotroph, Heterotroph	Sulfur oxidizing	Reysenbach et al. (2009)
Anoxybacillus flavithermus	Chemolithoautotroph	Arsenite oxidation	Jiang et al. (2015)

The consortia of microorganisms can improve growth, leaching process, acid production, and attachment to mineral surfaces (Rawlings and Johnson, 2007; Brune and Bayer, 2012). To design a consortium, temperature and pH also play major roles. The consortium so designed should have at least one iron-oxidizer and one sulfur-oxidizer (Rawlings and Johnson, 2007). In a consortium of *A. ferrooxidans* and *Leptospirillum ferrooxidans*, the optimum pH for the growth of *T. ferrooxidans* is within the range of 1.8–2.5, whereas *L. ferrooxidans* can grow at a pH of 1–2. In regard to temperature, strains of *T. ferrooxidans* can operate optimally within a range of 10°C–35°C (Siddiqui et al., 2009). However, strains of *Leptospirillum* can work within the range of 20°C–45°C. The consortium of *L. ferriphilum* and *Acidithiobacillus caldus* can operate in the range of 35°C–45°C (Rawlings and Johnson, 2007). Qiu et al. (2005) reported that the consortia of *A. ferrooxidans* and *A. thiooxidans* were more efficient in leaching of chalcopyrite than the pure cultures. They concluded that due to the consortia, the formation of inhibiting jarosite layers, which is the result of the formation of sulfuric acid from sulfur oxidation of *A. thiooxidans*, can be reduced. Liu et al. (2011) observed that the growth rate of *A. ferrooxidans* is increased if it is cocultured with the heterotroph *Acidiphilium acidophilum*.

Genomics, proteomics, and metabolomics of biomining bacteria are the major aspects to emphasize in the current and future impacts of biomining. Genomics is mainly concerned with the determination of the biodiversity of the biomining process. At least 56 genomes of extreme acidophilic bacteria; many representatives of psychro-tolerant, mesophilic, moderately thermophilic, and thermophilic microorganisms; and gram-positive and gram-negative bacteria have been sequenced (Cardenas et al., 2010). Initial studies were presented over a decade ago when the biomining bacterium *Acidithiobacillus ferrooxidans* ATCC 23270 was sequenced (Selkov et al., 2000). Researchers have used this genome information with bioinformatics tools to find genes involved in phosphate, sulfur, and iron metabolism and quorum sensing (Ramirez et al., 2002, 2004). Gene mining of the acidophilic biomining bacteria were also performed to identify and predict the role of small regulatory RNAs (srRNAs) in gene regulation (Shmaryahu and Holmes, 2007; Shmaryahu et al., 2009). Amouric et al. (2009) revealed the mechanisms involved in Fe(II) regulation, S oxidation in *A. ferrooxidans*. It is also known that acidophiles are extremely resistant to metals and metalloids. Hence, the genome information was also exploited to predict metal resistance genes in *A. ferrooxidans* (Holmes et al., 2001). Quatrini et al. (2005a,b, 2007) performed bioinformatics and experimental analysis of iron homeostasis and its potential regulation in *A. ferrooxidans*. This approach also has been extended to other bioleaching microorganisms (Osorio et al., 2008a,b). Navarro et al. (2009) and Baker-Austin et al. (2005) used combined genomic and experimental approaches to reveal the copper resistance mechanisms in *A. ferrooxidans* and in *Ferroplasma acidarmanus*, respectively. Metagenomics is another approach where microbial communities of an environment can be analyzed. This approach is useful for analyzing the microbial population dynamics during stages of biomining using next-generation sequencing technologies (Martinez et al., 2015).

Proteomics is another approach that allows the identification and localization of the corresponding genes available in the genomic sequence. It has also importance to understand the microbe-mineral interaction. Generally, the biomining bacteria are known to have metal resistance activity, and proteomics study can reveal the mechanism behind it. EPS production is known to play an important role in biomining for attachment to solid surfaces. Proteomic study also revealed the changes that occur during biofilm formation process (Martinez et al., 2015). Metabolomics is mainly concerned with the discovery of unique metabolite markers for assessing the microbial activity within the process of biomining and its future industrial application (Martinez et al., 2015).

LITHIC BACTERIA IN BIOMINING

Rock is the combination of different minerals that are rich in essential elements such as P, Fe, S, Mg, and Mo. Bacteria inhabiting such environments can dissolve those minerals and utilize them as sources of nutrients and energy by adopting different mechanisms. The principal mechanism is colonization, which involves physical penetration of the rock surface, causing disaggregation of the mineral and dissolution mediated by organic agents produced by the cells (Drever and Stillings, 1997; Konhauser, 2007). For colonization in mineral-rich environments, bacteria mainly produce exopolysaccharides (EPS), which is one of the phenomena for understanding the process of biomining. With this method, bacteria can attach to exposed mineral surfaces, then coat them with EPS, and finally disrupt mineral grains (Welch et al., 1999). Heterotrophic bacteria can produce organic acids causing enhanced EPS release for attachment to a mineral-rich environment. The organic acid and organic ligands produced by those bacteria in such conditions when growth is limited by the deficiency of essential nutrient. The organic acid promotes the chemical dissolution of the underlying minerals (Konhauser, 2007). Furthermore, organic ligands such as siderophore can chelate metal ions and bind to atoms on the mineral surface by forming complexes with metal ions and metals or metalloids (Drewniak et al., 2010), which are the important phenomenon of biomining. Among the lithic bacterial community, chemolithoautotrophic and heterotrophic bacteria are mainly involved in biomining. Bacteria belonging to the genera *Bacillus*, *Pseudomonas*, *Micrococcus*, *Brevibacterium*, *Arthrobacter*, which are reported as major participants in bioleaching or biomining, were also isolated from various lithobiontic environments and may be used for biomining potentials (Hungate et al., 1987; Groth et al., 1999; Fajardo-Cavazos and Nicholson, 2006; Dong et al., 2007; Baskar et al., 2009; Radwan et al., 2010; Campos et al., 2011). Additionally, *A. ferrooxidans*, which is a major participant in bioleaching or biomining, thrives well in a mineral-rich environment that is similar to the lithobiontic environment. According to the available previous reports, rock-inhabiting bacteria can solubilize phosphorus from rock-phosphate (Panhwar et al., 2011) and potassium from feldspar (Anjanadevi et al., 2016). The rock-weathering bacteria, such as those from the genera *Ensifer*, *Pseudomonas*, and *Bacillus*, have a greater ability to release Fe, K, and Si by producing acids and siderophores (Chen et al., 2015).

ACKNOWLEDGMENTS

The authors thank anonymous reviewers for useful suggestions for improving this chapter.

REFERENCES

Abdulla, H. 2009. Bioweathering and biotransformation of granite rock minerals by actinomycetes. *Microbial Ecology* 58(4):753–761.

Abdulla, H., May, E., Bahgat, M., and Dewedar, A. 2008. Characterisation of actinomycetes isolated from ancient stone and their potential for deterioration. *Polish Journal of Microbiology* 57(3):213–220.

Acharya, C., Kar, R. N., and Sukla, L. B. 2001. Bacterial removal of sulphur from different coals. *Fuel* 80(15):2207–2216.

Acharya, R. 1990. Bacterial leaching: A potential for developing countries. *Genetic Engineering and Biotechnology Monitor* 27:57–58.

Alting, S. A., and Chaerun, S. K. 2010. Bacterial bioleaching of sulfide mineral ores by mixotrophic bacterial consortia. *Proceedings of the Third International Conference on Mathematics and Natural Sciences.*

Amouric, A., Appia-Ayme, C., Yarzabal, A., and Bonnefoy, V. 2009. Regulation of the iron and sulfur oxidation pathways in the acidophilic *Acidithiobacillus Ferrooxidans*. *Advanced Materials Research* 71–73:163–166.

Anjanadevi, I. P., John, N. S., John, K. S., Jeeva, M. L., and Misra, R. S. 2016. Rock inhabiting potassium solubilizing bacteria from Kerala, India: Characterization and possibility in chemical K fertilizer substitution. *Journal of Basic Microbiology* 56(1):67–77.

Baglin, E. G., Noble, E. G., Lampshire, D. L., and Eisele, J. A. 1992. Solubilization of manganese from ores by heterotrophic micro-organisms. *Hydrometallurgy* 29:131–144.

Baker-Austin, C., Dopson, M., Wexler, M. Sawers, R. G., and Bond, P. L. 2005. Molecular insight into extreme copper resistance in the extremophilic archaeon *Ferroplasma acidarmanus* Fer1. *Microbiology* 151:2637–2646.

Baskar, S., Baskar, R., Lee, N., and Theophilus, P. K. 2009. Speleothems from mawsmai and krem phyllut caves, Meghalaya, India: Some evidences on biogenic activities. *Environmental Geology* 57:1169–1185.

Bayat, O., Sever, E., Bayat, B., Arslan, V., and Poole, C. 2009. Bioleaching of zinc and iron from steel plant waste using *Acidithiobacillus ferrooxidans*. *Applied Biochemistry and Biotechnology* 152:117–126.

Bell, R. A. 1993. Cryptoendolithic algae of hot semiarid lands and deserts. *Journal of Phycology* 29(2):133–139.

Beller, H. R., Chain, P. S., Letain, T. E., Chakicherla, A., Larimer, F. W., et al. 2006. The genome sequence of the obligately chemolithoautotrophic, facultatively anaerobic bacterium *Thiobacillus denitrificans*. *Journal of Bacteriology* 188:1473–1488.

Best, M. G. 2003. *Igneous and Metamorphic Petrology,* Second Edition. Malden, MA: Blackwell Science.

Bhatnagar, A., and Bhatnagar, M. 2005. Microbial diversity in desert ecosystems. *Current Science* 89(1):91–100.

Bhattacharjee, K., and Joshi, S. R. 2016. A selective medium for recovery and enumeration of endolithic bacteria. *Journal of Microbiological Methods* 129:44–54.

Birgitta, E. K., Anna, O., Yngve, A., Johanna, A., Arvid, O. J., et al. 2004. Microbial leaching of uranium and other trace elements from shale mine tailings at Ranstad. *Geoderma* 122:177–194.

Brandl, H., Barmettler, F., Castelberg, C. and Fabbri, C. 2016. Microbial mobilization of rare earth elements (REE) from mineral solids: A mini review. *AIMS Microbiology* 3(2):190–204.

Brierley, C. L. 1984. Microbiological mining: Technology status and commercial opportunities. *The World Biotech Report* 1:599–609.

Broady, P. A. 1981. The ecology of chasmolithic algae at costal locations of Antarctica. *Phycologia* 20:259–272.

Brune, K. D., and Bayer, T. S. 2012. Engineering microbial consortia to enhance biomining and bioremediation. *Frontiers in Microbiology* 3:203.

Campos, V. L., León, C., Mondaca, M. A., Yañez, J., and Zaror, C. 2011. Arsenic mobilization by epilithic bacterial communities associated with volcanic rocks from Camarones River, Atacama Desert, northern Chile. *Archives of Environmental Contamination and Toxicology* 61(2):185–192.

Cardenas, J. P., Valdés, J., Quatrini, R., Duarte, F., and Holmes, D. S. 2010. Lessons from the genomes of extremely acidophilic bacteria and archaea with special emphasis on bioleaching microorganisms. *Applied Microbiology and Biotechnology* 88(3):605–620.

Cary, S. C., McDonald, I. R., Barrett, J. E., and Cowan, D. A. 2010. On the rocks: The microbiology of Antarctic dry valley soils. *Nature Reviews Microbiology* 8:129–138.

Chen, W., Wang, Q., He, L., and Sheng, X. 2015. Changes in the weathering activity and populations of culturable rock-weathering bacteria from the altered purple siltstone and the adjacent soil. *Geomicrobiology Journal* 33(8):724–733.

Clark, D. A., and Norris, P. R. 1996. *Acidimicrobium ferrooxidans* gen. nov., sp. nov.: Mixed-culture ferrous iron oxidation with *Sulfobacillus* species. *Microbiology* 142:785–790.

Cockell, C. S., and Stokes, M. D. 2004. Ecology: Widespread colonization by polar hypoliths. *Nature* 431:414.

Cockell, C. S., Lee, P., Broady, P., Lim, D. S. S., Osinski, G. R., et al. 2005. Effects of asteroid and comet impacts on habitats for lithophytic organisms—A synthesis. *Meteoritics and Planetary Science* 40:1901–1914.

Cockell, C. S., McKay, C. P., Warren-Rhodes, K., and Horneck, G. 2008. Ultraviolet radiation-induced limitation to epilithic microbial growth in arid deserts—Dosimetric experiments in the hyperarid core of the Atacama Desert. *Journal of Photochemistry and Photobiology B: Biology* 90(2):79–87.

Corkhill, C. L., Wincott, P. L., Lloyd, J. R., and Vaughan, D. J. 2008. The oxidative dissolution of arsenopyrite (FeAsS) and enargite (Cu3 AsS4) by *Leptospirillum ferrooxidans*. *Geochimica et Cosmochimica Acta* 72:5616–5633.

Cottrell, M. T., and Kirchman, D. L. 2000. Community composition of marine bacterioplankton determined by 16S rRNA gene clone libraries and fluorescence in situ hybridization. *Applied and Environmental Microbiology* 66:5116–5122.

Cowan, D. A., Pointing, S. B., Stevens, M. I., Cary, S. C., Stomeo, F., et al. 2011. Distribution and abiotic influences on hypolithic microbial communities in an Antarctic Dry Valley. *Polar Biology* 34:307.

Das, A. P., Swain, S., and Pradhan, N. 2003. Bioremediation and bioleaching potential of multimetal resistant microorganism. *International Seminar on Mineral Processing Technology (mpt-2013), at CSIR-immt.*, Bhubaneswar, India.

DiRuggiero, J., Wierzchos, J., Robinson, C. K., Souterre, T., Ravel, J., et al. 2013. Microbial colonisation of chasmoendolithic habitats in the hyper-arid zone of the Atacama Desert. *Biogeosciences* 10:2439–2450.

Dong, H., Rech, J. A., Jiang, H., Sun, H., and Buck, B. J. 2007. Endolithic cyanobacteria in soil gypsum: Occurrences in Atacama (Chile), Mojave (United States), and Al-Jafr Basin (Jordan) Deserts. *Journal of Geophysical Research* 112(G2):1–11.

Dopson, M., and Lindstrom, E. B. 1999. Potential Role of *Thiobacillus caldus* in Arsenopyrite Bioleaching. *Applied and Environmental Microbiology* 65(1):36–40.

Drever, J. I., and Stillings, L. L. 1997. The role of organic acids in mineral weathering. *Colloids and Surfaces A: Physicochemical and Engineering Aspects* 120:167–181.

Drewniak, L., Matlakowska, R., Rewerski, B., and Sklodowska, A. 2010. Arsenic release from gold mine rocks mediated by the activity of indigenous bacteria. *Hydrometallurgy* 104:437–442.

Ehlers, G. E., and Blatt, H. 1997. *Petrology, Igneous Sedimentary and Metamorphic*. CBS publishers and distribution, 4596/1-A new delhi-11000, New Delhi, India.

Ehrlich, H. L. 1997. Microbes and metals. *Applied Microbiology and Biotechnology* 48:687–692.

Ehrlich, H. L., and Newman, D. K. 2009. *Geomicrobiology,* Fifth Edition. Boca Raton, FL: CRC Press.

Escobar, B., Huenupi, E., Godoy, I., and Wiertz, J. V. 2000. Arsenic precipitation in the bioleaching of enargite by Sulfolobus BC at 70°C. *Biotechnology Letters* 22:205–209.

Etienne, S., and Dupont, J. 2002. Fungal weathering of basaltic rocks in a cold oceanic environment (Iceland): Comparison between experimental and field observations. *Earth Surface Processes and Landforms* 27(7):737–748.

Ettenauer, J. D., Jurado, V., Piñar, G., Miller, A. Z., Santner, M., et al. 2014. Halophilic microorganisms are responsible for the rosy discolouration of saline environments in three historical buildings with mural paintings. *PLoS One* 9(8):e103844.

Fajardo-Cavazos, P., and Nicholson, W. 2006. *Bacillus* endospores isolated from granite: Close molecular relationships to globally distributed *Bacillus* spp. from endolithic and extreme environments. *Applied and Environmental Microbiology* 72(4):2856–2863.

Farbiszewska-Kiczma, J., Farbiszewska, T., and Bąk, M. 2004. Bioleaching of metals from polish black shale in neutral medium. *Physicochemical Problems of Mineral Processing* 38:273–280.

Fike, D. A., Cockell, C., Pearce, D., and Lee, P. 2002. Heterotrophic microbial colonization of the interior of impact-shocked rocks from Haughton impact structure, Devon Island, Nunavut, Canadian High Arctic. *International Journal of Astrobiology* 1(4):311–323.

Friedmann, E. I. 1971. Light and scanning electron microscopy of the endolithic desert algal habitat. *Phycologia* 10:411–428.

Friedmann, E. I., Lipkin, Y., and Ocampo-Paus, R. 1967. Desert algae of the Negev (Israel). *Phycologia* 6:185–196.

Garcia-Pichel, F. 2006. Plausible mechanisms for the boring on carbonates by microbial phototrophs. *Sedimentary Geology* 185:205–213.

Gaylarde, C. C., Gaylarde, P. M., and Neilan B. A. 2012. Endolithic phototrophs in built and natural Stone. *Current Microbiology* 65:183–188.

Gerrath, J. F., Gerrath, J. A., Mathes, U., and Larson, D. W. 2000. Endolithic algae and cyanobacteria from cliffs of the Niagara Escarpment, Ontario, Canada. *Canadian Journal of Botany* 78(6):807–815.

Golubic, S., Friedmann, E. I., and Schneider, J. 1981. The lithobiontic ecological niche, with special reference to microorganisms. *Journal of Sedimentary Research* 51(2):475–478.

Groth, I., Vetterman, R., Schuetze, B., Schumann, P., and Sa'iz-Jimenez, C. 1999. Actinomycetes in Karstic caves of northern Spain Altamira and Tito Bustillo. *Journal of Microbiological Methods* 36:115–122.

Grund, S. C., Hanusch, K., and Wolf, H. U. 2008. Arsenic and arsenic compounds. *Ullmann's Encyclopedia of Industrial Chemistry*. doi:10.1002/14356007.a03_113.pub2

Hassanien, A. G., Desouky, O. A. N., and Hussien, S. S. E. 2014. Bioleaching of some rare earth elements from Egyptian monazite using *Aspergillus ficuum* and *Pseudomonas aeruginosa*. *Walailak Journal of Science and Technology* 11:809–823.

Hillgartner, H., Dupraz, C., and Hug, W. 2001. Microbially induced cementation of carbonate sands: Are micritic meniscus cements good indicators of vadosedia genesis? *Sedimentology* 48:117–131.

Hirsch, P., Eckhard, F. E. W., and Palmer, Jr. R. J. 1995. Methods for the study of rock inhabiting microorganisms—A mini review. *Journal of Microbiological Methods* 23:143–167.

Hirsch, P., Mevs, U., Kroppenstedt, R. M., Schumann, P., and Stackebrandt, E. 2004. Cryptoendolithic actinomycetes from Antarctic sandstone rock samples: *Micromonospora endolithica* sp. nov. and two isolates related to *Micromonospora coerulea* Jensen 1932. *Systematic and Applied Microbiology* 27(2):166–174.

Holmes, D. S., Barreto, M., Valdes, J., Dominguez, C., Arriagada, C., et al. 2001. Genome sequence of *Acidithiobacillus ferrooxidans*: Metabolic reconstruction, heavy metal resistance and other characteristics. In *Biohydrometallurgy: Fundamentals, Technology and Sustainable Development*, (Eds.) V. Ciminelli and O. Garcia, pp. 237–251. Amsterdam, the Netherlands: Elsevier.

Hoppert, M., Flies, C., Pohl, W., Gunzl, B., and Schneider, J. 2004. Colonization strategies of lithobiontic microorganisms on carbonate rocks. *Environmental Geology* 46(3–4):421–428.

Horath, T., and Bachofen, R. 2009. Molecular characterization of an endolithic microbial community in dolomite rock in the Central Alps (Switzerland). *Microbial Ecology* 58:290–306.

Hughes, K. A., and Lawley, B. 2003. A novel Antarctic microbial endolithic community within gypsum crusts. *Environmental Microbiology* 5(7):555–565.

Hungate, B., Danin, A., Pellerin, N., Stemmler, J., Kjellander, P., et al. 1987. Characterization of manganese-oxidizing (MnII → MnIV) bacteria from Negev Desert rock varnish: Implications in desert varnish formation. *Canadian Journal of Microbiology* 33:939–943.

Jacobsen, S. B. 2003. How old is the planet earth? *Science* 300:1513–1514.

Jain, N., and Sharma, D. K. 2004. Biohydrometallurgy for nonsulfidic minerals—A review. *Geomicrobiology Journal* 21:135–144.

Jiang, D., Li, P., Jiang, Z., Dai, X., Zhang, R., et al. 2015. Chemolithoautotrophic arsenite oxidation by a thermophilic *Anoxybacillus flavithermus* strain TCC9-4 from a hot spring in Tengchong of Yunnan, China. *Frontiers in Microbiology* 6:360. doi: 10.3389/fmicb.2015.00360

Johnson, D. B., Grail, B. M., and Hallberg, K. B. 2013. A new direction for biomining: Extraction of metals by reductive dissolution of oxidized ores. *Minerals* 3:49–58.

Konhauser, K. 2007. *Introduction to Geomicrobiology.* Oxford, UK: Blackwell Publishing.

Kuhlman, K. R., Venkat, P., LaDuc, M. T., Kuhlman, G. M., and McKay, C. P. 2008. Evidence of a microbial community associated with rock varnish at Yungay, Atacama Desert, Chile. *Journal of Geophysical Research* 113(G4).

Leduc, L. G., and Ferroni, G. D. 1994. The chemolithotrophic bacterium *Thiobacillus ferrooxidans. FEMS Microbiology Reviews* 14:103–120.

Li, S., Shi, Y., Zhang, Q., Liao, X., Zhu, L., et al. 2013. Phylogenetic diversity of endolithic bacteria in Bole granite rock in Xinjiang. *Acta Ecologica Sinica* 33:178–184.

Liu, H., Yin, H., Dai, Y., Dai, Z., Liu, Y., et al. 2011. The co-culture of *Acidithiobacillus ferrooxidans* and *Acidiphilium acidophilum* enhances the growth, iron oxidation, and CO_2 fixation. *Archives of Microbiology* 193:857–866.

Makita, M., Esperón, M., Pereyra, B., López, A., and Orrantia, E. 2004. Reduction of arsenic content in a complex galena concentrate by *Acidithiobacillus ferrooxidans. BMC Biotechnology* 4:22.

Martinez, P., Vera, M., and Bobadilla-Fazzini, R. A. 2015. Omics on bioleaching: Current and future impacts. *Applied Microbiology and Biotechnology* 99(20):8337–8350.

Michel, C., Beny, C., Delorme, F., Poirier, L., Spolaore, P., et al. 2009. New protocol for the rapid quantification of exopolysaccharides in continuous culture systems of acidophilic bioleaching bacteria. *Applied Microbiology and Biotechnology* 82:371–378.

Mitchell, R., and Gu J. D. 2000. Changes in biofilm microflora of limestone caused by atmospheric pollutants. *International Biodeterioration and Biodegradation* 46:299–303.

Munoz, J. A., Blázquez, M. L., González, F., Ballester, A., Acevedo, F., et al. 2006. Electrochemical study of enargite bioleaching by mesophilic and thermophilic microorganisms. *Hydrometallurgy* 84:175–186.

Nagpal, S., Dahlstrom, D., and Oolman, T. 1993. Effect of carbon dioxide concentration on the bioleaching of a pyrite-arsenopyrite ore concentrates. *Biotechnology and Bioengineering* 41(4):459–464.

Navarro, C. A., Orellana, L. H., Mauriaca, C., and Jerez, C. A. 2009. Transcriptional and functional studies of *Acidithiobacillus ferrooxidans* genes related to survival in the presence of copper. *Applied and Environmental Microbiology* 75:6102–6109.

Nienow, J. A., and Friedmann, E. I. 1993. Terrestial lithophytic (rock) communities. In *Antarctic Microbiology*, E. I. Friedmann and A. B. Thistle (Eds.), pp. 343–412. New York, NY: John Wiley and Sons.

Omelon, C. R. 2016. Endolithic microorganisms and their habitats. In *Their World: A Diversity of Microbial Environments*, C. J. Hurst (Ed.), pp. 171–202. Switzerland: Springer International Publishing.

Orell, A., Remonsellez, Arancibia, R., and Jerez, C. A. 2013. Molecular characterization of copper and cadmium resistance determinants in the biomining thermoacidophilic archaeon *Sulfolobus metallicus*. *Archaea* 2013:289236.

Osorio, H., Martinez, V., Nieto, P., Holmes, D., and Quatrini, R. 2008a. Microbial iron management mechanisms in extremely acidic environments: Comparative genomics evidence for diversity and versatility. *BMC Microbiology* 8:203.

Osorio, H., Martinez, V., Veloso, F. A., Pedroso, I., Valdes, J., et al. 2008b. Iron homeostasis strategies in acidophilic iron oxidizers: Studies in *Acidithiobacillus* and *Leptospirillum*. *Hydrometallurgy* 94:175–179.

Panhwar, Q. A., Radziah, O., Zaharah, A. R., Sariah, M., and Razi, I. M. 2011. Role of phosphate solubilizing bacteria on rock phosphate solubility and growth of aerobic rice. *Journal of Environmental Biology* 32(5):607–612.

Pollmann, K., Kutschke, S., Matys, S., Kostudis, S., Hopfe, S., et al. 2016. Novel biotechnological approaches for the recovery of metals from primary and secondary resources. *Minerals* 6:54.

Pradhan, D., Pal, S., Sukla, L. B., Chaudhury, G. R., and Das, T. 2008. Bioleaching of low-grade copper ore using indigenous microorganisms. *Indian Journal of Chemical Technology* 15:588–592.

Qiu, M., Xiong, S., Zhang, W., and Wang, G. 2005. A comparison of bioleaching of chalcopyrite using pure culture or a mixed culture. *Minerals Engineering* 18:987–990.

Quatrini, R., Jedlicki, E., and Holmes, D. S. 2005a. Genomic insights into the iron uptake mechanisms of the biomining microorganism *Acidithiobacillus ferrooxidans*. *Journal of Industrial Microbiology and Biotechnology* 32:606–614.

Quatrini, R., Lefimil, C., Holmes, D. S., and Jedlicki, E. 2005b. The ferric iron uptake regulator (Fur) from the extreme acidophile *Acidithiobacillus ferrooxidans*. *Microbiology* 151:2005–2015.

Quatrini, R., Martinez, V., Osorio, H., Veloso, F., Pedroso, I., et al. 2007. Iron homeostasis strategies in acidophilic iron oxidizers: Comparative genome analysis. *Advanced Materials Research* 20–21:439–442.

Radwan, S., Mahmoud, H., Khanafer, M., Al-Habib, A., and Al-Hasan, R. 2010. Identities of epilithic hydrocarbon-utilizing diazotrophic bacteria from the Arabian Gulf Coasts, and their potential for oil bioremediation without nitrogen supplementation. *Microbial Ecology* 60(2):354–363.

Ramirez, P., Guiliani, N., Valenzuela, L., Beard, S., and Jerez, C. A. 2004. Differential protein expression during growth of *Acidithiobacillus ferrooxidans* on ferrous iron, sulfur compounds, or metal sulfides. *Applied and Environmental Microbiology* 70:4491–4498.

Ramirez, P., Toledo, H., Guiliani, N., and Jerez, C. A. 2002. An exported rhodanese-like protein is induced during growth of *Acidithiobacillus ferrooxidans* in metal sulfides and different sulfur compounds. *Applied and Environmental Microbiology* 68:1837–1845.

Rawlings, D. E. 2002. Heavy metal mining using microbes. *Annual Review of Microbiology* 56:65–91.

Rawlings, D. E. 2005. Characteristics and adaptability of iron- and sulfur-oxidizing microorganisms used for the recovery of metals from minerals and their concentrates. *Microbial Cell Factories* 4:13.

Rawlings, D. E., Dew, D., and Plessis, C. D. 2003. Biomineralization of metal containing ores and concentrates. *Trends in Biotechnology* 21(1):38–44.

Rawlings, D. E., and Johnson, D. B. 2007. *Biomining.* Heidelberg, Germany: Springer.

Rawlings, D. E., and Silver, S. 1995. Mining with microbes. *Nature Biotechnology* 13:773–778.

Reysenbach, A. L., Hamamura, N., Podar, M., Griffiths, E., Ferreira, S., et al. 2009. Complete and draft genome sequences of six members of the Aquificales. *Journal of Bacteriology* 191:1992–1993.

Rhind, T., Ronholm, J., Berg, B., Mann, P., Applin, D., et al. 2014. Gypsum-hosted endolithic communities of the Lake St. Martin impact structure, Manitoba, Canada, spectroscopic detectability and implications for Mars. *International Journal of Astrobiology* 13:366–377.

Rohwerder, T., Gehrke, T., Kinzler, K., and Sand, W. 2003. Bioleaching review part A: Progress in bioleaching: Fundamentals and mechanisms of bacterial metal sulfide oxidation. *Applied Microbiology and Biotechnology* 63:239–248.

Roy, S., and Roy, M. 2015. Bioleaching of heavy metals by sulfur oxidizing bacteria: A review. *International Research Journal of Environmental Sciences* 4(9):75–79.

Schippers, A., Hedrich, S., Vasters, J., Drobe, M., Sand, W., et al. 2014. Biomining: Metal recovery from ores with microorganisms. *Advances in Biochemical Engineering/Biotechnology* 141:1–47.

Selkov, E., Overbeek, R., Kogan, Y., Chu, L, Vonstein, V., et al. 2000. Functional analysis of gapped microbial genomes: Amino acid metabolism of *Thiobacillus ferrooxidans*. *Proceedings of the National Academy of Sciences USA* 97:3509–3514.

Shabani, M. A., Irannajad, M., Azadmehr, A. R., and Meshkini, M. 2013. Bioleaching of copper oxide ore by *Pseudomonas aeruginosa*. *International Journal of Minerals, Metallurgy and Materials* 20(12):1130–1133.

Shin, D., Kim, J., Kim, B. S., Jeong, J., and Lee, J. C. 2015. Use of phosphate solubilizing bacteria to leach rare earth elements from monazite-bearing ore. *Minerals* 5:189–202.

Shmaryahu, A., and Holmes, D. S. 2007. Discovery of small regulatory RNAs in the extremophile *Acidithiobacillus* genus suggests novel genetic regulation. *Advanced Materials Research* 20–21:535–538.

Shmaryahu, A., Lefimil, C., Jedlicki, E., and Holmes, D. S. 2009. Small regulatory RNA genes in Acidithiobacillus ferrooxidans: Case studies of 6S RNA and frr. *Advanced Materials Research* 71–73:191–194.

Siddiqui, M. H., Kumar, A., Kesari, K. K., and Arif, J. M. 2009. Biomining—A useful approach toward metal extraction. *American-Eurasian Journal of Agronomy* 2(2):84–88.

Sigler, W. V., Bachofen, R., and Zeyer, J. 2003. Molecular characterization of endolithic cyanobacteria inhabiting exposed dolomite in central Switzerland. *Environmental Microbiology* 5:618.

Staley, J. T. 1968. Prosthecomicrobium and ancalomicrobium: New prosthecate freshwater bacteria. *Journal of Bacteriology* 95(5):1921–1942.

Stevens, T. O. 1995. Optimization of media for enumeration aerobic heterotrophic bacteria from the subsurface. *Journal of Microbiological Methods* 21(3):293–303.

Stivaletta, N., and Barbieri, R. 2009. Endoliths in terrestrial arid environments: Implications for astrobiology. In *From Fossils to Astrobiology: Cellular Origin, Life in Extreme Habitats and Astrobiology*, J. Seckbach and M. Walsh (Eds.), pp. 319–333. Dordrecht, the Netherlands: Springer Science, Business Media B.V.

Stivaletta, N., López-García, P., Boihem, L., Millie, D. F., and Barbieri, R. 2010. Biomarkers of endolithic communities within gypsum crusts (Southern Tunisia). *Geomicrobiology Journal* 27(1):101–110.

Styriakova, I., Štyriak, I., Nandakumar, M.P., and Mattiasson, B. 2003. Bacterial destruction of mica during bioleaching of kaolin and quartz sands by *Bacillus cereus*. *World Journal of Microbiology and Biotechnology* 19(6):583–590.

Su, J. F., Zheng, S. C., Huang, T. L., Ma, F., Shao, S. C., et al. 2016. Simultaneous removal of Mn(II) and nitrate by the manganese-oxidizing bacterium *Acinetobacter* sp. SZ28 in anaerobic conditions. *Geomicrobiology Journal* 33(7):586–591.

Sukla, L. B., Esther, J., Panda, S., and Pradhan, N. 2014. Biomineral processing: A valid eco-friendly alternative for metal extraction. *Research and Reviews: Journal of Microbiology and Biotechnology* 3(4):1–10.

Suzuki, I. 2001. Microbial leaching of metals from sulfide minerals. *Biotechnology Advances* 19:119–132.

Tanaka, T., Yan, L., and Burgess, J. G. 2003. *Microbulbifera renaceous* sp. nov., a new endolithic bacterium isolated from the inside of red sandstone. *Current Microbiology* 47(5):412–416.

Taylor-George, S., Palmer, F., Staley, J. T., Borns, D., Curtiss, B., et al. 1983. Fungi and bacteria involved in desert varnish formation. *Microbial Ecology* 9:227–245.

Vandamme, P., Pot, B., Gillis, M., De Vos, P., Kersters, K., et al. 1996. Polyphasic taxonomy: A consensus approach to bacterial systematic. *Microbiological Reviews* 60:407–438.

Vitek, P., Camara-Gallego, B., Edwards, H. G. M., Jehlicka, J., Ascaso, C., et al. 2013. Phototrophic community in gypsum crust from the Atacama Desert studied by Raman spectroscopy and microscopic imaging. *Geomicrobiology Journal* 30:1–12.

Warren-Rhodes, K. A., McKay, C. P., Boyle, L. N., Wing, M. R., Kiekebusch, E. M., et al. 2013. Physical ecology of hypolithic communities in the central Namib Desert: The role of fog, rain, rock habitat, and light. *Journal of Geophysical Research: Biogeosciences* 118(4):1451–1460.

Weirich, G., and Schweisfurth, R. 1985. Extraction and culture of microorganisms from rock. *Geomicrobiology Journal* 4:1–20.

Welch, S. A., Barker, W. W., and Banfield, J. F. 1999. Microbial extracellular polymers and plagioclase dissolution. *Geochimica et Cosmochimica Acta* 63:1405–1419.

Wierzchos, J., Camara, B., de Los Rios, A., Davila, A. F., Sanchez Almazo, I. M., et al. 2011. Microbial colonisation of Ca-sulfate crusts in the hyperarid core of the Atacama Desert: Implications for the search for life on Mars. *Geobiology* 9:44–60.

Wierzchos, J., Davila, A. F., Artieda, O., Cámara, B., de los Ríos, A., et al. 2013. Ignimbrite as a substrate for endolithic life in the hyper-arid Atacama Desert: Implications for the search for life on Mars. *Icarus* 224(2):334–346.

Wong, F. K., Lacap, D. C., Lau, M. C., Aitchison, J. C., Cowan, D. A., et al. 2010. Hypolithic microbial community of quartz pavement in the high-altitude tundra of central Tibet. *Microbial Ecology* 60(4):730–739.

Wynn-Williams, D. D. 2000. Cyanobacteria in deserts—Life at the limit? In *The Ecology of Cyanobacteria*, B. A. Whitton and M. Potts (Eds.), pp. 341–366. the Netherlands: Kluwer Academic Publishers.

Zhao, H., Wang, J., Gan, X., Qin, W., Hu, M., et al. 2015. Bioleaching of chalcopyrite and bornite by moderately thermophilic bacteria: An emphasis on their interactions. *International Journal of Minerals, Metallurgy, and Materials* 22:777.

4 Microbial Surfactants
Recent Trends and Future Perspectives

Anila Fariq and Azra Yasmin

CONTENTS

INTRODUCTION

Surfactants are ubiquitous amphipathic compounds that are usually organic in nature and have the ability to reduce the surface tension of a liquid and the interfacial tension among the liquids. They possess a hydrophobic moiety, that is, via a tail, as well as a hydrophilic moiety, that is, via a head. The hydrophilic part is usually polar in nature; the hydrophobic part is nonpolar. Surfactants are soluble in both water and organic compounds because of their dual nature: the polar part has affinity for water and the nonpolar has affinity for organic compounds (Mishra et al., 2009). Most of the surfactants are derived chemically from nondegradable petroleum products (Liu et al., 2011). They are widely used as cleaning agents, and they have diverse applications in various industrial processes like dispersion, emulsification, wetting, foaming, and so on (Noudeh et al., 2010). These chemical surfactants are highly persistent in nature, and their excessive use in large quantities is becoming the potential source of environmental pollution. Certain surfactants cause the release of toxic pollutants like polychlorinated biphenyls (PCBs) when their concentrations are high in soil (Venhuis et al., 2004).

Natural surfactants are "surface-active" compounds of animal and plant origin. They also include surface-active compounds of microbial origin, that is, biosurfactants (Holmberg, 2001; Paraszkiewicz and Dlugoński, 2003). Natural surfactants from plants and animals are present in small amounts, and the cost of their yield is much higher than the cost of chemical synthesis. However, biosurfactants are surface-active metabolites that are produced by microbes during the stationary phase of their growth and could provide sustainable alternatives to their chemical counterparts. They are amphiphilic compounds with diverse chemical structures and properties but are comprised mainly of hydrophobic moieties, such as fatty acids or their derivatives, and hydrophilic moieties, such as amino acids, sugars, or long-chain peptides (Techaoei et al., 2007; Thies et al., 2016). Among the microbes, bacteria are the key producers of most of the biosurfactants (Kitamoto et al., 2002). The biosurfactant-producing bacteria are widely present among different genera such as *Bacillus, Rhodococcus, Arthrobacter*, and *Pseudomonas* (Pruthi and Cameotra, 1997; Suwansukho et al., 2008). They were initially found in fermentative bacteria as extracellular amphipathic compounds (Kitamoto et al., 2009). Biosurfactants are of great interest because of their diverse and environment-friendly nature; their cheap production by fermentation utilizing low-cost substrates; and their promising applications in the recovery of crude oil, health care, and the food industries and in remediation of metal and organic environmental pollutants (Desai and Banat, 1997).

According to Zion research report, the global biosurfactants market stood at 150 tons in 2014 in terms of volume, and it was worth around $13.5 million in 2014. The market is expected to reach up to $17.5 million by 2020, growing at a compound annual rate of 4% by 2020 (http://www.marketresearchstore.com/report/microbial-biosurfactants-market-z37354).

WHY DO MICROBES PRODUCE BIOSURFACTANTS?

With the help of biosurfactants, microbes keep a proficient association with the environment. Bacterial cells correspond with their surroundings with the aid of their envelopes (Burgos-Diaz et al., 2011). Surfactants such as rhamnolipid biosurfactants have the ability to retain open channels in biofilm by altering cell–cell and cell–surface interactions (Davey et al., 2003). Rhamnolipids not only maintain the structure and nutritional balance of the biofilm, but they also prohibit the invading bacteria from inhabiting the open spaces in the resident biofilm (Espinosa-Urgel, 2003). Several roles of biosurfactants are inimitable to the producing microorganisms, so it is not promising to generalize their functions (Cameotra et al., 2010).

Biosurfactants help in regulating the cell surface properties of producing organisms according to their desire through adhesion to and de-adhesion from surfaces.

The interface is modified by a biosurfactant when it is produced by bacteria and thus permits bacteria in attachment or detachment. By lowering the interface tension, biosurfactants are efficiently involved in the mobilization of hydrophobic substrates and allow their biodegradation (Ron and Rosenberg, 2001; Van Hamme et al., 2006). Under low cell density and limited agitation conditions, adhesion is observed to be the preliminary property for *A. calcoaceticus* RAG-1 to grow on liquid hydrocarbons (Rosenberg and Ron, 1997, 1999). Zhang and Miller (1994) reported that the presence of cell-bound rhamnolipid in *P. aeruginosa* increases the cell surface hydrophobicity. On the other hand, Rosenberg et al. (1988) found a decrease in cell surface hydrophobicity of *Acinetobacter* due to presence of its cell-bound emulsifier.

Because of the various physiological roles that biosurfactant-producing microbes play, they are found in diverse environments (Walter et al., 2010). They are capable of assimilating hydrophobic as well as soluble substrates (Carrillo et al., 1996) because of their wide adaptability to hostile environmental conditions. Many hydrocarbon-degrading bacterial communities are also efficient biosurfactant producers (Ganesh and Lin, 2009). Hydrophobic environments are appropriate habitats for potential biosurfactant-producing bacteria (Tambekar and Gadakh, 2013).

Screening of biosurfactant-producing microbes can be done by using various analytical techniques like surface and interfacial tension (Lin, 1996), Hemolysis (Mulligan et al., 1984), emulsification assay (Cooper and Goldenberg, 1987), CTAB agar plate (Siegmund and Wagner, 1991), oil spreading assay (Morikawa et al., 2000), drop collapse assay (Jain et al., 1991), and so on.

CLASSIFICATION OF BIOSURFACTANTS

Classification of biosurfactants is done on the basis of their chemical composition, molecular weight, or their microbial origin. The hydrophilic portion of a biosurfactant is mainly composed of various amino acids; peptides; anions/cations; and mono-, di-, or polysaccharides. The hydrophobic part consists of saturated, unsaturated, or hydroxylated fatty acids (Desai and Banat, 1997). Different properties of biosurfactants are altered by their structural orientation both on their surfaces and interfaces (Chen et al., 2010).

The molecular weight of biosurfactants usually ranges from 500 to 1500 Da, and their critical micelle concentration (CMC) values are generally in the range of 1–200 mg/L (Burgos-Diaz et al., 2011). Biosurfactants are generally divided into low-molecular-weight molecules and high-molecular-weight polymers. Low-molecular-mass biosurfactants reduce surface and interfacial tension proficiently, while high-molecular-mass biosurfactants do not lower surface tension but are effective in stabilizing emulsions (Rosenberg, 2006). Glycolipids and lipopeptides are classified as low-molecular-weight biosurfactants; however, polymeric biosurfactants are classified as high-molecular-weight surfactants (Table 4.1).

TABLE 4.1

Classification of Microbial Surfactants

Biosurfactant Class	Type of Biosurfactant	Structure	Microbial Source	References
Glycolipids	Rhamnolipids	Rhamnose molecules attached with one or two molecules of β-hydroxydecanoic acid	*Pseudomonas aeruginosa*	Jarvis and Johnson (1949)
	Sophorolipids	Dimeric carbohydrates linked to a long-chain hydroxy fatty acid and 6–9 various hydrophobic sophorosides	*T. petrophilum* and *T. apicola*	Cooper et al. (1983)
	Trehalose lipids	Nonreducing disaccharide	*Rhodococcus erythropolis*	Ristau and Wagner (1983)
	Mannosyl erythritol lipids	4-O-β-D-mannopyranosyl-D-erythritol linked to two chains of fatty acyl esters	*Pseudozyma* sp. and *Ustilago* sp.	Arutchelvi and Doble (2010)
Lipopeptides	Iturin	7 amino acids linked to a C14–C17 fatty acid	*Bacillus subtilis*	Kim et al. (2010)
	Surfactin	7 amino acid cyclic peptide linked to a C13–C16 fatty acid	*Bacillus subtilis*	Ron and Rosenberg (2001)
	Fengycin	10 amino acids linked to a C14–C18 fatty acid	*Bacillus subtilis*	Steller et al. (1999)
	Viscosin	9 amino acids linked to a 3-hydroxy fatty acid	*Pseudomonas fluorescens*	Alsohim et al. (2014)
	Amphisin	11 amino acids linked to a 3-hydroxy fatty acid	*Pseudomonas fluorescens*	Groboillot et al. (2011)
	Serrawettins	Nonionic cyclodepsipeptide	*Serratia marcescens*	Chan et al. (2013)
Polymeric biosurfactants	Emuslan	Lipopolysaccharide; molecular weight 1000 kDa	*Acinetobacter calcoaceticus*	Smyth et al. (2010)
	Alasan	Polysaccharide protein complex; Molecular weight 1000 kDa	*Acinetobacter radioresistens*	Smyth et al. (2010)

PRODUCTION OF BIOSURFACTANTS IN MICROBES

The production of biosurfactants is highly dependent on the nature of each biosurfactant and the microorganisms that produce it. Biosurfactants are produced through a fermentation process in the following possible ways: (a) production of biosurfactant related to growth, (b) production of biosurfactant in limiting conditions, (c) production of biosurfactant by resting cells, and (d) production allied with the precursor augmentation (Rodrigues and Teixeira, 2008). Biosurfactant production is directly proportional to substrate utilization (Desai and Desai, 1993). Diverse metabolic pathways exploit particular enzymes for the synthesis of hydrophobic and hydrophilic moieties of biosurfactants (Figure 4.1). Primary enzymes involved in the synthesis of biosurfactants are regulatory enzymes. Biosurfactant production is regulated by four mechanisms: induction, repression, regulation of nitrogen, and limitation of multivalent ions (Desai and Banat, 1997). Lipopeptide biosurfactants synthesis is generally controlled by an induction mechanism (Kluge et al., 1988; Ullrich et al., 1991; Besson and Michel, 1992).

Induction of trehalolipidis synthesis was reported when hydrocarbons were added to the growth medium of *Rhodococcus erythropolis* (Rapp et al. 1977, 1979).

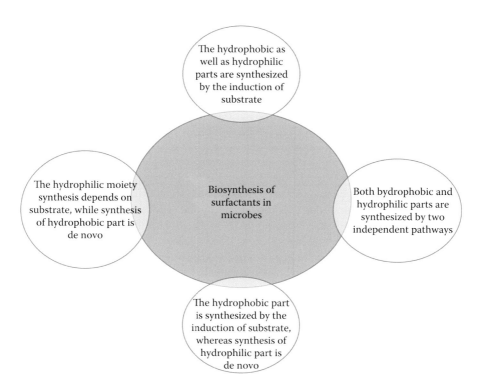

FIGURE 4.1   Regulation of biosurfactant synthesis in microbes.

Glycolipid synthesis was also observed on the media containing alkanes in *P. aeruginosa* SB-30 (Chakrabarty, 1985).

Acinetobacter calcoaceticus (Göbbert et al., 1984) and *Arthrobacter paraffineus* (Duvnjak et al., 1982) showed reduction in biosurfactant production due to organic acids and D-glucose. Repression in rhamnolipids synthesis by *P. aeruginosa* (Hauser et al., 1954, 1958) and liposan by *C. lipolytica* (Cirigliano and Carman, 1984) has been observed with the addition of acetate, tri-carboxylic acids, and D-glucose to their growth media, respectively.

Biosurfactant synthesis is also affected by the regulation of nitrogen and metal ions. Various studies have shown the onset of rhamnolipid synthesis in the lower nitrogen concentrations. In *P. aeruginosa*, synthesis of rhamnolipid has been observed in the stationary phase and in limited nitrogen conditions (Guerra-Santos et al., 1984; Ramana and Karanth, 1989). Inhibition of rhamnolipid synthesis has been reported in *Pseudomonas* sp. strain DSM-2874 by the addition of nitrogenous substrate in the resting cells (Syldatk et al., 1985). In another study, *R. erythropolis* showed synthesis of glycolipid in a nitrogen-deficient environment (Ristau and Wagner, 1983). Under amino acid-starved conditions, synthesis of emulsan has been observed in *A. calcoaceticus* RAG (Rubinovitz et al., 1982).

Higher yield of biosurfactant is obtained in the absence of multivalent cations (Guerra-Santos et al., 1984; Syldatk et al., 1985). A study revealed that synthesis of rhamnolipid is increased under lower salt conditions in *P. aeruginosa* DSM 2659 (Guerra-Santos et al., 1986). Many studies have shown the production of biosurfactant in iron deficient conditions by *P. fluorescens* (Persson et al., 1990a,b) and *P. aeruginosa* (Guerra-Santos et al., 1984, 1986), whereas salts of manganese and iron increased production of biosurfactant in *B. subtilis* (Cooper et al., 1981) and *Rhodococcus* sp. (Abu-Ruwaida et al., 1991).

The genetic makeup of biosurfactant-producing microbes plays a fundamental role in the production of biosurfactants. Various studies have discussed the metabolic pathways, enzymes, and operons involved in the extracellular production of biosurfactants. For example, nonribosomal peptide synthetases (NRPSs) are accountable for lipopeptide production; distant microbial species and plasmid-encoded-rhlA, B, R, and I genes of rhl quorum sensing system in *Pseudomonas* species are vital for the biosynthesis of glycolipid biosurfactants (Das et al., 2008).

Production of rhamnolipid is mediated by the genes encoded in plasmid. During the biosynthesis of rhamnolipids rhlA, B, R, and I genes are transcribed in 5′-rhlABRI-3′ direction in heterologous hosts (Ochsner et al., 1995). Koch et al. (2002) reported that the amphisin synthetase gene responsible for the production of amphisin in *Pseudomonas* sp. DSS73 is controlled by a two-component regulatory system: GacA response regulator and GacS sensor kinase.

The production of biosurfactants varies greatly with culture conditions, for example, the bioavailability of various raw materials necessary for growth of producing strains such as carbon, nitrogen, and oxygen; the C:N ratio; the limited amount of essential elements like phosphorus and sulfur; and so on. Environmental parameters like temperature, pH, aeration, agitation, oxygen availability, and divalent cations also affect the composition and type of biosurfactant as well as the growth and activity of producing strains (Singh et al., 2004; Salihu et al., 2009).

The production and type of biosurfactant is greatly influenced by carbon sources. Various carbon substrates like hydrocarbons, carbohydrates, vegetable and frying oils, and so on, have been used for the biosynthesis of biosurfactants (Salihu et al., 2009). Haba et al. (2003) reported the production of a rhamnolipids mixture, by *Pseudomonas aeruginosa* 47T2 by utilizing waste frying oil as a carbon substrate, with extensive antimicrobial properties and lowered surface tension up to 32.8 mN/m.

Various renewable substrates and industrial wastes can also be utilized for the production of biosurfactants. Scientists have been searching for suitable and inexpensive substrates that can produce a high yield and good-quality biosurfactants. These substrates include pineapple processing waste, potato, sugar beet, cassava, sorghum, soybean cake, canola meal, coconut cake, sawdust, corn cobs, tea waste, and so on, (Pandey et al., 2000). Govindammal and Parthasarathi (2013) investigated the economical production of rhamnolipid by *Pseudomonas fluorescens* with pineapple juice as a substrate. The lowest surface tension of isolate was recorded to be 25.4 mN/m, and the highest yield of biosurfactant was obtained 9.43 g/L in pineapple juice medium.

One of the important factors necessary for the growth of microbes involved in the production of biosurfactant is nitrogen. Meat extract, urea, ammonium nitrate, yeast extract, malt extract, sodium nitrate, peptone, and ammonium sulfate have been used extensively as sources of nitrogen for biosurfactant synthesis. Salt concentrations of media also influence the growth and cellular activities of biosurfactant-producing strains (Fakruddin, 2012).

Maximum production of biosurfactant was reported in *P. aeruginosa* using nitrates as the sole source of nitrogen, and the highest yield of biosurfactant was recorded by *Arthrobacter paraffineus* using urea and salts of ammonium as nitrogen sources (Adamczak and Odzimierz Bednarski, 2000). Makkar and Cameotra (1997) demonstrated the production of biosurfactant by *Bacillus subtilis* at 45°C using 2% sucrose as a carbon source and 4% NaCl at a pH range of 4.5–10.5. Maximum yield was obtained when nitrate ions or urea were used as nitrogen source.

Abouseoud et al. (2007) demonstrated production of rhamnolipid by *Pseudomonas fluorescens* using olive oil as a carbon substrate and ammonium nitrate as a nitrogen source, with high stability at a broad pH range, salinity at 10% NaCl, and temperature up to 120°C. Ilori et al. (2005) demonstrated production of biosurfactant by *Aeromonas* spp. using soybean as a nitrogen source and glucose as a carbon source. The biosurfactant obtained showed maximum activity at 40°C, 5% NaCl concentration, and a pH of 8.0.

Maqsood et al. (2011) determined the effects of ferrous sulfate, ferrous chloride, and ferrous ammonium sulfate on rhamnolipid production by *Pseudomonas aeruginosa*: 3.81 g/L rhamnolipid was recorded in a manitol medium with 0.008 g/L of ferrous sulfate; however, 1.85 g/L of rhamnolipid was obtained with 0.004 g/L ferrous chloride in medium. Sahoo et al. (2011) reported enhanced production of biosurfactants by *Pseudomonas aeruginosa* OCD1 with the addition of $MnSO_4$ and $ZnSO_4$ in the culture media. Response surface methodology was applied to determine the optimum environmental conditions for the maximum production of surfactin. The highest yield of surfactin was observed at 37.4°C and with a pH of 6.755, an agitation speed of 140 rpm, and 0.75 vvm aeration.

RECENT TRENDS AND APPLICATIONS OF BIOSURFACTANTS

FOOD SECTOR

The primary aim of the food industry is to offer safe products with organoleptic properties. Food additives are used to transform the characteristic properties of food and thus enhance and retain their nutritional value, texture, quality, taste, and appearance. Because of their inherent antiadhesive, antimicrobial, emulsification, solubilizing, and wetting properties, biosurfactants provide new prospects for meeting the growing demands of "green" and natural additives in the food-processing industries. Microbial-derived surfactants can potentially be utilized as key elements in the food industries either as food additives or for the treatment of food-contact surfaces. Waste from food industries can be used as substrates for biosurfactant production, thus reducing waste treatment costs. A number of reports demonstrated reduction in food pathogens using biosurfactants, which has raised interest in using biosurfactants as additives (Nitschke and Silva, 2016).

A limitation in the use of peptides like bacteriocins in food preservation is their intrinsic sensitivity to proteolytic enzymes. This problem can be resolved, however, by using ring-structure biosurfactants such as lipopeptides because they are well known for their antiadhesive, antimicrobial, antiviral, and antitumor activities. Lipopeptides such as surfactins are exploited in the baking industry to retain stability, texture, and volume and to emulsify fat to regulate the accretion of fat globules. Some lipopeptides from *Enterobacteriaceae* with high emulsification capabilities and enhanced viscosity at low pH have been used in the food industry. Various food biopreservatives like antimicrobial compounds have been used frequently to avoid food spoilage. High-molecular-weight biosurfactants are particularly attractive because of their structural and functional heterogeneity. High-molecular-weight biosurfactants have gained attention because a large number of reactive groups are present in each molecule, which means that they can facilitate emulsification by adhering with oil droplets, thereby providing steric stability to the emulsions in processed foods (Garti and Leser 1999; Bach and Gutnick 2006).

Gutierrez et al. (2007) demonstrated production of glycoproteins emulsifiers from *Halomonas* species with a remarkably high content of protein and uronic acids. These glycoproteins effectively emulsified a wide range of food oils in adverse pH and temperature conditions. In another study, Campos et al. (2013) showed innocuous biosurfactant production from *Candida utilis* using glucose and canola waste frying oil and its successful application in the formulation of a mayonnaise. Therefore, biosurfactants can be potentially utilized as bioemulsifiers in food industry.

Biosurfactants are potential antibiofilm agents. Biofilms consist of complex microbial communities that are held together by an extracellular matrix characteristically containing exopolysacchrides, nucleic acids, or proteins. Bacterial biofilms are a major cause of food contamination, which can cause food-borne diseases and also leads to food spoilage. Biofilm may destroy the overall quality and safety of the food products because it affects the sanitization of surfaces in contact with food. For example, *Listeria monocytogenes* biofilms attach to metal, rubber, and glass surfaces. *Escherichia coli* and *Staphylococcus aureus* form biofilms on polypropylene mesh.

These biofilms cause chronic diseases, and they have established resistance to sanitation. A few species of the family Enterobacteriaceae are also involved in cell adhesion and biofilm formation (Adetunji et al., 2014). Salmonellosis is the second most common cause of food-borne illness worldwide. It may form a biofilm with a risk of food contamination (Corcoran et al., 2014).

Sabaté and Audisio (2013) reported antagonistic effects of three surfactin-producing *Bacillus subtilis* strains against seven *Listeria monocytogenes* strains. These surfactin biosurfactants showed anti-Listeria activity and inhibited pathogenic activity at a wide range of pH, at different temperatures, and in the presence of proteolytic enzymes. This study suggests that surfactin biosurfactants are a new way to inhibit *L. monocytogenes* in the food industry.

Another problem in the food industry is auto-oxidation of lipids, which decreases food quality and the safety of food products, produces toxic compounds, and develops off-flavors. Antioxidants are food additives used to prevent lipid oxidation and thus enhance food shelf life. Some biosurfactants have been found to be potential antioxidant agents. Antioxidant activity of a lipopeptide surfactant from *B. subtilis* was revealed to be able to scavenge free radicals and could be used as an unconventional natural antioxidant (Yalcin and Cavusoglu, 2010).

Marzban et al. (2016) isolated antimicrobial glycolipid biosurfactant with antimicrobial potential from a marine bacterium *Buttiauxella* sp. using a low-cost substrate: molasses. This biosurfactant exhibited high antimicrobial activity against some pathogens such as *E. coli*, *Bacillus subtilis*, *Bacillus cereus*, *Candida albicans*, *Aspergillus niger*, and *Salmonella enterica*.

The studies mentioned in this chapter depicted the potential of biosurfactants in the food industry as antimicrobial agents, bioemulsifiers, and antibiofilm agents. They could be substitutes for conventional counterparts currently in use.

HEALTH SECTOR

Biosurfactants present promising molecules in therapeutic applications. These biosurfactants may interact with the cell membranes of other organisms and their surroundings because of their surface activities, which mean that they may be used as key elements in drug delivery systems and in cancer therapeutics. A few glycolipids and lipopeptides show selective inhibition of proliferation in cancer cells, and they may disrupt cell membranes, thus causing lysis by affecting their apoptosis pathways (Gudiña et al., 2013).

Biosurfactants like trehalose lipids serve as immunomodulating, antitumor, and anticancer agents. They may inhibit fibrin clot formation, activate fibrin clot lysis, and also act as antiadhesives of biofilms in prosthetic materials and dental plaques.

A glycolipid biosurfactant, trehalose lipid tetraester (THL), which is produced by *Nocardia farcinicam* was evaluated for *in vitro* antitumor activity on human cancer cells. It exhibited antiproliferative activity and arbitrated cell death by the initiation of DNA fragmentation. This study suggested that THL could be potentially applied in biomedicine as a therapeutic agent (Christova et al., 2014). Another study demonstrated that the antitumor activity of a surfactin produced by *Bacillus subtilis* and a glycoprotein produced by *Lactobacillus paracasei* revealed a decrease in the viability of breast cancer cells and inhibited cell proliferation (Duarte et al., 2014).

A wide range of biosurfactants from *Bacillus subtilis* strains showed potent antimicrobial, antiviral, hemolytic, antitumor, blood anticoagulant, and fibrinolytic activities (Kikuchi and Hasumi, 2002; Cameotra and Makkar, 2004; Kim et al., 2006; Henry et al., 2011; Sriram et al., 2011). Ghribi et al. (2012) investigated the antimicrobial activity of biosurfactant produced by *Bacillus subtilis* SPB1. The biosurfactant obtained showed efficient activity against *Klebsiella pneumoniae, Staphylococcus aureus, Staphylococcus xylosus, Enterococcus faecalis,* and so on. Antimicrobial activities of polylysine and surfactin were also reported by Huang et al. (2011) against *Salmonella enteritidis*. Shah et al. (2005) speculated about the antiviral activity of sphorolipids against human immunodeficiency virus. Saini et al. (2008) demonstrated viscosin obtained from *Pseudomonas libanensis* M9-3 repressed the relocation of the metastatic prostate cancer cell line. Biosurfactant obtained from *Lactobacillus paracasei* showed antiadhesive activity against *S. epidermidis, S. agalactiae, and S. aureus.* (Gudiña et al., 2010).

These studies demonstrated potential applications of biosurfactants in biomedicine, but their use is still limited due to lack of knowledge about their toxicity for humans and because of the absence of clinical data to validate their use in biomedical and health-related areas.

Environment Sector

Environmental pollution has resulted from the overproduction and extensive use of persistent and toxic hydrocarbons. Biosurfactants present an effective method of bioremediation of an environment polluted by hydrocarbons. Two mechanisms involved in the bioremediation of hydrocarbons using biosurfactants include bioavailability of substrates and cell surface interaction (Mulligan and Gibbs, 2004). The surface area of insoluble substrates is increased by biosurfactants, which result in an increase in their bioavailability and mobility. Bioremediation of hydrocarbons is enhanced by biosurfactants through emulsification, mobilization, and solubilization (Deziel et al., 1996; Nievas et al., 2008).

Biosurfactants tend to lower the surface and interface tension at the concentrations below CMC; at this stage, mobilization of hydrophobic substrates occurs. At the concentrations above CMC, micelles formation occurs by the aggregation of biosurfactant molecules and the solubilization of oil (Urum et al., 2004). High-molecular-weight biosurfactants cause the emulsification of fats and oils. When droplets of oil are suspended in water, emulsification occurs (Pacwa-Plociniczak et al., 2011). Biosurfactants can be used for the recovery of residual oil trapped in pores by lowering the surface tension between oil and water or oil and rock (Sen, 2008). Salehizadeh and Mohammadizad (2009) reported that lipopolysaccharide biosurfactant from *Alcaligenes* sp. MS-103 has the potential to be used in oil recovery.

Because of their recalcitrant nature and toxicity, even at lower concentrations, heavy metals pose a serious threat for all living organisms in an ecosystem. Biosurfactants present an efficient solution for the removal of metals from metal-contaminated soils.

Biosurfactants form complexes with metals and are desorbed in soil solution. Micelles of biosurfactants can also remove metals from soil surfaces by binding their polar heads with metals and mobilizing them in water (Mulligan and Gibbs, 2004; Singh and Cameotra, 2004; Juwarkar et al., 2007; Aşçi et al., 2008).

Di-rhamnolipid from the *Pseudomonas aeruginosa* strain BS2 was investigated as a washing agent for the bioremediation of metals from metal-contaminated soils. Results showed higher leaching behavior of different metals like cadmium, nickel, lead, copper, and chromium by biosurfactants compared to tap water; hence, biosurfactants could be used efficiently for the removal of metals from contaminated soils (Juwarkar et al., 2007).

Heavy metal-resistant, biosurfactant-producing bacteria can also be used to enhance the phytoremediation potential of plants growing in heavy metal-polluted soils. Sheng et al. (2008) demonstrated that root colonization of the biosurfactant-producing *Bacillus* sp. J119 strain with tomato plants could promote its growth and enhance its cadmium uptake in cadmium-contaminated soils.

AGRICULTURE SECTOR

In agriculture, wettability of soil is enhanced by biosurfactant-mediated hydrophilization. Increased wettability means that fertilizers can be evenly distributed in soil, and caking of fertilizers can be prevented (Makkar and Rockne, 2003). Fengycin biosurfactants with antifungal activity may act as biocontrol agents of different plant diseases (Kachholz and Schlingmann, 1987). Wei et al. (2010) reported that Fengycin production by *Bacillus subtilis* F29-3 had antifugal activity against filamentous fungi. Stanghellini and Miller (1997) reported that rhamnolipids from *Pseudomonas aeruginosa* were promising biocontrol agents for the control of zoosporic plant pathogens: they showed zoosporicidal activity against *Plasmopara, Pythium*, and *Phytophora* species, which were found to cause root rot fungal infections in cucumbers and peppers (Stanghellini et al., 1996).

Mulligan (2005) showed that lipopeptide was a potential biopesticide with insecticidal activity against *Drosophila melanogaster*. Biosurfactants can be used as eco-friendly and inexpensive alternatives for conventional pesticides that have undesirable toxic effects and are costly (Fakruddin, 2012).

FUTURE PERSPECTIVES

Few biosurfactants have been reported as alternative medicines, and probiotic biosurfactants have been less exploited in the health and medicine sector so far. They exhibit excellent antimicrobial, antibiofilm, antiadhesive, and antitumor activities (Table 4.2). Probiotics consist of indigenous human microflora and possess immense health benefits. Therefore, probiotic-derived biosurfactants are safe to use and offer new prospects in the medical field (Fariq and Saeed, 2016).

Because of the versatility and biochemical characters of biosurfactants, they have been gaining attention in the field of bionanotechnology, specifically for the design of new functional structures such as mannosylerythritol lipid (MEL) biosurfactants, which have self-assembling properties that have been used in carbohydrate ligand systems.

TABLE 4.2
Applications of Probiotic Biosurfactants

Probiotic Strain	Biosurfactant Produced	Applications	References
Corynebacterium xerosis	Coryxin	Antibiofilm agents against *Staphylococcus aureus, S. mutans, E. coli,* and *P. aeruginosa*	Dalili et al. (2015)
Citrobacter, Enterobacter	Fengycins, surfactins, kurstakins, iturins	Pharmaceutical, cosmetic, and biocontrol potential	Mandal et al. (2013)
Lactococcus lactis	Xylolipids	Antibacterial activity	Saravanakumari and Mani (2010)
Lactobacillus sp.	Surlactin	Antiadhesive of uropathogens	Velraeds et al. (1996)
L. paracasei	Glycoprotein	Antitumor activity	Duarte et al. (2014)

MEL-containing liposomes performed DNA encapsulation, gene transfection, and membrane fusion activities. Biosurfactant-mediated synthesis of various nanoparticles has been reported in many studies (Rodrigues, 2015). Biosurfactants aid in the stabilization of nanoparticles. A study reported stabilization of silver nanoparticles in the liquid phase up to three months by *Pseudomonas aeruginosa*–derived biosurfactant (Farias et al., 2014).

Nano vectors can be used for delivery of foreign DNA mammalian cells in gene therapy, drug delivery, and gene transfection. Nano vectors containing a biosurfactant enhance the effectiveness of gene transfection *in vitro* and *in vivo* because biosurfactants mediate a new pathway for gene delivery into the target cells by fusing with the plasma membranes (Nakanishi et al., 2009).

Other possibilities that have not yet been explored are using probiotic biosurfactants as vectors for drug delivery systems, and in nano-biotechnology for synthesizing nano devices for drugs and diagnostics. Integration of nano-biotechnology using biosurfactant stabilizers will pave new pathways for drug delivery systems and nano-diagnostics.

CHALLENGES IN BIOSURFACTANT COMMERCIALIZATION

A major limitation in the commercialization of biosurfactants is optimization of the fermentation process to scale up their production. Second, recovery of purified biosurfactants is cost-intensive. Using renewable substrates offers a sustainable, cost-reducing strategy for the production of biosurfactants on a commercial scale. But downstreaming of biosurfactant production still poses a question. Using statistical methods like surface response methodology for process optimization prior to commercialization of biosurfactant production may aid in reduction of actual production and optimization costs. Using metagenomics approaches for detection of biosurfactant-producing bacteria presents a suitable method for the identification of noncultivable biosurfactant producers. Genetic engineering of biosurfactant-producing microbes may lead to hyperproducing recombinant strains, which may produce high yields at low cost and use renewable substrates. Despite a few limitations, biosurfactants seem to promise a green approach and possess immense potential in health and medicine, food processing industries, and environmental sustainability.

REFERENCES

Abouseoud, M., R. Maachi, and A. Amrane. 2007. Biosurfactant production from olive oil by Pseudomonas fluorescens. *Communicating Current Research and Educational Topics and Trends in Applied Microbiology* 1:340–347.

Abu-Ruwaida, A. S., I. M. Banat, S. Haditirto, and A. Khamis. 1991. Nutritional requirements and growth characteristics of a biosurfactant-producing Rhodococcus bacterium. *World Journal of Microbiology and Biotechnology* 7(1):53–60.

Adamczak, M., and W. Odzimierz Bednarski. 2000. Influence of medium composition and aeration on the synthesis of biosurfactants produced by Candida antarctica. *Biotechnology Letters* 22(4):313–316.

Adetunji, V. O., A. O. Adedeji, and J. Kwaga. 2014. Assessment of the contamination potentials of some foodborne bacteria in biofilms for food products. *Asian Pacific Journal of Tropical Medicine* 7:S232–S237.

Alsohim, A. S., T. B. Taylor, G. A. Barrett, J. Gallie, X.-X. Zhang, et al. 2014. The biosurfactant viscosin produced by Pseudomonas fluorescens SBW25 aids spreading motility and plant growth promotion. *Environmental Microbiology* 16(7):2267–2281.

Arutchelvi, J., and M. Doble. 2010. Mannosylerythritol lipids: Microbial production and their applications. In Chavez, G. S. (ed.), *Biosurfactants*, pp. 145–177. Berlin, Germany: Springer.

Aşçı, Y., M. Nurbaş, and Y. Sağ Açıkel. 2008. A comparative study for the sorption of Cd (II) by soils with different clay contents and mineralogy and the recovery of Cd (II) using rhamnolipid biosurfactant. *Journal of Hazardous Materials* 154(1):663–673.

Bach, H., and D. L. Gutnick. 2006. Novel polysaccharide–protein-based amphipathic formulations. *Applied Microbiology and Biotechnology* 71(1):34.

Besson, F., and G. Michel. 1992. Biosynthesis of iturin and surfactin by Bacillus subtilis: Evidence for amino acid activating enzymes. *Biotechnology Letters* 14(11):1013–1018.

Burgos-Diaz, C., R. Pons, M. J. Espuny, F. J. Aranda, J. A. Teruel, et al. 2011. Isolation and partial characterization of a biosurfactant mixture produced by *Sphingobacterium* sp. isolated from soil. *Journal of Colloid and Interface Science* 361(1):195–204.

Cameotra, S. S., and R. S. Makkar. 2004. Recent applications of biosurfactants as biological and immunological molecules. *Current Opinion in Microbiology* 7(3):262–266.

Cameotra, S. S., and R. S. Makkar. 2010. Biosurfactant-enhanced bioremediation of hydrophobic pollutants. *Pure and Applied Chemistry* 82(1):97–116.

Cameotra, S. S., R. S. Makkar, J. Kaur, and S. K. Mehta. 2010. Synthesis of biosurfactants and their advantages to microorganisms and mankind. In Sen, R. (ed.), *Biosurfactants*, pp. 261–280. New York, NY: Springer.

Campos, J. M., T. L. Montenegro Stamford, L. A. Sarubbo, J. M. de Luna, et al. 2013. Microbial biosurfactants as additives for food industries. *Biotechnology Progress* 29(5):1097–1108.

Carrillo, P. G., C. Mardaraz, S. I. Pitta-Alvarez, and A. M. Giulietti. 1996. Isolation and selection of biosurfactant-producing bacteria. *World Journal of Microbiology and Biotechnology* 12(1):82–84.

Chakrabarty, A. M. 1985. Genetically-manipulated microorganisms and their products in the oil service industries. *Trends in Biotechnology* 3(2):32–39.

Chan, X. Y., C. Y. Chang, K. Wai Hong, K. K. Tee, W. Fong Yin, et al. 2013. Insights of bio-surfactant producing Serratia marcescens strain W2. 3 isolated from diseased tilapia fish: A draft genome analysis. *Gut Pathogens* 5(1):29.

Chen, M. L., J. Penfold, R. K. Thomas, T. J. P. Smyth, A. Perfumo, R. Marchant, I. M. Banat, et al. 2010. Solution self-assembly and adsorption at the air–water interface of the monorhamnose and dirhamnose rhamnolipids and their mixtures. *Langmuir* 26(23):18281–18292.

Christova, N., S. Lang, V. Wray, K. Kaloyanov, S. Konstantinov, et al. 2014. Production, structural elucidation and in vitro antitumor activity of trehalose lipid biosurfac-tant from Nocardia farcinica strain. *Journal of Microbiology Biotechnology* 2(4): 439–447.

Cirigliano, M. C., and G. M. Carman. 1984. Isolation of a bioemulsifier from *Candida lipo-lytica*. *Applied and Environmental Microbiology* 48(4):747–750.

Cooper, D. G., and B. G. Goldenberg. 1987. Surface-active agents from two *Bacillus* species. *Applied and Environmental Microbiology* 53(2):224–229.

Cooper, D. G., C. R. Macdonald, S. J. B. Duff, and N. Kosaric. 1981. Enhanced production of surfactin from *Bacillus subtilis* by continuous product removal and metal cation addi-tions. *Applied and Environmental Microbiology* 42(3):408–412.

Cooper, D. G., and D. A. Paddock. 1983. *Torulopsis* petrophilum and surface activity. *Applied and Environmental Microbiology* 46(6):1426–1429.

Corcoran, M., D. Morris, N. De Lappe, J. O'connor, P. Lalor, et al. 2014. Commonly used disinfectants fail to eradicate Salmonella enterica biofilms from food contact surface materials. *Applied and Environmental Microbiology* 80(4):1507–1514.

Dalili, D., M. Amini, M. Ali Faramarzi, M. Reza Fazeli, M. Reza Khoshayand, et al. 2015. Isolation and structural characterization of Coryxin, a novel cyclic lipopeptide from *Corynebacterium xerosis* NS5 having emulsifying and anti-biofilm activity. *Colloids and Surfaces B: Biointerfaces* 135:425–432.

Das, P., S. Mukherjee, and R. Sen. 2008. Genetic regulations of the biosynthesis of microbial surfactants: An overview. *Biotechnology and Genetic Engineering Reviews* 25(1):165–186.

Davey, M. E., N. C. Caiazza, and G. A. O'Toole. 2003. Rhamnolipid surfactant production affects biofilm architecture in *Pseudomonas aeruginosa* PAO1. *Journal of Bacteriology* 185(3):1027–1036.

Desai, J. D., and I. M. Banat. 1997. Microbial production of surfactants and their commercial potential. *Microbiology and Molecular Biology Reviews* 61(1):47–64.

Desai, J. D., and A. J. Desai. 1993. Production of biosurfactants. *Surfactant Science Series* 17:65–65.

Deziel, E., G. Paquette, R. Villemur, F. Lepine, and J. Bisaillon. 1996. Biosurfactant pro-duction by a soil *Pseudomonas* strain growing on polycyclic aromatic hydrocarbons. *Applied and Environmental Microbiology* 62(6):1908–1912.

Duarte, C., E. J. Gudiña, C. F. Lima, and L. R. Rodrigues. 2014. Effects of biosurfactants on the viability and proliferation of human breast cancer cells. *AMB Express* 4(1):40.

Duvnjak, Z., D. G. Cooper, and N. Kosaric. 1982. Production of surfactant by *Arthrobacter paraffineus* ATCC 19558. *Biotechnology and Bioengineering* 24(1):165–175.

Espinosa-Urgel, M. 2003. Resident parking only: Rhamnolipids maintain fluid channels in biofilms. *Journal of Bacteriology* 185(3):699–700.

Farias, C. B., A. F. Silva, R. D. Rufino, J. M. Luna, J. E. Gomes Souza, et al. 2014. Synthesis of silver nanoparticles using a biosurfactant produced in low-cost medium as stabilizing agent. *Electronic Journal of Biotechnology* 17(3):122–125.

Fariq, A., and A. Saeed. 2016. Production and biomedical applications of probiotic biosurfac-tants. *Current Microbiology* 72(4):489–495.

Ganesh, A., and J. Lin. 2009. Diesel degradation and biosurfactant production by Gram-positive isolates. *African Journal of Biotechnology* 8(21), 5847–5854.

Garti, N., and M. E. Leser. 1999. Natural hydrocolloids as food emulsifiers. *Design and Selection of Performance Surfactants* 2:104–145.

Ghribi, D., L. Abdelkefi-Mesrati, I. Mnif, R. Kammoun, I. Ayadi, et al. 2012. Investigation of antimicrobial activity and statistical optimization of *Bacillus subtilis* SPB1 biosurfactant production in solid-state fermentation. *Journal of Biomedicine and Biotechnology.* 2012:373682. doi: 10.1155/2012/373682

Göbbert, U., S. Lang, and F. Wagner. 1984. Sophorose lipid formation by resting cells of *Torulopsis bombicola. Biotechnology Letters* 6(4):225–230.

Govindammal, M., and R. Parthasarathi. 2013. Biosurfactant production using pineapple juice as medium by Pseudomonas fluorescens isolated from mangrove forest soil. *Indian Streams Research Journal* 2:1–10.

Groboillot, A., F. Portet-Koltalo, F. Le Derf, M. J. G. Feuilloley, N. Orange, et al. Poc. 2011. Novel application of cyclolipopeptide amphisin: Feasibility study as additive to remediate polycyclic aromatic hydrocarbon (PAH) contaminated sediments. *International Journal of Molecular Sciences* 12(3):1787–1806.

Gudiña, E. J., V. Rangarajan, R. Sen, and L. R. Rodrigues. 2013. Potential therapeutic applications of biosurfactants. *Trends in Pharmacological Sciences* 34(12):667–675.

Gudiña, E. J., V. Rocha, J. A. Teixeira, and L. R. Rodrigues. 2010. Antimicrobial and antiadhesive properties of a biosurfactant isolated from *Lactobacillus paracasei* ssp. *paracasei* A20. *Letters in Applied Microbiology* 50(4):419–424.

Guerra-Santos, L., O. Käppeli, and A. Fiechter. 1984. Pseudomonas aeruginosa biosurfactant production in continuous culture with glucosee as carbon source. *Applied and Environmental Microbiology* 48(2):301–305.

Guerra-Santos, L. H., O. Käppeli, and A. Fiechter. 1986. Dependence of *Pseudomonas aeruginosa* continous culture biosurfactant production on nutritional and environmental factors. *Applied Microbiology and Biotechnology* 24(6):443–448.

Gutierrez, T., B. Mulloy, K. Black, and D. H. Green. 2007. Glycoprotein emulsifiers from two marine Halomonas species: Chemical and physical characterization. *Journal of Applied Microbiology* 103(5):1716–1727.

Haba, E., A. Pinazo, O. Jauregui, M. J. Espuny, M. Rosa Infante, et al. 2003. Physicochemical characterization and antimicrobial properties of rhamnolipids produced by *Pseudomonas aeruginosa* 47T2 NCBIM 40044. *Biotechnology and Bioengineering* 81(3):316–322.

Hauser, G., and M. L. Karnovsky. 1954. Studies on the production of glycolipide by *Pseudomonas aeruginosa. Journal of Bacteriology* 68(6):645.

Hauser, G., and M. L. Karnovsky. 1958. Studies on the biosynthesis of L-rhamnose. *Journal of Biological Chemistry* 233(2):287–291.

Henry, G., M. Deleu, E. Jourdan, P. Thonart, and M. Ongena. 2011. The bacterial lipopeptide surfactin targets the lipid fraction of the plant plasma membrane to trigger immune-related defence responses. *Cellular Microbiology* 13(11):1824–1837.

Holmberg, K. 2001. Natural surfactants. *Current Opinion in Colloid and Interface Science* 6(2):148–159.

Huang, X., J. Suo, and Y. Cui. 2011. Optimization of antimicrobial activity of surfactin and polylysine against *Salmonella enteritidis* in milk evaluated by a response surface methodology. *Foodborne Pathogens and Disease* 8(3):439–443.

Ilori, M. O., C. J. Amobi, and A. C. Odocha. 2005. Factors affecting biosurfactant production by oil degrading *Aeromonas* spp. isolated from a tropical environment. *Chemosphere* 61(7):985–992.

Jain, D. K., D. L. Collins-Thompson, H. Lee, and J. T. Trevors. 1991. A drop-collapsing test for screening surfactant-producing microorganisms. *Journal of Microbiological Methods* 13(4):271–279.

Jarvis, F. G., and M. J. Johnson. 1949. A glyco-lipide produced by *Pseudomonas aeruginosa*. *Journal of the American Chemical Society* 71(12):4124–4126.

Juwarkar, A. A., A. Nair, K. V. Dubey, S. K. Singh, and S. Devotta. 2007. Biosurfactant technology for remediation of cadmium and lead contaminated soils. *Chemosphere* 68(10):1996–2002.

Kachholz, T., and M. Schlingmann. 1987. Possible food and agricultural application of microbial surfactants: an assessment. In: Kosaric, N., W. L. Cairns, N. C. C. Grey, (eds.), *Biosurfactant and Biotechnology*, New York, Marcel Dekker. 25:183–208.

Kikuchi, T., and K. Hasumi. 2002. Enhancement of plasminogen activation by surfactin C: Augmentation of fibrinolysis in vitro and in vivo. *Biochimica et Biophysica Acta (BBA)-Protein Structure and Molecular Enzymology* 1596(2):234–245.

Kim, P. I., J. Ryu, Y. H. Kim, and Y.-T. Chi. 2010. Production of biosurfactant lipopeptides iturin A, fengycin and surfactin A from *Bacillus subtilis* CMB32 for control of *Colletotrichum gloeosporioides*. *Journal of Microbiology and Biotechnology* 20(1):138–145.

Kim, S. D., S. K. Park, J. Y. Cho, H. J. Park, J. H. Lim, et al. 2006. Surfactin C inhibits platelet aggregation. *Journal of Pharmacy and Pharmacology* 58(6):867–870.

Kitamoto, D., H. Isoda, and T. Nakahara. 2002. Functions and potential applications of glycolipid biosurfactants—From energy-saving materials to gene delivery carriers. *Journal of Bioscience and Bioengineering* 94(3):187–201.

Kitamoto, D., T. Morita, T. Fukuoka, M.-A. Konishi, and T. Imura. 2009. Self-assembling properties of glycolipid biosurfactants and their potential applications. *Current Opinion in Colloid and Interface Science* 14(5):315–328.

Kluge, B., J. Vater, J. Salnikow, and K. Eckart. 1988. Studies on the biosynthesis of surfactin, a lipopeptide antibiotic from Bacillus subtilis ATCC 21332. *FEBS Letters* 231(1):107–110.

Koch, B., T. H. Nielsen, D. Sørensen, J. Bo Andersen, C. Christophersen, et al. 2002. Lipopeptide production in *Pseudomonas* sp. strain DSS73 is regulated by components of sugar beet seed exudate via the Gac two-component regulatory system. *Applied and Environmental Microbiology* 68(9):4509–4516.

Lin, S.-C. 1996. Biosurfactants: Recent advances. *Journal of Chemical Technology and Biotechnology* 66(2):109–120.

Liu, T., J. Hou, Y. Zuo, S. Bi, and J. Jing. 2011. Isolation and characterization of a biosurfactant-producing bacterium from Daqing oil-contaminated sites. *African Journal of Microbiology Research* 5(21):3509–3514.

Makkar, R. S., and K. J. Rockne. 2003. Comparison of synthetic surfactants and biosurfactants in enhancing biodegradation of polycyclic aromatic hydrocarbons. *Environmental Toxicology and Chemistry* 22(10):2280–2292.

Mandal, S. M., S. Sharma, A. K. Pinnaka, A. Kumari, and S. Korpole. 2013. Isolation and characterization of diverse antimicrobial lipopeptides produced by *Citrobacter* and *Enterobacter*. *BMC Microbiology* 13(1):152.

Maqsood, M. I., A. Jamal, and H. Abdul Azeem. 2011. Effects of iron salts on *Rhamnolipid Biosurfactant* production. *Biologia (Pakistan)* 57(1–2):121–132.

Marzban, A., G. Ebrahimipour, and A. Danesh. 2016. Bioactivity of a novel glycolipid produced by a *Halophilic Buttiauxella* sp. and improving submerged fermentation using a response surface method. *Molecules* 21(10):1256.

Matsuyama, T., T. Tanikawa, and Y. Nakagawa. 2011. Serrawettins and other surfactants produced by Serratia. In Chavez, G. S. (ed.), *Biosurfactants*, pp. 93–120. Berlin, Germany: Springer.

Fakruddin, M. 2012. Biosurfactant: Production and application. *Journal of Petroleum and Environment Biotechnology* 3(124):2. doi: 10.4172/2157-7463.1000124

Microbial Biosurfactants Market (Rhamnolipids, Sophorolipids, Mannosylerythritol Lipids (MEL) and Other) for Household Detergents, Industrial & Institutional Cleaners, Personal Care, Oilfield Chemicals, Agricultural Chemicals, Food Processing, Textile and Other Applications—Global Industry Perspective, Comprehensive Analysis and Forecast 2014–2020 report at http://www.marketresearchstore.com/report/microbial-biosurfactants-market-z37354.

Mishra, M., P. Muthuprasanna, K. Surya Prabha, P. Sobhita Rani, I. A. Satish, et al. 2009. Basics and potential applications of surfactants: A review. *International Journal of PharmTech Research*. 1(4):1354–1365.

Morikawa, M., Y. Hirata, and T. Imanaka. 2000. A study on the structure–function relationship of lipopeptide biosurfactants. *Biochimica et Biophysica Acta (BBA)-Molecular and Cell Biology of Lipids* 1488(3):211–218.

Mulligan, C. N. 2005. Environmental applications for biosurfactants. *Environmental Pollution* 133(2):183–198.

Mulligan, C. N., D. G. Cooper, and R. J. Neufeld. 1984. Selection of microbes producing biosurfactants in media without hydrocarbons. *Journal of Fermentation Technology* 62(4):311–314.

Mulligan, C. N., and B. F. Gibbs. 2004. Types, production and applications of biosurfactants. *Proceedings-Indian National Science Academy Part B* 70(1):31–56.

Nakanishi, M., Y. Inoh, D. Kitamoto, and T. Furuno. 2009. Nano vectors with a biosurfactant for gene transfection and drug delivery. *Journal of Drug Delivery Science and Technology* 19(3):165–169.

Nievas, M. L., M. G. Commendatore, J. L. Esteves, and V. Bucalá. 2008. Biodegradation pattern of hydrocarbons from a fuel oil-type complex residue by an emulsifier-producing microbial consortium. *Journal of Hazardous Materials* 154(1):96–104.

Nitschke, M., and S. S. E. Silva. 2016. Recent food applications of microbial surfactants. *Critical Reviews in Food Science and Nutrition Just-Accepted* doi: 10.1080/10408398.2016.1208635

Noudeh, G. D., M. H. Moshafi, P. Kazaeli, and F. Akef. 2010. Studies on bioemulsifier production by *Bacillus licheniformis* PTCC 1595. *African Journal of Biotechnology* 9(3) https://www.ajol.info/index.php/ajb/article/view/77915.

Ochsner, U. A., J. Reiser, A. Fiechter, and B. Witholt. 1995. Production of *Pseudomonas aeruginosa* rhamnolipid biosurfactants in heterologous hosts. *Applied and Environmental Microbiology* 61(9):3503–3506.

Pacwa-Płociniczak, M., G. A. Płaza, Z. Piotrowska-Seget, and S. S. Cameotra. 2011. Environmental applications of biosurfactants: Recent advances. *International Journal of Molecular Sciences* 12(1):633–654.

Pandey, A., C. R. Soccol, and D. Mitchell. 2000. New developments in solid state fermentation: I-bioprocesses and products. *Process Biochemistry* 35(10):1153–1169.

Paraszkiewicz, K., and J. Dlugoński. 2003. Microbial biosurfactants–Synthesis and application (Pol). *Biotechnologia* 4:82–91.

Persson, A., G. Molin, N. Andersson, and J. Sjöholm. 1990a. Biosurfactant yields and nutrient consumption of *Pseudomonas fluorescens* 378 studied in a microcomputer controlled multifermentation system. *Biotechnology and Bioengineering* 36(3):252–255.

Persson, A., G. Molin, and C. Weibull. 1990b. Physiological and morphological changes induced by nutrient limitation of Pseudomonas fluorescens 378 in continuous culture. *Applied and Environmental Microbiology* 56(3):686–692.

Pruthi, V., and S. S. Cameotra. 1997. Production and properties of a biosurfactant synthesized by *Arthrobacter protophormiae*—An Antarctic strain. *World Journal of Microbiology and Biotechnology* 13(1):137–139.

Ramana, K. V., and N. G. Karanth. 1989. Factors affecting biosurfactant production using Pseudomonas aeruginosa CFTR-6 under submerged conditions. *Journal of Chemical Technology and Biotechnology* 45(4):249–257.

Rapp, P., H. Bock, E. Urban, F. Wagner, W. Gebetsberger, et al. 1977. Use of trehalose lipids in enhanced oil recovery. *DESCHEMA Monograph Biotechnology* 81:177–185.

Rapp, P., H. Bock, V. Wray, and F. Wagner. 1979. Formation, isolation and characterization of trehalose dimycolates from *Rhodococcus erythropolis* grown on n-alkanes. *Microbiology* 115(2):491–503.

Ristau, E., and F. Wagner. 1983. Formation of novel anionic trehalosetetraesters from *Rhodococcus erythropolis* under growth limiting conditions. *Biotechnology Letters* 5(2):95–100.

Rodrigues, L. R. 2015. Microbial surfactants: Fundamentals and applicability in the formulation of nano-sized drug delivery vectors. *Journal of Colloid and Interface Science* 449:304–316.

Rodrigues, L. R., and J. A. Teixeira. 2008. Biosurfactants production from cheese whey. *Advances in Cheese Whey Utilization* 2008:81–104.

Ron, E. Z., and E. Rosenberg. 2001. Natural roles of biosurfactants. *Environmental Microbiology* 3(4):229–236.

Rosenberg, E., and E. Z. Ron. 1997. Bioemulsans: Microbial polymeric emulsifiers. *Current Opinion in Biotechnology* 8(3):313–316.

Rosenberg, E., and E. Z. Ron. 1999. High-and low-molecular-mass microbial surfactants. *Applied Microbiology and Biotechnology* 52(2):154–162.

Rosenberg, E., C. Rubinovitz, R. Legmann, and E. Z. Ron. 1988. Purification and chemical properties of *Acinetobacter calcoaceticus* A2 biodispersan. *Applied and Environmental Microbiology* 54(2):323–326.

Rosenberg, M. 2006. Microbial adhesion to hydrocarbons: Twenty-five years of doing MATH. *FEMS Microbiology Letters* 262(2):129–134.

Rubinovitz, C., D. L. Gutnick, and E. Rosenberg. 1982. Emulsan production by *Acinetobacter calcoaceticus* in the presence of chloramphenicol. *Journal of Bacteriology* 152(1):126–132.

Sabaté, D. C., and M. C. Audisio. 2013. Inhibitory activity of surfactin, produced by different Bacillus subtilis subsp. subtilis strains, against Listeria monocytogenes sensitive and bacteriocin-resistant strains. *Microbiological Research* 168(3):125–129.

Sahoo, S., S. Datta, and D. Biswas. 2011. Optimization of culture conditions for biosurfactant production from *Pseudomonas aeruginosa* OCD1. *Journal of Advanced Scientific Research* 1(2):32–36.

Saini, H. S., B. E. Barragán-Huerta, A. Lebrón-Paler, J. E. Pemberton, R. R. Vázquez, et al. 2008. Efficient purification of the biosurfactant viscosin from *Pseudomonas libanensis* strain M9-3 and its physicochemical and biological properties. *Journal of Natural Products* 71(6):1011–1015.

Salehizadeh, H., and S. Mohammadizad. 2009. Microbial enhanced oil recovery using biosurfactant produced by *Alcaligenes faecalis*. *Iranian Journal of Biotechnology* 7(4):216–223.

Salihu, A., I. Abdulkadir, and M. N. Almustapha. 2009. An investigation for potential development on biosurfactants. *Biotechnology and Molecular Biology Reviews* 4(5):111–117.

Saravanakumari, P., and K. Mani. 2010. Structural characterization of a novel xylolipid biosurfactant from *Lactococcus lactis* and analysis of antibacterial activity against multidrug resistant pathogens. *Bioresource Technology* 101(22):8851–8854.

Sen, R. 2008. Biotechnology in petroleum recovery: The microbial EOR. *Progress in Energy and Combustion Science* 34(6):714–724.

Shah, V., G. F. Doncel, T. Seyoum, K. M. Eaton, I. Zalenskaya, et al. 2005. Sophorolipids, microbial glycolipids with anti-human immunodeficiency virus and sperm-immobilizing activities. *Antimicrobial Agents and Chemotherapy* 49(10):4093–4100.

Sheng, X., L. He, Q. Wang, H. Ye, and C. Jiang. 2008. Effects of inoculation of biosurfactant-producing Bacillus sp. J119 on plant growth and cadmium uptake in a cadmium-amended soil. *Journal of Hazardous Materials* 155(1):17–22.

Siegmund, I., and F. Wagner. 1991. New method for detecting rhamnolipids excreted by *Pseudomonas* species during growth on mineral agar. *Biotechnology Techniques* 5(4):265–268.

Singh, P., and S. S. Cameotra. 2004. Potential applications of microbial surfactants in biomedical sciences. *TRENDS in Biotechnology* 22(3):142–146.

Smyth, T. J. P., A. Perfumo, S. McClean, R. Marchant, and I. M. Banat. 2010. Isolation and analysis of lipopeptides and high molecular weight biosurfactants. In *Handbook of Hydrocarbon and Lipid Microbiology*, pp. 3687–3704. Berlin, Germany: Springer.

Sriram, M. I., S. Gayathiri, U. Gnanaselvi, P. S. Jenifer, S. Mohan Raj, et al. 2011. Novel lipopeptide biosurfactant produced by hydrocarbon degrading and heavy metal tolerant bacterium *Escherichia fergusonii* KLU01 as a potential tool for bioremediation. *Bioresource Technology* 102(19):9291–9295.

Stanghellini, M. E., D. H. Kim, S. L. Rasmussen, and P. A. Rorabaugh.1996. Control of root rot of peppers caused by *Phytophthora capsici* with a nonionic surfactant. *Plant Disease* 80(1):1113–1116.

Stanghellini, M. E., and R. M. Miller. 1997. Biosurfactants: Their identity and potential efficacy in the biological control of zoosporic plant pathogens. *Plant Disease* 81(1):4–12.

Steller, S., D. Vollenbroich, F. Leenders, T. Stein, B. Conrad, et al. 1999. Structural and functional organization of the fengycin synthetase multienzyme system from *Bacillus subtilis* b213 and A1/3. *Chemistry and Biology* 6(1):31–41.

Suwansukho, P., V. Rukachisirikul, F. Kawai, and A. H-Kittikun. 2008. Production and applications of biosurfactant from *Bacillus subtilis* MUV4. *Sonklanakarin Journal of Science and Technology* 30(2):87.

Syldatk, C., S. Lang, U. Matulovic, and F. Wagner. 1985. Production of four interfacial active rhamnolipids from n-alkanes or glycerol by resting cells of *Pseudomonas* species DSM 2874. *Zeitschrift für Naturforschung C* 40(1–2):61–67.

Tambekar, D. H., and P. V. Gadakh. 2013. Biochemical and molecular detection of biosurfactant producing bacteria from soil. *International Journal of Life Sciences Biotechnology Pharma Research* 2:204–211.

Techaoei, S., P. Leelapornpisid, D. Santiarwarn, and S. Lumyong. 2007. Preliminary screening of biosurfactant producing microorganisms isolated from hot spring and garages in northern Thailand. *KMITL Science and Technology Journal* 7(S1):38–43.

Thies, S., S. C. Rausch, F. Kovacic, A. Schmidt-Thaler, S. Wilhelm, et al. 2016. Metagenomic discovery of novel enzymes and biosurfactants in a slaughterhouse biofilm microbial community. *Scientific Reports* 6:27035.

Ullrich, C., B. Kluge, Z. Palacz, and J. Vater. 1991. Cell-free biosynthesis of surfactin, a cyclic lipopeptide produced by *Bacillus subtilis*. *Biochemistry* 30(26):6503–6508.

Urum, K., and T. Pekdemir. 2004. Evaluation of biosurfactants for crude oil contaminated soil washing. *Chemosphere* 57(9):1139–1150.

Van Hamme, J. D. Ajay Singh, and O. P. Ward. 2006. Physiological aspects: Part 1 in a series of papers devoted to surfactants in microbiology and biotechnology. *Biotechnology Advances* 24(6):604–620.

Velraeds, M. M. C., H. C. van der Mei, G. Reid, and H. J. Busscher. 1996. Physicochemical and biochemical characterization of biosurfactants released by *Lactobacillus* strains. *Colloids and Surfaces B: Biointerfaces* 8(1–2):51–61.

Venhuis, S. H., and M. Mehrvar. 2004. Health effects, environmental impacts, and photochemical degradation of selected surfactants in water. *International Journal of Photoenergy* 6(3):115–125.

Walter, V., C. Syldatk, and R. Hausmann. 2010. Screening concepts for the isolation of biosurfactant producing microorganisms. In Sen, R. (ed.), *Biosurfactants*, pp. 1–13. New York, NY: Springer.

Wei, Y.-H., L.-C. Wang, W.-C. Chen, and S.-Y. Chen. 2010. Production and characterization of fengycin by indigenous *Bacillus subtilis* F29-3 originating from a potato farm. *International Journal of Molecular Sciences* 11(11):4526–4538.

Yalcin, E., and K. Cavusoglu. 2010. Structural analysis and antioxidant activity of a biosurfactant obtained from *Bacillus* subtilis RW-I. *Turkish Journal of Biochemistry-Turk Biyokimya Dergisi* 35(3):243–247.

Zhang, Y. M., and R. M. Miller. 1994. Effect of a *Pseudomonas* rhamnolipid biosurfactant on cell hydrophobicity and biodegradation of octadecane. *Appllied Environmental Microbiology*, 60:2101–2106.

5 *In Vitro* Cultivation of AMF Using Root Organ Culture
Factory of Biofertilizers and Secondary Metabolites Production

Sanjeev Kumar and Shivani Yadav

CONTENTS

INTRODUCTION

The introduction of green techniques with high-input agriculture and the continuing degradation of natural resources have raised issues with sustainable farming. Yields of several crops have now become constant in several regions for 15 to 20 years. Problems associated with the overuse of high-input agricultural practices can be overcome by using biological organisms. Therefore, more sustainable alternatives will be needed to overcome these constraints. Several reports have suggested using mycorrhizal biofertilizers as efficient inoculums for organic agriculture. Arbuscular mycorrhizal fungi are the major obligate symbiotic fungi for more than 80% of terrestrial plants. Mycorrhizal fungi are responsible for the exchange of nutrients and protect the plant from adverse environmental condition. They also create a symbiotic association with root fungi called mycorrhizal fungi, which enhances the adaptation of both of associated partners. These interactions of plants with fungi in the soil can

95

be used as a bioferlitilizer or phosphate uptake biofertilizer, and they increase the efficiency of the absorption of other essential nutrients from soil to plant (Marshner and Dell, 1994).

During the last decade, germplasm collection of mycorrhizal fungal species/isolate based on pot culture has been shown not to be fit for preservation and multiplication due to the high risk of contaminants. The isolation and multiplication of mycorrhizal fungi in pot culture has limited use as potential biofertilizers. A major weakness of pot culture lies in the contamination of pure culture, which is difficult to maintain in longer culture conditions. Additionally, mass multiplication of mycorrhizal cultures in greenhouses needs a sophisticated growth chamber and longer storage time. The pot culture required for mass multiplication of field-collected mycorrhizal spores has an increased chance of cross contamination between strains/culture. Thus, continuous monitoring and characterization is needed. However, the recent emergence of *in vitro* culture and the increased number of mycorrhizal species grown under root organ culture offer enormous possibilities for mycorrhizal fungi entering into a new era of quality management, mostly for germplasm collection and biofertilizer production (Declerck et al., 2005). *In vitro* cultivation of arbuscular mycorrhizal (AM) fungi has the capacity to provide high-quality, contaminant-free AMF inoculums for research into potential sources of biofertilizers. Therefore, an adequate supply of AM fungal strains and fungal DNA is required for continuous quality control. Several reports suggest multiplication of mycorrhizal fungi in pot culture used for taxonomic, molecular, and biochemical study may be more prone to error because of the cross contamination between pot cultures. Identification and description of AM fungal spores are mainly collected from field soil and pot culture, and these spores change with age due to the effect of different environmental stresses. During last decades, the improvement of technologies related to the cultivation of excised roots allowed the successful cultivation of some AM fungal strains under *in vitro* condition. These improved methods led to an increase in the number of AM species/isolates have been made available in root organ culture. In depth and specific characterization of mycorrhizal fungi for organic farming continues to rely on the successful cultivation of a maximum number of mycorrhizal species/strains grown under root organ culture. During the last decade, germplasm collection of AM fungal species/isolates in pot culture has not been fit for preservation and multiplication due to the high risk of contaminants. Declerck et al. (2000) suggest that the increasing number of mycorrhizal species grown under root organ culture with longer maintenance time using subculturing tools can mean greater demand in industrial biofertilizer production and can also be one of the powerful tools of mycorrhizal research. Two germplasm banks have been established for the propagation, characterization, and maintenance of AM germplasm in living cultures: the International Culture Collection of (Vesicular) Arbuscular Mycorrhizal Fungi (INVAM, http:/invam.caf.wvu.edu/) in the United States and the International Bank of Glomeromycota (BEG, http:/www.kent.ac.uk/bio/beg) in Europe. In addition, the Centre for Mycorrhiza Culture Collection (CMCC, http:/ ycorrhizae.org.in/index.php) has been established by TERI in New Delhi, India, for conservation and multiplication of AM fungal strains collected from terrestrial ecosystem. A literature survey analysis revealed that there are more than 21 mycorrhizal fungi grown under root organ culture and are suggested as an efficient system for biofertilizer

TABLE 5.1
List of AMF Species Reported in Root Organ Culture

S. Number	AMF Species	References
1	*Rhizophagus intraradices*	Chabot et al. (1992); Karandashov et al. (1999)
2	*Funneliformis mosseae*	Dalpé, unpublished data
3	*Rhizophagus proliferus*	Declerck et al. (2000)
4	*Rhizophagus versiforme*	Diop et al. (1994)
5	*Rhizophagus fasciculatus*	Declerck et al. (1998)
6	*Claroideoglomus eutincatum*	Schreiner and Koide (1993); Pawlowska et al. (1999)
7	*Glomu sclarum*	de Souza and Barbara (1999)
8	*Claroideoglomus caledonium*	Karandashov et al. (1999)
9	*Glomus macrocarpum*	Declerck et al. (1998)
10	*Glomus cerebriforme*	Samson et al. (2000)
11	*Glomus constrictum*	Mathur and Vyas (1995)
12	*Claroideoglomus lamellosum*	Y. Dalpé, unpublished data
13	*Glomus fistulosum*	Nuutila et al. (1995); Gryndler et al. (1998)
14	*Glomus cerebriforme*	Samson et al. (2000)
15	*Glomus deserticola*	Mathur and Vyas (1995)
16	*Gigaspora margarita*	Miller-Wideman and Watrud (1984); Karandashov et al. (1999)
17	*Gigaspora gigantea*	Gadkar et al. (1997)
18	*Gigaspora rosea*	Forbes et al. (1998)
19	*Acaulospora rehmii*	Dalpé and Declerck (2002)
20	*Scutellospora reticula*	de Souza and Declerck (2003)
21	*Scutellospora calospora*	Kandula et. al. (2006)

Source: Modified from Declerck, S. et al., The monoxenic culture of arbuscular mycorrhizal fungi as a tool for germplasm collections. *In Vitro Culture of Mycorrhizas*, Declerck, S., Strullu, D. G., and Fortin, A. (Eds.), Springer Verlag, pp. 17–29, 2005; and Fortin, J. A. et al., *Canadian Journal of Botany*, 80, 1–20, 2002.

production (Table 5.1). Many mycorrhizal species/strains have been grown under root organ culture but are not identified correctly; however, they are used as efficient and reliable sources of mycorrhizal strain for long-term culturing as well as biofertilizer production (Declerck et al., 1996; Strullu et al., 1997; Declerck et al., 1998).

PREPARATION OF TRANSFORMED ROOT ORGAN CULTURES OF *DAUCUS CAROTA* AND COLONIZATION WITH SPORES

Trap culture, hydroponics, and aeroponics culture are soil-less methods for the production of clean mycorrhizal spores. Root organ culture allows successful large-scale cultivation of mycorrhizal spores that can be used as a direct inoculum for soil

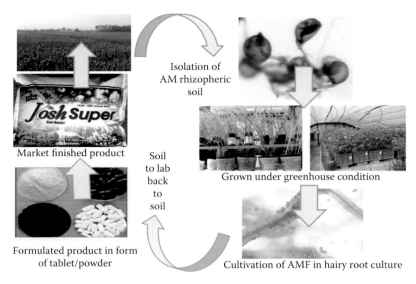

FIGURE 5.1   Mycorrhizal technology-based biofertilizers from root organ-based culture.

application, as shown in Figure 5.1. These cultivation methods can provide an efficient technology for large-scale production (IJdo et al. 2011). It is well known that mycorrhiza are obligate symbiosis fungi, and therefore the excised root required as host partner of AM symbiosis was first suggested by Mosse and Hepper (1975). Isolation of healthy AM spores from pot culture using the wet sieving method is described by Gerdemann and Nicolson (1963). Fresh, healthy mycorrhizal spores can be isolated from approximately 100 g of rhizospheric soil from trap culture kept in 1–2 L plastic beakers. After repeated decantation of soil suspension with sieving, lower-gravity mycorrhizal spores can be separated from the soil. Globular to subglobular 50–500 μm diameter spores can be recognized in sieving under a Sterio microscope. The soil is suspended in about 500 mL to 1 L of tap water, and the soil macro-aggregate is crushed by hand. After 10–30 seconds of settling down of the soil particles, the upper layer of soil suspension is passed through different sieves 300BSS, 100BSS, and 60BSS. This procedure is repeated until the upper layer of soil suspension is transparent. AM fungal spores are collected on 100 BSS and used for inoculation on minimal (M) media plate. Some smaller spores are also collected on 300BSS. However larger spores such as *Gigaspora margarita* can be obtained on 60 BSS fractions. AM spores must be surface-sterilized by mixing with Chloramine-T with Tween 20 (0.1% v/v) for 10 minutes. Moreover, spores can be washed with different antibiotic solutions and then rinsed several times with Mili Q water. The surface-sterilized mycorrhizal spores can transfer aseptically on Ri-T-DNA transformed carrot hairy root and maintained routinely on minimal medium (M) called white medium (Becard and Fortin, 1988) or MSR medium (Strullu and Romand, 1986). Every 15 weeks, media containing spores and root can be clonally subcultured into two compartment petri plates (St-Arnaud et al., 1996). The two compartments, containing sucrose-deficient minimal media, allow the spores to proliferate in the absence of roots (Doner and

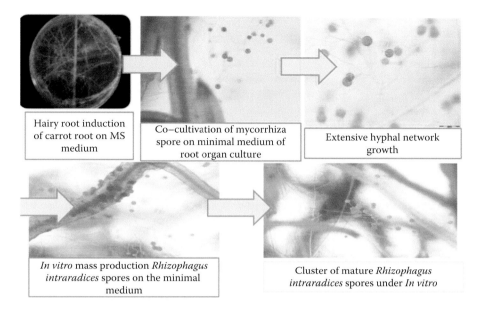

Hairy root induction of carrot root on MS medium

Co–cultivation of mycorrhiza spore on minimal medium of root organ culture

Extensive hyphal network growth

In vitro mass production *Rhizophagus intraradices* spores on the minimal medium

Cluster of mature *Rhizophagus intraradices* spores under *In vitro*

FIGURE 5.2 Different patterns of development of *Rhizophagus intraradices* (Mycorrhizal fungi) cultivate in dual culture of *Ri-T DNA* transformed carrot.

Bécard, 1991). Initiation and propagation of isolated roots required pregermination of sterile seed on solid and liquid media. After clonally subcultured roots are inoculated with soil living bacteria *Agrobacterium rhizogenes*. Infection of excised roots (hairy root) with *A. rhizogenes* (soil-borne bacterium with Ri plasmid) have the potential to proliferate on growing media (Becard and Fortin, 1988). Roots with a cluster of 10–50 mycorrhizal spores from one compartment of old root cultures were cut and transferred to the new receiver-operating characteristic (ROC) medium plates with fresh roots, as shown in Figure 5.2. Three months after continuous subculture, the media plate can be incubated at 26°C, and the new sporulation is visible in the ROC medium plates, as shown in Figure 5.2. Spores from ROC plate are cut out with a sterile scalpel and transferred to a 15 mL Falcon tube that is filled with 15 mL citrate buffer; then the spores are incubated for 60 minutes at 37°C with horizontal shaking at 250 U/min. Spores can be left at room temperature for 10 minutes to allow sediment to collect at the bottom of tube. The supernatant is then discarded, and the spores can be washed with autoclaved Mili Q water and then filtered with sieve (300 and 100 BSS). After 5 minutes, the spores can be collected from sieve and placed in a fresh tube and then be washed again with Mili Q water. Collected spores can be stored at −20°C for small-scale nursery application.

NEW INSIGHT OF ROOT ORGAN CULTURE

AM fungal isolates propagated in pot culture have been used routinely for inoculum production. However, the identification and description of AM fungal spores are done mainly with spores collected from field soil and pot culture, and differences are evident because of different environmental stresses. Improvements in the technologies related to the cultivation of excised roots allowed the successful cultivation of some AM fungal strains, leading to an increase in the number of AM species/isolates that have been made available in root organ culture. Holistic investigation on mycorrhizal species for systematic and biodiversity studies depend on the flourishing cultivation of a maximum number of mycorrhizal species grown under root organ culture. Several reports describe root organ culture as an efficient system for multiple type characterization and biofertilizer production (Table 5.1). Simon et al. (1992) found that biochemical and molecular characterization of AM fungi is more precise and accurate for fungi grown under *in vitro* condition compared with AM fungi grown in pot culture. Therefore, *in vitro* culture is an efficient and reliable artificial system; it is a suitable method for investigating basic and practical aspects of AM symbiosis and complements experimental approaches. Growth of extraradical mycelium under root organ culture has led mainly to the production of arbuscule-like structures (ALSs) (Bago et al., 1998), unique and clear visualization of plant infection process (Elmeskaoui et al., 1995), sporulation dynamics (Declerck et al., 1996), hyphal morphology (Bago et al., 1998), and spore ontogeny (de Souza and Barbara, 1999). Monoexenic culture of AM fungi provides substantial quantity of contamination-free fungal material that is suitable for taxonomic and evolutionary studies (Fortin et al., 2002). Recent development of root organ cultures and the availability of successive generations of contamination-free spores could strengthen molecular, biochemical, and microscopy studies in AM fungi. For example, Rhody et al. (2003) and Ferrol et al. (2000) described monophyly of AM fungi grown in pot culture using three β-Tublin and five H^+-ATP genes, respectively. In contrast, Corradi et al. (2004) reported monophyly studies of AM fungi grown in root organ culture using two β-tublin and one H^+-ATP genes and suggested that the presence of additional forms of β-tublin and H^+-ATP genes most likely originated from contaminants.

It is also known that the availability of contamination-free fungal material in successive generations of particular AM fungi grown under *in vitro* conditions is not only suitable for molecular analysis but also for biochemical and morphological analysis. Bentivenga and Morton (1994) investigated fatty acid profiles in successive generations of AM fungal isolates colonized with different hosts and suggested that fatty acids profile can be considered stable potential taxonomic characters rather than spore-based identification. Most reports mislead detection and identification of AM fungi from spores and colonized root used as starting sample for molecular analysis (Sanders et al., 1996; Redecker et al., 1997). Clapp et al. (2001) observed more intraspecific variation in the LSU region than in the SSU of ribosomal DNA of *Glomus intraradices* grown in *in vitro* conditions, which earlier investigations based on pot culture had not confirmed. They also found all sequences obtained using SSU rDNA clustered with known *Rhizophagus intraradices*. No sequences fell outside the *Glomeraceae* of *Glomus* group A (Schüßler et al., 2001). In a subsequent study by Schüßler et al. (2003), the researchers observed that DNA originating from pot culture contained a high risk of contaminated sequences and thus led to misidentification of mycorrhizal fungi using phylogenetic analysis. It was further observed by Declerck et al. (2000) and Koch et al. (2004) that AM fungi monoexenic culture was indisputably beneficial for the long-term maintenance of controlled, contamination-free medium, which revealed a more complete picture of comparative study originating from molecular, morphological, and biochemical data sets.

CONSTRAINTS RELATED TO MYCORRHIZAL INOCULUMS: PRODUCTION AND APPLICATION

AMF are obligate symbionts, and few species of AMF able to multiply in *in vitro* condition, away from their host plants. Therefore, the method has been executed for only a few AM fungal species (Berruti et al., 2016). This limited feature creates challenges for the large-scale production of AMF. There are mainly three types of mycorrhizal incocula. The first is field-collected AM spores, which are found in low numbers, parasitized with microbes and fungi, lack suitable information for taxonomic characters, and hinder a more accurate identification used as inoculums. Crude inoculum can be used for inoculation of known strains of AMF with specific host called trap culture. Trap cultures are helpful for inducing sporulation of specific mycorrhizal community that are undetected in initial extraction of spores from field soil (Morton et al., 1995). Therefore, trapping is necessary to obtain contamination-free, healthy mycorrhizal spores that can be used as inoculum for the establishment of monosporal culture. Bever et al. (1996) and Koske et al. (1997) observed that trap cultures tended to encourage preferential sporulation of some species when different when create selection pressure. However, when mycorrhizal species/isolates originated from trap culture are not correctly identified, it is very difficult to calculate infectivity potential to check the efficiency of inoculated biofertilizers. This is because trap cultures have the potential risk of contamination from unwanted weed or pathogen, as suggested by Berruti et al. (2016). Inert material used during trap culture can be optimized for mycorrhizal spores multiplication and finally can serve as a source of inoculum. Both approaches for inoculant production using direct field sampling and multiplication in trap culture are tedious and time consuming, and require skilled taxonomists for correct separation of pure mycorrhizal spore (Kumar and Chaurasia, 2016). In addition, collection and identification of AM fungal spores from trap culture also prejudice knowledge of other fungal species present in a soil sample. Morton (1993) reported that collection of AM spores by the sieving and decanting methods led to differences in (1) washing protocol to remove spores on or in roots, (2) sizes of sieve openings can be required for capture of spores, and (3) centrifugation protocol.

ROOT ORGAN CULTURE AS AN EXCELLENT SOURCE OF SECONDARY METABOLITE PRODUCTION

Recent application of root organ culture is not limited to biofertilizer application; it can also play an important role for mass scaling of secondary metabolites. Plant secondary metabolites are molecules known to take part in the adaptation of plants in adverse environments and are also important sources of valuable biological product

TABLE 5.2
List of AMF Species Identified as a Potential Source of Secondary Metabolite Production

Plant Name	Family	Secondary Metabolites	Types of Mycorrhiza Association	References
Hordeum vulgare	Poaceae	Isoprenoid cyclohexenone derivatives	*Rhizophagus intraradices*	Fester et al. (1999)
Triticum aestivum	Poaceae	Isoprenoid cyclohexenone derivatives	*Rhizophagus intraradices*	Fester et al. (1999)
Castanospermum australe	Fabaceae	Alkaloid castanospermine	*Rhizophagus intraradices*	Abu-Zeyad et al. (1999)
Mentha arvensis	Lamiaceae	Essentail oil	*Rhizophagus fasiculatus*	Gupta et al. (2002)
Coriandrum sativum	Apiaceae	Essential oil	*Rhizophagus macrocarpum* and *Rhizophagus fasciculatus*	Kapoor et al. (2002)
Ocimum basilicm	Lamiaceae	Essential oil	*Gigaspora rosea*	Copetta et al. (2006)
Origanum spp.	Lamiaceae	Essential oil	*Funneliformis mosseae*	Khaosaad et al. (2006)
Artemisia annua	Asteraceae	Terpenoids complex	*Glomus macrocarpum* and *R. fascic fasciculatus*	Kapoor et al. (2007)
Inula ensifolia	Asteraceae	Thymol derivative	*Rhizophagus clarus*	Zubek et al. (2010)
Arnica montana	Asteraceae	Phenolic acids	*Rhizophagus intoradices*	Jurkiewicz et al. (2010)
Mentha viridis	Lamiaceae	Essential oil	*Claroideoglomus etunicatum*	Karagiannidis et al. (2012)
Santolina chamaecyparissus	Asteraceae	Essential oil	*Claroideoglomus lamellosum*	Karagiannidis et al. (2012)
Curcuma longa	Zingiberaceae	Flavonoids, phenolic contents	*Glomus, Gigaspora* and *Acaulospora* sp.	Dutta and Neog (2016)
Brassica juncea	Brassicaceae	Phenol, flavonoids	*Funneliformis mosseae, R. fasciculatus,* and *G. macrocarpum*	Sarwat et al. (2016)

with high medicinal property. Several studies have suggested roles and applications of mycorrhiza for secondary metabolite production, as shown in Table 5.2. Moreover, different efficient and reliable protocol for *in vitro* production of bioferftilizers using root organ culture have been widely studied; however, very few methods of large-scale cultivation of secondary metabolites under hairy root organ culture have led to commercial success. Therefore, T-DNA transformed root is extremely differentiated and can produce a wide range of stable secondary metabolites; however, secondary metabolites generated from conventional plant cell cultures are not genetically and biochemically stable. Because of this instability, secondary metabolite production from conventional cell culture methods is very low. Bennett (1984) suggested that secondary metabolites play an important role in regulating crucial defense mechanisms by creating antifeedent and antitoxicity activity during stress conditions. Mycorrhizal association increases absorption of nutrients like P, C, and N and also indirectly produce bioactive compounds (Toussaint, 2008; Pedone-Bonfim et al., 2015). An investigation by Mandal et al. (2013) in sweet leaf concluded that jasmonic acid and polysaccharides are more plentiful in mycorrhizal plants than in nonmycorrhizal plants. Chen et al. (2016) investigated the role of elicitor for activation of photosynthesis and energy metabolism. They identified a G protein–regulated signal transduction pathway toward secondary metabolism production, as shown in Figure 5.3. Many reports suggest that the plant is a reservoir of massive multiplication for the biosynthesis of secondary metabolites and also increases accumulation inside cell or tissue when it interacts with symbiotic fungi (Zhi-lin et al., 2007). The production and effectiveness of secondary metabolites containing high medicinal property were tested by Zubek et al. (2015) in a pot culture experiment consisting of *Viola tricolor* L. (heartsease, wild pansy) as a host plant associated with mycorrhizal fungi. They concluded that there was no significant difference of secondary metabolites production when *Viola tricolor* was inoculated with *Funneliformis mosseae*;

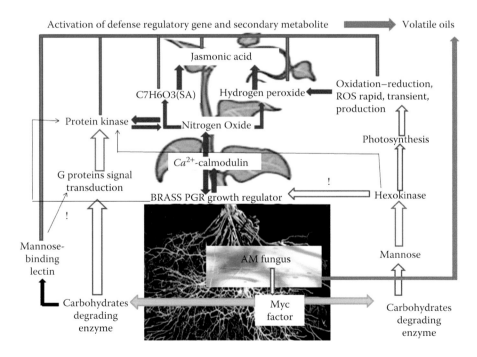

FIGURE 5.3 A mechanistic model of secondary metabolite production activated by elicitor originated from symbiotic fungi. (Modified from Chen, F. et al., *Scientific Reports*, 6, 34735, 2016.)

however, higher metabolite production was observed when the same plant was colonized with *Rhizophagus irregularis*. Bona et al. (2017) noted increased concentration of citric acid in a tomato plant grown under field condition when associated with AM fungi. Copetta et al. (2006) studied the accumulation of essential oil in shoot and root biomass of *Ocimum basilicum L. var. Genovese* when colonized by three AM fungi, *Funelliformis mosseae* BEG 12, *Gigaspora margarita* BEG 34, and *Gigasporarosea* BEG 9. *Arnica montana* is a very rare medicinal plant that produces phenolic acid in roots. Jurkiewicz et al. (2010) clearly showed enhanced concentration of phenolic acids in shoots and sesquiterpene in roots and shoots of *Arnica montana* colonized with *Rhizophagus intraradices*. Abu-Zeyad et al. (1999) studied positive the correlation between AM fungal infection and the castanospermine content of seeds of field-grown trees. Castanospermine is an alkaloid with high medicinal value because it inhibits the AIDS virus. Mycorrhizal colonization significantly enhances root colonization, plant height, dry matter, and oil content in a plant compared with a noncolonized plant (Gupta et al., 2002). Azadirachtin is an important active bioactive ingredient and medicinal property extracted from kernel of neem seeds. Venkateswarlu et al. (2008) reported significantly more concentration of azadirachtin in the kernel of the neem seed when the nursery seedling was colonized by *Rhizophagus fasciculatus* and *Funneliformis mosseae*; it resulted in increased plant height, dry weight, root colonization, and phosphorus content. Mycorrhizal inoculations represent an efficient and sustainable approach for improving plant productivity and also enhancing the biosynthesis of secondary metabolites (phenolic content) in artichoke leaves and flower heads, which was further confirmed by Ceccarelli et al. (2010). A report by Kapoor et al. (2016) suggested that the increased uptake of phosphorus in mycorrhizal plants has been largely attributed to the enhancement of terpenoid production, and Srivastava et al. (2016) observed that the transformed root of *Ocimum basilicum* can be used as factory of secondary metabolite (Rosmarinic acid) when colonized with *Rhizophagus irregularis*.

CONCLUSION

Symbiosis interactions of plants with fungi enhance production and accumulation of several secondary metabolites like terpenoids, alkaloids, and phenols that have high medicinal value. Studies suggest that mycorrhizal fungi enhance plant growth and development, stimulate plant resistance, reduce absorption of heavy metals, and promote plant sustainability under metal stress; they can also be used as biotic elicitors for secondary metabolite production in plants. Moreover, cultivation of mycorrhizal fungi under *in vitro* conditions may provide high-quality, contamination-free AMF inoculums having several industrial applications.

ACKNOWLEDGMENTS

The author is grateful to the honorable chancellor, Mr. Ashok Mital, of Lovely Professional University, India, for providing the lab infrastructure of Mycorrhiza. This research was supported by funds provided by Lovely Professional University, India.

REFERENCES

Abu-Zeyad, R., A. G. Khan, and C. Khoo. 1999. Occurrence of arbuscular mycorrhiza in Castanospermumaustrale A. Cunn. and C. Fraser and effects on growth and production of castanospermine. *Mycorrhiza* 9:111–117.

Bago, B., et al. 1998. Branched absorbing structures (BAS): A feature of the extraradical mycelium of symbiotic arbuscular mycorrhizal fungi. *New Phytologist* 139:375–388.

Becard, G., and J. A. Fortin. 1988. Early events of vesicular-arbuscular mycorrhizal formation on Ri T-DNA trans-formed roots. *New Phytologist* 108:211–221.

Bécard, G., et al. 1991. Identification and quantification of trehalose in vesicular arbuscular mycorrhizal fungi by in vivo 13C NMR and HPLC analyses. *New Phytologist* 118(4):547–552.

Bentivenga, S. P., and J. B. Morton. 1994. Stability and heredity of fatty acid methyl ester profile in *Glomalean* endomycorrhizal fungi. *Mycological Research* 98:1419–1426.

Berruti, A., E. Lumini, R. Balestrini, and V. Bianciotto. 2016. Arbuscular mycorrhizal fungi as natural biofertilizers: Let's benefit from past successes. *Frontiers in Microbiology* 6:1559.

Bever, J. D., et al. 1996. Host-dependent sporulation and species diversity of arbuscular mycorrhizal fungi in a mown grassland. *Journal of Ecology* 84(1):71–82.

Bona, E., et al. 2017. Arbuscular mycorrhizal fungi and plant growth-promoting pseudomonads improve yield, quality and nutritional value of tomato: A field study. *Mycorrhiza* 27(1):1–11.

Ceccarelli, N., et al. 2010. Mycorrhizal colonization impacts on phenolic content and antioxidant properties of artichoke leaves and flower heads two years after field transplant. *Plant and Soil* 335(1–2):311–323.

Chabot, S., G. Bécard, and Y. Piché. 1992. Life cycle of *Glomus intraradices* in root organ culture. *Mycologia* 84(3):315–321.

Chen, F., C.-G. Ren, T. Zhou, Y.-J. Wei, and C.-C. Dai. 2016. A novel exopolysaccharide elicitor from endophytic fungus Gilmaniella sp. AL12 on volatile oils accumulation in Atractylodes lancea. *Scientific Reports* 6:34735.

Clapp, J. P., A. Rodriguez, and J. C. Dodd. 2001. Inter-and intra-isolate rRNA large subunit variation in *Glomus coronatum* spores. *New Phytologist* 149(3):539–554.

Copetta, A., G. Lingua, and G. Berta. 2006. Effects of three AM fungi on growth, distribution of glandular hairs, and essential oil production in *Ocimum basilicum* L. var. Genovese. *Mycorrhiza* 16 (7):485–494.

Corradi, N., G. Kuhn, and I. R. Sanders. 2004. Monophyly of β-tubulin and H⁺-ATPase gene variants in *Glomusintraradices*: Consequences for molecular evolutionary studies of AM fungal genes. *Fungal Genetics and Biology* 41:262–273.

Dalpé, Y., and S. Declerck. 2002. Development of *Acaulospora rehmii* spore and hyphal swellings under root-organ culture. *Mycologia* 94:850–855.

de Souza, F. A., and R. L. L. Barbara. 1999. Ontogeny of *Glomus clarum* in Ri T-DNA transformed roots. *Mycologia* 91(2):343–350.

de Souza, F. A. and S. Declerck. 2003. Mycelium development and architecture, and spore production of *Scutellospora reticulata* in monoxenic culture with Ri T-DNA transformed carrot roots. *Mycologia* 95:1004–1012.

Declerck, S., S. Cranenbrouck, Y. Dalpé, S. Séguin, A. Grandmougin-Ferjani, et al. 2000. *Glomus proliferum* sp. nov: A description based on morphological, biochemical, molecular and monoxenic cultivation data. *Mycologia* 92:1178–1187.

Declerck, S., S. Séguin, and Y. Dalpé. 2005. The monoxenic culture of arbuscular mycorrhizal fungi as a tool for germplasm collections. *In Vitro Culture of Mycorrhizas*. Declerck, S., Strullu, D. G., and Fortin, A. (Eds.), SpringerVerlag, pp. 17–29.

Declerck, S., D. Strullu, and C. Plenchette. 1996. *In vitro* mass- production of the arbuscular mycorrhizal fungus, *Glomus versiforme*, associated with *Ri T*-DNA transformed carrot roots. *Mycological Research* 10:1237–1242.

Declerck, S., D. G. Strullu, and C. Plenchette. 1998. Monoxenic culture of the intraradical forms of Glomus sp. isolated from a tropical ecosystem: A proposed methodology for germplasm collection. *Mycologia* 90(4):579–585.

Diop, T. A., C. Plenchette, and D. G. Strullu. 1994. Dual axenic culture of sheared-root inocula of vesicular-arbuscular mycorrhizal fungi associated with tomato roots. *Mycorrhiza* 5:17–22.

Doner, L. W., and G. Bécard. 1991. Solubilization of gellan gels by chelation of cations. *Biotechnol Techniques* 5:25–28.

Dutta, S. C., and B. Neog. 2016. Accumulation of secondary metabolites in response to antioxidant activity of turmeric rhizomes co-inoculated with native arbuscular mycorrhizal fungi and plant growth promoting rhizobacteria. *Scientia Horticulturae* 204:179–184.

Elmeskaoui, A., J. P. Damont, M. J. Poulin, Y. Piché, and Y. Desjardins. 1995. A tripartite culture system for endomycorrhizal inoculation of micro propagated strawberry plantlets *in vitro*. *Mycorrhiza* 5:313–319.

Ferrol, N., J. M. Barea, and C. Azcón-Aguilar. 2000. The plasma membrane H$^+$-ATPase gene family in the arbuscular mycorrhizal fungus *Glomus mosseae*. *Current Genetics* 37(2):112–118.

Fester, T., W. Maier, and D. Strack. 1999. Accumulation of secondary compounds in barley and wheat roots in response to inoculation with an arbuscular mycorrhizal fungus and co-inoculation with rhizosphere bacteria. *Mycorrhiza* 8(5):241–246.

Forbes, P. J., S. Millam, J. E. Hooker, and L. A. Harrier. 1998. Transformation of the arbuscular mycorrhiza *Gigasporarosea* by particle bombardment. *Mycological Research* 102:497–501.

Fortin, J. A., G. Bécard, S. Declerck, Y. Dalpé, M. St-Arnaud, et al. 2002. Arbuscular mycoorhiza on root-organ cultures. *Canadian Journal of Botany* 80:1–20.

Gadkar, V., A. Adholeya, and T. Satyanarayana. 1997. Randomly amplified polymorphic DNA using the M13 core sequence of the vesicular-arbuscular mycorrhizal fungi *Gigaspora margarita* and *Gigaspora gigantea*. *Canadian Journal of Microbiology* 43:795–798.

Gerdemann, J. W., and T. Hs Nicolson. 1963. Spores of mycorrhizal Endogone species extracted from soil by wet sieving and decanting. *Transactions of the British Mycological Society* 46(2):235–244.

Gryndler, M., H. Hrselova, I. Chvatalova, and M. Vosatka. 1998. *In vitro* proliferation of *Glomus fistulosum* intraradical hyphae from mycorrhizal root segments in maize. *Mycological Research* 102:1067–1073.

Gupta, M. L., et al. 2002. Effect of the vesicular–arbuscular mycorrhizal (VAM) fungus Glomus fasciculatum on the essential oil yield related characters and nutrient acquisition in the crops of different cultivars of menthol mint (Menthaarvensis) under field conditions. *Bioresource Technology* 81(1):77–79.

IJdo, M., S. Cranenbrouck, and S. Declerck. 2011. Methods for large-scale production of AM fungi: Past, present, and future. *Mycorrhiza* 21(1):1–16.

Jurkiewicz, A., et al. 2010. Optimization of culture conditions of Arnica montana L.: Effects of mycorrhizal fungi and competing plants. *Mycorrhiza* 20(5):293–306.

Kapoor, R., V. Chaudhary, and A. K. Bhatnagar. 2007. Effects of arbuscularmycorrhiza and phosphorus application on artemisinin concentration in *Artemisia annua* L. *Mycorrhiza* 17(7):581–587.

Kapoor, R., B. Giri, and K. G. Mukerji. 2002. Mycorrhization of coriander (Coriandrumsativum L) to enhance the concentration and quality of essential oil. *Journal of the Science of Food and Agriculture* 82(4):339–342.

Karagiannidis, N., T. Thomidis, and E. Panou-Filotheou. 2011. Effects of *Glomus lamellosum* on growth, essential oil production and nutrients uptake in selected medicinal plants. *Journal of Agricultural Science* 4(3):137.

Karagiannidis, N., et al. 2012. Response of three mint and two oregano species to *Glomus etunicatum* inoculation. *Australian Journal of Crop Science* 6(1):164.

Karandashov, V. E., I. N. Kuzovkina, E. George, and H. Marschner. 1999. Monoxenic culture of arbuscular mycorrhizal fungi and plant hairy roots. *Russian Journal of Plant Physiology* 46:87–92.

Khaosaad, T., et al. 2006. Arbuscular mycorrhiza alter the concentration of essential oils in oregano (Origanum sp., Lamiaceae). *Mycorrhia* 16(6):443–446.

Koch, A. M., et al. 2004. High genetic variability and low local diversity in a population of arbuscular mycorrhizal fungi. *Proceedings of the National Academy of Sciences of the United States of America* 101(8):2369–2374.

Koske, R. E., J. N. Gemma, and N. Jackson. 1997. A preliminary survey of mycorrhizal fungi in putting greens. *Journal of Turf Grass Science* 73(2):8.

Kowalchuk, G. A., F. A. De Souza, J. A. Van Veen. 2002. Community analysis of arbuscular mycorrhizal fungi associated with *Ammophila arenaria* in Dutch coastal sand dunes. *Molecular Ecology* 11:571–581.

Kumar, S., and P. Chaurasia. 2016. Mycorrhizal diversity: Methods and constraints? *Indian Journal of Science and Technology* 9(37).

Marshner, H., and B. Dell. 1994. Nutrient uptake in Mycorrhizal symbiosis. *Plant and Soil* 59:89–102.

Mathur, N., and A. Vyas. 1995. *In vitro* production of *Glomus deserticola* in association with *Ziziphus nummularia*. *Plant Cell Reports* 14:735–737.

Miller-Wideman, M. A., and L. Watrud. 1984. Sporulation of *Gigaspora margarita* in root culture of tomato. *Canadian Journal of Microbiology* 30:642–646.

Morton, J. B. 1993. Problems and solutions for the integration of glomalean taxonomy, systematic biology, and the study of endomycorrhizal phenomena. *Mycorrhiza* 2:97–109.

Mosse, B., and C. Hepper. 1975. Vesicular-arbuscular mycorrhizal infections in root organ cultures. *Physiological Plant Pathology* 5(3):215–218.

Nuutila, A. M., M. Vestberg, and V. Kauppinen. 1995. Infection of hairy roots of strawberry (*Fragaria×Ananassa* Duch.) with arbuscular mycorrhizal fungus. *Plant Cell Reports* 14:505–509.

Pawlowska, T. E., D. D. Douds, and I. Charvat. 1999. In vitro propagation and life cycle of the arbuscular mycorrhizal fungus *Glomus etunicatum*. *Mycological Research* 103:1549–1556.

Pedone-Bonfim, M. V. L., F. S. B. da Silva, and L. C. Maia. 2015. Production of secondary metabolites by mycorrhizal plants with medicinal or nutritional potential. *Acta Physiologiae Plantarum* 37(2):1–12.

Redecker, D., et al. 1997. Restriction analysis of PCR-amplified internal transcribed spacers of ribosomal DNA as a tool for species identification in different genera of the order Glomales. *Applied and Environmental Microbiology* 63(5):1756–1761.

Rhody, D., et al. 2003. Differential RNA accumulation of two β-tubulin genes in arbuscular mycorrhizal fungi. *Mycorrhiza* 13(3):137–142.

Samson, J., Y. Dalpé, and Y. Piché. 2000. Isolement *in vitro* de deux nouvelles souches de *Glomus*en co-culture avec des racines de carotte transformées. In *Proceedings of ColloqueMycorhizes*, Rivière-du-loup, Que, p. 24.

Sanders, I. R., J. P. Clapp, and A. Wiemken. 1996. The genetic diversity of arbuscular mycorrhizal fungi in natural ecosystems–a key to understanding the ecology and functioning of the mycorrhizal symbiosis. *New Phytologist* 133(1):123–134.

Sarwat, M., et al. 2016. Mitigation of NaCl stress by arbuscular mycorrhizal fungi through the modulation of osmolytes, antioxidants and secondary metabolites in mustard (*Brassica juncea* L.) plants. *Frontiers in Plant Science* 7:2040.

Schreiner, R. P., and R. T. Koide. 1993. Stimulation of vesicular-arbuscular mycorrhizal fungi by mycotrophic and nonmycotrophic plant root systems. *Applied and Environmental Microbiology* 59:2750–2752.

Schüβler, A., D. Schwarzott, and C. Walker. 2001. A new fungal phylum, the Glomeromycota phylogeny and evolution. *Mycological Research* 105:1413–1421.

Schüßler, A., D. Schwarzott, and C. Walker. 2003. Glomeromycota rRNA genes the diversity of myths? *Mycorrhiza* 13:233–236.

Simon, L., M. Lalonde, and T. D. Bruns. 1992. Specific amplification of 18S fungal ribosomal genes from vesicular-arbuscular mycorrhizal fungi colonizing roots. *Applied Environmental Microbiology* 58:291–295.

Srivastava, S., X. A. Conlan, D. M. Cahill, and A. Adholeya. 2016. *Rhizophagus irregularis* as an elicitor of rosmarinic acid and antioxidant production by transformed roots of Ocimum basilicum in an in vitro co-culture system. *Mycorrhiza* 26(8):919–930.

St-Arnaud, M., et al. 1996. Enhanced hyphal growth and spore production of the arbuscular mycorrhizal fungus *Glomus intraradices* in an in vitro system in the absence of host roots. *Mycological Research* 100(3):328–332.

Strullu, D. G., T. Diop, and C. Plenchette. 1997. Constitution of in vitro collections: A proposed life cycle of Glomus. *Comptes Rendus de l'Académiedes Sciences-Series III-Sciences de la Vie* 320:41–47.

Strullu, D. G., and C. Romand. 1986. Méthode d'obtention d'endomycorhizes à vésicules et arbuscules en conditions axéniques. *Comptes rendus de l'Academie des Sciences. Serie III. Sciences de la Vie* 303:245–250.

Venkateswarlu, B., et al. 2008. Mycorrhizal inoculation in neem (*Azadirachta indica*) enhances azadirachtin content in seed kernels. *World Journal of Microbiology and Biotechnology* 24(7):1243–1247.

Zhi-lin, Y., D. Chuan-chao, and C. Lian-qing. 2007. Regulation and accumulation of secondary metabolites in plant-fungus symbiotic system. *African Journal of Biotechnology* 6(11):1266–1271.

Zubek, S., et al. 2010. Arbuscular mycorrhizal fungi alter thymol derivative contents of Inulaensifolia L. *Mycorrhiza* 20(7):497–504.

Zubek, S., et al. 2015. Enhanced concentrations of elements and secondary metabolites in Viola tricolor L. induced by arbuscular mycorrhizal fungi. *Plant and Soil* 390(1–2):129–142.

6 Microbial Fuel Cell
Green Bioenergy Process Technology

Ajay Kumar, Joginder Singh, and Chinnappan Baskar

CONTENTS

INTRODUCTION

Energy crises force people to think about renewable sources of energy for the sustainability of the life on the earth (Painuly, 2001). Until now, our economy is driven by nonrenewable sources of energy such as coal, petrol, and natural gas, but these sources have an adverse effect on the environment and human health (Akella et al., 2009). To overcome this problem, researchers are thinking about alternative sources that are derived from biomasses by exploiting microbes such as bioethanol, biobutanol, biodiesel, biohydrogen, and bioelectricity generated by microbial fuel cells (MFCs) (Churasia et al., 2016; Gottumukkala et al., 2017; Sudhakar et al., 2017; Wenzel et al., 2017). An MFC is a bioreactor that is used to produce sustainable green electricity by oxidation of organic matter like glucose, acetate, lactate, and so on, by the action of bacteria. Two kinds of microbial cells are reported in the literature, namely, single-chamber microbial cell and two-chamber microbial cell (Cheng et al. 2006a). Two-chamber microbial cells are designed containing two compartments, one is an anode chamber, associated with single bacterium or consortium of bacteria, and the other is cathode chamber (Saba et al., 2017). MFCs have the capacity to generate

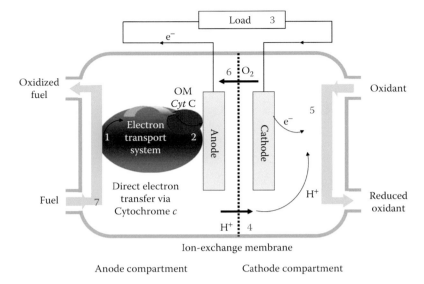

FIGURE 6.1 Diagrammatic representation of two-chamber microbial fuel cell. (From Kim, B.H. et al., *Applied Microbiology and Biotechnology*, 76(3), 485, 2007.)

bioelectricity by using the broad range of organic substrates and biomass (Li et al., 2016; Ma et al., 2016). In a laboratory system model, a proton exchange membrane (PEM) is used to separate both the anode and cathode chambers. The diagram in Figure 6.1 shows a two-chamber microbial fuel cell.

The process of bioelectricity generation by two-chamber MFCs involves the following steps:

1. Oxidation of fuel, such as organic waste and biomass
2. Transfer of electron to electrode as generated by metabolic activity of the microbes
3. Resistance
4. Diffusion of proton
5. Cathodic reaction
6. Diffusion of oxygen governed by Fick's law of diffusion
7. Flow of nonideal fuel

WORKING MECHANISM OF MICROBIAL FUEL CELL

During the operating condition of the microbial fuel cells, a bacterial reaction can be carried out at a temperature range from 15°C to 60°C. Different kinds of biodegradable organic matter such as carbohydrate, protein, volatile acids, and alcohol and recalcitrant compound like cellulose can be in MFCs (Logan et al., 2006). Intermediate can be a cytochrome, flagella, or a mediator (Mathuriya and Yakhmi, 2016). Figure 6.2 shows bioelectricity production by the action of microbes.

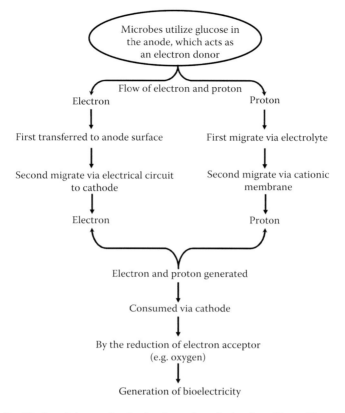

FIGURE 6.2 Bioelectricity production by the action of microbes. (From Chaturvedi, V. and Verma, P., *Bioresources and Bioprocessing*, 3(1), 38, 2016.)

Glucose + 6 Water → 6 Carbon dioxide + 24H$^+$ + 24e (E = 0.014 V)

(Intermediate)$_{ox}$ + e → (Intermediate)$_{rd}$

$6O_2$ + 24H$^+$ + 24e → 12H$_2$O (E = 1.23 V)

FUEL CELL DESIGN

Two-chamber microbial fuel cells are fabricated by a two-chamber designing system in which a polymeric proton exchange membrane is used to separate bacteria in an anode chamber from those in the cathode chamber (Figure 6.3). Aqueous cathodes are used in most of the MFCs, and dissolved oxygen is provided to the electrode by bubbling water with air (Liu and Logan, 2004).

1. *Anode compartment*: The materials that are chemically stable and conductive in reactor solution are generally preferred for the formation of anode. The most favorable metal anode is made up of noncorrosive stainless steel,

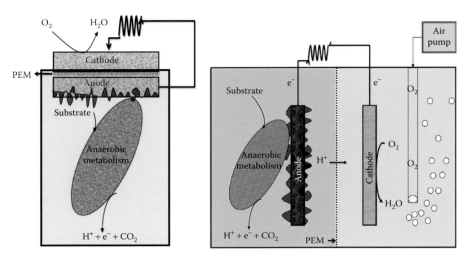

FIGURE 6.3 Schematic representation of single- and dual-chambered MFC. (From Mohan, S.V. et al., *Renewable and Sustainable Energy Reviews*, 40, 779–797, 2014.)

but due to the toxic effect of copper ion, it is not useful for an electrode. For the construction of an electrode, carbon (such as carbon paper, graphite, granular graphite matrix, etc.) is the most versatile material (Cheng et al. 2006b).

2. *Microbial culture*: Numerous microorganisms have the capability to produce the electricity. Many new strains of bacteria have been identified for their versatility and mechanism of current generation in microbial fuel cells (Logan, 2009). Bacteria like *Clostridium butyricum*, *Enterococcus faecium*, and so on, and fungus like *Saccharomyces cerevisiae* were used to operate MFCs. One unique benefit of using photosynthetic bacteria in MFCs is the elimination of carbon dioxide from the atmosphere due to photosynthesis coupled with bioelectricity generation (Rosenbaum et al., 2010). The most commonly employed microorganisms for energy generation in MFCs are listed in Table 6.1. Mixed cultures of microbial population have also been used in MFCs, for example, natural microbial community, domestic wastewater, sediments from oceans and lakes, as well as brewery wastewater (Rabaey et al., 2005; Feng et al., 2008).

3. *Substrates*: A range of organic substrates can be used for anaerobic digestion by microbes in bioelectricity production (Table 6.2).

4. *Redox mediators*: A mediator is a compound with low redox potential that is added to the growth media at a specific concentration and extracts the electrons from the metabolic reactions of the microbes and supplies those electrons to the anode electrode (Sevda and Sreekrishnan, 2012, Figure 6.4). In MFCs, ferricyanide (hexacyanoferrate) is the most commonly used soluble mediator employed for the cathodic reactions. It has comparatively more redox potential and rapid reduction kinetics on the cathode compared to oxygen. Also, in the solution, its concentration is not limited by the solubility as in the case of oxygen.

TABLE 6.1

List of Microorganisms Involved in the Process of Energy Generation in MFC

S. Number	Microorganism	References
1	*Geobacter*	Lovley et al. (1993); Rotaru et al. (2011); Nevin et al. (2008)
2	*Shewanella*	Watson and Logan (2010); Wang et al. (2013)
3	*Anabaena; Nostoc*	Tanaka et al. (1985); Yagishita et al. (1997, 1998)
4	*Clostridium sp.; Pseudomonas luteola; Ochrobactrum pseudogrignonense*	Zhao et al. (2012)
5	*Leptolyngbya sp. JPMTW1*	Maity et al. (2014)
6	*Shewanella oneidensis; Geobacter sulfurreducens*	Gorby (2006)
7	*Escherichia coli*	Nandy et al. (2016); Park et al. (2016)
8	*Escherichia coli; Pseudomonas aeruginosa; Brevundimonas diminuta*	Wang et al. (2017)

TABLE 6.2

Various Substrates Being Employed as Substrate for Generation of Electricity in MFC

S. Number	Substrate	References
1	Domestic wastewater	Choi and Ahn (2013)
2	Swine wastewater	Min et al. (2005)
3	Oil wastewater	Jiang et al. (2013); Choi and Liu (2014)
4	Waste sludge	Ge et al. (2013); Choi and Ahn (2014)
5	Fruit and vegetable wastes	Logroño et al. (2015)
6	Food waste leachate	Choi and Ahn (2015)
7	Glucose, acetate, propionate, and butyrate	Ahn and Logan (2010)
8	Volatile fatty acids	Choi and Ahn (2015)
9	Wastewater sludge	Passos et al. (2016)
10	Milk industry effluent	Pant et al. (2016)

$$\left[\text{Fe(CN)6}\right]^{3-} + e^- \rightarrow \left[\text{Fe(CN)6}\right]^{4-} \ (E'^0 = 0.358 \text{ V})$$

$$O_2 + 4[\text{Fe(CN)6}]^{4-} + 4H^+ \rightarrow [\text{Fe(CN)6}]^{3-} + 2H_2O$$

5. *Cathode compartment*: For the fabrication of the cathode, both conventional carbon-based electrodes as well as novel electrodes are used, including graphite, carbon cloth, carbon paper (CP), carbon nanotube platinum (CNT/Pt)-coated CP, and so on (Mashkour and Rahimnejad, 2015).

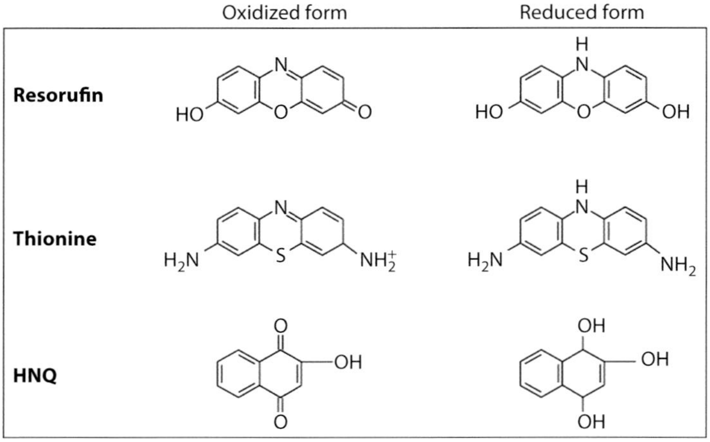

FIGURE 6.4 Redox mediators. (From Drapcho, C.M. et al., *Biofuels Engineering Process Technology*, McGraw-Hill, New York, NY, 2008.)

Ferricyanide ($K_3[Fe(CN)_6]$), oxygen is the most suitable electron acceptor for the MFC and has an impact on the performance of cathode (Rismani-Yazdi et al., 2008).

6. *Exchange membrane*: Teflon and ultrax are used as used as proton exchange membrane because they have the lowest resistance. Liu et al. (2004) reported that they could eliminate the membrane by using pressed carbon paper as the separator.

Diffusion of the oxygen through the membrane is estimated as

$$W = JA = -DA\frac{dC}{dx}$$

where:
   W is the rate of oxygen transfer through the membrane
   D is the binary diffusion coefficient, m^2/s
   dC/dx is the concentration gradient across membrane, mol/cm^3-cm

ELECTRON TRANSFER MECHANISM

For the microbial fuel cell operations, only those microbes with high electron discharge capacity and those that are electrochemically active are considered. Lin et al. (2014) and Mohan et al. (2014) describe the two modes of electron transfer: (1) direct electron transfer (DET), which involves physical contact of bacterial cell membrane, and (2) mediated electron transfer (MET) via redox mediators based on electron carrier involvement (Figure 6.5).

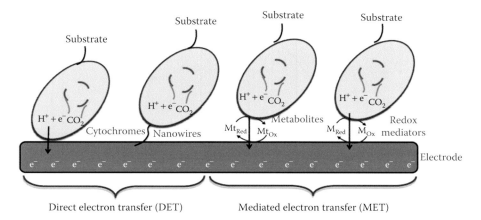

FIGURE 6.5 Electron transfer mechanism from the microbial metabolism to the anode. (From Mohan, S.V. et al., *Renewable and Sustainable Energy Reviews*, 40, 779–797, 2014.)

POWER GENERATION

Using an empirical Monod type equation, voltage was modeled as the function of substrate concentration (Lin et al., 2014)

$$P = P_{max} \frac{S}{K_s} + S$$

where:
P_{max} is the maximum power
K_s is the half saturation constant

Multimeter is used to measure the load in MFC. Voltage measurements are converted to current values using Ohm's law:

$$V = IR$$

where:
V is the voltage (V)
I is the current (A)
R is the resistance

The power output from an MFC is calculated as

$$P = IV$$

where P is the power (W).
Power density is calculated based on anode surface area as follows:

$$PD_A = \frac{IV}{A_A}$$

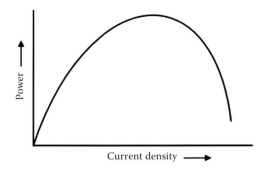

FIGURE 6.6 Typical power–current curve (polarization curve). (From Rismani-Yazdi, H. et al., *Journal of Power Sources*, 180(2), 683–694, 2008.)

where:
   PD_A is the power density based on area (W/m²)
   A_A is the anode surface area (m²)

Internal resistance of the microbial fuel cell is calculated either by the polarization slope method (*V–I* curve) or by the power density peak method (Figure 6.6). The slope of the voltage–current curve represents the internal resistance in the polarization slope method, while the external resistance at which the MFC power output reaches maximum amount is considered as the internal resistance of system (Logan, 2009).

As long as the substrate is supplied, MFCs can produce current (Logan et al., 2006; Rismani-Yazdi et al., 2008). The theoretical ideal voltage, E_{emf} (V), attainable from an MFC can be thermodynamically predicted by the Nernst equation:

$$E_{emf} = E_{emf}^0 - \frac{RT}{nF} \ln(\Pi) \tag{6.1}$$

where:
   $E_{emf}^0(V)$ is the standard cell electromotive force
   R is the ideal gas constant (8.314 Jmol⁻¹ K⁻¹)
   T is the absolute temperature (K)
   n is the number of electrons transferred in the reaction (dimensionless)
   F is the Faraday's constant (96,485 C mol⁻¹)
   Π is the chemical activity of products divided by those of reactants (dimensionless)

The cell emf is calculated as follows:

$$E_{emf} = E_{cat} - E_{an} \tag{6.2}$$

where the minus sign is a result of the definition of the anode potential as a reduction reaction (although an oxidation reaction is occurring).

TABLE 6.3
Maximum Power Density in Various MFCs Using Microbes

Strain	Reactor Type	Fuel Used	Power Density (mW/m^2)	References
Clostridial isolate	Two chamber	Complex Medium	–	Prasad et al. (2006)
P. aeruginosa	Two chamber	Palm oil mill effluent	4140	Islam et al. (2016)
Pseudomonas putida	Single chamber	Acetate	86.1	Khater et al. (2017)
Mesophilic bacteria	Two chamber	Landfill leachate	1513	Sonawane et al. (2017)
Cellulose-degrading bacteria (CDB)	Two chamber	Rice straw	145	Hassan et al. (2014)
Exoelectrogenic bacteria	Single chamber	Phenol	31.3	Song et al. (2014)

Rabaey and Verstraete (2005) reported that by transferring electron from a reduced substrate (at a low potential) to an electron acceptor (at a high potential), bacteria gain energy. The energy gained can be calculated as follows:

$$\Delta G = -nF\Delta E$$

where:
  n is the number of electrons exchanged
  F is Faraday's constant (96485 Coulomb/mol)
  ΔE is the potential difference between electron donor and acceptor

Maximum power densities in various MFCs using pure culture are presented in Table 6.3.

APPLICATIONS OF MICROBIAL FUEL CELLS

BIOELECTRICITY GENERATION

The main feature of an MFC is the utilization of organic carbohydrate substrates from biomass obtained from agricultural, industrial, and municipal wastes for the production of bioelectricity. Another advantage of MFCs is the direct conversion of fuel molecules into electricity without the production of heat (Du et al., 2007). MFC technology can be used as a potential sustainable source of energy. MFC technology can also be applied toward the construction of bio-batteries. The primary and basic design of an MFC can be modified in different ways to provide a base for further construction of new ideas and applications.

WASTEWATER MANAGEMENT

Wastewater effluent from industrial, municipal, and other sources acts as a prime source for energy harvesting. It is also a suitable substrate for bioremediation.

Microbial fuel technology proves to be an ideal solution to wastewater management (Gajda et al., 2016; Parkash, 2016). The three primary parameters on which the efficiency of MFC technology are based are maximum power density, Coulombic efficiencies, and chemical oxygen demand (COD).

DRAWBACKS OF MICROBIAL FUEL CELLS

Several factors influence the performance of the microbial fuel cell (Gil et al., 2003):

1. Fuel oxidation rate
2. Rate of electron transfer to the electrode by the microbes
3. Circuit resistance
4. Proton transfer to the cathode by the membrane
5. Oxygen supply and reduction at the cathode

Various drawbacks of MFCs and possible solutions to enhance the efficiency of MFCs are shown in Figure 6.7.

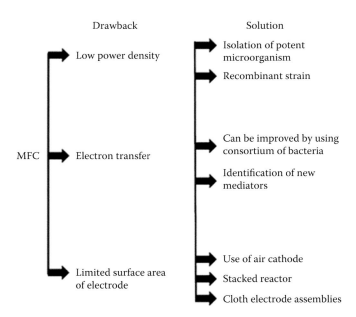

FIGURE 6.7   Drawbacks and possible solutions to enhance the efficiency of MFC. (From Chaturvedi, V. and Verma, P., *Bioresources and Bioprocessing*, 3(1), 38, 2016.)

LIFE CYCLE ASSESSMENT OF MICROBIAL FUEL CELLS

Life cycle assessment (LCA) is a tool to assess the environmental impacts of a product, process, or activity throughout its life cycle: from the extraction of raw materials through processing, transport, use, and disposal. The materials used for the construction of microbial fuel cells have had some negative consequences for the environment. Materials such as carbon, graphite, and platinum used for designing electrodes are being investigated for their impact on the environment, as reported by Foley et al. (2010).

CONCLUSION

Microbial fuel cells have emerged as a sustainable source of energy. They utilize domestic sewage waste for the production of bioelectricity and hence decrease the amount of energy needed for the treatment of sewage waste. With the depletion of nonrenewable sources of energy, scientists and engineers are developing more efficient uses for MFCs to lessen growing pressure on the environment. There is hope for successful implementation of this technology in the future.

REFERENCES

Ahn, Y., and B. E. Logan. 2010. Effectiveness of domestic wastewater treatment using microbial fuel cells at ambient and mesophilic temperatures. *Bioresource Technology* 101(2):469–475.

Akella, A. K., R. P. Saini, and M. P. Sharma. 2009. Social, economical and environmental impacts of renewable energy systems. *Renewable Energy* 34(2):390–396.

Bond, D. R., and D. R. Lovley. 2003. Electricity production by *Geobacter sulfurreducens* attached to electrodes. *Applied and Environmental Microbiology* 69(3):1548–1555.

Chaturvedi, V., and P. Verma. 2016. Microbial fuel cell: A green approach for the utilization of waste for the generation of bioelectricity. *Bioresources and Bioprocessing* 3(1):38.

Chaudhuri, S. K., and D. R. Lovley. 2003. Electricity generation by direct oxidation of glucose in mediatorless microbial fuel cells. *Nature Biotechnology* 21(10):1229–1232.

Cheng, S., H. Liu, and B. E. Logan. 2006. Increased performance of single-chamber microbial fuel cells using an improved cathode structure. *Electrochemistry Communications* 8(3):489–494.

Cheng, S., H. Liu, and B. E. Logan. 2006b. Increased power generation in a continuous flow MFC with advective flow through the porous anode and reduced electrode spacing. *Environmental Science and Technology* 40(7):2426–2432.

Choi, J., and Y. Ahn. 2013. Continuous electricity generation in stacked air cathode microbial fuel cell treating domestic wastewater. *Journal of Environmental Management* 130:146–152.

Choi, J., and Y. Ahn. 2015. Enhanced bioelectricity harvesting in microbial fuel cells treating food waste leachate produced from biohydrogen fermentation. *Bioresource Technology* 183:53–60.

Choi, J., and Y. Liu. 2014. Power generation and oil sands process-affected water treatment in microbial fuel cells. *Bioresource Technology* 169:581–587.

Churasia, A., J. Singh, and A. Kumar. 2016. Production of biodiesel from soybean oil biomass as renewable energy source. *Journal of Environmental Biology* 37(6):

Drapcho, C. M., N. P. Nhuan, and T. H. Walker. 2008. *Biofuels Engineering Process Technology*. New York, NY: McGraw-Hill.

Du, Z., H. Li, and T. Gu. 2007. A state of the art review on microbial fuel cells: A promising technology for wastewater treatment and bioenergy. *Biotechnology Advances* 25(5):464–482.

Feng, Y., X. Wang, B. E. Logan, and H. Lee. 2008. Brewery wastewater treatment using air-cathode microbial fuel cells. *Applied Microbiology and Biotechnology* 78(5):873–880.

Foley, J. M., R. A. Rozendal, C. K. Hertle, P. A. Lant, and K. Rabaey. 2010. Life cycle assessment of high-rate anaerobic treatment, microbial fuel cells, and microbial electrolysis cells. *Environmental Science and Technology* 44(9):3629–3637.

Gajda, I., J. Greenman, C. Melhuish, and I. A. Ieropoulos. 2016. Electricity and disinfectant production from wastewater: Microbial fuel cell as a self-powered electrolyser. *Scientific Reports* 6, 255–271.

Ge, Z., F. Zhang, J. Grimaud, J. Hurst, and Z. He. 2013. Long-term investigation of microbial fuel cells treating primary sludge or digested sludge. *Bioresource Technology* 136:509–514.

Gil, G.-C., I.-S. Chang, B. H. Kim, M. Kim, J.-K. Jang, et al. 2003. Operational parameters affecting the performance of a mediator-less microbial fuel cell. *Biosensors and Bioelectronics* 18(4):327–334.

Gorby, Y. A. 2006. Bacterial nanowires: Electrically conductive filaments and their implications for energy transformation and distribution in natural and engineered systems. In *Bio Micro and Nanosystems Conference, BMN'06*, pp. 20–20. San Francisco, CA: IEEE.

Gorby, Y. A., S. Yanina, J. S. McLean, K. M. Rosso, D. Moyles, et al. 2006. Electrically conductive bacterial nanowires produced by *Shewanella oneidensis* strain MR-1 and other microorganisms. *Proceedings of the National Academy of Sciences* 103(30):11358–11363.

Gottumukkala, L. D., K. Haigh, and J. Görgens. 2017. Trends and advances in conversion of lignocellulosic biomass to biobutanol: Microbes, bioprocesses and industrial viability. *Renewable and Sustainable Energy Reviews* 76:963–973.

Hassan, S. H. A., S. M. F. Gad El-Rab, M. Rahimnejad, M. Ghasemi, J.-H. Joo, et al. 2014. Electricity generation from rice straw using a microbial fuel cell. *International Journal of Hydrogen Energy* 39(17):9490–9496.

Islam, M. A., W. Woon Chee, E. Baranitharan, Y. Abu, K. Cheng Chin, et al. 2016. Evaluation of electricity generation and wastewater treatment from palm oil mill effluent using single and dual chamber microbial fuel cell. 100–106.

Jang, J. K., I. Seop Chang, and B. Hong Kim. 2004. Improvement of cathode reaction of a mediator less microbial fuel cell. *Journal of Microbiology and Biotechnology* 14(2):324–329.

Jang, J. K., Pham, T. H., Chang, I. S., Kang, K. H., Moon, H., Cho, K. S., and Kim, B. H. (2004). Construction and operation of a novel mediator-and membrane-less microbial fuel cell. *Process Biochemistry*, 39(8), 1007–1012.

Jang, J. K., I. Seop Chang, H. Moon, K. Hyun Kang, and B. Hong Kim. 2006. Nitrilotriacetic acid degradation under microbial fuel cell environment. *Biotechnology and Bioengineering* 95(4):772–774.

Jiang, Y., A. C. Ulrich, and Y. Liu. 2013. Coupling bioelectricity generation and oil sands tailings treatment using microbial fuel cells. *Bioresource Technology* 139:349–354.

Khater, D. Z., K. M. El-Khatib, and H. M. Hassan. 2017. Microbial diversity structure in acetate single chamber microbial fuel cell for electricity generation. *Journal of Genetic Engineering and Biotechnology*, 15(1):127–137.

Kim, B. H., I. Seop Chang, and G. M. Gadd. 2007. Challenges in microbial fuel cell development and operation. *Applied Microbiology and Biotechnology* 76(3):485.

Levin, D. B., L. Pitt, and M. Love. 2004. Biohydrogen production: Prospects and limitations to practical application. *International Journal of Hydrogen Energy* 29(2):173–185.

Li, S., C. Cheng, and A. Thomas. 2016. Carbon-based microbial-fuel-cell electrodes: From conductive supports to active catalysts. *Advanced Materials* 29(8): 1602547.

Lin, C.-W., C.-H. Wu, Y.-Hsuan Chiu, and S.-L. Tsai. 2014. Effects of different mediators on electricity generation and microbial structure of a toluene powered microbial fuel cell. *Fuel* 125:30–35.

Liu, H., and B. E. Logan. 2004. Electricity generation using an air-cathode single chamber microbial fuel cell in the presence and absence of a proton exchange membrane. *Environmental Science and Technology* 38(14):4040–4046.

Logan, B. E. 2009. Exoelectrogenic bacteria that power microbial fuel cells. *Nature Reviews Microbiology* 7(5):375–381.

Logan, B. E., B. Hamelers, R. Rozendal, U. Schröder, J. Keller, et al. 2006. Microbial fuel cells: Methodology and technology. *Environmental Science and Technology* 40(17):5181–5192.

Logroño, W., G. Ramírez, C. Recalde, M. Echeverría, and A. Cunachi. 2015. Bioelectricity generation from vegetables and fruits wastes by using single chamber microbial fuel cells with high Andean soils. *Energy Procedia* 75:2009–2014.

Lovley, D. R., S. J. Giovannoni, D. C. White, J. E. Champine, E. J. P. Phillips, et al. 1993. *Geobacter metallireducens* gen. nov. sp. nov., a microorganism capable of coupling the complete oxidation of organic compounds to the reduction of iron and other metals. *Archives of Microbiology* 159(4): 336–344.

Ma, J., H. Ni, D. Su, and X. Meng. 2016. Bioelectricity generation from pig farm wastewater in microbial fuel cell using carbon brush as electrode. *International Journal of Hydrogen Energy* 41(36):16191–16195.

Maity, J. P., C.-P. Hou, D. Majumder, J. Bundschuh, T. R. Kulp, et al. 2014. The production of biofuel and bioelectricity associated with wastewater treatment by green algae. *Energy* 78:94–103.

Mashkour, M., and M. Rahimnejad. 2015. Effect of various carbon-based cathode electrodes on the performance of microbial fuel cell. *Biofuel Research Journal* 2:296–300.

Mathuriya, A. S., and J. V. Yakhmi. 2016. Microbial fuel cells–Applications for generation of electrical power and beyond. *Critical Reviews in Microbiology* 42(1):127–143.

Min, B., J. R. Kim, S. E. Oh, J. M. Regan, and B. E. Logan. 2005. Electricity generation from swine wastewater using microbial fuel cells. *Water Research* 39(20):4961–4968.

Mohan, S. V., G. Velvizhi, J. A. Modestra, and S. Srikanth. 2014. Microbial fuel cell: Critical factors regulating bio-catalyzed electrochemical process and recent advancements. *Renewable and Sustainable Energy Reviews* 40:779–797.

Moon, H., I. S. Chang, and B. H. Kim. 2006. Continuous electricity production from artificial wastewater using a mediator-less microbial fuel cell. *Bioresource Technology* 97(4):621–627.

Moqsud, M. A., K. Omine, N. Yasufuku, M. Hyodo, and Y. Nakata. 2013. Microbial fuel cell (MFC) for bioelectricity generation from organic wastes. *Waste Management* 33(11):2465–2469.

Nandy, A., V. Kumar, and P. P. Kundu. 2016. Effect of electric impulse for improved energy generation in mediatorless dual chamber microbial fuel cell through electroevolution of *Escherichia coli*. *Biosensors and Bioelectronics* 79:796–801.

Nevin, K. P., H. Richter, S. F. Covalla, J. P. Johnson, T. L. Woodard, et al. 2008. Power output and columbic efficiencies from biofilms of *Geobacter sulfurreducens* comparable to mixed community microbial fuel cells. *Environmental Microbiology* 10(10):2505–2514.

Painuly, J. P. 2001. Barriers to renewable energy penetration: A framework for analysis. *Renewable Energy* 24(1):73–89.

Pant, D., G. Van Bogaert, Y. Alvarez-Gallego, L. Diels, and K. Vanbroekhoven. 2016. Evaluation of bioelectrogenic potential of four industrial effluents as substrate for low cost microbial fuel cells operation. *Environmental Engineering and Management Journal (EEMJ)* 51(8):1897–1904.

Park, I. H., P. Kim, and K. S. Nahm. 2016. The influence of active carbon supports toward the electrocatalytic behavior of Fe_3O_4 nanoparticles for the extended energy generation of mediatorless microbial fuel cells. *Applied Biochemistry and Biotechnology* 179(7):1170–1183.

Parkash, A. 2016. Microbial fuel cells: A source of bioenergy. *Journal of Microbal & Biochemical Technology* 8:247–255.

Passos, V. F., S. Aquino Neto, A. R. de Andrade, and V. Reginatto. 2016. Energy generation in a microbial fuel cell using anaerobic sludge from a wastewater treatment plant. *Scientia Agricola* 73(5):424–428.

Prasad, D., T. K. Sivaram, S. Berchmans, and V. Yegnaraman. 2006. Microbial fuel cell constructed with a micro-organism isolated from sugar industry effluent. *Journal of Power Sources* 160(2):991–996.

Rabaey, K., and Verstraete, W. (2005). Microbial fuel cells: novel biotechnology for energy generation. *TRENDS in Biotechnology*, 23(6), 291–298.

Rhoads, A., H. Beyenal, and Z. Lewandowski. 2005. Microbial fuel cell using anaerobic respiration as an anodic reaction and biomineralized manganese as a cathodic reactant. *Environmental Science and Technology* 39(12):4666–4671.

Rismani-Yazdi, H., S. M. Carver, A. D. Christy, and O. H. Tuovinen. 2008. Cathodic limitations in microbial fuel cells: An overview. *Journal of Power Sources* 180(2): 683–694.

Rosenbaum, M., Z. He, and L. T. Angenent. 2010. Light energy to bioelectricity: Photosynthetic microbial fuel cells. *Current Opinion in Biotechnology* 21(3):259–264.

Rosenbaum, M., F. Zhao, U. Schröder, and F. Scholz. 2006. Interfacing electrocatalysis and biocatalysis with tungsten carbide: A high-performance, noble-metal-free microbial fuel cell. *Angewandte Chemie International Edition* 45(40):6658–6661.

Rotaru, D. E. H., A. E. Franks, R. Orellana, C. Risso, and K. P. Nevin. 2011. *Geobacter*: The microbe electric's physiology, ecology, and practical applications. *Advances in Microbial Physiology* 59(1):1–101.

Saba, B., A. D. Christy, Z. Yu, A. C. Co, R. Islam, et al. 2017. Characterization and performance of anodic mixed culture biofilms in submersed microbial fuel cells. *Bioelectrochemistry* 113:79–84.

Sangeetha, T., and M. Muthukumar. 2013. Influence of electrode material and electrode distance on bioelectricity production from sago-processing wastewater using microbial fuel cell. *Environmental Progress and Sustainable Energy* 32(2):390–395.

Sevda, S., and T. R. Sreekrishnan. 2012. Effect of salt concentration and mediators in salt bridge microbial fuel cell for electricity generation from synthetic wastewater. *Journal of Environmental Science and Health, Part A* 47(6):878–886.

Sharma, Y., and B. Li. 2010. The variation of power generation with organic substrates in single-chamber microbial fuel cells (SCMFCs). *Bioresource Technology* 101(6):1844–1850.

Sonawane, J. M., S. B. Adeloju, and P. C. Ghosh. 2017. Landfill leachate: A promising substrate for microbial fuel cells. *International Journal of Hydrogen Energy* 42(37):23794–23798.

Song, T.-S., X.-Y. Wu, and C. C. Zhou. 2014. Effect of different acclimation methods on the performance of microbial fuel cells using phenol as substrate. *Bioprocess and Biosystems Engineering* 37(2):133–138.

Sudhakar, M. P., A. Jegatheesan, C. Poonam, K. Perumal, and K. Arunkumar. 2017. Biosaccharification and ethanol production from spent seaweed biomass using marine bacteria and yeast. *Renewable Energy* 105:133–139.

Tanaka, K., R. Tamamushi, and T. Ogawa. 1985. Bioelectrochemical fuel-cells operated by the cyanobacterium, *Anabaena variabilis. Journal of Chemical Technology and Biotechnology* 35(3):191–197.

Tharali, A. D., N. Sain, and W. Jabez Osborne. 2016. Microbial fuel cells in bioelectricity production. *Frontiers in Life Science* 9(4):252–266.

Tommasi, T., G. Paolo Salvador, and M. Quaglio. 2016. New insights in microbial fuel cells: Novel solid phase anolyte. *Scientific Reports* 6:1–7.

Wang, G., L. Wei, C. Cao, M. Su, and J. Shen. 2017. Novel resolution-contrast method employed for investigating electron transfer mechanism of the mixed bacteria microbial fuel cell. *International Journal of Hydrogen Energy* 42(16):11614–11621.

Wang, H., F. Qian, G. Wang, Y. Jiao, Z. He, et al. 2013. Self-biased solar-microbial device for sustainable hydrogen generation. *ACS Nano* 7(10):8728–8735.

Watson, V. J., and B. E. Logan. 2010. Power production in MFCs inoculated with *Shewanella oneidensis* MR-1 or mixed cultures. *Biotechnology and Bioengineering* 105(3):489–498.

Wei, J., P. Liang, X. Cao, and X. Huang. 2011. Use of inexpensive semicoke and activated carbon as biocathode in microbial fuel cells. *Bioresource Technology* 102(22):10431–10435.

Wei, L., H. Han, and J. Shen. 2012. Effects of cathodic electron acceptors and potassium ferricyanide concentrations on the performance of microbial fuel cell. *International Journal of Hydrogen Energy* 37(17):12980–12986.

Wenzel, J., L. Fuentes, A. Cabezas, and C. Etchebehere. 2017. Microbial fuel cell coupled to biohydrogen reactor: A feasible technology to increase energy yield from cheese whey. *Bioprocess and Biosystems Engineering* 40(6):807–819.

Yagishita, T., S. Sawayama, K.-I. Tsukahara, and T. Ogi. 1997. Behavior of glucose degradation in *Synechocystis* sp. M-203 in bioelectrochemical fuel cells. *Bioelectrochemistry and Bioenergetics* 43(1):177–180.

Yagishita, T., S. Sawayama, K.-I. Tsukahara, and T. Ogi. 1998. Performance of photosynthetic electrochemical cells using immobilized *Anabaena variabilis* M-3 in discharge/culture cycles. *Journal of Fermentation and Bioengineering* 85(5):546–549.

Zhang, Y., G. Mo, X. Li, W. Zhang, J. Zhang, et al. 2011. A graphene modified anode to improve the performance of microbial fuel cells. *Journal of Power Sources* 196(13):5402–5407.

Zhao, G., F. Ma, L. Wei, H. Chua, C.-C. Chang, et al. 2012. Electricity generation from cattle dung using microbial fuel cell technology during anaerobic acidogenesis and the development of microbial populations. *Waste Management* 32(9):1651–1658.

Zhou, M., M. Chi, J. Luo, H. He, and T. Jin. 2011. An overview of electrode materials in microbial fuel cells. *Journal of Power Sources* 196(10):4427–4435.

7 Expanding Avenues for Probiotic Yeast *Saccharomyces boulardii*

Santosh Anand, Kumar Siddharth Singh, and Dipesh Aggarwal

CONTENTS

INTRODUCTION

The beneficial effects of edible microbes were known long before the term "probiotics" was even coined. Many of the probiotics were being used unknowingly as part of traditional food and fermented food products. Probiotics are live microbes that, when administered in sufficient quantities, confer a health benefit to the host.

To date, many probiotics have been isolated from fermented food products and dairy products. Many of these beneficial probiotics were later identified to be normal inhabitants of a healthy gut and consequently isolated from human, swine, and other animal sources (Reid et al., 2003). Early research into probiotics has advanced from mere isolation to the formulation of more than 200 different fermented products. Consequently, clinical antidotes against particular gastrointestinal disorders were determined for probiotics and prebiotic matrices. Later, different mechanisms of action of probiotics were determined using a combination of biophysical and advanced molecular techniques.

Initial work on probiotics was limited to its health benefits, and probiotics were thought to promote general well-being. Multiple-drug-resistant (MDR) strains are emerging very fast and are outrunning the rate of discovery of new antibiotics. This has led to a search for alternative therapies that pose fewer side effects than antibiotics and pose no risks. Probiotics are becoming an increasingly popular choice as an alternative therapy, and their use has changed from prophylactic to therapeutic management of many gastrointestinal disorders such as irritable bowel syndrome, diarrhea, liver disease, and even obesity (Ringel et al., 2012). They are also used to augment the reestablishment of normal gut microbiota after an antibiotic treatment.

The discovery of probiotics has also expanded to other sources such as fruits, cereals and even spices. Today, there are an enormous number of identified probiotics and fermented products, but the exact efficacy and dosage level is not properly defined. Because of strain-to-strain differences and strain-host specificity, the use of only a few probiotics in clinical practice has been adopted (Ringel et al., 2012). Despite these limitations, extraordinary strides have been made in probiotics research, and many reports are very promising. The number of known probiotics has now become enormous, and they consist of bacteria of different phyla and yeast.

Much literature on bacterial probiotics is already available, but the same amount of study on yeasts is largely missing. Historically, yeasts have been an important part of food products. The name "yeast" arises from the foam produced during beer fermentation and the carbon dioxide produced for the leavening of bread dough. Apart from its most frequent use in food items, it has also been used to antagonize pathogenic bacteria by employing different mechanisms. It has also been used as biocontrol agents for preventing spoilage of raw and processed food products and agricultural produce (Hatoum et al., 2012). Many yeasts like *Torulaspora delbrueckii*, *Kluyveromyces lactis*, *K. lodderae*, *K. marxianus*, and *Yarrowia lipolytica* have been found to have probiotic properties such as tolerance to harsh gastrointestinal conditions and other probiotic attributes (Vandenplas et al., 2009). But most studies have focused on *Saccharomyces boulardii* and its efficacy in the management of many gastrointestinal disorders. *Saccharomyces boulardii* is the most popular and widely studied probiotic yeast. It plays a role in the management of different types of diarrhea and gastrointestinal complications, has an expanding range of applications in treating conditions such as inflammatory bowel disease (IBD), candidiasis, and blastocystosis. First discovered in 1923 by Henri Boulard from the skins of lychee (a Southeast Asian fruit), research on *S. boulardii* progressed into estimation of its biotherapeutic properties (Sazawal et al., 2006). With emerging evidence for its high efficacy in the prevention of gastrointestinal disorders, the research gained rapid momentum into its isolation from various food matrices. This probiotic acts through various mechanisms and is thus effective against both acute and chronic gastrointestinal disorders. This chapter describes the clinical efficacy of *S. boulardii*, including its mechanism of action, novel avenues in food, and future directions.

CLASSIFICATION OF *SACCHAROMYCES BOULARDII* AND GENOMIC FEATURES

The classification of yeasts is based traditionally on their ecological origin, growth characteristics, substrate utilization, product production, and modes of sexual reproduction. Thus, the identity of strains has a high degree of ambiguity, and subtle differences exist between members of the same group. But with the advent of modern molecular biology techniques, even little differences can be identified; thus, molecular taxonomy has contributed a lot to the correct classification of traditionally used yeasts. *Saccharomyces boulardii* was initially classified as a different species of yeast due to its distinct physiological properties and phenotypic differences with *Saccharomyces cerevisiae* (baker's yeast). Some of these differences are growth optimum at higher temperature (37°C), tolerance to low pH, phenotypic differences (asporogenous), copy number differences in subtelomeric genes, nutrient utilization (no galactose uptake), loss of certain genomic identifiers (Ty1/2 elements), different microsatellite markers, and an inability to mate with many *S. cerevisiae* strains (McFarland et al., 1994; Mitterdorfer et al., 2002). Extraordinary advances in modern molecular taxonomy have been made since the discovery of this yeast. Evidence from genomic and proteomic comparisons have identified this yeast as a member of the *S. cerevisiae* family, and it now has been conclusively identified as a probiotic strain of *S. cerevisiae* correctly referred to as *Saccharomyces cerevisiae var. boulardii* (Edwards-Ingram et al., 2007).

Clustered regularly interspaced palindromic repeat (CRISPR) is a novel approach to manipulating genes into bacterial hosts very precisely. This technique holds enormous potential and has recently been applied to manipulate fungal hosts too (Krappmann et al., 2017). The power to manipulate the yeast genome efficiently is significant because most bacterial hosts lag behind in the proper post-translational modifications required for expressing eukaryotic proteins. *S. boulardii* has myriad types of health benefits, and it has been found to reside longer in the gut compared to *S. cerevisiae*. Thus, this yeast holds great potential in producing novel biomolecules directly in the gut; however, it does not have reliable auxotrophic strains for its controlled genetic manipulation. Being CRISPR-compliant, *S. boulardii* is a very attractive focus for study, and many auxotrophic strains have been developed (Liu et al., 2016).

S. BOULARDII IN GASTROINTESTINAL DISORDERS

Saccharomyces boulardii has been found to be very effective in the treatment of different types of diarrhea. Diarrhea is defined as having three or more liquid stools in a day, or such defecation is more frequent than usual for a particular person (WHO, 2013). Traveler's diarrhea is an acute diarrheal condition affecting about 40 million people worldwide annually; it is caused by various pathogenic microbes such as *Escherichia coli, Campylobacter, Shigella, Aeromonas, Salmonella*, and *Plesiomonas*. Although, symptomatic treatments like mainstream antibiotics form the main line of therapy, they leave the patient devoid of useful commensals. *S. boulardii* has been reported to be highly effective against traveler's diarrhea both alone and in combinations with other probiotics such as *Lactobacillus acidophilus* and *Bifidobacterium bifidum*. Also, it confers antagonistic pressure against pathogenic microbes using various mechanisms, and it aids in the proper development of an evolving gut microbiota in the host (Kelesidis et al., 2012).

Antibiotic-associated diarrhea (AAD) is another condition that is becoming more frequent because of the steep rise in the use of antibiotics, more frequent hospitalizations, and deteriorating health of many people worldwide. AAD leads to loss of normal gut microbiota, and it disturbs the general dynamics of the gut. Absence of gut commensals just after an antibiotic treatment course leads to removal of protective biological cover (McFarland, 2014). Undigested food fibers are metabolized by gut commensals into host-beneficial products such as vitamins, biotin, and secondary metabolites. In the absence of these commensals, these undigested food fibers accumulate in the intestine and oversensitize the gut. Also, trigger diarrheal symptoms commonly called as AAD (Young et al., 2004). *S. boulardii* has been found to be very helpful in managing AAD and establishment of normal gut microbiota (McFarland, 2014). Many researchers have proposed that the use of alternative therapy such as probiotics is urgently required for management of gastrointestinal infections and would help in reducing the rate of emergence of MDR microbes.

Also, the intestinal dysbiosis that is caused by various infections, gastrointestinal disorders, and the use of harsh antibiotics leads to the disappearance of useful gut microbes. These gut microbes are required for production of valuable metabolites such as short chain fatty acids (SCFAs), secondary metabolites, and vitamins and for electrolyte balance. They also provide protection against opportunistic pathogens and help in maintenance of the normal mucus layer. The reestablishment of the normal gut microbiome after such disturbed conditions has been found to be very effectively managed by *S. boulardii* (More et al., 2015). Next we discuss in detail some of the specific effects of *S. boulardii* in different clinical conditions.

EFFECT ON *HELICOBACTER PYLORI*

Helicobacter pylori (*H. pylori*) is a highly prevalent, gram-negative, spiral-shaped pathogen associated with chronic gastritis and peptic ulcer, and it is a risk factor for gastric malignancies. The rate of *H. pylori* infection in the population of industrialized countries is estimated to be at 20%–50%. In developing countries, the rate is as high as 80%, most probably due to unhygienic habits and the uncontrolled use of antibiotics, especially in childhood (Ruggiero, 2014). It is considered to be the major causative agent of chronic gastritis and duodenal ulcer; it also leads to the development of gastric cancer and mucosa-associated lymphoid tissue (MALT) lymphoma (Muhan et al., 2016). The most prescribed therapy, consisting of three approaches—a proton-pump inhibitor, clarithromycin, and amoxicillin/nitroimidazole—has been used for decades for *H. pylori* eradication (Malfertheiner et al., 2007). However, eradication rates have continued to decline, and failure rates currently exceed 20% in several countries due to development of antibiotic-resistant strains (Vitor and Vale, 2011). Probiotics as an adjunctive therapy has evolved into important gut-modulating agents that can exert antagonistic effects against *H. pylori* both *in vitro* and *in vivo* (Gotteland et al., 2006). This mode of preventive therapy is desirable because most probiotics do not have side effects and have complimentary benefits in terms of maintaining normal gut health.

In a meta-analysis for efficacy of *S. boulardii* supplementation in the management of *H. pylori* infection, the addition of *S. boulardii* significantly increased the eradication rate, but it still fell short of the desired level of success. However, *S. boulardii* significantly decreased the side effects of the standard triple therapy, which led to better patient compliance (Szajewska et al., 2005). Recently, in a randomized double-blind, placebo-controlled clinical trial, 28 asymptomatic primary school children with positive *H. pylori* stool antigen (HpSA) were given lyophilized *S. boulardii*–containing capsules; the control group received placebo capsules containing lactose and wheat starch powder. The children were followed weekly and were reinvestigated by HpSA testing four to eight weeks after the said treatment. On comparison with 24 children, mean HpSA titer reduced from 0.40 ± 0.32 to 0.21 ± 0.27 in the study group; no such difference was reported in the control group. The study showed a positive effect of *S. boulardii* on the reduction of *H. pylori* in the human gastrointestinal system, but it was incapable of its eradication when used as single-line therapy (Namkin et al., 2016).

EFFECT ON *CLOSTRIDIUM DIFFICILE*

Clostridium difficile is a gram-positive anaerobic bacterium and the major causative agent of colitis and diarrhea. *C. difficile* infection is mediated by two potent exotoxins, toxin A and toxin B (Pothoulakis and Lamont, 2001). *C. difficile*–associated disease (CDAD) is one of the most common nosocomial infections worldwide. The beneficial effects of *S. boulardii* in CDAD have been studied using both *in vitro* and *in vivo* models (Sezer et al., 2009; Karen et al., 2010). Vancomycin and metronidazole form the standard line of therapy used to tackle *C. difficile* infection. *S. boulardii* in combination with antibiotic therapy has been found effective for treating *C. difficile* diarrhea and colitis (Surawicz et al., 2000; McFarland, 2010). In a randomized, placebo-controlled trial of 124 patients suffering from *C. difficile* infection, *S. boulardii* at a dose of 500 mg/day was given with or without antibiotics (Mcfarland et al., 1994). Results revealed a significant reduction in reoccurrence of infection in those treated with *S. boulardii* (34.6% compared to 64.7% for the placebo).

Kabbani et al. (2017) examined the effects of the probiotic *S. boulardii* CNCM I-745 strain in combination with the antibiotics amoxicillin and clavulanate on the microbiota and gut conditions of healthy humans. Stool samples and questionnaires on gastrointestinal symptoms were taken from subjects. The changes in microbiota composition of stool specimens were analyzed using 16s rRNA gene pyrosequencing. Antibiotic treatment was found to be associated with marked microbiota changes and alteration in the presence of different genera. *S. boulardii* CNCM I-745 treatment mitigated antibiotic-induced dysbiosis and reduced antibiotic-associated diarrhea. Another strain of *S. boulardii* was also found to prevent *C. difficile* outbreak associated with cecal inflammation in hamsters (Koon et al., 2016). In a recent systematic review and meta-analysis by Lau and Chamberlain (2016), 26 randomized controlled trials (RCTs) involving 7,957 patients were analyzed. Use of this probiotic significantly reduced the risk of developing CDAD by 60.5% (relative risk (RR) = 0.395; 95% confidence interval (CI), 0.29–0.53; $p < 0.001$). Probiotics proved beneficial in both adults and children (59.5% and 65.9% reduction, respectively), especially among hospitalized patients. *Lactobacillus*, *Saccharomyces* and mixture of other probiotics were found to be beneficial in lowering the risks of developing CDAD symptoms (63.7%, 58.5%, and 58.2% reduction).

EFFECT ON DIARRHEA-CAUSING PATHOGENS

Pathogenic varieties of *E. coli* such as enterotoxigenic *E. coli* (ETEC), enterohemorrhagic *E. coli* (EHEC), and enteropathogenic *E. coli* (EPEC) and other pathogens such as *Vibrio cholerae* are prime causative agents of diarrhea. ETEC, EPEC, and *Vibrio cholerae* are known to cause secretory diarrhea, while EHEC secreting Shiga toxin is associated with hemorrhagic diarrhea, colitis, and hemolytic uremic syndrome (bloody diarrhea) at severe stages (Nataro and Kaper, 1998). *S. boulardii* was found to inhibit the effect of *V. cholerae* toxin and secretions (Czerucka et al., 1994). *S. boulardii* inhibits signaling pathways activated by bacterial invasion and mitigates secretion of IL-8 in response to *V. cholerae* infection in cells (Buts et al., 2006). It was also found to improve gut barrier function and inhibit the pro-inflammatory cytokine profile in EHEC-infected T84 cells (Dalmasso et al., 2006a). This yeast was also found to decrease bacterial translocation toward mesenteric lymph nodes and bring improvement in the pro-inflammatory cytokine profile in ETEC-infected porcine intestinal cells. Rotavirus, a genus of double-stranded RNA virus in the family Reoviridae, is the leading cause of diarrheal diseases mainly among small children. Rotavirus infects mature enterocytes induced via an oxidative stress-dependent mechanism (Buccigrossi et al., 2014). *S. boulardii* was found to prevent chloride ion secretion inhibition of reactive oxygen species formation and to reestablish the balance of the GSH/GSSH redox system (Stier and Bischoff, 2016).

EFFECT ON FUNGAL INFECTIONS

Candida infection includes adhesion, morphogenesis, and biofilm formation and the secretion of proteases, phospholipases, and endotoxins. *S. boulardii* was found to have antagonistic effects against *Candida* infection. Immunologically, *S. boulardii* hinders production of pro-inflammatory cytokines (interferon-γ, IL-1β, TNF-α) and stimulates anti-inflammatory cytokines IL-4 and IL-10 (Fidan et al., 2009). Earlier, it has been shown that both live *S. boulardii* cells and their culture extract containing metabolites like phenylethanol, caproic, caprylic, and capric acid weaken adhesion, and inhibit succeeding hyphae and biofilm formation (Krasowska et al., 2009). Administration of *S. boulardii* was found to decrease the colonization and severity of DSS-induced clinical scores and histological inflammation in a BALB/c mouse model of colitis. *S. boulardii* exhibited antagonistic effects through down-regulation of TNF-α and TLR2 and upregulation of TLR4. TNF-α reduction due to *S. boulardii* is mediated via TLR2, which is involved in yeast recognition (Jawhara and Poulain, 2007). In an *in vitro* experiment, Murzyn et al. (2010) observed that both *S. boulardii* and its extract significantly inhibited *C. albicans* adhesion to Caco-2 and intestine 407 epithelial cell lines. The pro-inflammatory cytokine IL-8 gene expression by *C. albicans* infected Caco-2 cells was suppressed by the addition of extract. In a meta-analysis of randomized controlled trials, Hu et al. (2016) found that *S. boulardii* was effective in reducing the risk of Candida colonization in preterm neonates and in preventing invasive fungal sepsis in preterm neonates.

EFFICACY OF *S. BOULARDII* IN ANTIBIOTIC-ASSOCIATED DIARRHEA

Antibiotic-associated diarrhea (AAD) refers to inflammation of the intestine and the passing of loose, watery stools; it results from an imbalance in the colonic microbiota caused by antibiotic therapy (Guarino et al., 2008). Today, bacterial preparations containing probiotic lactic acid bacteria and yeast is given for AAD, which may help in maintaining homeostasis of the gut microbiome, enhancing immune responses, and lowering colonic pH to favor the growth of nonpathogenic bacteria. As a formulation, *S. boulardii* has been used for long time, and it has an excellent safety profile for many people. Earlier, Kotowska et al. (2005) found a decrease in the frequency of AAD in *S. boulardii* (500 mg/day) supplemented group (3.4%, $p < 0.05$), compared to 17.3% in the placebo group, in enrolled 269 children taking antibiotics treatment. Similarly, the effectiveness of *S. boulardii* was assessed in a meta-analysis of RCTs in adults and children, and involved 1,076 subjects. The yeast was well tolerated, and a significant protective effect of *S. boulardii* was found (pooled RR = 0.43, 95% confidence incidence 0.23–0.78) (Szajewska et al., 2005). Although many meta-analysis results and evidence suggest that *S. boulardii* may reduce the comparative risk of AAD by approximately 60% (McFarland, 2006; Szajewska et al., 2006), the quality of the data is still weak. Recently, in a randomized, double-masked, placebo-controlled trial, 2,444 patients were screened. Analyses included data from 246 patients aged 60 years and 231 patients aged 56.5 years, randomized to the placebo group and *S. boulardii* group, respectively, with 19 and 21 AADs in the respective groups ($p = 0.87$). The hazard ratio of AAD in the *S. boulardii* group compared with the placebo group was 1.02 (95% confidence interval, 0.55–1.90; $p = 0.94$). Nine serious adverse events were recorded in the *S. boulardii* group, and three serious adverse events were recorded in the placebo group. No evidence for *S. boulardii* effect was found in preventing AAD in a population of hospitalized patients (Ehrhardt et al., 2016).

EFFICACY OF *S. BOULARDII* IN ACUTE DIARRHEA

Acute diarrhea is a known cause of morbidity and mortality worldwide. Probiotics such as *S. boulardii*, as complementary therapies, seem to be capable therapeutic agents. Acute diarrhea is a result of infections in the gastrointestinal tract due to bacteria, viruses, or protozoa; malabsorption disorders; systemic infections; nutritional deficiency; allergies; and intolerances to food substances or drugs (Guandalini, 2000). A number of randomized, placebo-controlled studies showed the efficacy of *S. boulardii* in the prevention of acute diarrhea (Riaz et al., 2012). In October 2011, the World Gastroenterology Organization (WGO) published its evidence-based recommendations about probiotics like *S. boulardii*, *L. reuteri* ATCC 55730, *L. rhamnosus* GG, and *L. casei* DN-114 001 in the treatment of acute diarrhea; they are useful in reducing the severity and duration of diarrhea by 24 hours (Guarner et al., 2008). Also, Dinleyici et al. (2012), in their systematic review and meta-analysis, found that *S. boulardii* can significantly reduce the duration of diarrhea by approximately 24 hours and that of hospitalization by approximately 20 hours, with strong evidence that this probiotic has a clinically significant benefit. Recently, Das et al. (2016) conducted a double-blind, RCT to study the efficacy and safety of *S. boulardii* in acute childhood rotavirus diarrhea. The trial included children age 3 months to 5 years with acute watery diarrhea and rotavirus positive ($n = 60$) with intervention ($n = 30$, receiving *S. boulardii* 500 mg/day for 5 days), and control ($n = 30$) groups. Diarrhea duration was significantly decreased in the intervention group (60 vs. 89; 95% CI: -41.2 to -16.8).

MECHANISMS OF ACTION OF *SACCHAROMYCES BOULARDII*

Probiotics may confer their beneficial effects on the host by employing a myriad of mechanisms. The mode of action may be luminal/trophic, such as adhesion-mediated competitive exclusion, secretion of antimicrobial agents, strengthening gut barrier functions, and disrupting the quorum-sensing and signaling of pathogens. It might also be using immunological routes such as potentiation of the host immune system and modulation of the level of cytokines in the host to regulate the host-pathogen interactions (Antoine, 2010). Adhesion to gut mucosa is considered to be an important factor for high probiotic potential in a strain. Probiotics having high gut adhesion potential can compete for binding sites and are effective prophylactic measures for preventing pathogen colonization. Some innovative studies using whole probiotics and surface adhesion proteins of probiotics to inhibit pathogen adhesion have also been done. These techniques reduce pathogen load and have a high potential as an alternative to microbial interference therapy (Asahara et al., 2010; Yadav et al., 2013).

Immunomodulation of the host by probiotics also involves defensive training for foreign invasion to the host. This results in suppression of pro-inflammatory and upregulation of anti-inflammatory cytokines and thus heightens the host's immune response in the event of any infection. Probiotics secrete many agents that upregulate the expression of tight junction proteins in the epithelial cell lining. They also lead to overproduction of mucin proteins and thus a thickened mucus layer, which in turn leads to a robust gut barrier and effective pathogen evasion. Probiotics might secrete small molecules, organic acids, and so on, that act as antimicrobial agents and minimize the microbial load. Quorum-sensing cross-talk is important for the pathogenic profile and morphogenesis of certain pathogens. Probiotics' secretions have been found to interfere with this type of cell signaling, ultimately resulting in infection control. The beneficial effects of probiotics may not depend necessarily on their high gut residence time. This has been observed specifically in some probiotics such as *Lactobacillus casei* and *S. boulardii*, which colonize the gut only transiently and modulate the behavior of normal gut inhabitants while in the gut (Zanello et al., 2009). *S. boulardii* acts via different mechanisms and has been found to deploy few or all adaptations to act effectively.

INTERFERENCE WITH PATHOGEN ADHESION

Pathogens inside the gut lumen deploy various invasive adaptations to colonize the host. Adhesion is usually the first step in this process, and strategies disrupting this step can effectively prevent infection. Probiotics have been found to decrease pathogen adhesion in many studies. Although the exact mechanisms are not known, many probiotic surface adhesion proteins have been implicated. These surface adhesion proteins are thought to compete with pathogens for the adhesion sites present on the gut. Few studies have specifically shown the involvement of these surface adhesion proteins in minimizing the pathogen adhesion (Provencio et al., 2009).

Similarly, the probiotic yeast *S. boulardii*, when used as live whole cells or even as a culture extract, has been found to inhibit colonization and biofilm formation of *Candida albicans* (Krasowska et al., 2009). The high efficacy of culture extract in this case suggests that the surface proteins and/or carbohydrates or secreted proteins are involved in exclusion of the pathogen. In another study, the cell wall and whole cell fraction of *S. boulardii* have also been found to inhibit pathogen (*Clostridium difficile*) adhesion to intestinal cell lines. This decrease was found to be dose dependent and was caused by the presence of a serine protease in *S. boulardii* preparations (Tasteyre et al., 2002). Another study reported that pathogenic bacteria (*S. typhimurium* and *E. coli* O157) adhere to the *S. boulardii* surface and are effectively excluded from binding to the gut mucosa (Martins et al., 2013). This is possible due to unique characteristics of *S. boulardii*, such as having a mannose-rich surface that is capable of binding bacteria as decoys for host mucosa (Tiago et al., 2012). This exclusion of pathogen from the gut results in less opportunity for manifestation of a pathogenic profile and disturbance of normal cytokine profile in the host. Out of all these observations, one must remember that *S. boulardii* remains in the gut only temporarily; thus, the sole contribution of steric hindrance in its exclusion of pathogens is less likely, and the effects are mostly due to its secreted factors.

GUT BARRIER FUNCTION

Mammalian gut has a single-cell epithelial lining with basolateral polarity covered by a special mucus layer, which is a two-layered gel made up of glycoproteins and carbohydrate components. The mucus layer forms the first line of defense acting as a physical barrier to foreign microbes. It has a tightly packed inner layer impervious to most microbes and a loosely packed outer layer that acts as the site for binding of most microbes. The outer layer is continuously removed by peristalsis taking away the microbial load from the gut. The gut barrier consists of this mucus layer, which harbors secretory IgA and host-secreted antimicrobial peptides. It also includes many connecting proteins that seal the epithelial cells together to form complexes recognized as tight junctions, desmosomes, and adherens junctions and regulate intestinal permeability (Stier et al., 2016).

Due to its gel-like nature, the mucus layer is a dynamic entity; it allows the exchange of small molecules, nutrients, water, electrolytes, and signaling molecules between the intestinal lumen, microbes, and the host. This allows the pathogens to show their pathogenic profile, and some of the pathogens (*Helicobacter pylori*) are even able to breach the gut barrier by penetrating through the inner mucus layer. With an infection in the gut leading to diarrhea, the pathogenic profile mostly manifests as disturbed solute exchange systems and water retention/uptake mechanisms regulated by various transporters like chloride transporters. Some manifest as a weakening of the normal epithelial lining, such as the modulation in the permeability of tight junctions and even physical damage to the cell lining. Some might also lead to defective mucus layer integrity originating from disturbed expression of mucin proteins from the host gut (Namkin et al., 2016).

Probiotics have been found to ameliorate the negative effects in many cases of a gut barrier breach by intestinal pathogens (*H. pylori, C. albicans, S. aureus, P. aeruginosa,* and *E. coli*) and to restore normal gut barrier function. *S. boulardii* has been found to improve intestinal permeability in Crohn's disease patients who have disturbed mucosal integrity (Garcia et al., 2008). This probiotic yeast was also shown to preserve gut barrier function of cultured intestinal cells infected with EPEC. This was observed as an improvement in transepithelial resistance, the distribution profile of tight junction proteins (ZO-1), and the permeability of inulin (Czerucka et al., 2000). During infection, the intestinal permeability can rise abruptly due to caspase-3 mediated apoptosis caused by disturbed calcium influx after pathogenic stimulus. *S. boulardii* has been found to prevent EHEC induced apoptosis in cultured intestinal cells by inhibiting the production and secretion of TNF-α. *S. boulardii* has also been shown to prevent pathogen invasion by inhibiting activation of an ERK1/2 pathway that leads to development of a pathogenic profile. In case of infection by *C. difficile*, it has been observed that *S. boulardii* increases the production of secretory IgA, ultimately strengthening the gut barrier (Ohland and MacNaughton, 2010).

S. boulardii inhibited the activation of NF-κB associated pathways activated by bacterial invasion and phosphorylation of all three MAP kinases (ERK1/2, p38, and JNK), and mitigated secretion of IL-8 in response to infection in cells. It also upregulated the distribution of transmembrane tight junctions (Buts et al., 2006).

S. boulardii has also been associated with strengthening of the epithelial cell lining by reorganization of protein complexes like tight junctions following the $\alpha2\beta1$ integrin signaling pathway. This reorganization is very helpful in mitigating diseases like IBD and other pathogen-associated infectious diseases (Canonici et al., 2011). *S. boulardii* has also been found to activate many enzymes of host brush-border epithelia such as maltase, sucrase, lactase, trehalase, alkaline phosphatase, and aminopeptidases using its cell wall component polyamines—spermine, putrescine, and spermidine (Buts et al., 2010). It also stimulates the host to secrete more IgA and express more immunoglobulin receptors. *S. boulardii* also secretes a leucine aminopeptidase (a zinc-metalloprotease family enzyme) in the intestinal lumen that provides protection from foreign antigens when the intestinal gut barrier is compromised. All these mechanisms play an essential role in action of *S. boulardii* for maintenance of host gut health.

SMALL MOLECULES

Probiotics exert their host protective effects using many mechanisms. One of the prominent mechanisms is production of certain biochemicals that inhibit growth of pathogenic microbes. These might bring changes in pH using SCFAs (like lactic acid and acetic acid); create nutrient deprivation; produce antimicrobials such as hydrogen peroxide, nitric oxide, and bacteriocins; and induce the secretion of defensins from the host (Vandenplas et al., 2009).

Enteral tube feeding in critically ill human patients has been found to contribute to high incidences of diarrhea and an imbalance in the composition of healthy gut microbiota. One of the many causes for this could be deficiency of luminal SCFAs. SCFAs form the major by-product of anaerobic microbial metabolism in the colon and contribute to electrolyte and water absorption by host mucosa and to the stimulation of growth and differentiation of enterocytes and enteric neurons. *S. boulardii* has been found to decrease the incidence of diarrhea in such patients by up to 83%. This protective effect stems from higher production of total SCFA (butyrate, acetate, and propionate) due to administration of *S. boulardii,* as evident in the stool of such patients (Schneider et al., 2005). A similar type of protective effects due to *S. boulardii* mediated production of SCFAs has also been observed in the case of rat and pig populations.

C. albicans is a systemic fungal pathogen that affects the gastrointestinal tract and is fast becoming drug resistant. The major virulence factor associated with *C. albicans* is its rapid morphogenesis between hyphae, pseudohyphae, and yeast forms, which is important for its adhesion and invasion of host mucosa. Alternative approaches for control of this pathogen include use of *S. boulardii*, which has been shown to inhibit the manifestation of the pathogenic profile of this pathogen. This has been achieved primarily by secretion of capric acid from *S. boulardii*, which inhibits adhesion, filamentous growth, and biofilm formation of *C. albicans*. Capric acid causes activation of cAMP pathways and Hog1 kinase cascade, which reduces virulence-linked genes of *C. albicans*. Metabolites such as capric acid were found to downregulate the gene expression of CSH1, INO1, and HWP1 genes, which encode proteins that are directly linked with surface hydrophobicity and the formation of the receptor components of fungal cell wall, thus facilitating adhesion and biofilm formation (Murzyn et al., 2010).

ANTIMICROBIAL MOLECULES

It has been shown *in vitro* that *S. boulardii* decreases the multiplication of pathogens such as *Shigella*, *C. albicans*, *E. coli*, *S. aureus*, *S. typhimurium*, and *E. histolytica*. *S. boulardii* secreted factors present in its conditioned medium can dramatically modify *C. difficile* receptors and inhibit binding of toxin A to brush-border receptors (Pothoulakis et al., 1993). This was later found to be due to production of a 54 kDa serine protease that lyses the toxin A and its receptor of *C. difficile*. This also increases the immunoglobulin-A levels in response to inactivated toxin A (Im and Pothoulakis, 2012). Another study has shown that this 54 kDa protease regulates secretion of water and electrolytes during *C. difficile* infection but that it has no effect on the underlying cellular damage. This protease also interferes with the binding between the toxin A and toxin B of *C. difficile* to their receptors on the epithelial cell lining. This protease has been found to show similar protective effects during infection by *Shigella* and *E. histolytica*. *S. boulardii* also induces structural changes in *H. pylori* cells with cellular damage (Vandenplas et al., 2009).

S. boulardii produces another protein of size 120 kDa, which is non-enzymatic; it neutralizes cholera toxin-induced cAMP secretions from cultured intestinal cells (Czerucka et al., 1994). This leads to restoration of a healthy gut profile, which is usually tightly regulated for cAMP secretions. During infection by *E. coli* O55B5, it has been found that *S. boulardii* can minimize the toxicity of its surface lipopolysaccharide (LPS) endotoxins by the release of a protein phosphatase (of size 63 kDa) that has a high dephosphorylation activity. This phosphatase targets two sites on the LPS and dephosphorylates it, rendering it inactive (Buts et al., 2006). Culture supernatant fractions (of size 3 kDa) from *S. boulardii* were found to minimize the inflammatory profile of LPS-activated dendritic cell population and inhibit T-cell proliferation (Thomas et al., 2009).

IMMUNOMODULATION

Disease conditions in the gut are clearly manifested as a disturbance of the immune profile in the host mucosa. Apart from weak gut barrier function, this is observed as a striking increase in pro-inflammatory cytokines and a striking decrease in anti-inflammatory cytokines. These symptoms are effectively alleviated by probiotics because they improve the immune profile of the host and interfere with pathogenic signals that stimulate the inflammatory profile. Apart from its trophic effects and protective function, *S. boulardii* also has immunomodulatory properties due to its complex carbohydrate and nucleic acid composition (Vandenplas et al., 2009). This yeast has been found to help in the establishment of normal gut microbiota in different types of diarrhea and even in IBD.

Toxins from pathogenic microbes such as *C. difficile*, EPEC, *Shigella*, and EHEC stimulate the NFκB pathway by activating the ERK 1/2 and p38 kinases. *S. boulardii* was found to inhibit pro-inflammatory TNF-α transcription and associated apoptosis in EHEC-infected T84 cells (Dalmasso et al., 2006b). *S. boulardii* was also able to reduce the degree of protein phosphorylation by EPEC, including Src homology 2 domain containing protein (SHC), an upstream regulatory protein of the MAPK pathway (Czerucka et al., 2000). Badia et al. (2012) observed downregulation in gene expression of pro-inflammatory cytokines TNFα, IL-6, and GM-CSF and of chemokines CCL2, CCL20, and CXCL8 during ETEC infection. This leads to expression of pro-inflammatory cytokines such as interleukin-8 from the host cell and further increase in inflammation. *S. boulardii* produces a small (<1 kDa), water-soluble, and heat-stable factor referred to as *S. boulardii* anti-inflammatory factor (SAIF). This factor was found to protect the host intestinal cells by blocking the activation of NFκB and gene expression of pro-inflammatory cytokine IL8 (Sougioultzis et al., 2006). Metabolites of *S. boulardii* were also found to inhibit toxin A–induced Erk1/2 and JnK/SAPK activation along with mucosal inflammation (Chen et al., 2006).

With pathogenic stimulus in the gut, nitric oxide (NO) is produced from L-arginine by an inducible NO synthase (iNOS). This NO leads to an elevated pro-inflammatory profile showing cytotoxicity, edema, vasodilatation, and triggering of cytokine-mediated inflammation networks. During a study on castor oil–induced diarrhea in rats, *S. boulardii* was found to minimize the diarrheal symptoms, and its protective function was found to be antagonized by L-arginine. It was then speculated that because L-arginine is a natural substrate for NO production, iNOS systems must play a role in this interaction. It was later confirmed that the iNOS was indeed involved, and the protective effect of *S. boulardii* was due to its inhibition of iNOS (Girard et al., 2005).

IBD is a disorder of the gut and has significant contribution from the immunological imbalance in the gut. Apart from usual inflammation mediators such as toll-like receptors, a novel target such as a nuclear receptor—peroxisome proliferator activated receptor gamma (PPAR-γ) has been identified that plays a definitive role in IBD and microbe-induced inflammation. *S. boulardii* was found to block the TNF-α regulated PPAR-γ and IL-8 by interfering with the activation of NF-κB (Lee et al., 2008). This is a novel mechanism by which *S. boulardii* might show its protective effect.

S. boulardii was also found to decrease the pro-inflammatory response in intraepithelial lymphocytes caused by infection by pathogenic *E. coli* and *C. albicans* (Fidan et al., 2009). This would help in better management of such infections and faster recovery of patients. In another study, lymphocytes were transferred to severe combined immunodeficiency (SCID) mice, which were fed daily with *S. boulardii*. It was observed that *S. boulardii* influenced the migration of T-cells toward mesenteric lymph nodes, which prevents further progression of inflammation. This shows *S. boulardii* can be used as an effective therapy in patients suffering from IBD (Dalmasso et al., 2006).

QUORUM SENSING

The maintenance of normal gut microbiota, gut health, and manifestation of the pathogenic profile is the result of interactions between the microbiota, host, and the pathogens. The intercellular signaling by microbes is usually accomplished using small molecules and specific biomolecules called quorum-sensing molecules. *S. boulardii* was observed to interfere with MAP kinases and NF-κB signal transduction pathways that play an important role in *C. difficile* toxin-associated pathogenesis (Na et al., 2005). As mentioned earlier, *C. albicans* pathogenicity and biofilm formation depends primarily on its morphogenesis and quorum sensing. A report has shown the involvement of a common quorum-sensing molecule called "farnesol" in preventing biofilm formation of *C. albicans* (Ramage et al., 2002).

The cross talk between *Citrobacter rodentium* (pathogen) and the host is required for its adhesion and subsequent pathogenesis. *S. boulardii* has been shown to minimize *C. rodentium* adherence to the host by interfering with its adhesion (Tir receptor) and translocation apparatus (EspB protein). This ultimately leads to lower pathogenesis, which is manifested by improvement in intestinal barrier integrity and amelioration of the disturbed inflammatory profile during infection by *C. rodentium* (Wu et al., 2008). EHEC infection primarily leads to disturbed intestinal permeability and overproduction of a pro-inflammatory cytokine (IL-8) by manipulating cell signal transduction pathways. *S. boulardii* was found to decrease the severity of EHEC infection by a mechanism not involving competitive adhesion. It interferes with bacterial factors that disturb the signal transduction pathways for maintaining tight-junction permeability of the epithelial lining (Dahan et al., 2003).

S. BOULARDII AS A NUTRACEUTICAL

Saccharomyces boulardii (*S. boulardii*) is a unique, nonpathogenic yeast supplement that has been utilized worldwide as a probiotic to support gastrointestinal health. It is a unique biotherapeutic yeast that can survive gastric acidity and is unaffected and uninhibited by most antibiotics. It does not colonize the human intestinal tract but exerts its beneficial effect on the host as it moves through the gastrointestinal tract (Mitterdorfer et al., 2001). Dairy products serve as an ideal system for delivery of probiotic organisms to the human gastrointestinal tract. Dairy products have the necessary carbohydrate components such as lactose (may act as prebiotics) and the growth promoting favorable environment that enhances the shelf life. Although widely used as baker's yeast in food, other yeasts such as the probiotic *S. boulardii* have been underutilized outside the hospital setting. *S. boulardii* has many probiotic properties suitable for promoting a healthy gut and shows drastic effects in prophylaxis and therapy of intestinal dysbiosis such as diarrhea.

So far, use of this yeast as a dietary adjunct for humans has been limited, despite its being the integral part of many dairy related products. Host food components efficiently utilized by probiotics and accelerating their growth are called prebiotics and are generally carbohydrates such as lactose, inulin, fructo-oligosaccharides (FOSs), mannan-oligosaccharides (MOSs), cellulose, and so on. Pharmaceutical preparations containing *S. boulardii* are available in the market mainly in the form of capsules or lyophilized powder. Various formulations containing *S. boulardii* alone or in combination with other probiotic microorganisms and some prebiotics are available; see Table 7.1.

TABLE 7.1

Dietary Supplements Products Containing *S. boluardii* in Adjunct with or without Other Probiotics

S. Number	Commercial Product/Company	Formulation	Probiotic	Prebiotic	Amount per Serving (CFU)
1	NutriCology®	Capsules	*S. boulardii*	—	9 billion (450 mg)
2	Biotics Research Corporation	Capsules	*S. boulardii*	—	4 billion (235 mg)
3	Boula®	Capsules	*S. boulardii*	—	5 billion (250 mg)
4	Cytoplan	Capsules	*S. boulardii*	—	5 billion (250 mg)
5	Jarrow Formulas®	Capsules	*S. boulardii*	MOS-200 mg	5 billion (250 mg)
6	OptiBac Probiotics	Capsules	*S. boulardii*	—	5 billion (250 mg)
7	Douglas Laboratories	Capsules	*S. boulardii*	FOS and inulin	3 billion (300 mg)
8	Swanson®	Capsules	*S. boulardii*	MOS-200 mg	5 billion (250 mg)
9	Now Foods	Capsules	*S. boulardii*	Organic inulin (FOS)	10 billion
10	Kirkman®	Capsules	*L. rhamnosus*	Inulin, microcrystalline cellulose	5.6 billion
			L. acidophilus		4.0 billion
			B. bifidum		4.0 billion
			L. casei		800 million
			Streptococcus thermophilus		600 million
			L. plantarum		3.6 billion
			S. boulardii		1.5 billion

APPLICATIONS IN FOOD AND FUTURE DIRECTIONS

Probiotic microorganisms are incorporated in food as dietary adjuncts to maintain a healthy gastrointestinal balance to increase human health (Czerucka et al., 2007). The use of yeast as a probiotic food supplement is still restricted and is not completely elucidated. To date, *S. boulardii* is the main recognized probiotic yeast. As mentioned earlier, *S. boulardii* is generally administered in lyophilized powder, and its application as a food additive has been reported only in a limited number of cases, such as in the fermentation of vegetable raw materials (Campbell et al., 2016) and incorporation into yogurt (Karaolis et al., 2013).

S. boulardii exerts beneficial health effects via many mechanisms, such as production of antibacterial toxins, induction of probiotics' growth, increased production of important immunological factors, augmentation of intestinal cells, and increased production of digestive enzymes (sucrase, lactase, and maltase) and SCFAs, and also by decreasing pro-inflammatory cytokines (McFarland, 2010). The expression of large repertoire of mechanisms by *S. boulardii* would warrant suitable growth microenvironment. More than other food matrices, raw fruits and vegetables may represent the ideal vehicle for functional health ingredients because of the richness of their nutrients and their microstructure comprised of many sites (e.g., intercellular spaces, stomas, lenticels, capillaries, naturally occurring irregularities, and tissue lesions), which favor microbial internalization and protection (Di Cagno et al., 2013).

Survival of the health-promoting microorganism throughout the commercial life of the product is very important. Functional foods need to be both viable and safe for consumption till the end of their shelf life. *S. boulardii* is not part of the normal intestinal microbiota, but it is not susceptible to bile salts and pancreatic fluids (Czerucka et al., 2007). Its ability to survive in the gut combined with its resistance to common antibiotic treatments makes this organism an excellent alternative for application in novel functional foods. However, clinical application of *S. boulardii* is restricted due to its sensitivity to acidic environments leading to deceased bioavailability (Thomas et al., 2014). Several researchers had investigated different techniques for improving the bioavailability of *S. boulardii*, such as microencapsulation or immobilization in matrix. It was also shown that encapsulation of *S. boulardii* in alginate microspheres was associated with increased intestinal delivery (Graff et al., 2008). Even after encapsulation, the microorganism has to be viable and the coating should be able to overcome pressure variations *in vivo*.

Many encapsulation matrices are available that mostly deliver the bioactive agent/microbe in a controlled manner to the host. Out of many such formulations, pH responsive encapsulation matrices have become popular. They allow controlled delivery of the probiotic directly into the intestine and rescue them from the deleterious effects of the gastric acids. Some examples of these matrices are gelatin, chitosan, carrageenan, alginate, starch, pectin/cellulose derivatives and other synthetic monomers. Of these, biological matrices (chitosan, carrageenan, etc.) are now preferred over chemical matrices due to their biodegradability, biocompatibility, less immunogenicity, and greater safety. Apart from the matrices, the performance of the controlled release formulation depends heavily on the techniques used for encapsulation. Among the various encapsulation techniques like chemical crosslinking, emulsification, spray drying, ionotropic gelation, chemical coacervation and layer by layer (LbL) method, the LbL technique is one of the easiest and facilitates creation of functional surfaces envisaged for *S. boulardii*. The yeast was encapsulated by LbL using oppositely charged polyelectrolytes, chitosan, and dextran sulfate to protect from degradation during its gastrointestinal transit. Thus, encapsulation ensures better bioavailability of the probiotic in the intestine, making it more effective in the prevention and treatment of several gastrointestinal diseases (Thomas et al., 2014).

RISKS ASSOCIATED WITH USE OF *S. BOULARDII* AS A PROBIOTIC

S. boulardii is usually a nonpathogenic yeast, but sometimes, with a very low probability, it can cause invasive infection (Kollaritsch et al., 1993; Doron and Snydman, 2015). The risk of fungemia due to *S. boulardii* administration is estimated to be 1 in 5.6 million users (Stier and Bischoff, 2016). Fungemia cases are mainly associated with ill, immunocompromised persons and patients on central venous catheters (Whelan and Myers, 2010). Roy et al. (2012) reported seven cases within 15 months of *Saccharomyces* fungemia in tertiary care hospitals related to the use of probiotics and recommended avoiding the use of probiotics containing *S. boulardii* in critically ill or vulnerable patients, especially those on central venous catheters. Although there is theoretical risk of epithelial penetration, followed by systemic translocation by the administrated probiotics or host's colonic microflora, earlier studies showed origination of fungemia from digestive tract translocation, contamination of the central venous line, or air contamination during opening of the packet (Hennequin et al., 2000; Herek et al., 2004). *S. boulardii* can be effectively treated with antimycotic drugs like caspofungin, fluconazole, and amphotericin B, although treatment failure with some drugs was reported (Burkhardt et al., 2005; Atici et al., 2017). Physicians should be careful in recommending *S. boulardii* for patients having a history of long-term hospital stay and HIV patients and critically ill patients in ICUs.

CONCLUSION

S. boulardii has been used successfully in the management of different types of diarrhea; it has prevented pathogenesis and has even helped in alleviating IBD. Its identity as a separate species has been challenged frequently, and it has been declared as a unique probiotic strain in the *S. cerevisiae* family itself courtesy of advanced molecular phylogeny. Recent research has elucidated various underlying mechanisms for its mitigation of diarrhea and gastrointestinal infections, many of which are unique to it. *S. boulardii* has myriad effects that manifest via trophic, luminal, and inflammatory cross-talk between microbiota and the host gut. The temporary gut residence time, antibiotic resistance, multifactorial mechanisms of action, and few reports of pathogenicity by this probiotic suggest its dynamic role in maintaining host gut health. A careful analysis must be made for the expectations from this yeast and the health profile of the patient receiving it as treatment.

Many novel modes of delivery, such as encapsulation, have been developed to increase the gut residence time of this yeast and may have enormous implications on the way the yeast benefits the host. The research on this probiotic yeast has focused mainly on managing gastrointestinal complications, but novel avenues emerge due to its compliance to genetic modifications by CRISPR. This genetic capability and its positive cross-talk with normal gut microbiota should prove essential in developing it as a genetically modified biotherapeutic agent targeting specific diseases. The research on this complex probiotic yeast has many open avenues, and additional ways that it can benefit humanity will surely be discovered.

REFERENCES

Antoine, J. M. 2010. Probiotics: Beneficial factors of the defence system. *Proc Nutr Soc* 69, no. 3: 429–433.

Asahara, T., K. Shimizu, T. Takada, S. Kado, N. Yuki, et al. 2010. Protective effect of lactobacillus casei strain shirota against lethal infection with multi-drug resistant salmonella enterica serovar typhimurium Dt104 in mice. *J Appl Microbiol* 110(1):163–173.

Atici, S., A. Soysal, K. Karadeniz Cerit, S. Yilmaz, B. Aksu, et al. 2017. Catheter-related *Saccharomyces Cerevisiae Fungemia* following *Saccharomyces Boulardii Probiotic* treatment: In a child in intensive care unit and review of the literature. *Med Mycol Case Rep* 15:33–35.

Badia, R., G. Zanello, C. Chevaleyre, R. Lizardo, F. Meurens, et al. 2012. Effect of *Saccharomyces Cerevisiae* var. Boulardii and beta-galactomannan oligosaccharide on porcine intestinal epithelial and dendritic cells challenged *in vitro* with *Escherichia Coli* F4 (K88). *Vet Res* 43:4.

Buccigrossi, V., G. Laudiero, C. Russo, E. Miele, M. Sofia, et al. 2014. Chloride secretion induced by rotavirus is oxidative stress-dependent and inhibited by *Saccharomyces Boulardii* in human enterocytes. *PLoS One* 9(6):e99830.

Burkhardt, O., T. Kohnlein, M. Pletz, and T. Welte. 2005. *Saccharomyces Boulardii* induced sepsis: Successful therapy with voriconazole after treatment failure with fluconazole. *Scand J Infect Dis* 37(1):69–72.

Buts, J. P., and N. De Keyser. 2010. Interaction of *Saccharomyces Boulardii* with intestinal brush border membranes: Key to probiotic effects? *J Pediatr Gastroenterol Nutr* 51(4):532–533.

Buts, J. P., N. Dekeyser, C. Stilmant, E. Delem, F. Smets, and E. Sokal. 2006. *Saccharomyces Boulardii* produces in rat small intestine a novel protein phosphatase that inhibits *Escherichia Coli* endotoxin by dephosphorylation. *Pediatr Res* 60(1):24–29.

Campbell, C., A. K. Nanjundaswamy, V. Njiti, Q. Xia, and F. Chukwuma. 2016. Value-added probiotic development by high-solid fermentation of sweet potato with *Saccharomyces Boulardii*. *Food Sci Nutr* 4:532–533.

Canonici, A., C. Siret, E. Pellegrino, R. Pontier-Bres, L. Pouyet, et al. 2011. *Saccharomyces Boulardii* improves intestinal cell restitution through activation of the alpha2beta1 integrin collagen receptor. *PLoS One* 6(3):e18427.

Chen, X., E. G. Kokkotou, N. Mustafa, K. R. Bhaskar, S. Sougioultzis, M. et al. 2006. *Saccharomyces boulardii* inhibits Erk1/2 mitogen-activated protein kinase activation both *in vitro* and *in vivo* and protects against clostridium difficile toxin a-induced enteritis. *J Biol Chem* 281(34):24449–24454.

Czerucka, D., S. Dahan, B. Mograbi, B. Rossi, and P. Rampal. 2000, *Saccharomyces boulardii* preserves the barrier function and modulates the signal transduction pathway induced in *Enteropathogenic Escherichia Coli*-infected T84 cells. *Infect Immun* 68(10):5998–6004.

Czerucka, D., T. Piche, and P. Rampal. 2007. Review article: Yeast as probiotics— *Saccharomyces Boulardii*. *Aliment Pharmacol Ther* 26(6):767–778.

Czerucka, D., I. Roux, and P. Rampal. 1994. *Saccharomyces Boulardii* inhibits secretagogue-mediated adenosine 3′,5′-Cyclic monophosphate induction in intestinal cells. *Gastroenterology* 106(1):65–72.

Dahan, S., G. Dalmasso, V. Imbert, J. F. Peyron, P. Rampal, and D. Czerucka. 2003. *Saccharomyces boulardii* interferes with *enterohemorrhagic Escherichia Coli*-induced signaling pathways in T84 cells. *Infect Immun* 71(2):766–773.

Dalmasso, G., F. Cottrez, V. Imbert, P. Lagadec, J. F. Peyron, et al. 2006a. *Saccharomyces Boulardii* inhibits inflammatory bowel disease by trapping T cells in mesenteric lymph nodes. *Gastroenterology* 131(6):1812–1825.

Dalmasso, G., A. Loubat, S. Dahan, G. Calle, P. Rampal, and D. Czerucka. 2006b. *Saccharomyces Boulardii* prevents Tnf-Alpha-Induced apoptosis in ehec-infected T84 cells. *Res Microbiol* 157(5):456–465.

Das, S., P. K. Gupta, and R. R. Das. 2016. Efficacy and safety of *Saccharomyces Boulardii* in acute rotavirus diarrhea: Double blind randomized controlled trial from a developing country. *J Trop Pediatr* 62(6):464–470.

Di Cagno, R., R. Coda, M. De Angelis, and M. Gobbetti. 2013. Exploitation of vegetables and fruits through lactic acid fermentation. *Food Microbiol* 33(1):1–10.

Dinleyici, E. C., M. Eren, M. Ozen, Z. A. Yargic, and Y. Vandenplas. 2012. Effectiveness and safety of *Saccharomyces Boulardii* for acute infectious diarrhea. *Expert Opin Biol Ther* 12(4):395–410.

Doron, S., and D. R. Snydman. 2015. Risk and safety of probiotics. *Clin Infect Dis* 60(2):S129–S134.

Edwards-Ingram, L., P. Gitsham, N. Burton, G. Warhurst, I. Clarke, et al. 2007. Genotypic and physiological characterization of *Saccharomyces Boulardii*, the probiotic strain of *Saccharomyces Cerevisiae*. *Appl Environ Microbiol* 73(8):2458–2467.

Ehrhardt, S., N. Guo, R. Hinz, S. Schoppen, J. May, M. Reiser, M. P. Schroeder et al. 2016. *Saccharomyces Boulardii* to prevent antibiotic-associated diarrhea: A randomized, double-masked, placebo-controlled trial. *Open Forum Infect Dis* 3(1):ofw011.

Fidan, I., A. Kalkanci, E. Yesilyurt, B. Yalcin, B. Erdal, et al. 2009. Effects of *Saccharomyces Boulardii* on cytokine secretion from intraepithelial lymphocytes infected by *Escherichia Coli* and candida albicans. *Mycoses* 52(1):29–34.

Garcia, V., E. M. De Lourdes De Abreu Ferrari, H. Oswaldo Da Gama Torres, A. Guerra Pinto, A. Carolina Carneiro Aguirre, et al. 2008. Influence of *Saccharomyces Boulardii* on the intestinal permeability of patients with crohn's disease in remission. *Scand J Gastroenterol* 43(7):842–848.

Girard, P., Y. Pansart, and J. M. Gillardin. 2005. Inducible nitric oxide synthase involvement in the mechanism of action of *Saccharomyces Boulardii* in castor oil-induced diarrhoea in rats. *Nitric Oxide* 13(3):163–169.

Gotteland, M., O. Brunser, and S. Cruchet. 2006. Systematic review: Are probiotics useful in controlling gastric colonization by helicobacter pylori? *Aliment Pharmacol Ther* 23(8):1077–1086.

Graff, S., S. Hussain, J. C. Chaumeil, and C. Charrueau. 2008. Increased intestinal delivery of viable *Saccharomyces Boulardii* by encapsulation in microspheres. *Pharm Res* 25(6):1290–1296.

Guandalini, S., L. Pensabene, M. A. Zikri, J. A. Dias, L. G. Casali, et al. 2000. *Lactobacillus Gg* administered in oral rehydration solution to children with acute diarrhea: A multi-center European trial. *J Pediatr Gastroenterol Nutr* 30(1):54–60.

Guarino, A., F. Albano, S. Ashkenazi, D. Gendrel, J. H. Hoekstra, et al. 2008. European Society for Paediatric Gastroenterology, Hepatology, and Nutrition/European Society for Paediatric Infectious Diseases evidence-based guidelines for the management of acute gastroenteritis in children in Europe: Executive summary. *J Pediatr Gastroenterol Nutr* 46(5):619–621.

Guarner, F., A. C. Khan, J. Carisch, R. Eliakim, A. Gangl, et al. 2008. Probiotics and prebiotics. *World Gastroenterology Organisation Practice Guideline*, pp. 1–21.

Guarner, F. 2007. Prebiotics in inflammatory bowel diseases. *Br J Nutr* 98(1):S85–S89.

Guarner, F., A. G. Khan, J. Garisch, R. Eliakim, A. Gangl, et al. 2011. World Gastroenterology Organisation global guidelines: Probiotics and prebiotics. *J Clin Gastroenterol* 46(6):468–481.

Hatoum, R., S. Labrie, and I. Fliss. 2012. Antimicrobial and probiotic properties of yeasts: From fundamental to novel applications. *Front Microbiol* 3:421.

Hennequin, C., C. Kauffmann-Lacroix, A. Jobert, J. P. Viard, C. Ricour, et al. 2000. Possible role of catheters in *Saccharomyces Boulardii Fungemia*. *Eur J Clin Microbiol Infect Dis* 19(1):16–20.

Herek, O., I. G. Kara, and I. Kaleli. 2004. Effects of antibiotics and *Saccharomyces Boulardii* on bacterial translocation in burn injury. *Surg Today* 34(3):256–260.

Hu, H. J., G. Q. Zhang, Q. Zhang, S. Shakya, and Z. Y. Li. 2016. Probiotics prevent candida colonization and invasive fungal sepsis in preterm neonates: A systematic review and meta-analysis of randomized controlled trials. *Pediatr Neonatol* 15(1):17–21.

Im, E., and C. Pothoulakis. 2012. Recent advances in *Saccharomyces Boulardii* research. *Gastroenterol Clin Biol* 34(1):S62–S70.

Jawhara, S., and D. Poulain. 2007. *Saccharomyces Boulardii* decreases inflammation and intestinal colonization by candida albicans in a mouse model of chemically-induced colitis. *Med Mycol* 45(8):691–700.

Kabbani, T. A., K. Pallav, S. E. Dowd, J. Villafuerte-Galvez, R. R. Vanga, et al. 2017. Prospective randomized controlled study on the effects of *Saccharomyces Boulardii* Cncm I-745 and amoxicillin-clavulanate or the combination on the gut microbiota of healthy volunteers. *Gut Microbes* 8(1):17–32.

Karaolis, C., G. Botsaris, I. Pantelides, and D. Tsaltas. 2013. Potential application of *Saccharomyces Boulardii* as a probiotic in goat's yoghurt: Survival and organoleptic effects. *IJFST* 48(7):1445–1452.

Karen, M., O. Yuksel, N. Akyurek, E. Ofluoglu, K. Caglar, et al. 2010. Probiotic agent *Saccharomyces Boulardii* reduces the incidence of lung injury in acute necrotizing pancreatitis induced rats. *J Surg Res* 160(1):139–144.

Kelesidis, T., and C. Pothoulakis. 2012. Efficacy and safety of the probiotic *Saccharomyces Boulardii* for the prevention and therapy of gastrointestinal disorders. *Therap Adv Gastroenterol* 5(2):111–125.

Kollaritsch, H., H. Holst, P. Grobara, and G. Wiedermann. 1993. Prevention of traveler's diarrhea with *Saccharomyces Boulardii*. Results of a placebo controlled double-blind study. *Fortschr Med* 111(9):152–156.

Koon, H. W., B. Su, C. Xu, C. C. Mussatto, D. H. Tran, et al. 2016. Probiotic *Saccharomyces Boulardii* Cncm I-745 prevents outbreak-associated clostridium difficile-associated cecal inflammation in hamsters. *Am J Physiol Gastrointest Liver Physiol* 311(4):G610–G623.

Kotowska, M., P. Albrecht, and H. Szajewska. 2005. *Saccharomyces Boulardii* in the prevention of antibiotic-associated diarrhoea in children: A randomized double-blind placebo-controlled trial. *Aliment Pharmacol Ther* 21(5):583–590.

Krappmann, S. 2016. Crispr-Cas9, the new kid on the block of fungal molecular biology. *Medical Mycology* 55(1):16–23.

Krappmann, S., 2017. CRISPR-Cas9, the new kid on the block of fungal molecular biology. *Med Mycol* 55:16–23.

Krasowska, A., A. Murzyn, A. Dyjankiewicz, M. Lukaszewicz, and D. Dziadkowiec. 2009. The antagonistic effect of *Saccharomyces Boulardii* on candida albicans filamentation, adhesion and biofilm formation. *FEMS Yeast Res* 9(8):1312–1321.

Lau, C. S., and R. S. Chamberlain. 2016. Probiotics are effective at preventing *Clostridium* difficile-associated diarrhea: A systematic review and meta-analysis. *Int J Gen Med* 9:27–37.

Lee, S. Y., Y. W. Shin, and K. B. Hahm. 2008. Phytoceuticals: mighty but ignored weapons against *Helicobacter pylori* infection. *J Dig Dis* 9(3):129–139.

Liu, J. J., K. Kong, I. I., G. C. Zhang, L. N. Jayakody, H. Kim, et al. 2016. Metabolic engineering of probiotic *Saccharomyces Boulardii*. *Appl Environ Microbiol* 82(8):2280–2287.

Malfertheiner, P., F. Megraud, C. O'Morain, F. Bazzoli, E. El-Omar, et al. 2007. Current concepts in the management of helicobacter pylori infection: The maastricht Iii consensus report. *Gut* 56(6):772–781.

Martins, F. S., A. T. Vieira, S. D. Elian, R. M. Arantes, F. C. Tiago, et al. 2013. Inhibition of tissue inflammation and bacterial translocation as one of the protective mechanisms of *Saccharomyces Boulardii* against salmonella infection in mice. *Microbes Infect* 15(4):270–279.

McFarland, L. V. 1996. *Saccharomyces Boulardii* is not *Saccharomyces Cerevisiae*. *Clin Infect Dis* 22(1):200–201.

McFarland, L. V. 2006. Meta-analysis of probiotics for the prevention of antibiotic associated diarrhea and the treatment of *Clostridium* difficile disease. *Am J Gastroenterol* 101(4):812–822.

McFarland, L. V. 2010. Systematic review and meta-analysis of *Saccharomyces Boulardii* in adult patients. *World J Gastroenterol* 16(18):2202–2222.

McFarland, L. V. 2014. Use of probiotics to correct dysbiosis of normal microbiota following disease or disruptive events: A systematic review. *BMJ Open* 4(8):e005047.

McFarland, L. V., C. M. Surawicz, R. N. Greenberg, R. Fekety, G. W. Elmer, et al. 1994. A randomized placebo-controlled trial of *Saccharomyces Boulardii* in combination with standard antibiotics for *Clostridium* difficile disease. *JAMA* 271(24):1913–1918.

Mitterdorfer, G., W. Kneifel, and H. Viernstein. 2001. Utilization of Prebiotic Carbohydrates by Yeasts of Therapeutic Relevance. *Lett Appl Microbiol* 33(4):251–255.

Mitterdorfer, G., H. K. Mayer, W. Kneifel, and H. Viernstein. 2002. Clustering of *Saccharomyces Boulardii* strains within the species S. *Cerevisiae* using molecular typing techniques. *J Appl Microbiol* 93(4):521–530.

More, M. I., and A. Swidsinski. 2015. *Saccharomyces Boulardii* Cncm I-745 supports regeneration of the intestinal microbiota after diarrheic dysbiosis: A review. *Clin Exp Gastroenterol* 8:237–255.

Muhan, L. Ü., S. Yu, J. Deng, Q. Yan, C. Yang, et al. 2016. Efficacy of probiotic supplementation therapy for *Helicobacter pylori* eradication: a meta-analysis of randomized controlled trials. *PLoS One* 11(10):e0163743.

Muñoz-Provencio, D., M. Llopis, M. Antolín, I. De Torres, F. Guarner, et al. 2009. Adhesion properties of *Lactobacillus casei* strains to resected intestinal fragments and components of the extracellular matrix. *Arch Microbiol* 191(2):153–161.

Murzyn, A., A. Krasowska, P. Stefanowicz, D. Dziadkowiec, and M. Lukaszewicz. 2010. Capric acid secreted by *S. Boulardii* inhibits C. albicans filamentous growth, adhesion and biofilm formation. *PLoS One* 5(8):e12050.

Namkin, K., M. Zardast, and F. Basirinejad. 2016. *Saccharomyces Boulardii* in helicobacter pylori eradication in children: A randomized trial from Iran. *Iran J Pediatr* 26(1):e3768.

Nataro, J. P., and J. B. Kaper. 1998. Diarrheagenic *Escherichia Coli*. *Clin Microbiol Rev* 11(1):142–201.

Ohland, C. L., and W. K. Macnaughton. 2010. Probiotic bacteria and intestinal *Epithelial Barrier* function. *Am J Physiol Gastrointest Liver Physiol* 298(6):G807–G819.

Pothoulakis, C., C. P. Kelly, M. A. Joshi, N. Gao, C. J. O'Keane, et al. 1993. *Saccharomyces Boulardii* inhibits *Clostridium* difficile toxin a binding and enterotoxicity in rat ileum. *Gastroenterology* 104(4):1108–1115.

Pothoulakis, C., and J. T. Lamont. 2001. Microbes and microbial toxins: Paradigms for microbial-mucosal interactions Ii. The integrated response of the intestine to *Clostridium* difficile toxins. *Am J Physiol Gastrointest Liver Physiol* 280(2):G178–G183.

Ramage, G., S. P. Saville, B. L. Wickes, and J. L. Lopez-Robot. 2002. Inhibition of candida albicans biofilm formation by farnesol, a quorum-sensing molecule. *Appl Environ Microbiol* 68(11):5459–5463.

Reid, G., J. Jass, M. Tom Sebulsky, and J. K. McCormick. 2003. Potential uses of probiotics in clinical practice. *Clin Microbiol Rev* 16(4):658–672.

Riaz, M., S. Alam, A. Malik, and S. M. Ali. 2012. Efficacy and safety of *Saccharomyces Boulardii* in acute childhood diarrhea: A double blind randomised controlled trial. *Indian J Pediatr* 79(4):478–482.

Ringel, Y., E. M. M. Quigley, and H. C. Lin. 2012. Using probiotics in gastrointestinal disorders. *Am J Gastroenterol* 1(1):34–40.

Roy, U., L. G. Jessani, S. M. Rudramurthy, R. Gopalakrishnan, S. Dutta, et al. 2012. Seven cases of *Saccharomyces Fungaemia* related to use of probiotics. *Mycoses* 79(4):478–482.

Ruggiero, P. 2014. Use of probiotics in the fight against helicobacter pylori. *World J Gastrointest Pathophysiol* 5(4):384–391.

Sazawal, S., G. Hiremath, U. Dhingra, P. Malik, S. Deb, and R. E. Black. 2006. Efficacy of probiotics in prevention of acute diarrhoea: A meta-analysis of masked, randomised, placebo-controlled trials. *Lancet Infect Dis* 6(6):374–382.

Schneider, S. M., F. Girard-Pipau, J. Filippi, X. Hebuterne, D. Moyse, et al. 2005. Effects of *Saccharomyces Boulardii* on fecal short-chain fatty acids and microflora in patients on long-term total enteral nutrition. *World J Gastroenterol* 11(39):6165–6169.

Sezer, A., U. Usta, and I. Cicin. 2009. The effect of *Saccharomyces Boulardii* on reducing irinotecan-induced intestinal mucositis and diarrhea. *Med Oncol* 26(3):350–357.

Sougioultzis, S., S. Simeonidis, K. R. Bhaskar, X. Chen, P. M. Anton, et al. 2006. *Saccharomyces Boulardii* produces a soluble anti-inflammatory factor that inhibits Nf-Kappab-Mediated Il-8 gene expression. *Biochem Biophys Res Commun* 343(1):69–76.

Stier, H., and S. C. Bischoff. 2016. Influence of *Saccharomyces Boulardii* Cncm I-745 on the gut-associated immune system. *Clin Exp Gastroenterol* 9:269–279.

Surawicz, C. M., L. V. McFarland, R. N. Greenberg, M. Rubin, R. Fekety, et al. 2000. The search for a better treatment for recurrent *Clostridium* difficile disease: Use of high-dose vancomycin combined with *Saccharomyces Boulardii*. *Clin Infect Dis* 31(4):1012–1017.

Szajewska, H., A. Horvath, and M. Kolodziej. 2006. Systematic review with meta-analysis: *Saccharomyces Boulardii* supplementation and eradication of helicobacter pylori infection. *Aliment Pharmacol Ther* 41(12):1237–1245.

Szajewska, H., and J. Mrukowicz. 2005. Meta-analysis: Non-pathogenic yeast *Saccharomyces Boulardii* in the prevention of antibiotic-associated diarrhoea. *Aliment Pharmacol Ther* 22(5):365–372.

Tasteyre, A., M. C. Barc, T. Karjalainen, P. Bourlioux, and A. Collignon. 2002. Inhibition of *in vitro* cell adherence of *Clostridium difficile by Saccharomyces boulardii*. *Microb Pathog* 32(5):219–225.

Thomas, M. B., M. Vaidyanathan, K. Radhakrishnan, and A. M. Raichur. 2014. Enhanced viability of probiotic *Saccharomyces boulardii* encapsulated by layer-by-layer approach in pH responsive chitosan–dextran sulfate polyelectrolytes. *J Food Eng* 12(136):1–8.

Thomas, S., I. Przesdzing, D. Metzke, J. Schmitz, A. Radbruch, and D. C. Baumgart. 2009. *Saccharomyces Boulardii* inhibits lipopolysaccharide-induced activation of human dendritic cells and T-cell proliferation. *Clin Exp Immunol* 156(1):78–87.

Tiago, F. C., F. S. Martins, E. L. Souza, P. F. Pimenta, H. R. Araujo, et al. 2012. Adhesion to the yeast cell surface as a mechanism for trapping pathogenic bacteria by *Saccharomyces Probiotics*. *J Med Microbiol* 61(Pt 9):1194–1207.

Vandenplas, Y., O. Brunser, and H. Szajewska. 2009. *Saccharomyces Boulardii* in childhood. *Eur J Pediatr* 168(3):253–265.

Vitor, J. M., and F. F. Vale. 2011. Alternative therapies for helicobacter pylori: Probiotics and phytomedicine. *FEMS Immunol Med Microbiol* 63(2):153–164.

Whelan, K., and C. E. Myers. 2010. Safety of probiotics in patients receiving nutritional support: A systematic review of case reports, randomized controlled trials, and nonrandomized trials. *Am J Clin Nutr* 91(3):687–703.

Wu, X., B. A. Vallance, L. Boyer, K. S. Bergstrom, J. Walker, et al. 2008. *Saccharomyces Boulardii* ameliorates citrobacter rodentium-induced colitis through actions on bacterial virulence factors. *Am J Physiol Gastrointest Liver Physiol* 294(1):G295–G306.

Yadav, A. K., A. Tyagi, J. K. Kaushik, A. C. Saklani, S. Grover, et al. 2013. Role of surface layer collagen binding protein from indigenous *Lactobacillus plantarum* 91 in adhesion and its anti-adhesion potential against gut pathogen. *Microbiol Res* 168(10):639–645.

Young, V. B., and T. M. Schmidt. 2004. Antibiotic-associated diarrhea accompanied by large-scale alterations in the composition of the fecal microbiota. *J Clin Microbiol* 42(3):1203–1206.

Zanello, G., F. Meurens, M. Berri, and H. Salmon. 2009. *Saccharomyces Boulardii* effects on gastrointestinal diseases. *Curr Issues Mol Biol* 11(1):47–58.

8 Mechanism of Microbial Heavy Metal Accumulation from a Polluted Environment and Bioremediation

Vineet Kumar

CONTENTS

INTRODUCTION

Throughout the twenty-first century, human activity (such as energy and fuel production, metalliferous surface finishing industry, pesticide and fertilizer industry, industrial effluent and sludge, leatherworking, combustion of fossil fuels, mining, agriculture, metallurgy, electroplating, faulty waste disposal, photography, electrolysis, metal surface treatments, and military operations) have directly or indirectly discharged industrial waste containing heavy metals into rivers, lakes, and drains. These heavy metals eventually find their way into the human body through the food chain. Such heavy metal accumulation causes health hazards (including potential carcinogenicity) even in very minute concentrations of about 1 mg/L (Sarkar et al., 2016). At present, heavy metal pollution is a major environmental problem because metal ions persist due to their nondegradable and recalcitrant nature. Hence, their toxic effects also last (Tchounwou et al., 2012). Therefore, bioconcentration and subsequent biomagnification of heavy metals (and the high levels of toxicity they impart to biological organisms, both macro and micro) indicate the necessity for the elimination of toxic metals from the environment (Govarthanan et al., 2014). It is imperative to reduce or remove heavy metal contamination in order to prevent or reduce the possibility of uptake in the food chain. In recent years, various physiochemical reactions such as oxidation and reduction, chemical precipitation, filtration, flocculation, activated charcoal, coagulation, electrochemical treatment, evaporation, ion-exchange, and reverse osmosis have been found to be capable of removing heavy metals, but high level chemicals, high energy consumption, and generation of huge amounts of toxic sludge and other secondary pollutants are some disadvantages associated with such techniques (Barakat, 2011). Compared to conventional remediation techniques, bioremediation is an innovative, eco-friendly, and promising technology for removal and/ or recovery of heavy metals from polluted soil and water, and for reestablishing the natural condition of soil and water (U.S. EPA, 2012). Bioremediation uses primarily microorganisms (bacteria, fungi, yeast, and cynobacteria) or microbial processes to degrade and/or transform environmental pollutants into harmless or less toxic forms. Microorganisms use these hazardous substances as a sole source of C (carbon), N (nitrogen), and (P) phosphorus for the degradation process; thus, these substances act as growth substrates (Rani et al., 2009; Azubuike et al., 2016). Microorganisms have developed different detoxifying mechanisms such as biosorption, bioaccumulation, bioleaching, and biotransformation for their survival in heavy-metal-contaminated habitats (Ianeva, 2009). Microorganisms have a high surface area–to–volume (SA:V) ratio because of their small size and therefore provide a large contact area that can interact with various metal ions and other materials in the surrounding environment. These materials then move into and out of the cell by diffusion and active transport. The removal of metal ions is done through mechanisms employed to derive energy from metals-redox reactions to deal with toxic metals through enzymatic and nonenzymatic processes. Metal accumulation has received a lot of attention during the last two decades because of the potential use of microorganisms for removing heavy metals from contaminated media.

Microorganisms use heavy metals as terminal electron acceptors or reduce them through the detoxification mechanism from the polluted environment. This chapter presents insights into the use of microbes for the removal of heavy metals from soil and water contaminated with industrial waste. The various factors affecting heavy metal bioremediation process are also discussed.

BIOREMEDIATION OF HEAVY METALS BY MICROORGANISMS

Heavy metals are elements with metallic properties (stability as cations, ligand specificity, conductivity, etc.) and an atomic number greater than 20. However, heavy metals with a density greater than 5.0 g/cm^3 are generally categorized in three classes: toxic metals (e.g., mercury [Hg], chromium [Cr], lead [Pb], zinc [Zn], copper [Cu], nickel [Ni], cadmium [Cd], arsenic [As], cobalt [Co], tin [Sn]), precious metals (e.g., lead [Pb], platinum [Pt], silver [Ag], gold [Au], ruthenium [Ru]), and radionuclides (e.g., uranium [U], thorium [Th], radium [Ra], americium [Am]). Among them, the most common heavy metal contaminants are Pb^{2+}, Cr^{2+}/Cr^{3+}, Cd^{2+}, Ni^{2+}/Ni^{4+}, Zn^{2+}, Cu^{2+}, and Hg^{2+} (Bishop, 2002). Heavy metals cannot be broken down by chemical and biological processes; they can only transform from one oxidation state to another so that they become water-soluble, precipitated, and less toxic. Hence, the remediation of environment niches (i.e., soil, sediments, and water) contaminated with heavy metals and metalloids can be achieved through biologically encoded changes in the oxidation state. The use of microorganisms to remediate heavy-metal-contaminated sites is a sustainable tool to restore the natural state of the polluted site that is cost effective. Bioremediation as a treatment method uses living microorganisms to transform the toxic pollutants to harmless or less toxic forms with less input of energy, chemicals, and time. Generally, microbes use heavy metals as terminal electron acceptors by changing their physical and chemical states or by reducing them from the contaminated environment (U.S. EPA, 2012; Azubuike et al., 2016). Thus, the bioremediation strategy of heavy metals depends on the active metabolizing and tolerance capabilities of microorganisms. Microorganisms are omnipresent in heavy-metal-polluted environments and can easily convert heavy metals into nontoxic forms through biosorption, biomineralization, bioaccumulation, bioleaching, and biotransformation. Microorganisms also mobilize heavy metals from the polluted sites by chelation, leaching, redox transformation, and methylation mechanisms. Different defense systems in microorganisms such as compartmentalization, complex formation, exclusion, and synthesis of binding proteins and peptides reduce the metals' stress. Bioremediation may also involve aerobic or anaerobic processes. Aerobic processes often involve introduction of oxygen atoms into the reactions mediated by monooxygenases, dioxygenases, hydroxylases, oxidative dehalogenases, or chemically reactive oxygen atoms generated by ligninases or peroxidases. Anaerobic processes involve initial activation reactions followed by oxidative catabolism mediated by anoxic electron acceptors. The major mechanisms of heavy metal bioremediation and detoxification by microorganisms are illustrated in Figure 8.1.

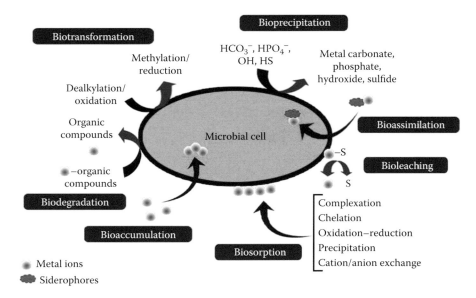

FIGURE 8.1 Mechanism of microbial heavy metal bioremediation from contaminated sites.

There are mainly two types of bioremediation, *in situ* or *ex situ* bioremediation, and classification depends on several factors such as geographical location and geology of the polluted site, depth of pollution, degree of pollution, and the type and concentration of pollutants. *In situ* bioremediation involves treating pollutants where they are located. In this process, microorganisms come into direct contact with the pollutants and use them as substrates for their energy source. *Ex situ* bioremediation involves physically extracting media (i.e., soil and sediment) from a polluted site and moving it to another location for treatment (U.S. EPA, 2012). However, *in situ* and *ex situ* bioremediation techniques have specific benefits and costs.

MOBILIZATION

Microorganisms can mobilize heavy metals at contaminated sites through autotrophic and heterotrophic leaching, methylation, and chelation by siderophores and metabolites, which can result in volatilization (Figure 8.1). Such processes can lead to dissolution of insoluble metal compounds and minerals, including phosphates, sulfides, oxides, and more complex mineral ores, and desorption of metal species from exchange sites on, for example, clay minerals or organic matter in the soil (White et al., 1995; Akhtar et al., 2013). The technique used to reduce the mobilization of heavy metals from polluted sites by changing the physiochemical state of the toxic metals is called immobilization (Vivaldi, 2001).

BIOLEACHING

Bioleaching is the process of dissolving sulfide minerals and extracting metals by the production of less toxic metals by unmediated, discharging bacteria. The bacteria genus most involved in bioleaching is *Thiobacillus*, a gram-negative, rod shaped, non-spore-forming bacteria that grows under aerobic conditions. Most thiobacilli are chemolitho-autotrophic species that use the CO_2 from the atmosphere as their carbon source for the synthesis of new cell material (Gadd, 2000). The energy derives from the oxidation of reduced or partially reduced sulfur compounds, including elemental sulfur (S), sulfides (S^{2-}), and thiosulfate ($S_2O_3^{2-}$), with the final oxidation product being sulfate (SO_4^{2-}). Bacterial leaching is carried out in an acidic environment (pH 1.5–3.0) by acidophilic bacteria species *Thiobacillus ferrooxidans* and *T. thiooxidans*. In this acidic environment, most metal ions are soluble. Other thiobacilli can oxidize S and S^{2-}, but they grow only at higher pH levels, at which metal ions are not soluble. The bioleaching process using acidophilic sulfur-oxidizing bacterial species *Acidithiobacillus ferrooxidans*, *Acidithiobacillus thiooxidans,* and *Leptospirillum ferrooxidans* has been used for successful removal of metals from sediment, soil, and sludge. Generally autotrophic leaching is carried out by these acidophilic bacteria species, which fix CO_2 and obtain energy from the oxidation of ferrous iron or reduced sulfur compounds, which causes the solubilization of metals because of the resulting production of Fe^{3+} and H_2SO_4. This in turn results in solubilization of other metal compounds. Microorganisms can acidify their surrounding environment by proton (H^+) efflux via plasma membrane H^+-ATPase pumps, maintenance of charge balance, or as a result of respiratory CO_2 accumulation (Gadd, 2004). Acidification can also lead to metal release via a number of obvious routes such as competition between H+ and the metal ions or in a sorbed form, resulting in the release of free metal cations. In heterotrophic leaching, heterotrophic microorganisms (i.e., bacteria and fungi) that require organic compounds for their growth and energy supply may contribute to metal leaching as a result of the efflux of organic acids and siderophores (Gadd, 2000). In soil, metal mobilization by heterotrophic miroorganisms is more important than autotrophic leaching for, for example, phosphate- and sulfate-containing minerals, because this leads to release of these important nutrients. Heterotrophic leaching may be mostly appropriate for wastes of high pH because most *Thiobacilli* cannot solubilize effectively above pH 5.5. Leaching is also carried out by fungi (i.e., *Aspergillus* and *Penicillium*). Leaching by this group of organisms is mediated by the production of organic acids (e.g., citrate, lactate, oxalate, gluconate, and fumarate), which are excreted into the culture and may chelate toxic metal ions, resulting in the formation of metalloorganic molecules. These organic acids also help in the solubilization of metal ions and leaching from their surfaces.

METAL TRANSFORMATIONS

Biotransformation is a process leading to the change of the structure of the original chemical compound to such a degree that its original characteristic properties change as well. The biotransformation process modifies not only the physical and chemical properties of compounds (i.e., solubility and bioavailability) but also the toxicity level of the pollutants. Microorganisms can facilitate (bio)transformation of heavy metals through chemical reactions such as methylation, dealkylation, oxidation, and reduction. Biotransformation processes lead to metal volatilization into the environment (Gadd, 2010).

Biomethylation

Methylation of Hg^{2+}, As^{5+}, Te, Sn, Se, and Pb^{2+} can be mediated by a range of bacteria and fungi under aerobic (presence of oxygen) and anaerobic (absence of oxygen) conditions (Gadd, 2004). In this process, methyl groups ($-CH_3$) are transferred to metal by microbial enzymatic action, and a given microorganism may transform a number of different metals and metalloids. Methylation generally increases the toxicity of metal as a result of increased lipophilicity, thus increasing permeation across plasma membrane. However, volatilization facilitates heavy metal diffusion away from the cell, and in this way the toxicity of a metal is effectively decreased. Metal volatilization has been observed with Pb^{2+}, Hg^{2+}, Sn^{2+}, Se^{2+}, and As^{5+}. For example, Hg^{2+} is readily oxidized to the volatile and very toxic forms methylmercury (CH_3Hg^+) and dimethylmercury ($[CH_3]_2Hg$), which can then diffuse away from the cell. Methylation of metals has been known to eliminate significant level of metal from polluted soils, sediments, surface waters, industrial effluent, and sewage. Microbial methylation of Se, resulting in volatilization, has been used successfully for *in situ* bioremediation of Se-containing soil, sediment, and water at Kesterson Reservoir, California, (Thompson-Eagle and Frankenberger, 1992). Several bacterial and fungal species can methylate arsonic compounds such as arsenite [As(III), AsO_2^-], arsenate [As(V), AsO_4^{3-}], and methylarsonic acid ($CH_3H_2AsO_3$) to volatile dimethyl-($[CH_3]_2HAs$) or trimethylarsine ($[CH_3]_3As$). The mechanisms of methylation of metals and metalloids are carried out by the activity of S-adenosylmethionine, methylcobalamin or N-methyltetrahydrofolate.

Redox Transformations

Microorganisms can mobilize various metals, metalloids, and organometallic compounds in the environment by oxidation-reduction processes (Lovley, 2000; Gadd, 2004). Anaerobic dissimilatory metal-reducing bacteria and archaea can reduce a variety of metals (i.e., Fe^{3+}, Mn^{4+}, Se^{4+}, and Cr^{6+}) to a lower redox state by using them as terminal electron acceptors in anaerobic respiration. While Fe and Mn increase their solubility upon reduction, the solubility of other metals such as U^{6+} to U^{4+} and Cr^{6+} to Cr^{3+} decreases, resulting in immobilization (Smith and Gadd, 2000). The dissimilatory reduction of Fe, Cr, U, Au, and some other metals and metalloids is performed by various groups of microorganisms present in polluted environments and is widely used for toxic waste management.

IMMOBILIZATION

Immobilization reduces the external free metal ions in soil and water. In some circumstances, it may also promote solubilization by shifting the equilibrium to release more metal ions into the medium (Gadd, 2000, 2004). Immobilized living biomass takes the form of bacterial biofilms on inert supports and is used in fixed bed reactors, fluidized beds, trickle filters, rotating biological contactors, and air-lift bioreactors for the treatment of heavy-metal-containing effluent. For instance, binding of metal ions to polysaccharides, proteins, and humic substances can immobilize the metal even further, thus preventing its intake into a bacterial cell. These substances thus detoxify metals merely by complex formation or by forming an effective barrier surrounding the cell.

METAL PRECIPITATION

Microorganisms may immobilize heavy metals efficiently through their precipitation either as the result of dissimilatory reduction or by interaction with the product of microbial metabolism. In the presence of toxic metals, fungi, bacteria, and algae produce sulfide (S^{2-}), carbonate (CO_3), hydroxide ($-OH$), and phosphate ($-PO_4^{3-}$), which may interact with heavy metals to form highly insoluble metal precipitates. This strategy has attracted a lot of attention in the remediation of heavy-metal-polluted sites. Dissimilatory sulfate reduction and the subsequent precipitation of metal sulfides have been identified as the most important reactions in the removal of heavy metals from industrial effluent. On the basis of cellular metabolism of microbes, metal precipitation may be either dependent or independent. In the cellular-dependent process, the removal of metals from solution is often associated with the active defense system of the microorganisms. In the presence of toxic metals, microorganisms react to produce several compounds that favor the precipitation process. However, precipitation may be a consequence of the chemical interaction between the microbial cell surface and metal ions. Initially, it was thought that, at higher pH values, metals may accumulate inside the cells or on the cell walls by sorption–precipitation. Sulfur- and sulfate-reducing bacteria are geochemically significant in reductive precipitation of U^{6+} and Cr^{6+}, a process mediated by multiheme cytochrome c proteins. The action of sulfate-reducing bacteria forms H_2S, which precipitates with Zn^{2+}, Cu^{2+}, Ni^{4+}, and so on. Moreover, sulfate-reducing bacteria lower the sulfate concentration and cause an increase in pH. In the cellular-independent process, the metal uptake may take place both in the solution and on the cell surface of the microorganisms after a chemical interaction between the metal and cell surface.

BIOSORPTION

The term *biosorption* can describe any system where a sorbate (e.g., an atom, molecular ion, molecule) interacts with a biosorbent (i.e., a solid surface of a biological matrix) and results in accumulation at the sorbate–biosorbent interface and thus in a reduction in the solution sorbate's concentration. Biosorption can be defined as the microbial uptake of organic and inorganic compounds, both soluble and insoluble, by physiochemical mechanisms, that is, adsorption (Fomina and Gadd, 2014). This process seems to be more feasible for large-scale application compared to other microbe-mediated methods.

INTRACELLULAR AND EXTRACELLULAR IMMOBILIZATION BY METAL-BINDING COMPOUNDS

An array of specific and nonspecific metal-binding compounds is produced by microorganisms to facilitate metal immobilization. The metal immobilization can be divided into two types: (1) intracellular metal immobilization and (2) extracellular metal immobilization. Intracellular immobilization of metals involves two processes: vacuoles compartmentalization and complexation by cytoplasmic peptides such as GSH, phytochelatins, and metallothioneins (Gadd, 2000). Metallothionein (MT) is a metal-binding protein that can modulate the intracellular concentrations and bind both the essential and nonessential metals. In extracellular immobilization, extracellular polymeric substances (EPSs), mixtures of polysaccharides, mucopolysaccarides, and proteins, are produced by bacteria, fungi, and algae that bind with heavy metals.

MECHANISM OF MICROBIAL METAL ACCUMULATION

Living and dead cells of microorganisms are capable of accumulating metal, metalloids, and radionuclides; there may be differences, however, in the mechanisms involved in metal accumulation. Accumulation of heavy metals and metalloids can occur either by metabolism-independent (passive sorption) or by intracellular, metabolism-dependent active uptake. Both processes can occur in the same organism.

METABOLISM-INDEPENDENT BIOSORPTION (PASSIVE ACCUMULATION)

The term "biosorption" is frequently used for the range of processes by which microbial biomasses remove heavy metals and other substances from solution. The term can also be used in a stricter sense to mean uptake by living or dead biomass of microorganisms via physiochemical mechanisms such as ion exchange, adsorption, and complexation, although, in living biomass, metabolic processes may also influence and/or contribute to the biosorption process (White et al., 1995). Generally, the metabolism-independent biosorption process using dead biomasses is the result of a physiochemical interaction between the metals and functional groups such as hydroxyl ($-OH$), carboxyl ($-COOH$), phosphate ($-PO_4^{3-}$), sulfhydryl (thiol) ($-SH$), sulfate ($-SO_4^{2-}$), amide (R-$CONH_2$), amino ($-NH_2$), and carbonyl ($-RCHO$) present on the microbial cell surface (Fomina and Gadd, 2014). Among them, $-OH$, $-NH_2$, $-PO_4^{3-}$, are the most important functional groups in biomass that can participate in biosorption. This type of biosorption is relatively fast and usually reversible (White et al., 1995). Some distinctive mechanisms involved in the biosorption process include ion exchange, covalent bonding, microprecipitation, complexation, chemisorption, adsorption–complexation in pores and on surfaces, heavy metal hydroxide condensation, and these do not depend on cellular metabolism. Numerous mechanisms, each working independently, contribute to the overall uptake of metals, and more than one process may contribute to metal uptake in any one system. The uptake of heavy metal by microbial biomass was calculated using the following equation:

$$Q = \frac{(C_i - C_f)V}{W}$$

where:
  Q is the metal ions uptake capacity of microorganism (g g^{-1})
  C_i and C_f are the initial and final metal ion concentrations, respectively, during,
      before, and after adsorption (g L^{-1})
  V is the volume of solution (L)
  W is the quantity of the adsorbent (g)

The removal ratio of a metal was evaluated as follows:

$$\text{Removal ratio } (\%) = \frac{C_0 - C_e}{C_0} \times 100$$

where:
  C_0 and C_e are the initial and residual metal concentrations (mg L^{-1}), respectively
  X is the biomass concentration (g L^{-1})

The Langmuir, Freundlich, and Langmuir-Freundlich equations/models are the most frequently used isotherm models to describe the metal biosorption mechanism. The Langmuir isotherm model is based on the assumptions that the highest adsorption occurs on the saturated monolayer of a surface containing a finite number of identical sites, the energy of adsorption is constant, and there is no migration of adsorbate molecules in the surface plane. On the basis of these assumptions, the Langmuir isotherm model represented by the following equation:

$$q_e = \frac{q_m b C_e}{1 + b C_e}$$

where:
  q_e is the quantity of equilibrium metal ions adsorbed a (mg g^{-1})
  q_m is the mass of completely adsorbed solute required to saturate a unit mass of
      adsorbent (mg g^{-1})
  b is the equilibrium adsorption constant related to the affinity of binding sites
      (L mg^{-1})
  C_e is the equilibrium concentration (mg L^{-1})

The Freundlich model is basically empirical and was developed for heterogeneous surfaces. This model is as follows:

$$q_e = \frac{k(C_e)1}{n}$$

where:
  k and n are the equilibrium constants indicative of adsorption capacity and
      adsorption intensity, respectively.

The Langmuir–Freundlich model is represented by the following equation:

$$q_e = \frac{q_m b C_e^m}{1 + b C_e^m}$$

where:

q_e is the quantity of metal ions adsorbed at equilibrium (mg g^{-1})

q_m is the mass of completely adsorbed solute required to saturate a unit mass of adsorbent (mg g^{-1})

b is the equilibrium adsorption constant related to the affinity of binding sites (L mg^{-1})

C_e is the equilibrium concentration (mg L^{-1})

m is the Langmuir–Freundlich parameter

Values for $m \gg 1$ indicate heterogeneous adsorbent, while values closer to or even 1.0 indicate a material with relatively homogenous binding sites.

Ion Exchange

The cell walls of microorganisms contain mainly polysaccharides, lipids, and proteins, and bivalent metal ions exchange with the counter ions of the polysaccharides. For example, the alginates of marine algae occur as salts of Na$^+$, K$^+$, Ca^{2+}, and Mg^{2+} (Rubinelli et al., 2002). These ions can exchange with counter ions such as Zn^{2+} Co^{2+}, Cd^{2+}, Cu^{2+}, resulting in the biosorptive heavy-metal uptake from multimetal solutions.

Complexation

The removal of metal ions from a solution may also take place via complex formation between the metal ions and the active functional groups present on the microbial cell surface. Aksu et al. (1992) hypothesized that biosorption of Cu^{2+} ions by Z. ramigera and C. vulgaris takes place through both adsorption and formation of coordination bonds between metal ions and −NH$_2$ and −COOH groups of cell wall polysaccharides. Complexation was found to be the only mechanism responsible for Ca, Mg, Cd, Zn, Cu, and Hg binding by Pseudomonas syringae.

Biosorption of Heavy Metals by Bacteria

The −COOH, amine, phosphonate, sulfonate and −OH groups are the major groups responsible for binding of metal ions in bacteria cell walls. Three main mechanisms for the metal binding of bacterial cell walls are (1) ion-exchange reactions with teichoic acid and peptidoglycan, (2) precipitation through nucleation reactions, and (3) complexation with oxygen and nitrogen ligands (White et al., 1995; Gadd, 2000). The bacterial cell wall consists of an array of polysaccharides and proteins, and hence offers a number of active sites capable of binding different metal ions. Generally, two types of bacteria exist in nature: gram positive and gram negative. The Gram-positive bacteria cell wall is comprised of a thick and multiple layer of peptidoglycan, a complex organic polymer composed of N-acetylglucosamine (NAG) and N-acetylmuramic acid (NAM) units cross-linked by short peptides. Spanning the stack of peptidoglycan is teichoic acid. These give the gram-positive cell wall an overall negative charge because of the presence of phosphodiester bonds between the teichoic acid monomers. However, the −COOH group of the peptidoglycan molecules is the major metal binding site in gram-positive bacteria.

Gram-negative bacteria consist of a thin layer of peptidoglycan composed of only 20% in the periplasmic space between the inner and outer lipid membranes. The outer membrane (OM) consists of lipopolysaccharides on its outer leaflet and facilitates non-vesicle-mediated transport through channels (e.g., porins) or specialized transporters. The highly charged nature of LPS (lipopolysaccharide) confers an overall negative charge on the gram-negative cell wall. But gram-negative bacterial cell membranes are lower in these components and are poorer metal absorbers. Microbial extracellular polymers that form slime layers or capsules also have metal-binding capacity. They are mainly composed of glycoproteins, LPSs, and polysaccharides, which may be associated with polysaccharides, lipids, and proteins. Table 8.1 summarizes some studies on biosorption of different heavy metals by living and dead biomass of bacteria.

TABLE 8.1
Heavy Metals Biosorption by Living and/or Nonliving Biomass Bacteria

Microbial Biomass	Heavy Metal	Functional Group	Mechanism	References
Acinetobacter haemolyticus	Cr^{6+}	–COOH, –OH, and $CONH_2$–R	Complexation	Ahmad et al. (2013)
Aeromonas hydrophila	Pb^{2+}	COOH, –OH, and $-NH_2$	—	Hasan et al. (2009)
Arthrobacter sp.	Eu^{3+}	–OH, C=O, and $-NH_2$	Adsorption	Cadogan et al. (2015)
Bacillus cereus, Bacillus pumilis	Cr^{6+}	—	—	Sultan et al. (2012)
Bacillus sphaericus	Cu^{2+}, Ni^{2+}, and Cr^{6+}	—	Ion exchange, precipitation	Al-Daghistani (2012)
Bacillus thuringiensis	Eu^{3+}	–COOH, $-PO_3$, and –OH	Ion exchange	Pan et al. (2017)
Halomonas sp. TA-04	Cr^{6+}	—	Ion exchange	Focardi et al. (2012)
Mesorhizobium amorphae CCNWGS0123	Cu^{2+}	O–H, N–H, C–H, C=O, –NH, –CN, C–N, C–O, amide-I, –II, –III	Precipitation	Mohamad et al. (2012)
Micrococcus sp.	Cr, Ni	—	—	Congeevaram et al. (2007)
Pseudomonas plecoglossicida	Cd^{2+}	–NH, –OH, –CH, and –CONH	Ion exchange, electrostatic interaction	Guo et al. (2012)
Pseudomonas aeruginosa and Bacillus subtilis	Cr^{6+}	—	—	Tarangini et al. (2009)

(Continued)

TABLE 8.1 (*Continued*)

Heavy Metals Biosorption by Living and/or Nonliving Biomass Bacteria

Microbial Biomass	Heavy Metal	Functional Group	Mechanism	References
Pseudomonas alcaligene, Pseudomonas resinovorans	As^{5+}	$-OH$, $-COOH$, and NH_2	Chemisorption	Banerjee et al. (2016)
Pseudomonas putida	Al^{3+}	$-OH$, $-COOH$, and $-PO_3$	Adsorption	Boeris et al. (2016)
Pseudomonas putida V1.	Methymurcury	—	Ion exchange	Cabral et al. (2014)
Pseudomonas sp. G1	Cu^{2+}, Zn_{2+}	—	Adsorption	Wierzba (2010)
Pseudomonas sp. I3	Pb^{2+}	$-CH_2$, $C-O$, $C-N$, $N-H$, $-COO$ and $-SO_3$	Adsorption	Li et al. (2017)
Rhodosporidium fluviale	$Cs+$	—	Adsoprtion, ion exchange	Lan et al. (2014)
Sphaerotilus natans	Cd^{2+}, Cu^{2+}	—	—	Esposito et al. (2001)
Stenotrophomonas maltophilia	Cu^{2+}, Cd^{2+}, and Pb^{2+}	—	—	Parungao et al. (2007)
Streptomyces violaceoruber strain LZ-26-1	Cr^{6+}	—	—	Chen et al. (2014)
Yarrowia lipolytica	Ni^{2+}	$-OH$, $-COOH$, $C=O$, $-NH$	Ion exchange	Shinde et al. (2012)

Biosorption of Heavy Metals by Fungi and Yeast

Fungi and yeast are used in various industrial fermentation processes because they serve as an economical and endless supply of biomass for the removal of metals ions in polluted environments. Many fungi have high chitin content in their cell walls, and this polymer of N-acetyl glucosamine is an effective metal and radionuclide biosorbent. Fungal phenolic polymers and melanins contain peptides, phenolic units, fatty acids, carbohydrates, and aliphatic hydrocarbons; therefore, they possess many potential binding sites for metal ions. The oxygen-containing groups in these substances, including $-H$, $-COOH$, carbonyl, methoxyl, and phenolic groups, may be particularly important in the binding of metal ions. In addition, nitrogen-containing groups such as $-NH_2$ groups are considered to be important metals binding sites. The $-NH_2$ groups of chitin were found to be a main site of thorium (Th) uptake in *Rhizopus arrhizus*. Many fungi and yeast have excellent biosorbents of heavy metals; examples include *Trichoderma harzianum, T. virens, T. autroviride,* and *Aspergillus niger, Rhizopus, Aspergillus, Streptoverticullum, Sacchromyces, Penicillium spp.,* and

Rhizopus arrhizus. Table 8.2 summarizes some studies on biosorption of various heavy metals by living and dead biomass of fungi and yeast. In contrast, the cell walls of fungi, especially the filamentous ones, are composed of polysaccharides such as β-glucan, chitin and chitosan, glycoproteins, lipids, melanins, D-galactosamine polymers, and polyuronides. The chemical groups $-RCONH_2$, PO_4^{3-}, $-NH_2$, $-SH$, $-COOH$, $-OH$, and amine are considered good metal binding sites (Vimala and Das, 2011).

Biosorption of Heavy Metals by Algae

Algae (microalgae, cynobacteria, unicellular algae, and macroalgae) are photoautotrophic organisms adapted to a wide range of environmental conditions such as soil, fresh- and saltwater habitats, as well as domestic and industrial wastes dumping sites. They have a high SA:V ratio available for contact with the surrounding nutrients. In

---

TABLE 8.2

Heavy Metals Biosorption by Living and/or Nonliving Biomass of Fungi and Yeast

Microbial Biomass	Heavy Metal	Functional Group	Mechanism	References
Aspergillus flavus	Pb^{2+}, Cu^{2+}	—	—	Akar and Tunali (2006.)
Aspergillus niger	Cr^{6+}	$-COOH$, $-C-H$, $-N-H$, and $O-H$	Precipitation	Mondal et al. (2017)
Aspergillus niger	Zn^{2+}, Co^{2+}, and Cd^{2+}	—	—	Hajahmadi et al. (2015)
Aspergillus niger, Penicillium austurianum, Saccharomyces cerevisiae, Trichoderma reesi	Pb^{2+}	—	Precipitation	Awofolu et al. (2006)
Aspergillus niger, Penicillium chrysogenum and Rhizopus oryzae	Zn^{2+}, Cu^{2+}	—	—	Tahir et al. (2017)
Aspergillus terreus	Sr^{2+}	—-	—-	Khani et al. (2012)
Aspergillus sp.	Cr^{6+}, Ni^{2+}	—	—	Congeevaram et al. (2007)
Botrytis cinerea	Zn^{2+}	$-OH$, $-NH$	Precipitation	Tunali and Akar (2006)
Cicer arientinum	Fe^{3+}	$-OH$, $-COOH$, and $-NH$	Adsorption	Ahalya et al. (2006)
Cladophora hutchinsiae	U^{6+}	$-OH$, $-NH_2$, $C=O$, $=C-H$	—	Bagda e al. (2017)
Fusarium spp.	Zn^{2+}	—	—	Velmurugan et al. (2010)

(Continued)

TABLE 8.2 (*Continued*)
Heavy Metals Biosorption by Living and/or Nonliving Biomass of Fungi and Yeast

Microbial Biomass	Heavy Metal	Functional Group	Mechanism	References
Mucor rouxii	Cu^{2+}	N–H, O–H, C =O, N–H	Precipitation	Shraboni et al. (2008)
Phanerochaete chrysosporium	Zn^{2+}, Cu^{2+}, and Ni^{2+},	—	—	Zouboulis et al. (2003)
Paecilomyces lilacinus	Cr^{6+}	—	—	Sharma and Adholeya (2011)
Phanerochaete chrysosporium, *Aspegillus awamori*, *Aspergillus flavus*, *Trichoderma viride*	Pb^{2+}, Cd^{2+}, Cu^{2+}, and Ni^{2+}		Complexation	Joshi et al. (2011)
Pichia jadinii and *Pichia anomala*	Cr^{6+}	—	Oxidation-reduction	Martorell et al. (2012)
Pycnoporus sanguineus	Pb^{2+}, Cu^{2+}, and Cd^{2+}		Precipitation	Zulfadhly et al. (2001)
Rhizopus and *Aspergillus* spp.	Cd^{2+}, Cr^{6+}	—	—	Zafar et al. (2007)
Saccharomyces cerevisiae	U^{6+}	–OH, N–H, C=O, $-PO_3$,	Complexation, precipitation	Wang et al. (2017)
Streptomyces ciscaucasicus	Zn^{2+}	–OH, –NH, –COOH, and C–O	Complexation	Li et al. (2010)
Streptomyces rimosus	Pb^{2+}	–COO, –C–O, –NH, –C=O, and –OH	Complexation	Selatnia et al. (2004)
Trichoderma asperellum	Cr^{6+}	—	Precipitation	Chang et al. (2016)
Trichoderma sp.	Ni^{2+}, Cd^{2+}	—	Precipitation	Nongmaithem et al. (2016)

algae, cell surface is the main metal binding site, and heavy metal sorption involves exchange of metal ions with surface-bound protons or cations. Other binding sites in algae are polysaccharides such as glycan, alginic acid, proteins, mannan, and xylans. The cell wall of algae are composed mainly of cellulose, while the cell wall of cyanobacteria (blue–green algae) is composed of peptidoglycan; some species also produce sheaths and EPSs, which are used for sorption. The potential metal-binding groups in the cell walls of algae consist of polysaccharides, lipids, and proteins, which offer several functional groups, such as –OH, $-NH_2$, –COOH, $-PO_3$, and –SH, that confer a negative charge on the cell surface and provide a high binding affinity for different metal ions. Biosorption of heavy metals by microalgae is generally a biphasic process. The first phase is adsorption by extracellular cell surface associated molecules, which depends on the pH of the medium, heavy metal species, biomass concentration, and type of algae. The second phase is absorption and accumulation of metal ions inside the cell. This is a slow and time-consuming process involving active transport through the cell membrane into the interior and binding to proteins and other intracellular components. It is a metabolic-dependent mechanism that is inhibited by low temperatures, metabolic inhibitors, absence of energy sources, and uncouplers and occurs only in living cells (Wilde and Benemann, 1993) (Table 8.3).

TABLE 8.3

Heavy Metals Biosorption by Living and/or Nonliving Biomass of Algae

Microbial Biomass	Heavy Metal	Functional Group	Mechanism	References
Chlamydomonas reinhardtii	Pb^{2+}, Cu^{2+}	—	Physical adsorption, ion exchange	Flouty and Estephane (2012)
Cladophora fracta	Cd^{2+}, Hg^{2+}, Cu^{2+}, and Zn^{2+}	—	—	Ji et al. (2012)
Cyanobacteria Microcystis	Sb^{3+}	$-COOH$, $-OH$, and $-NH_2$	Complexation	Sun et al. (2011)
Cyanobacteria microcystis	Sb^{3+}	$-COOH$, $-OH$, and $-NH_2$	Complexation	Wu et al. (2012)
Desmodesmus pleiomorphus	Zn^{2+}, Cd^{2+}	—	Precipitation	Monteiro et al. (2011)
Mixture and *Spirulina maxima*	Cu^{2+}, Zn^{2+}	—	Complexation, adsorption	Chan et al. (2014)
Oedogonium westti	Cd^{2+}, Cr^{6+}, Ni^{2+}, and Pb^{2+}	—	Physical adsorption, ion exchange	Shamshad et al. (2016)
Pelvetia canaliculata	Cr^{6+}	—	Ion exchange	Hackbarth et al. (2016)
Phormidium ambiguum, *Pseudochlorococcum typicum* and *Scenedesmus quadricauda var quadrispina*	Cd^{2+}, Pb^{2+}, and Hg^{2+}	—	Complexation, precipitation	Shanab et al. (2012)
Sargassum cymosum	Cr^{6+}	—	Ion exchange	Souza, et al. (2016)
Sargassum filipendula	Cu^{2+}, Ni^{2+}, and Pb^{2+}	—	Precipitation	Munaro et al. (2015)
Scenedesmus obliquus	Zn^{2+}, Cd^{2+}	—	Precipitation	Monteiro et al. (2011)
Spirogyra hyalina	Cd^{2+}, Hg^{2+}, Pb^{2+}, As, and Co	—	Complexation, adsorption	Nirmal Kumar and Oommen (2012)

(Continued)

TABLE 8.3 (*Continued*)
Heavy Metals Biosorption by Living and/or Nonliving Biomass of Algae

Microbial Biomass	Heavy Metal	Functional Group	Mechanism	References
Spirulina platensis	Cr^{6+}		Physical adsorption, ion exchange	Kwak et al. (2015)
Spirulina sp.	Cr^{3+}, Cd^{2+}, and Cu^{2+}	–CCOH, –OH, –PO₃ NH, and C=O	Physical adsorption, ion exchange	Chojnacka et al. (2005), Rezaei (2016)
Tetraselmis suecica	Cd^{2+}		Physical adsorption, ion exchange	Pérez-Rama et al. (2010)

METABOLIC-DEPENDENT INTRACELLULAR ACCUMULATION (ACTIVE UPTAKE)

Transport of heavy metal ions across a microbial cell membrane into the cytoplasm, known as intracellular accumulation, may be mediated by the same mechanism used to convey metabolically important ions such as K^+, Mg^+, and Na^+ (Gadd, 1990). This is referred to as bioaccumulation, or active uptake, and depends on metabolic energy of microorganisms and a variety of physical and chemical processes, for example, adsorption, precipitation, and complexation. Bioaccumulation of heavy metal is a slow metabolic-dependent removal mechanism that includes the influx of heavy metals across the bacterial membranes through ion channels, ion pumps, carrier-mediated transport, endocytosis, and lipid permeation (Gadd, 1990, 2010). After uptake into cells, metals may be compartmentalized and/or converted into more innocuous forms by binding or precipitation (Gadd, 1990). Generally, bioaccumulation occurs when an organism absorbs a toxic substance at a rate greater than that at which the substance is lost.

The organism used for accumulating heavy metal ions should have a tolerance to one or more metals at elevated concentration and must exhibit enhanced transformation abilities. Heavy metal accumulation by microorganisms can be studied by the expression of metal-binding cysteine-rich peptides such as phytochelatins (PCs), glutathione (GSH), and metallothioneins (MTs) (Gadd, 2010) that bind metal ions (such as Cd^{2+}, Pb^{2+}, Hg^{2+}, and Cu^{2+}) and sequester them in biologically inactive forms. The production of these novel metal-detoxifying proteins is induced by the presence of metal ions. In eukaryotic microorganisms, for example, fungi and yeasts, a majority of intracellular Co^{2+}, Mn^{1+}, Zn^{2+}, Mg^{2+}, and K^+ is located in the vacuole, where there may be binding to low-molecular-weight polyphosphate. In this process, heavy metals form complexes with specific proteins like MTs.

Accumulation of Metals in Bacteria

Heavy metals such as Cu^{2+}, Ni^{2+}, Zn^{2+}, and Cd^{2+} are required by bacteria in trace amounts as enzyme cofactors and as structural components of proteins. Bacterial cells are constantly exposed to stressful environments and have the ability to resist those stresses, which is necessary for their survival. The capability of microorganisms to grow in the presence of high metal concentrations might result from specific mechanisms of resistance such as alteration of solubility and toxicity, efflux systems, precipitation, or extracellular complexation of metals. Metal resistance genes are located on plasmids, chromosomes, or transposons. However, some heavy metal resistance systems are usually chromosomal-based and are more complex than plasmid systems, which are usually toxic-ion efflux pumps. The main processes for regulating the intracellular concentrations of inorganic cations and anions are membrane transport systems. Under certain condition, metal ions can be accumulated by uptake systems with high substrate specificity. Bacteria have several resistance mechanisms by which they can mobilize, immobilize, or transform metals, thus reducing the metals' toxicity and allowing the bacteria to tolerate heavy metal ion uptake. The major mechanisms are physical sequestration, exclusion, complexation, detoxification, and so on (Figure 8.1). Generally, bacterial cells take up the heavy metal cations of similar size, structure, and valence with the same mechanism. They possess two types of metal ion uptake systems: one is fast and unspecific, and is driven by the chemiosmotic gradient across the cytoplasmic membrane; the other type is slower, exhibits high substrate specificity, and is coupled with ATP hydrolysis. Sometimes, crystallization and precipitation of heavy metals takes place because of bacteria-mediated reactions or due to the production of specific metabolites. Several bacteria have developed a cytosolic sequestration mechanism for defense from heavy metal toxicity. In this process, metal ions might also become compartmentalized or converted into more innocuous forms after entering the bacterial cell. This detoxification mechanism in bacteria facilitates accumulation of metals in high concentrations. In addition, certain bacteria utilize methylation as an alternative for metal resistance or detoxification mechanism. In addition, microorganisms can eliminate several heavy metals from the metal-polluted soils by reducing them to a lower redox state. Bacterial species that catalyze such reducing reactions are referred to as dissimilatory metal-reducing bacteria, and they exploit metals as terminal electron acceptors in anaerobic respiration; most of them use Fe^{3+} and S^0 as terminal electron acceptors. Metal-chelating agents, called siderophores, secreted by bacteria and fungi have an important role in the acquisition of several heavy metals (Figure 8.2).

Accumulation of Metals in Fungi and Yeast

Some metals are essential to fungi and yeast; others are toxic even in minute quantities. However, some highly adapted fungi have evolved metal resistance systems to enable them to grow at lethal concentrations of heavy metals. The viable and nonviable biomass of fungi exhibited the ability to accumulate metal ions, and conditions such as pH level, initial metal concentration, exposure time, and biomass concentration have an influential effect on metal uptake. Bioaccumulation of heavy metals in fungi and yeast encompasses a combination of several processes like complication, electrostatic attraction, ion exchange, van der Waals forces, covalent binding, precipitation, and adsorption. Fungi and yeast can also produce MTs, GSH, and PCs in response to the presence of toxic metals; some of these are metal-specific and may bind to the intracellular content of metals, thereby conferring resistance to the

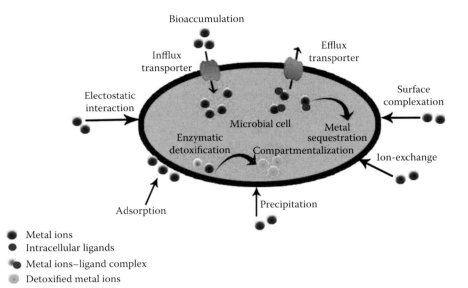

FIGURE 8.2   Heavy metal uptake and detoxification processes inside living bacteria cells.

metals. In addition, mechanisms such as excretion or compartmentalization, and exclusion of toxic heavy metals from cells by ion-selective metal transporters have been proposed for reducing heavy metal toxicity in fungi. Fungal vacuoles also play important roles in regulation of cytosolic concentrations of metal ions, metal detoxification, and storage of metabolites, and they may detoxify potentially toxic metal ions. A schematic of heavy metal accumulation in fungi is illustrated in Figure 8.3.

Accumulation of Metals in Algae

Algae are abundant and are well adapted to a wide range of habitats such as domestic and industrial effluents, fresh- and saltwater, constructed wetlands, and salt marshes. They have a significant ability to uptake and accumulate heavy metals from their surrounding environment. Heavy metals enter microalgae cells via micronutrient transporters. Once in the cell, algae respond to heavy metals by the synthesis of low-molecular-weight compounds such as carotenoids and GSH, and the induction of several antioxidants, as well as enzymes (i.e., glutathione peroxidase, superoxide dismutase, ascorbate peroxidase, and catalase). In algae, heavy metal detoxification may be achieved by binding to specific intracellular compounds and/or transport of the metals to specific cellular compartments. Algal tolerance to heavy metal seems to be highly dependent, however, on the defense responses against the possible oxidative damages, active efflux of metal ions by primary ATPase pumps, and the exudation capacity of chelating compounds. The metal-binding proteins in plants and algae were generally assumed to be MTs, and they play a key role in metal-binding ligands. Heavy metal ions can cause cell membrane depolarization and cell cytoplasm acidification. A schematic of heavy metal accumulation in algae is presented in Figure 8.3.

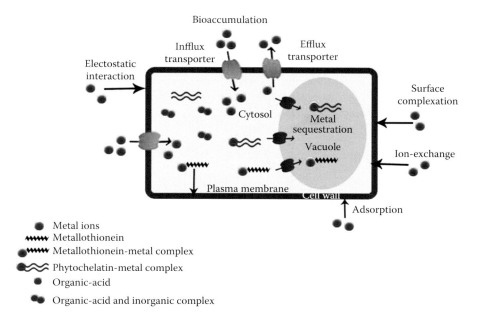

Metal ions
Metallothionein
Metallothionein-metal complex
Phytochelatin-metal complex
Organic-acid
Organic-acid and inorganic complex

FIGURE 8.3 Heavy metal uptake and detoxification processes inside living fungi and algae cells.

FACTORS AFFECTING THE BIOREMEDIATION OF HEAVY METALS

Microorganisms can detoxify and transform numerous heavy metals because of their metabolic activity and their capacity to adapt to extreme environments. Application of bioremediation technologies through biostimulation and bioaugmentation approaches with microorganisms is frequently successful. However, the scope and rate of microbial remediation of pollutants depends on the concentration and chemical structure of pollutants, their availability to microorganisms, the number and type of microorganisms available for detoxifying or transforming heavy metals, and the physiochemical properties of the environment to which the pollutants are released. Factors that influence the rate of microbial remediation of heavy metals can be classified as either biological (related to microorganisms and their nutritional requirements) or environmental (related to the environment).

BIOLOGICAL FACTORS

Heavy Metal Interaction with Soil Organic Matter

The fate of pollutants in the media (soil, sediment, and water) depends on the media properties and physiochemical characteristics of the pollutants. Heavy metals persist in the environment for long periods, and the soil serves as a large sink for them. Soil organic matter, soil type, and mineral fraction affect the adsorption of heavy metal ions to the solid surface. Sufficient soil organic matter reduces the bioavailability of metals and decreases bioaccumulation in living biosphere, which in turn results in long-term pollution in soils. Metal ions can bind to other organic and inorganic chemical components of the soil matrix, protecting the metals from chemical as well as biological transformation. In this case, the soil acts as a filter, and defensive microorganisms and plant roots prevent groundwater pollution. Absorption is an analogous process in which a pollutant penetrates into the bulk mass of the soil matrix. Both adsorption and absorption reduce the availability of heavy metals to most microorganisms, and their metabolized rate is proportionally reduced; nonadsorbed molecules are bioavailable and thus are exposed to degradation and transformation.

Nutrient Availability

Nutrient availability affects the microbial transformation and detoxification process of heavy metals, including direct inhibition of the proliferation process and enzymatic activities of pollutant-degrading organisms. This inhibition can occur, for example, if there is competition between microorganisms for limited nutrients, antagonistic interactions between microorganisms, or the predation of microorganisms by bacteriophages and protozoans for their growth and survival. In addition, microorganisms require minerals such nitrogen (N), phosphate (P), and potassium (K) as nutrients for cellular metabolism and successful growth in polluted sites. In contaminated sites, organic carbon levels are often high because of the nature of the pollutants, and easily available nutrients can become rapidly depleted during microbial growth. Therefore, it is common practice to supplement contaminated land with nutrients and thus stimulate the *in situ* microbial communities and enhance biodegradation of the pollutants.

Bioavailability of Heavy Metals

The fractions of a chemical pollutant in soil that can be taken up or altered by living organisms is called bioavailability. Two important factors determine the amount of bioavailable pollutant: mass transfer and intrinsic activity of cell. Bioavailability differs between species and organisms, so it can be defined in terms of specific organisms as the extent to which a pollutant is free to move into or onto a specific organism. The *in situ* microbial transformation of inorganic pollutants is a function of the bioavailability of the a specific pollutant and the catabolic activity of microbes.

Toxicity of End Products

The principle of bioremediation is to degrade or to transform hazardous compounds to less hazardous forms using living microorganisms or microbial consortia. It should be noted that in some instances, however, the metabolites formed during biodegradation and biotransformation processes are more toxic that the parent compound. Thus, it is important to ensure that the toxic pollutants are suitably detoxified at the end of the degradation process.

Environmental Factors

Environmental factors, such as pH, temperature, oxygen, and moisture availability, vary from location (site) to location (site) and can influence the process of metal remediation by inhibiting the growth of indigenous pollutant-degrading and/or pollutant-transforming microorganisms. Among environmental factors, pH is one of the most significant for bioremediation of environmental pollutants. Bioremediation can occur under a wide range of pH, but a pH between 6.5 and 8.5 is generally optimal for biodegradation and/or biotransformation of pollutants in most terrestrial and aquatic ecosystems.

Temperature has also a considerable effect on heavy metal remediation from contaminated sites. The solubility of heavy metals increases with temperature, which ultimately increases the bioavailability of heavy metals to microorganisms. In addition, oxygen solubility decreases with increasing temperature, which reduces the metabolic activity of aerobic microorganisms. Bioremediation of heavy metals can proceed under both aerobic and anaerobic conditions; most work has tended to focus on the dynamics of aerobic metabolism of heavy metals, partly because of the ease of study and the culture of aerobic microorganisms relative to anaerobic microorganisms. Moisture is also required for all biological processes to help transport waste products, food, water, and nutrients in and out of the microbial cell. Moisture influences the rate of contaminant metabolized by microorganisms because it influences the kind and amount of soluble materials that are available as well as the osmotic pressure and pH of terrestrial and aquatic systems.

CONCLUSION

Heavy metals are a great concern because of increased industrial activity, which is increasing the amount of heavy metals in the environment. Heavy metal exposure causes several, often fatal consequences to organs and tissues through mechanisms such as oxidative stress and that often lead to cell death. Existing and traditional treatment methods, such as oxidation reduction, chemical precipitation, ion exchange, filtration, reverse osmosis, evaporation, membrane technology, and electrochemical treatment, are used for the removal of heavy metals from soil and water. These methods are not sufficient, however, to eradicate the problem, and the disadvantages of their use include high cost, incomplete removal of heavy metals, and production of more toxic sludge during treatment. There is obviously a need to develop effective bioremediation techniques for detoxifying heavy metals completely. Recent technology using microbes and their enzymes for the detoxification and biotransformation of heavy metals is better for the environment. Bioremediation using microbes that have the ability to accumulate and transform heavy metals means better-quality soil and water. Depending on the type of heavy metals, different mechanisms of bioremediation have been implemented by microorganisms. It can be said that microbial bioremediation technology has given us a platform that directs us toward the elimination of heavy metal contamination in an eco-friendly manner.

REFERENCES

Ahalya N, Kanamadi RD, Ramachandra TV. 2006. Biosorption of iron(III) from aqueous solutions using the husk of *Cicer arientinum*. *Indian Journal of Chemical Technology* 13: 122–127.

Ahmad WA, Ahmad WHW, Karim NA, Raj ASS, Zakaria ZA. 2013. Cr(VI) reduction in naturally rich growth medium and sugarcane bagasse by *Acinetobacter haemolyticus*. *International Biodeterioration and Biodegradation* 85: 571–576.

Akar T, Tunali S. 2006. Biosorption characteristics of Aspergillus flavus biomass for removal of Pb(II) ions from an aqueous solution. *Bioresource Technology* 97: 1780–1787.

Akhtar MS, Chali B, Azam T. 2013. Bioremediation of arsenic and lead by plants and microbes from contaminated soil. *Research in Plant Sciences* 1.3: 68–73.

Aksu Z, Sag Y, and Kutsal T. 1992. The biosorption of Cu (II) by C. Vulgaris and Z. ramigera. *Environmetal Technology* 13: 579–586.

Al-Daghistani HI. 2012. Bio-remediation of Cu, Ni and Cr from rotogravure wastewater using immobilized, dead, and live biomass of indigenous thermophilic *Bacillus* species. *The International Journal of Microbiology* 10(1). DOI: 10.5580/2a7f.

Awofolu O, Okonkwo J, Roux-Van Der Merwe R, Badenhorst J, Jordaan E. 2006. A new approach to chemical modification protocols of *Aspergillus niger* and sorption of lead ion by fungal species. *Electronic Journal of Biotechnology* 9(4): 340–348.

Azubuike CC, Chikere CB, Okpokwasili GC. 2016. Bioremediation techniques–classification based on site of application: Principles, advantages, limitations and prospects. *World Journal of Microbiology and Biotechnology* 32: 180.

Bagda E, Tuzen M, Sari A. 2017. Equilibrium, thermodynamic and kinetic investigations for biosorption of uranium with green algae (*Cladophora hutchinsiae*). *Journal of Environmental Radioactivity* 175–176: 7–14.

Banerjee A, Sarkar P, Banerjee S. 2016. Application of statistical design of experiments for optimization of As(V) biosorption by immobilized bacterial biomass. *Ecological Engineering* 86: 13–23.

Barakat MA. 2011. New trends in removing heavy metals from industrial wastewater. *Arabian Journal of Chemistry* 4: 361–377.

Bishop PL. 2002. *Pollution Prevention: Fundamentals and Practice*. Tsinghua University Press, Beijing, China.

Boeris PS, del Rosario Agustín M, Acevedo DF, Lucchesi GI. 2016. Biosorption of aluminum through the use of non-viable biomass of *Pseudomonas putida*. *Journal of Biotechnology* 236: 57–63.

Cabral L, Giovanella P, Kerlleman A, Gianello C, Bento FM, Camargo FAO. 2014. Impact of selected anions and metals on the growth and in vitro removal of methylmercury by *Pseudomonas putida* V1. *International Biodeterioration and Biodegradation* 91: 29–36.

Cadogan EI, Lee C, Popuri SR. 2015. Facile synthesis of chitosan derivatives and Arthrobacter sp. Biomass for the removal of europium(III) ions from aqueous solution through biosorption. *International Biodeterioration and Biodegradation* 102: 286–297.

Chan A, Salsali H, McBean E. 2014. Heavy metal removal (copper and zinc) in secondary effluent from wastewater treatment plants by microalgae. *ACS Sustainable Chemical Engineering* 2: 130–137.

Chang F, Tian C, Liu S, Ni J. 2016. Discrepant hexavalent chromium tolerance and detoxification by two strains of *Trichoderma asperellum* with high homology. *Chemical Engineering Journal* 298: 75–81.

Chen Z, Zou L, Zhang H, Chen Y, Liu P, Li X. 2014. Thioredoxin is involved in hexavalent chromium reduction in *Streptomyces violaceoruber* strain LZ-26-1 isolated from the Lanzhou reaches of the Yellow River. *International Biodeterioration and Biodegradation* 94: 146–151.

Chojnacka K, Chojnacki A, Gorecka H. 2005. Biosorption of Cr(III), Cd(II) and Cu(II) ions by blue-green algae *Spirulina* sp. *Chemosphere* 59: 75–84.

Congeevaram S, Dhanarani S, Park J, Dexilin M, Thamaraiselvi K. 2007. Biosorption of chromium and nickel by heavy metal resistant fungal and bacterial isolates. *Journal of Hazardous Materials* 146: 270–277.

Esposito A, Pagnanelli F, Lodi A, Solisio C, Veglio F. 2001. Biosorption of heavy metals by *Sphaerotilus natans*: An equilibrium study at different pH and biomass concentrations. *Hydrometallurgy* 60: 129–141.

Flouty R, Estephane G. 2012. Bioaccumulation and biosorption of copper and lead by a unicellular algae *Chlamydomonas reinhardtii* in single and binary metal systems. *Journal of Environmental Management* 111: 106–114.

Focardi S, Pepi, M., Landi, G., Gasperini, G., Ruta, M., et al. 2012. Hexavalent chromium reduction by whole cells and cell free extract of the moderate halophilic bacterial strain *Halomonas* sp. TA-04. *International Biodeterioration and Biodegradation* 66: 63–70.

Fomina M, Gadd GM. 2014. Biosorption: Current perspectives on concept, definition and application. *Bioresource Technology* 160: 3–14.

Gadd GM. 1990. Heavy metal accumulation by bacteria and other microorganisms. *Experientia* 46: 834–840.

Gadd GM. 2000. Bioremedial potential of microbial mechanisms of metal mobilization and immobilization. *Current Opinion in Biotechnology* 11: 271–279.

Gadd GM. 2004. Microbial influence on metal mobility and application for bioremediation. *Geoderma* 122: 109–119.

Gadd GM. 2010. Metals, minerals and microbes: Geomicrobiology and bioremediation. *Microbiology* 156: 609–643.

Govarthanan M, Lee GW, Park JH, Kim JS, Lim SS, et al. 2014. Bioleaching characteristics, influencing factors of Cu solubilization and survival of *Herbaspirillum* sp. GW103 in Cu contaminated mine soil. *Chemosphere* 109: 42–48.

Guo J, Zheng XD, Chen QB, Zhang L, Xu XP. 2012. Biosorption of Cd(II) from aqueous solution by *Pseudomonas plecoglossicida*. *Current Microbiology* 65: 350–355.

Hackbarth FV, Maass D, Souza AAU, Vilar VJP, Souza SMAGU. 2016. Removal of hexavalent chromium from electroplating wastewaters using marine macroalga *Pelvetia canaliculata* as natural electron donor. *Chemical Engineering Journal* 290: 477–489.

Hajahmadi Z, Younesi H, Bahramifar N, Khakpour H, Pirzadeh K. 2015. Multicomponent isotherm for biosorption of Zn(II), CO(II) and Cd(II) from ternary mixture on to pretreated dried *Aspergillus niger* biomass. *Water Resources and Industry* 11: 71–80.

Hasan SH, Srivastava P, Talat M. 2009. Biosorption of Pb(II) from water using biomass of Aeromonas hydrophila: Central composite design for optimization of process variables. *Journal of Hazardous Materials* 168: 1155–1162.

Ianeva OD. 2009. Mechanisms of bacteria resistance to heavy metals. *Mikrobiol Z* 71(6): 54–65.

Ji L, Xie S, Feng J, Li Y, Chen L. 2012. Heavy metal uptake capacities by the common freshwater green alga *Cladophora fracta*. *Journal of Applied Phycology* 24: 979–983.

Joshi PK, Swarup A, Maheshwari S, Kumar R, Singh N. 2011. Bioremediation of heavy metals in liquid media through fungi isolated from contaminated sources. *Indian Journal of Microbiology* 51(4): 482–487.

Khani MH, Pahlavanzadek H, Alizadeh K. 2012. Biosorption of strontium from aqueous solution by fungus Aspergillus terreus. *Environmental Science and Pollution Research International* 19: 2408–2418.

Kwak HW, Kim MK, Lee JY, Yun H, Kim MH, et al. 2015. Preparation of bead-type biosorbent from water-soluble *Spirulina platensis* extracts for chromium (VI) removal. *Algal Research* 7: 92–99.

Lan T, Feng Y, Liao J, Li X, Ding C, et al. 2014. Biosorption behavior and mechanism of cesium-137 on Rhodosporidium fluviale strain UA2 isolated from cesium solution. *Journal of Environmental Radioactivity* 134: 6–13.

Lovley DR. 2000. Fe(III) and Mn(IV) reduction. In: Lovley, DR. (Ed.), Environmental Microbe –Metal Interactions. *American Society of Microbiology*, Washington, pp. 3–30.

Li D, Xu X, Yu H, Han X. 2017. Characterization of Pb^{2+} biosorption by psychrotrophic strain *Pseudomonas* sp. I3 isolated from permafrost soil of Mohe wetland in Northeast China. *Journal of Environmental Management* 1962: 8–15.

Li H, Lin Y, Guan W, Chang J, Xu L, et al. 2010. Biosorption of Zn(II) by live and dead cells of *Streptomyces ciscaucasicus* strain CCNWHX 72–14. *Journal of Hazardous Materials* 179: 151–159.

Martorell MM, Fernandez PM, Farina JI, Figueroa LIC. 2012. Cr (VI) reduction by cell-free extracts of *Pichia jadinii* and *Pichia anomala* isolated from textile-dye factory effluents. *International Biodeterioration and Biodegradation* 71: 80–85.

Mohamad OA, Hao X, Xie P, Hatab S, Lin Y, Wei G. 2012. Biosorption of copper(II) from aqueous solution using nonliving *Mesorhizobium amorphae* strain CCNWGS0123. *Microbes and Environments* 27: 234–241.

Mondal NK, Samanta A, Dutta S, Chattoraj S. 2017. Optimization of Cr (VI) biosorption onto *Aspergillus niger* using 3-level Box-Behnken design: Equilibrium, kinetic, thermodynamic and regeneration studies. *Journal of Genetic Engineering and Biotechnology*. Doi: 10.1016/j.jgeb.2017.01.006.

Monteiro CM, Castro PML, Malcat FX. 2011. Capacity of simultaneous removal of zinc and cadmium from contaminated media, by two microalgae isolated from a polluted site. *Environmental Chemistry Letter* 9: 511–517.

Munaro MT, Bertagnolli C, Kleinubing SJ, Silva MGC, Silva EA. 2015. Bioadsorç ao e dessorç~ao dos íons CU23, NI2þ e PB2þ pelo resíduo da extraç~ao do alginato da alga *Sargassum filipendula*. *Blucher Chemical Engineering Proceedings* 2: 1–10.

Nirmal Kumar JI, Oommen C. 2012. Removal of heavy metals by biosorption using freshwater alga Spirogyra hyaline. *Journal of Environmental Biology* 33(1): 27–31.

Nongmaithem N, Roy A, Bhattacharya PM. 2016. Screening of *Trichoderma* isolates for their potential of biosorption of nickel and cadmium. *Brazilian Journal of Biotechnology* 47(2016): 305–313.

Pan X, Wu W, Lü J, Chen Z, Li L, et al. 2017. Biosorption and extraction of europium by *Bacillus thuringiensis* strain. *Inorganic Chemistry Communications* 75(2017): 21–24.

Parungao MM, Tacata PS, Tanayan CRG, Trinidad LC. 2007. Biosorption of copper, cadmium and lead by copper-resistant bacteria isolated from Mogpog River, Marinduque. *Philippine Journal of Science* 136(2): 155–165.

Pérez-Rama M, Torres E, Suáre C, Herrero C, Abalde J. 2010. Sorption isotherm studies of Cd(II) ions using living cells of the marine microalga Tetraselmis suecica (Kylin) Butch. *Journal of Environmental Management* 91: 2045–2050.

Rani A, Souche YS, Goel R. 2009. Comparative assessment of *in situ* bioremediaticn potential of cadmium resistant acidophilic *Pseudomonas putida* 62BN and alkalophilic *Pseudomonas monteilli* 97AN strains on soybean. *International Biodeterioration and Biodegradation* 63: 62–66.

Rezaei H. 2016. Biosorption of chromium by using Spirulina sp. *Arabian Journal of Chemistry* 9(6): 846–853.

Rubinelli P, Siripornadulsil S, Gao-Rubinelli F, and Sayre RT. 2002. Cadmium- and iron-stress-inducible gene expression in the green alga *Chlamydomonas reinhardtii*: Evidence for H43 protein function in iron assimilation. *Planta* 215: 1–13.

Sarkar T, Masihul Alam M, Parvin N, Fardous Z, Chowdhury AZ, et al. 2016. Assessment of heavy metals contamination and human health risk in shrimp collected from different farms and rivers at Khulna-Satkhira region, Bangladesh. *Toxicology Reports* 3: 346–350.

Selatnia A, Boukazoula A, Kechid N, Bakhti MZ, Chergui A, Kerchich Y. 2004. Biosorption of lead (II) from aqueous solution by a bacterial dead *Streptomyces rimosus* biomass. *Biochemical Engineering Journal* 19: 127–135.

Shamshad I, Khan S, Waqas M, Asma M, Nawab J, et al. 2016. Heavy metal uptake capacity of fresh water algae (Oedogonium westti) from aqueous solution: A mesocosm research. *International Journal of Phytoremediation* 18: 4, 393–398.

Shanab S, Essa A, Shalaby E. 2012. Bioremoval capacity of three heavy metals by some microalgae species (Egyptian Isolates). *Plant Signaling and Behavior* 7: 3, 1–8.

Sharma S, Adholeya A. 2011. Detoxification and accumulation of chromium from tannery effluent and spent chrome effluent by *Paecilomyces lilacinus* fungi. *International Biodeterioration and Biodegradation* 65: 309–317.

Shinde N, Bankar A, Kumar A, Zinjarde S. 2012. Removal of Ni(II) ions from aqueous solutions by biosorption onto two strains of Yarrowia lipolytica. *Journal of Environmental Management* 102: 115–124.

Shraboni SM, Das SK, Sah T, Panda GC, Bandyopadhyoy T, Guha AK. 2008. Adsorption behavior of copper ions on *Mucor rouxii* biomass through microscopic and FTIR analysis. *Colloids and Surfaces B: Biointerfaces* 63: 138–145.

Smith WL, and Gadd GM. 2000. Reduction and precipitation of chromate by mixed culture sulphate-reducing bacterial biofilms. *Journal of Applied Microbiology* 88: 983–991.

Souza FB, Brandao HL, Hackbarth FV, Souza AAU, Boaventura RAR, et al. 2016. Marine macro-alga Sargassum cymosum as electron donor for hexavalent chromium reduction to trivalent state in aqueous solutions. *Chemical Engineering Journal* 283: 903–910.

Sultan S, Mubashar K, Faisal M. 2012. Uptake of toxic Cr(VI) by biomass of exo-polysaccharides producing bacterial strains. *African Journal of Microbiology Research* 6: 3329–3336.

Sun F, Wu F, Liao H, Xing B. 2011. Biosorption of antimony (V) by freshwater cyanobacteria Microcystis biomass. *Chemical Engineering Journal* 171: 1082–1090.

Tahir A, Lateef Z, Abdel-Megeed A, Sholkamy EN, Mostafa AA. 2017. In vitro compatibility of fungi for the biosorption of zinc(II) and copper(II) from electroplating effluent. *Current Science* 112(4): 839–844.

Tarangini K, Kumar A, Satpathy GR, Sangal VK. 2009. Statistical optimization of process parameters for Cr(VI) biosorption onto mixed cultures of *Pseudomonas aeruginosa* and Bacillus subtilis. *Soil, Air Water* 37: 319–327.

Tchounwou, PB, Yedjou CG, Patlolla AK, and Sutton DJ. 2012. Heavy Metals Toxicity and the Environment. *EXS* 101: 133–164.

Thompson-Eagle ET, Frankenberger WT. 1992. Bioremediation of soils contaminated with selenium. In R. Lal and B.A. Stewart, (Eds.) *Advances in Soil Science*, pp. 261–309. Springer, New York.

Tunali S, Akar T. 2006. Zn(II) biosorption properties of Botrytis cinerea biomass. *Journal of Hazardous Materials* 131: 137–145.

U.S. EPA. 2012. A citizen's guide to bioremediation. *EPA 542-F-12-003*.

Velmurugan P, Shim J, You Y, Choi S, Kamala-Kannan S, et al. 2010. Removal of zinc by live, dead, and dried biomass of *Fusarium* spp. isolated from the abandoned-metal mine in South Korea and its perspective of producing nanocrystals. *Journal of Hazardous Materials* 182: 317–324.

Vimala R, and Das N. 2011. Mechanism of Cd(II) adsorption by macrofungus *Pleurotus platypus*. Journal of Environmental Science 23(2): b288–293.

Vivaldi M. 2001. *Bioremediation: An Overview. Pure and Applied Chemistry* 73(7): 1163–1172.

Wang T, Zheng X, Wang X, Lu X, Shen Y. 2017. Different biosorption mechanisms of Uranium(VI) by live and heat-killed *Saccharomyces cerevisiae* under environmentally relevant conditions. *Journal of Environmental Radioactivity* 167: 92–99.

White C, Wilkinson SC, Gadd GM. 1995. The role of microorganisms in biosorption of toxic metals and radionuclides. *International Biodeterioration and Biodegradation* 35: 17–40.

Wierzba S. 2010. Heavy metals biosorption from aqueous solution by *Pseudomonas sp.* G1. *Proceedings of the ECOpole* 4: 85–89.

Wilde EW, and Benemann JR. 1993. Bioremoval of heavy metals by the use of microalgae. *Biotechnology Advances* 11: 781–812.

Wu F, Sun F, Wu S, Yan Y, Xing B. 2012. Removal of antimony(III) from aqueous solution by freshwater cyanobacteria Microcystis biomass. *Chemical Engineering Journal* 183: 172–179.

Zafar S, Aqil F, Ahmad I. 2007. Metal tolerance and biosorption potential of filamentous fungi isolated from metal contaminated agricultural soil. *Bioresource Technology* 98: 2557–2561.

Zouboulis AI, Matis KA, Loukidou M, Sebesta F. 2003. Metal biosorption by PAN-immobilized fungal biomass in simulated wastewaters. *Colloids and Surfaces A: Physicochemical and Engineering Aspects* 212: 185–195.

Zulfadhly Z, Mashitah MD, Bhatia S. 2001. Heavy metals removal in fixed-bed column by the macro fungus *Pycnoporus sanguineus*. *Environmental Pollution* 112: 463–470.

9 Enabling System Biology in Yeast for the Production of Advanced Biofuels

Arun Beniwal, Priyanka Saini,
Jagrani Minj, and Shilpa Vij

CONTENTS

INTRODUCTION

Since the beginning of civilization humans have used the microbial cell factory for the production of beverages and fermented foods. More recently, microbes have been cultivated to produce various valuable compounds and important chemicals like biofuel, which offers a widespread range of applications. Chaim Weizmann developed a process of acetone–butanol–ethanol (ABE) fermentation during World War I. It was used for the production of acetone for about 50 years, and it was recently revived in scientific community for 1-butanol production. Other old methods of fermentation were also given a second look and revived for the production of other valuable products.

Presently most biofuel produced in the United States is ethanol, which is mainly produced from corn. The production of the ethanol is strongly favored by current policy. After the adoption of the Renewable Fuel Standard (RFS), the blending of second-generation biofuels based on lignocellulosic feedstock was required from 2010 onward. The total amount of biofuel produced, now mandated by the RFS, is expected to surge from 15 billion liters in 2006 to approximately 136 billion liters in 2022 (Eisentraut, 2010). The RFS necessitates a rise in consumption of lignocellulosic-based ethanol from almost zero in 2010 to about 60.6 billion liters per year in 2022. The standard also calls for reducing greenhouse gases for the advanced biofuels of about 50%–60% compared to fossil fuels for making biofuel production more sustainable. These requirements in turn favor the growth of highly efficient biofuel technologies.

Recently, there has been substantial attention paid to the microbial cell factory–based production of the chemicals that were found naturally in plants and other organisms and also to the production of various humanmade chemicals, which, of course, have not been present in any organism (Mukhopadhyay et al., 2008).

Production of advanced biofuels, such as the alkanes, alkenes, and aromatics, by microorganisms always requires a significant retooling of the microorganisms' original metabolism. Great advances in phenotypic characterization using the latest tools have been made, and genome-editing tools have provided a step forward toward improving the characterization of the yeast cell factory. Despite the cutting-edge technology related to synthetic biology and systems biology, challenges remain for development of new microbial cell factories that can be used for the industrial production of valuable advanced chemicals (Figure 9.1). To ensure homeostasis in the

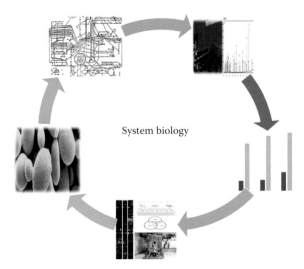

FIGURE 9.1 Steps in systems biology that achieve the desired production of the target biofuel. Complex biological systems such as whole yeast cells were analyzed with high throughput analytical techniques. A yeast cell factory must be selected and metabolically engineered for the production of advanced biofuel. The results obtained from metabolic engineering and new modeling approaches essentially must be evaluated using new molecular techniques. The cycle will be complete once the desired production level of the advanced biofuel has been achieved.

metabolic pathway when a cell factory is exposed to various environmental stress conditions, the yeast cells have developed regulations and multifaceted interactions between the different metabolic pathways (Saini et al., 2017). Therefore, the carbon flux must be redirected for the production of the desired metabolites. The engineering of the cell requires various rounds of what is called the design-build-test cycle by Nielsen and Keasling (2016). This cycle requires that the metabolic pathway be improved using genetic engineering for the production of desired compounds such as advanced biofuels (Langer, 2012; Caspeta et al., 2013).

ENGINEERING OF YEAST CELL METABOLISM

Beside the optimization of the desired pathway, the critical aspect during metabolic engineering is manipulating the metabolism of the host yeast cell factory for in a particular direction. The engineered pathway must function in the framework with the existing cellular metabolism. The metabolic and system biology engineers rely on the native pathways of a cell for catabolism of the sugar and for the generation of the necessary building blocks that are generally the starting metabolites for the desired pathway. These are also the source of the energy and the redox cofactors such as NADP, NADPH, and ATP (Chubukov et al., 2014).

The entire cell factory has the machinery necessary for sensing and adjusting the metabolism of the cell in respect to the increased demand of all these cofactors. The metabolic control of the cell is therefore optimized for the survival and production of the desired compounds. However, an increased demand on the cell to act as the carbon source and energy from the constructed, engineered metabolic pathway might create a challenge for the microbial cell factory. These situations require the necessary system-level approaches in the host cell that depend on the large-scale models (King et al., 2015; Wu et al., 2015). Today, stoichiometric metabolic models at the genome scale are repeatedly applied for examining the complete metabolic network. These models were also found to be helpful in understanding the reasons behind the alterations in central pathways and how they prompt the cell to the rest of the cellular metabolism (King et al., 2015).

ENGINEERING OF THE HOST CELL BY MAINTAINING THE LEVELS OF COFACTORS

The reduced metabolites formed by the cell factory, like the biofuels, depend on the reductive anabolic reaction pathways. These pathways need the NADH to act as the main electron donor. Most of the cell factories generate NADH as an energy metabolite during glycolysis. The major problem is the imbalance between the cofactors. Recently, Javidpour et al. (2014) modified a single step in the fatty acid anabolic pathway so that it accepted the cofactor NADH and not the cofactor NADPH. They reported a parallel upsurge in the formation of either the free fatty acids or the long chain methyl ketones. The specificity of the cofactor might possibly be changed in the fundamental biometabolism to generate NADPH instead of cofactor NADH; however, there are no reports of showing this result. One of main constraints for this method is thermodynamic stability because most of the microorganisms keep their ratio of the NADPH/NADP+ considerably more than the ratio of NADH/NAD+ (Chubukov et al., 2016). This behavior may be because higher energy is generally essential for regenerating NADPH compared with the cofactor NADH. So the newer algorithms should also account for the thermodynamic force while altering the cofactor specificity (King et al., 2014; Noor et al., 2014).

Biobutanol Production

The other commonly used biofuels are bioalcohols. The most important among them is ethanol. Along with methanol, ethanol is considered an alternative fuel for the various internal combustion engines. Ethanol is one of the biomass-based renewable fuels produced from different sugars using fermentation. The various substrates used for the fermentation are sugarcane, corn, sugar beet, barley, cheese whey, sweet sorghum, and agricultural residues (Kokkiligadda et al., 2016). Methanol is primarily produced by petrol and coal-based fuels. Consequently, ethanol is considered a superior fuel over methanol because it is a renewable source. It is used extensively as an alternative fuel in countries like Brazil. In spite of its advantages, the use of ethanol comes with important drawbacks for its use as an alternative for fuel. Ethanol corrodes the already existing pipelines because of its acetic acid, chloride ions, and polar nature. Metals such as aluminum and lead are susceptible to corrosive attack by dry ethanol. A small fraction of the corrosion is also caused by moisture absorbed by the ethanol, which in turn oxidizes the metal components (Si et al., 2014).

Biofuel produced from nonedible sources such as lignocellulosic biomass may be a possible solution for addressing the problems related to greenhouse emissions and nonenergy depletions. The yeast *S. cerevisiae* is most widely used strain for the production of ethanol from sugars. Advances in technology related to the fermentation sector have increased the production of bioethanol in the last two decades. However, fuel ethanol comes with several disadvantages, such as its incompatibility with gasoline, greater moisture content, and low energy density. Therefore, other advanced biofuels are considered as suitable alternatives for ethanol (Hong and Nielsen, 2012; Buijs et al., 2013).

Next-generation biofuels include butanols (Iso-butanol, 1- butanol, and 2- butanol), which are regarded as higher alcohols that possess various advantages over ethanol. First, the lower corrosiveness of butanol means that it can be used in current gasoline engines. Second, butanol possesses a higher miscibility with the mixture of the gasoline mixture. Third, butanol possesses a higher energy density compared with ethanol (Dürre, 2007). Butanol has a four-carbon structure, while ethanol has a one-carbon structure and methanol has a two-carbon structure. Butanol, as a fuel, is similar to ethanol because it blends easily with gasoline, it might be possible to blend it with diesel. Butanol contains more oxygen compared to biodiesel, which leads to a further declination of the soot. NOx emissions might be reduced because of the elevated heat of evaporation of butanol, which finally leads to a decreased combustion temperature. Thus, butanol may offer advantages compared with the extensively applied ethanol. Nevertheless, the major drawback of using butanol over ethanol is its lower levels of production. The yield of butanol during ABE fermentation is low compared to the *S. cerevisiae*–based process of ethanol fermentation. However, with the recent development of new technology in butanol fermentation process, an elevated level of butanol titer has been achieved.

n-Butanol is formed by a number of *Clostridium* species by means of the ABE fermentation route, which carries a production ratio of 1:3:6 and a butanol titer of 13 g/L. The ABE fermentation is mainly carried out using the strains *Clostridium acetobutylicum* and *C. beijerinckii.* However, fermentations using the clostridial strains are associated with several problems, including their slower growth rates on existing substrates, sporulation, their tendency to infections by bacteriophage, and strict anaerobic cultivations of the strains (de Jong et al., 2012). A recent hike in the price of blackstrap, a raw material used during ABE fermentation, is also responsible to some degree for the decline in the application of this fermentation process. Additional industrially applicable microorganisms have been metabolically engineered for the production of n-butanol. This process incorporates different variants of the existing pathway in clostridium or modulates the degradation pathways of ketoacid (Smith et al., 2010). During production of n-butanol, a titer to a concentration 15 g/L had been observed in *E. coli* strains. Industrial scale n-butanol fermentation using this important bacterium strain also suffers from an increased risk of bacteriophage infections and contamination with bacteria. In comparison to these *E. coli* strains, yeast *S. cerevisiae* offers substantial benefits in terms of accessible large-scale fermentation. The main reason for using this yeast strain is long experience working with this yeast *S. cerevisiae* in the fermentations process. This cell factory offers a high robustness during industrial-scale production, and a higher tolerance against different inhibitory compounds. Today, therefore, a wide-ranging interest in fermentation of butanol has increased because of its beneficial biofuel properties. Major yeast cell *S. cerevisiae* has been exploited as an advantageous cell factory for producing useful biofuel-like products, and it also produces secondary metabolites and advanced chemicals. *S. cerevisiae* is considered a facultative anaerobe cell factory that offers ease in handling, and it also has an innate tolerance to different by-products of fermentation, such as ethanol (Fischer et al., 2008). The ability of this yeast strain to lower the pH of the medium during the fermentation process decreases the contamination risk by other microbes such as bacteria, which generally possess less tolerance toward lower pH. For the above-mentioned reason, production of butanol using *S. cerevisiae* has been significantly attempted in recent years for the synthesis of advanced butanol. The various methods that have been worked out for engineering of *S. cerevisiae* using system biology and new molecular tools are summarized below.

Yeast *S. cerevisiae* for 1-Butanol Production

S. cerevisiae as a cell factory does not possess the ability to produce 1-butanol itself; however, it can produce an intermediate compound of the pathway involved in 1-butanol production in the case of bacteria *clostridium*. This important metabolite synthesized by a yeast cell is aceto-acetyl-CoA, which is produced from acetyl-CoA and plays an important part as a preliminary metabolite generated in the TCA cycle. Therefore, it acts as main precursor during synthesis of a number of vital biomolecules. For the production of both the laboratory scale and industrial scale

1-butanol by yeast *S.cerevisiae*, it is obligatory to introduce important metabolic enzymes from other microorganisms to convert aceto-acetyl-CoA into the desired metabolite 1-butanol (Figure 9.2). The organism first used for delivering the necessary enzyme was *Clostridium*. Steen et al. (2008) attempted to produce 1-butanol using overexpression of individual enzymes of the pathway during butanol production in clostridium. Overexpression of these genes in the metabolic pathway allows a higher degree of catalysis of aceto-acetyl-CoA into 1-butanol (Figure 9.2).

The study reported that significant obstacles in the heterologous pathway of butanol production need to be surmounted. These include the choice of the enzyme, balancing the intermediates formed in the metabolic pathway, verification of the gene expression and protein levels, and maintaining the viability of the host cell. The overexpressed enzymes from other organism such as *Ralstonieutropha, C. beijerinckii,* and *Streptomyces collinus* were also compared. Thiolase enzyme, which carries out the switching from acetyl-CoA biomolecule into aceto-acetyl-CoA from *Escherichia coli, R. eutropha, Clostridium beijerinckii,* and *S. cerevisiae*, improved the production of 1-butanol. The constructed strain producing thiolase (Erg10) from *S. cerevisiae*; crotonase (Crt), bifunctional butyraldehyde/butanol dehydrogenase (AdhE2), and 3-hydroxybutyryl-CoA dehydrogenase (Hbd) from the strain *C. beijerinckii*; and

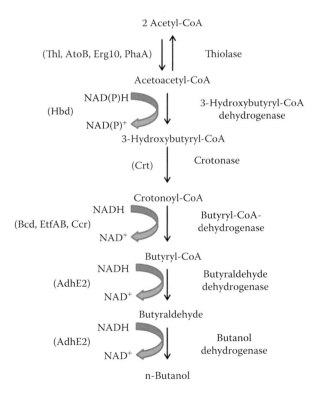

FIGURE 9.2 n-Butanol synthetic pathway showing isozymes present in different microorganisms were substituted.

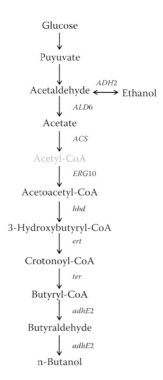

Glucose

Puyuvate

Acetaldehyde ⟷ Ethanol
ADH2

ALD6

Acetate

ACS

Acetyl-CoA

ERG10

Acetoacetyl-CoA

hbd

3-Hydroxybutyryl-CoA

ert

Crotonoyl-CoA

ter

Butyryl-CoA

adhE2

Butyraldehyde

adhE2

n-Butanol

FIGURE 9.3   n-Butanol pathway in engineered *Saccharomyces cerevisiae.*

crotonyl-CoA reductase (Ccr) from *S. collinus* exhibited the maximum productivity of about 2.5 mg/L when compared with the different constructed microbial cell factories (Yoshikuni et al., 2008) (Figure 9.3). The observed outcome, where the application of Ccr gene was found to be more efficient than that found in the clostridium species enzyme (etfA, bcd, and etfB), demonstrated that the chief enzyme of the pathway, that is, butyryl-CoA dehydrogenase, should be altered to augment the formation of 1-butanol in the course of heterologous pathway (Steen et al., 2008).

The study authors demonstrated the substitution of the isozymes in *S. cerevisiae*. Examination of the metabolic pathway intermediates and possible metabolic engineering points for enhancing the biosynthesis of n-butanol was also performed. They reported that, while comparing the generated strain with the parental producers of n-butanol such as *Clostridia* strains (10 g/L) and the other *E. coli* strains, metabolically engineered (0.5 g/L) strains provide a potential candidate for higher n-butanol concentration. The increases in concentration of the desired product will undoubtedly be essential for increasing the magnitude and offer a better precedence. Nevertheless, the quantity of formed 1-butanol was inadequate to validate the application of yeast *S. cerevisiae* as a key microbial strain for the formation of 1-butanol. Numerous attempts have been made to get increased yield of the 1-butanol, such as (1) increasing the available concentration of the cytosolic acetyl-CoA so that this metabolite can serve as a precursor of 1-butanol production, (2) using diverse alternative enzymes present in the metabolic pathway of 1-butanol biosynthesis, and (3) designing new metabolic pathways using newer molecular tools for production of butanol.

USING DIVERSE ALTERNATIVE ENZYMES PRESENT IN THE METABOLIC PATHWAY OF 1-BUTANOL BIOSYNTHESIS

One strategy for production of 1-butanol involves Ccr enzyme from *S. collinus*. This enzyme was further substituted with (Ter) crotonyl-CoA-specific trans-enoyl-CoA reductase enzyme from the strain *Treponema denticola*. The Ter enzyme offers the benefit of circumventing the overturn oxidation of the enzyme butyryl-CoA with crotonyl-CoA. Essentially, the Ter enzyme might be responsible for increased flux along the metabolic pathway of 1-butanol biosynthesis (Krivoruchko et al., 2013). Application of enzyme Ter in the 1-butanol production pathway collectively with the enzyme CoA-acylating aldehyde dehydrogenase of the *E. coli* strain (EcEutE) and butanol dehydrogenase (CaBdhB) enzyme of *C. acetobutylicum* efficiently enhances the 1-butanol production via reversed β-oxidation (Lian and Zhao, 2015).

INCREASING THE AVAILABLE CONCENTRATION OF CYTOSOLIC ACETYL-COA

Besides its important role as a main structural material for the cellular metabolism of a cell, acetyl-CoA is also the chief precursor molecule for the biological synthesis of a number of biofuel and other important molecules, such as n-butanol, alkanes, polyhydroxybutyrate (PHB), fatty acid ethyl esters (FAEEs), and isoprenoid-based drugs. Therefore, the main precursor during production of the 1-butanol is acetyl-CoA. Production of acetyl-CoA is the rate-limiting step in the metabolic pathway. In industrially important *E. coli*, metabolite acetyl-CoA is gradually produced from the key metabolite pyruvate using either pyruvate dehydrogenase (PDH) under the aerobic conditions or pyruvate formatelyase (PFL) under the anaerobic conditions.

However, in the yeast *S. cerevisiae*, the metabolism of this key metabolite acetyl CoA is mainly divided into numerous compartments, together with the peroxisomes, nucleus mitochondria, and cytosol. Metabolite acetyl-CoA is mostly formed inside the microbial cell in mitochondria; however, yeast *S. cerevisiae* is found to be deficient in the machinery responsible for exporting the acetyl-CoA of mitochondrial to cytosol, where the important biosynthesis of the preferred metabolites is generally found to occur (Strijbis and Distel, 2010). Acetyl-CoA is produced in the cytosol of the cell via PDH-bypass reaction, and the activation of the acetate is the main rate-limiting step of the reaction. This results in lower activity and also elevated energy demands of ACS (Shiba et al., 2007). Numerous advanced engineering methods have been used to boost the accessibility of acetyl-CoA in the yeast *S. cerevisiae*; for example, ACS mutant from the strain *Salmonella enterica* has been used with an augmented activity of acetyl-CoA (Chen et al., 2013; Krivoruchko et al., 2013).

Another method might be incorporation of the heterologous biosynthetic pathways of acetyl-CoA with a lower energy input requirement (Tang et al., 2013). These strategies have been particularly important in improving the production of n-butanol (Krivoruchkoet al., 2013), PHB (Kocharin et al., 2012), isoprenoids (Shiba et al., 2007), and fatty acids (Tang et al., 2013) in yeast *S. cerevisiae*. The presence of low concentrations of the cytosolic acetyl-CoA in yeast *S. cerevisiae* is inadequate for the synthesis of a number of important metabolites. This in turn is responsible for lower productivity of the butanol than in the bacterium *E. coli*, which has ability to produce acetyl-CoA gradually. Krivoruchko et al. (2013) increased the flux of cytosolic acetyl-CoA to improve the productivity of butanol production. This was performed through the incorporation of the genes acetyl-CoA acetyltransferase (ERG10), acetaldehyde dehydrogenase (ALD6), and alcohol dehydrogenase (ADH2), which are placed on plasmid. Different strains containing deletions in the citrate synthase (CIT2) or malate synthase (MLS1) genes were also constructed for improving the flux and for decreasing the leakage of the acetyl CoA through the important glyoxylate pathway. The study reported using the Ter strain in the 1-butanol pathway, and the desired strain was able to produce a maximum of 16.3 mg/L of butanol. *S. cerevisiae* also synthesized other metabolites like glycerol and ethanol with the biosynthesis of 1-butanol because they utilize similar intermediate metabolites of the pathway.

Advancements in molecular and system biology approaches were other strategies taken into account by different group of researchers for increasing the concentration of acetyl-CoA present in the cytosol for reducing or removing the competitive reactions for producing the by-products glycerol and ethanol. The double-deletion mutant that is missing the genes of the glycerol pathway (the GPD1 and GPD2 genes that encode the glycerol-3-phosphate dehydrogenases enzyme) represented a decline in the production of glycerol and consumption of NADH during conversion of dihydroxyacetone phosphate into metabolite glycerol-3-phosphate, which resulted in an augmentation in the production of 1-butanol to the concentration of nearly 14.1 mg/L. (Sakuragi et al., 2015). Moreover, the knockout of the genes of alcohol dehydrogenases (ADH1 and ADH4), which are responsible for the formation of ethanol, along with the knockout of the GPD1 and GPD2 genes redirected the glycolytic flux in the direction of the formation of acetyl-CoA. This also leads to an improved 1-butanol production.

Construction of Metabolic Pathway for 1-Butanol Production

Another alternative method for producing fuel alcohols is to exploit the degradation pathway of the amino acids that are released from the hydrolysis of n-protein. Along with the clostridium pathway of 1-butanol production, other pathways were also constructed for the production of 1-butanol in yeast *S. cerevisiae*. Branduardi et al. (2013) demonstrated that amino acids can also act as the substrate for butanol and isobutanol production. They developed a novel pathway for the 1-butanol production all the way through the glycine degradation pathway. They designed and constructed a novel metabolic pathway by expressing a number of genes. Glycine oxidase, malate synthase genes (MLS1and DAL7 genes), and β-isopropylmalate dehydrogenase gene were used for the enhanced production of the 1-butanol through the Ehrlich pathway. During the measurement of the kinetic parameters of growth using a key substrate amino acid glycine, the production in the medium of butanol and isobutanol was measured to be 92 and 58 mg/L, respectively.

Another recent approach was the design of a 1-butanol–producing metabolic route that plays a role in the endogenous threonine metabolism. The strategies used in this method of 1-butanol formation were overexpression of the genes related to catabolism of the threonine, and further deletion of genes responsible for affecting the flux of the pathway involved in the biosynthesis of 1-butanol (Si et al., 2014). The researcher overexpressed the endogenous threonine deaminase (*ILV1* or *CHA1*) genes, which are responsible for catalyzing the conversion of threonine to 2-keto-butyrate and cause an enhanced 1-butanol production. In addition, overexpression of three genes (*LEU1*, *LEU2*, and *LEU4*), encoded isopropyl-malate isomerase, β-isopropylmalate dehydrogenase, and α-isopropyl-malate synthase, respectively. These genes are playing necessary roles in the pathway of leucine biosynthesis. Furthermore, augmented production of 1-butanol production was also accomplished by knockout of the *ILV2* gene, which encodes enzyme acetolactate synthase, and gene *ADH1*, which encodes enzyme alcohol dehydrogenase and, overall, resulted in enhanced 1-butanol production of 242.8 mg/L.

FATTY ACID FOR THE PRODUCTION OF BIOFUEL IN *S. CEREVISIAE*

The microbial-based biosynthesis of fatty acids has recently received increased attention because it offers a way for renewable biofuel and oleo-chemical production (Lennen et al., 2013). There have been a number of reports on the bioengineering of the bacterium *E. coli* for the production of various important oleo-chemicals such as the alkanes that can directly be used as biofuels. However, for large-scale production, the yeast *S. cerevisiae* is the appropriate candidate due to its higher tolerance of the different harsh fermentation conditions and its widespread application for bioethanol production. Sustainable production of biofuels requires creation of cell factory platform strains. In these contexts, yeast *S. cerevisiae* is a promising candidate because the engineered strains can be easily implemented into the already established bioethanol plants (Mattanovich et al., 2014).

The fatty acid biosynthesis in yeast *S. cerevisiae* varies from that of the fatty acid present in the case of bacteria such as *E. coli*. In bacteria, the synthesis of free fatty acid is generally executed by a Type II fatty acid synthase (FAS) that is comprised of the separate, monofunctional enzymes, although in yeast *S. cerevisiae*, the biosynthesis of the fatty acids is present in two compartments, that is, the cytoplasm and the mitochondria (Zhou et al., 2014). The Type I FAS is responsible for carrying out synthesis in cytoplasm; the Type II FAS is responsible for the mitochondria-based biosynthesis. Mitochondrial-based Type II FAS has been found to be the single mitochondrial source for the octanoic acid. This acid is an important precursor of the cofactor lipoic acid, which is essential for preserving the function of numerous enzymes of mitochondrial complexes such as the pyruvate dehydrogenase enzyme (Hiltunen et al., 2009). Nevertheless, the majority of the storage and functional lipids are formed by type I FAS, which synthesizes fatty acid from acetyl-CoA and malonyl-CoA (Koch et al., 2014; Zhou et al., 2014). This difference is significant because it has consequences and because it is helpful for further engineering the pathway of fatty acid metabolism.

Zhou et al. (2016) demonstrated the higher level of FFA in yeast *S. cerevisiae*. The genetically modified strain produces FFA in a concentration of 10.4 g/L. The authors also constructed an engineered pathway using alcohol dehydrogenases and enzyme aldehyde reductases for exchanging of FFA with important alkanes and fatty alcohols in a concentration of 0.8 and 1.5 mg/L. Zhu et al., (2017) also demonstrated the application of Type I fatty acid synthases. This enzyme is normally responsible for the synthesis of long chain fatty acids. The enzyme is genetically engineered to synthesize the medium chain fatty acids and important valuable compounds like methyl ketones, which are components presently used in transportation fuels. Therefore, new system biology approaches along with synthetic biology will assist the efficient construction of microbial cell machinery for the synthesis of fatty acid–derived biofuels.

ISOPRENOID-DERIVED ADVANCED BIOFUEL

Isoprenoids are one of the biggest and most diverse groups of the products available naturally. These are a class of valuable compounds used widely as flavorings and in pharmaceuticals (Kirby et al., 2009). Isoprenoids are composed of more than 50,000 compounds, including a number of valuable primary metabolites, such as carotenoids, secondary metabolites, and sterols, that can be used in medicine (Breitmaier, 2006; Davies et al., 2015). Advanced biofuels have attracted a lot of attention because the changing global climate has compelled the growth of sources that are carbon-neutral.

The arrangement of general isoprenoids provides a number of advantages as fuel compounds. For instance, the branching at the methyl position is a collective structural attribute responsible for lowering the freezing point significantly. The cyclic structure of the isoprenoids is also responsible for the increased energy density and is usually considered an important feature for jet fuels (Lee et al., 2008; Peralta-Yahya, 2010). The branching means that a higher number of tertiary carbon atoms are available for stabilizing the induced radicals, and it is also responsible for increasing the octane number. Recently, some of the isoprenoids have been verified and formulated as possible diesel gasoline and jet fuels. The reason for their selection is their high energy content, high octane/cetane numbers, and cold weather properties (Peralta-Yahya et al., 2011; Mack et al., 2014).

The isoprenoids are mainly categorized into different groups based on the number of carbon atoms present in their structure: hemiterpenoids contain 5 carbon atoms (C5), monoterpenoids contain C10, sesquiterpenoids C15, and diterpenoids C20; the triterpenoids contain the highest number: C30. The C15 isoprenoids, bisabolane and farnesane, have a cetane number of 52 and 58, respectively. These cetane numbers fall in the range of biodiesel. The replacement of jet fuel requires a high-energy content and this can be attained with ring structures that are highly constrained. Constrained ring structures are found in isoprenoid pinene dimers. The two universal five-carbon building blocks for synthesizing the isoprenoids are isopentenyl diphosphate (IPP) and its isomer dimethylallyl diphosphate (DMAPP). These important precursors might be formed by two pathways: 2-methyl-d-erythrito-4-phosphate

(MEP) pathway, and the 1-deoxy-D-xylulose-5-phosphate (DXP) and the mevalonate (MVA) pathway.

The natural source of the isoprenoids is plants, but they generally do not manufacture enough to support large-scale industrial biofuel production. Large quantities of isoprenoids can be produced from algae, such as *Botryococcusbraunii*; however, their growth is slow and they produce a large quantity of fatty acids, producing an extract similar to a biocrude, which would further require cracking to produce biofuels. To increase the production quantities of isoprenoid, the mevalonate pathways and the deoxyxylulose-5-phosphate pathways can be overexpressed and deregulated in the yeast *S. cerevisiae* and bacterium *E. coli*, respectively. These were then introduced heterologously into these foreign microorganisms. Most of the target engineering has been done on the mevalonate pathway for increasing the production of isoprenoids. Engineering of this important pathway resulted in 40 g l^{-1} of the C15 amorphadiene in *S. cerevisiae* and 27 g l^{-1} of the amorpha-4,11-diene in *E. coli* (Tsuruta et al., 2009; Westfall et al., 2012).

Plants are the usual source of the farnesene and bisabolene, which are regarded as the sesquiterpene precursors of farnesane and bisabolane, respectively. With new genetic engineering techniques, the engineered cell platforms might possibly be the most convenient and the best cost-effective means for the production of these compounds. As biofuels, farnesane and bisabolane display superior cold properties, with measured cloud points of about −78°C and −25°C when compared with D2 diesel's cloud point of −3°C. The complex ring portion of the bisabolane translates into enhanced density (0.88 g/mL) of this fuel. This in turn creates an increased energy density per volume of fuel (Renninger and McPhee, 2008; Peralta-Yahya, 2010). However, in comparison with bisabolane, isoprenoid farnesane generally depicts lower density (0.77 g/mL) (Peralta-Yahya et al., 2011). Farnesane has been found to be best suited for the commercialization process. Amyris, the renewable products company based in Emeryville, California, used industrial yeast cell machinery *S. cerevisiae* PE-2 for the production of farnesene. This important compound is then hydrogenated chemically to form the desired farnesane (Renninger and McPhee, 2008; Rude et al., 2009; Ubersax et al., 2010).

JET FUELS

The global aviation industry has the goal of being carbon neutral or achieving negative growth by 2020. It has placed great emphasis on reducing the carbon dioxide (CO_2) emissions to about 50% relative to 2005 levels by the year 2050 (IATA, 2009). The U.S. Federal Aviation Administration (FAA) has as one of its objectives that nearly 1 billion gallons of renewable jet fuel will be consumed by the U.S. aviation industry starting in 2018. Therefore, a lot of emphasis has been placed on finding new advanced biofuels for the aviation industry that have considerably lower greenhouse gases emissions than new conventional fuels. By 2022, the target for the consumption of total biofuels is about 36 billion gallons per year. Corn ethanol, which is one of the main sources of ethanol production, can provide a maximum amount of 15 billion gallons of ethanol, with the remaining amount fulfilled by advanced biofuels. Minimum directives for 2022 for advanced biofuels are about 1 billion gallons for diesel from the biomass-based source and about 16 billion gallons for cellulose-based fuels, and nearly 4 billion gallons from the undifferentiated advanced category of biofuels (Winchester et al., 2013).

Jet fuels are generally manufactured to have a higher energy density (53.4 MJ/L) and equivalent net heat combustion. Appropriate biofuels or the precursors of the biofuels that can be put in the category of the jet fuels would be n-alkenes (n-olefins), n-alkanes, and different compounds of terpenes (sabinene, terpinene, and pinene). Microbes as cell factories produce hydrocarbons of diverse types such as the alkanes from fatty aldehyde decarbonylation and aliphatic isoprenoid compounds (Sukovich et al., 2010). Decarbonylation of fatty aldehyde is not very well understood right now, but it might present a clean route to the development of advanced diesel fuels from fatty acids. Three different pathways of alkane/alkene biosynthesis have been discovered recently, the first one and the one of greatest significance is the head-to-head condensation in *Shewanella oneidensis*. The fatty acids were condensed to the long chain alkenes (C23–C33) (Sukovich et al., 2010).

The proficient conversion of the emitted carbon dioxide either straight or by the biomass into the "drop-in compatible" hydrocarbon-based biofuels is the crucial target of the "biorenewable" research and development. A major step in this research is the transition of desirable intermediates of the metabolic pathway into hydrocarbons, such as olefins and alkanes. The pathway of fatty acid biosynthesis is for providing the biofuel precursors because it provides better efficiency and greater energy conservation (Atsumi et al., 2008). Some natural metabolic pathways in microbial cell factories can convert fatty acid intermediates into olefins and alkanes. Rude et al. (2011) reported that the P450 enzyme (OleTJE) from *Jeotgalicoccus* sp. catalyzes the transformation of derivatives of the fatty acid into the important terminal olefins such as 1-alkenes. This enzyme was discovered by application of the reverse genetic approach (Rude et al., 2011). The next and important metabolic route, discovered with the assistance of the subtractive genome analysis, is the transformation of the derivatives of fatty acid metabolism into different alkanes with carbon values from C13 to C17. Schirmer et al. (2010) obtained a titer of 300 mg/L of alkane after overexpression of the two specific genes from *Nostoc punctiforme* PCC73102 was performed in *E. coli*. This study also showed the distribution of pentadecene, pentadecane, tridecane, and the heptadecene in a ratio of 10:40:10:40. The authors also found that more than 80% of the desired product was found in the extracellular medium.

CHALLENGES IN SYSTEMS BIOLOGY

The field of systems biology possesses an exceptional range of prospects for constructing and understanding the metabolic pathways related to the biology of the yeast. The latest technical developments are in metabolomics methods; high-sensitivity proteomic, next-generation sequencing; and recent advancements in the field of fluxomics techniques. These developments make the systems biology protocols more commanding tools available for the synthetic biologist (Gardner et al., 2013). Complete genome engineering of the yeast cell factory for advanced biofuel production can benefit directly from the latest sequencing methods, which are used for characterization of the strain and lead to rapid progress in developing robust yeast cell factories.

Even with many successes finding stimulating new systems and techniques, the models that work well at the laboratory scale often do not show similar profiles in larger fermentation conditions. These strains are not sufficiently robust to bear the slight variations in the system parameters. The low-sample throughput obtained using the advanced-omics techniques strictly confines the effectiveness of the obtained data far from the hypotheses of the direct interest. Therefore, systems biology should reap some advantages from research hard work that highlights the method, data sharing, and reproducibility. Restrictions in reproducibility impede predictability.

Only a few laboratories implement both the computational and experimental, and also work together because of the difficulties performing both types of work. Therefore, the association between both computational and experimentalist specialists might turn out to be much more productive and also allow a more fruitful exchange of data. These data exchanges are particularly important for advancements in synthetic biology (Chubukov et al., 2016).

CONCLUSION

Numerous significant fuel production systems have been established in different yeast cell factories recently and include isobutanol production. While most recent studies were quite promising, extensive engineering will be required to increase the desired titers of the advanced biofuels. A number of studies focused on the cellular physiology, stress, and heterologous metabolic pathways, but there is an expectation that this information can be used to deduce the important pathway that has bottlenecks and to optimize the cellular circuit design. Regardless of the considerable advancement in the development of yeast cell factories for the increased biosynthesis of advanced biofuels at laboratory scale, there is an even higher demand for additional improvement of these yeast cell factories before these strains can meet the robust standards of the industry. The yield and productivity of advanced biofuel need to be economically viable so that it can compete with the existing ethanol-based fermentation in the near future. The systems biology approach can reveal a number of strategies that will be helpful in achieving the desired production and productivity levels. Thus, additional engineering approaches are also required to learn the tolerance toward the biofuel using complex biomass-based feedstock along with the productivity of the advanced biofuel. Therefore, systems biology holds promise as a significant technology for the development of future strains that are more efficient yeast cell machineries.

REFERENCES

Atsumi, S., and J. C. Liao. 2008. Metabolic engineering for advanced biofuels production from Escherichia coli. *Current opinion in Biotechnology* 19, no. 5: 414–419.

Branduardi, P., V. Longo, N. Maria Berterame, G. Rossi, and D. Porro. 2013. A novel pathway to produce butanol and isobutanol in Saccharomyces cerevisiae. *Biotechnology for Biofuels* 6, no. 1: 68.

Breitmaier, E. 2006. Terpenes: Importance, general structure, and biosynthesis. *Terpenes: Flavors, Fragrances, Pharmaca, Pheromones* (2006): 1–9. doi: 10.1002/9783527609949.ch1.

Buijs, N. A., V. Siewers, and J. Nielsen. 2013. Advanced biofuel production by the yeast Saccharomyces cerevisiae. *Current Opinion in Chemical Biology* 17, no. 3: 480–488.

Caspeta, L., and J. Nielsen. 2013. Economic and environmental impacts of microbial biodiesel. *Nature Biotechnology* 31, no. 9: 789–793.

Chen, Y., L. Daviet, M. Schalk, V. Siewers, and J. Nielsen. 2013. Establishing a platform cell factory through engineering of yeast acetyl-CoA metabolism. *Metabolic Engineering* 15: 48–54.

Chubukov, V., L. Gerosa, K. Kochanowski, and U. Sauer. 2014. Coordination of microbial metabolism. *Nature Reviews Microbiology* 12, no. 5: 327–340.

Chubukov, V., A. Mukhopadhyay, C. J. Petzold, J. D. Keasling, and H. Martín. 2016. Synthetic and systems biology for microbial production of commodity chemicals. *npj Systems Biology and Applications* 2: 16009.

Davies, F. K., R. E. Jinkerson, and M. C. Posewitz. 2015. Toward a photosynthetic microbial platform for terpenoid engineering. *Photosynthesis Research* 123, no. 3: 265–284.

de Jong, E. D., A. Higson, P. Walsh, and M. Wellisch. 2012. Bio-based chemicals value added products from biorefineries. Amsterdam, the Netherlands: IEA Bioenergy, Task 42 Biorefinery.

Dürre, P. 2007. Biobutanol: An attractive biofuel. *Biotechnology Journal* 2, no. 12: 1525–1534.

Eisentraut, A. (2010). Sustainable Production of Second-generation Biofuels: Potential and Perspectives in Major Economies and Developing Countries: Information Paper. OECD/IEA.

Fischer, C. R., D. Klein-Marcuschamer, and G. Stephanopoulos. 2008. Selection and optimization of microbial hosts for biofuels production. *Metabolic Engineering* 10, no. 6: 295–304.

Gardner, T. S. 2013. Synthetic biology: From hype to impact. *Trends in Biotechnology* 31, no. 3: 123.

Hiltunen, J. K., M. S. Schonauer, K. J. Autio, T. M. Mittelmeier, A. J. Kastaniotis, and C. L. Dieckmann. 2009. Mitochondrial fatty acid synthesis type II: More than just fatty acids. *Journal of Biological Chemistry* 284, no. 14: 9011–9015.

Hong, K.-K., and J. Nielsen. 2012. Metabolic engineering of Saccharomyces cerevisiae: A key cell factory platform for future biorefineries. *Cellular and Molecular Life Sciences* 69, no. 16: 2671–2690.

IATA, A. 2009. Global Approach to Reducing Aviation Emissions. *First Stop: Carbon Neutral Growth from 2020.*

Javidpour, P., J. H. Pereira, E.-B. Goh, R. P. McAndrew, S. M. Ma, et al. 2014. Biochemical and structural studies of NADH-dependent FabG used to increase the bacterial production of fatty acids under anaerobic conditions. *Applied and Environmental Microbiology* 80, no. 2: 497–505.

King, Z. A., and A. M. Feist. 2014. Optimal cofactor swapping can increase the theoretical yield for chemical production in *Escherichia coli* and *Saccharomyces cerevisiae*. *Metabolic Engineering* 24: 117–128.

King, Z. A., C. J. Lloyd, A. M. Feist, and B. O. Palsson. 2015. Next-generation genome-scale models for metabolic engineering. *Current Opinion in Biotechnology* 35: 23–29.

Kirby, J., and J. D. Keasling. 2009. Biosynthesis of plant isoprenoids: Perspectives for microbial engineering. *Annual Review of Plant Biology* 60: 335–355.

Koch, B., C. Schmidt, and G. Daum. 2014. Storage lipids of yeasts: A survey of nonpolar lipid metabolism in Saccharomyces cerevisiae, Pichia pastoris, and Yarrowia lipolytica. *FEMS Microbiology* R 38, no. 5: 892–915.

Kocharin, K., Y. Chen, V. Siewers, and J. Nielsen. 2012. Engineering of acetyl-CoA metabolism for the improved production of polyhydroxybutyrate in *Saccharomyces cerevisiae*. *Amb Express* 2, no. 1: 52.

Kokkiligadda, A., A. Beniwal, P. Saini, and S. Vij. 2016. Utilization of cheese whey using synergistic immobilization of β-galactosidase and *Saccharomyces cerevisiae cells* in dual matrices. *Applied Biochemistry and Biotechnology*, 179 (8): 1469–1484.

Krivoruchko, A., C. Serrano-Amatriain, Y. Chen, V. Siewers, and J. Nielsen. 2013. Improving biobutanol production in engineered *Saccharomyces cerevisiae* by manipulation of acetyl-CoA metabolism. *Journal of Industrial Microbiology and Biotechnology* 40, no. 9: 1051–1056.

Langer, E. 2012. Biomanufacturing outlook. *Pharmaceutical Technology* 36, no. 2: 54–56.

Lee, S. K., H. Chou, T. S. Ham, T. S. Lee, and J. D. Keasling. 2008. Metabolic engineering of microorganisms for biofuels production: From bugs to synthetic biology to fuels. *Current Opinion in Biotechnology* 19, no. 6: 556–563.

Lennen, R. M., and B. F. Pfleger. 2013. Microbial production of fatty acid-derived fuels and chemicals. *Current Opinion in Biotechnology* 24, no. 6: 1044–1053.

Lian, J., and H. Zhao. 2015. Recent advances in biosynthesis of fatty acids derived products in *Saccharomyces cerevisiae* via enhanced supply of precursor metabolites. *Journal of Industrial Microbiology and Biotechnology* 42, no. 3: 437–451.

Mack, J. H., V. H. Rapp, M. Broeckelmann, T. Soon Lee, and R. W. Dibble. 2014. Investigation of biofuels from microorganism metabolism for use as anti-knock additives. *Fuel* 117: 939–943.

Mattanovich, D., M. Sauer, and B. Gasser. 2014. Yeast biotechnology: Teaching the old dog new tricks. *Microbial Cell Factories* 13, no. 1: 34.

Mukhopadhyay, A., A. M. Redding, B. J. Rutherford, and J. D. Keasling. 2008. Importance of systems biology in engineering microbes for biofuel production. *Current Opinion in Biotechnology* 19, no. 3: 228–234.

Nielsen, J., and J. D. Keasling. 2016. Engineering cellular metabolism. *Cell* 164, no. 6: 1185–1197.

Noor, E., A. Bar-Even, A., Ed Reznik, W. Liebermeister, and R. Milo. 2014. Pathway thermodynamics highlights kinetic obstacles in central metabolism. PLoS Comput Biol 10, no. 2: e1003483.

Peralta-Yahya, P. P., and J. D. Keasling. 2010. Advanced biofuel production in microbes. *Biotechnology Journal* 5, no. 2: 147–162.

Peralta-Yahya, P. P., M. Ouellet, R. Chan, A. Mukhopadhyay, J. D. Keasling, and T. S. Lee. 2011. Identification and microbial production of a terpene-based advanced biofuel. *Nature Communications*, 2: 483.

Renninger, N. S., and D. J. McPhee. 2008. Fuel compositions comprising farnesane and farnesane derivatives and method of making and using same. U.S. Patent 7,399,323, issued July 15.

Rude, M. A., T. S. Baron, S. Brubaker, M. Alibhai, S. B. Del Cardayre, and A. Schirmer. 2011. Terminal olefin (1-alkene) biosynthesis by a novel P450 fatty acid decarboxylase from Jeotgalicoccus species. *Applied and Environmental Microbiology* 77, no. 5: 1718–1727.

Rude, M. A., and A. Schirmer. 2009. New microbial fuels: A biotech perspective. *Current Opinion in Microbiology* 12, no. 3: 274–281.

Saini, P., A. Beniwal, and S. Vij. 2017. Physiological response of *Kluyveromyces marxianus* during oxidative and osmotic stress. *Process Biochemistry*. doi:10.1016/j.procbio.2017.03.001.

Sakuragi, H., H. Morisaka, K. Kuroda, and M. Ueda. 2015. Enhanced butanol production by eukaryotic *Saccharomyces cerevisiae* engineered to contain an improved pathway. *Bioscience, Biotechnology, and Biochemistry* 79, no. 2: 314–320.

Schirmer, A., M. A. Rude, X. Li, E. Popova, and S. B. Del Cardayre. 2010. Microbial biosynthesis of alkanes. *Science* 329, no. 5991: 559–562.

Shiba, Y., E. M. Paradise, J. Kirby, D.-K. Ro, and J. D. Keasling. 2007. Engineering of the pyruvate dehydrogenase bypass in *Saccharomyces cerevisiae* for high-level production of isoprenoids. *Metabolic Engineering* 9, no. 2: 160–168.

Si, T., Y. Luo, H. Xiao, and H. Zhao. 2014. Utilizing an endogenous pathway for 1-butanol production in *Saccharomyces cerevisiae*. *Metabolic Engineering* 22: 60–68.

Smith, K. M., K.-M. Cho, and J. C. Liao. 2010. Engineering Corynebacterium glutamicum for isobutanol production. *Applied Microbiology and Biotechnology* 87, no. 3: 1045–1055.

Steen, E. J., R. Chan, N. Prasad, S. Myers, C. J. Petzold, et al. 2008. Metabolic engineering of *Saccharomyces cerevisiae* for the production of n-butanol. *Microbial Cell Factories* 7, no. 1: 36.

Strijbis, K., and B. Distel. 2010. Intracellular acetyl unit transport in fungal carbon metabolism. *Eukaryotic Cell* 9, no. 12: 1809–1815.

Sukovich, D. J., J. L. Seffernick, J. E. Richman, J. A. Gralnick, and L. P. Wackett. 2010. Widespread head-to-head hydrocarbon biosynthesis in bacteria and role of OleA. *Applied and Environmental Microbiology* 76, no. 12: 3850–3862.

Tang, X., H. Feng, and W. Ning Chen. 2013. Metabolic engineering for enhanced fatty acids synthesis in Saccharomyces cerevisiae. *Metabolic Engineering* 16: 95–102.

Tsuruta, H., C. J. Paddon, D. Eng, J. R. Lenihan, T. Horning, et al. 2009. High-level production of amorpha-4, 11-diene, a precursor of the antimalarial agent artemisinin, in *Escherichia coli. PLoS One* 4, no. 2: e4489.

Ubersax, J. A., and D. M. Platt. 2010. Genetically modified microbes producing isoprenoids. U.S. Patent Application 12/791,596, filed June 1.

Westfall, P. J., D. J. Pitera, J. R. Lenihan, D. Eng, F. X. Woolard, et al. 2012. Production of amorphadiene in yeast, and its conversion to dihydroartemisinic acid, precursor to the antimalarial agent artemisinin. *Proceedings of the National Academy of Sciences* 109, no. 3: E111–E118.

Winchester, N., D. McConnachie, C. Wollersheim, and I. A. Waitz. 2013. Economic and emissions impacts of renewable fuel goals for aviation in the US. *Transportation Research Part A: Policy and Practice* 58: 116–128.

Wu, S. G., L. He, Q. Wang, and Y. J. Tang. 2015. An ancient Chinese wisdom for metabolic engineering: Yin-Yang. *Microbial Cell Factories* 14, no. 1: 39.

Yoshikuni, Y., J. A. Dietrich, F. F. Nowroozi, P. C. Babbitt, and J. D. Keasling. 2008. Redesigning enzymes based on adaptive evolution for optimal function in synthetic metabolic pathways. *Chemistry and Biology* 15, no. 6: 607–618.

Zhou, Y. J., N. A. Buijs, V. Siewers, and J. Nielsen. 2014. Fatty acid-derived biofuels and chemicals production in *Saccharomyces cerevisiae. Frontiers in Bioengineering and Biotechnology* 2: 32.

Zhou, Y. J., N. A. Buijs, Z. Zhu, J. Qin, V. Siewers, and J. Nielsen. 2016. Production of fatty acid-derived oleochemicals and biofuels by synthetic yeast cell factories. *Nature Communications* 7: 11709.

Zhu, Z., Y. J. Zhou, A. Krivoruchko, M. Grininger, Z. K. Zhao, and J. Nielsen. 2017. Expanding the product portfolio of fungal type I fatty acid synthases. *Nature Chemical Biology* 13: 360–362.

10 Beneficial Effects of Dairy Foods Enriched with Prebiotics and Probiotics

Jagrani Minj, Priyanka Saini, Shayanti Minj,
Arun Beniwal, Deepansh Sharma,
Shriya Mehta, and Shilpa Vij

CONTENTS

INTRODUCTION

Dairy foods, especially fermented milk foods, are very promising food products among all the dairy products. The importance of these foods derive from the live probiotic bacteria in them. Today, development of new and innovative food products is an attractive area of research as consumers demand more and more beneficial foods. Innovation in product developments may be the incorporation of probiotics, prebiotics, fruits purees, or other additives. Many probiotic bacteria have been reported for their beneficial effects such as counteracting hypocholesterolemia, cancer, diabetes, hypertension, and diarrhea; their antimicrobial and antioxidative properties; and so on. Probiotic bacteria lactobacilli and bifidobacteria are mostly studied for their probiotic properties. Prebiotics are mainly the nondigestible dietary fibers. Prebiotics are reported for their action as nutritional components for probiotic bacteria. Probiotic bacteria utilize these nondigestable food ingredients into their diets in the colon where there is almost complete depletion of nutrients for the survival of any probiotic bacteria and this is called the synbiotic association. Mostly probiotic bacteria utilize the prebiotics, but some strains are very specific for specific prebiotics.

TYPES OF FERMENTED DAIRY PRODUCTS

Many dairy products enriched with probiotics and prebiotics are studied for their beneficial aspects. Among these dairy products, yogurt, dahi, lassi, fermented cheese, fermented beverages, and so on, are very popular. Research reports indicate that many countries are working in the field of functional foods that are mainly enriched with probiotics and prebiotics. Some of the developed and studied probiotic products are listed in Table 10.1.

TABLE 10.1
Some Classified Probiotic Dairy Products Developed Worldwide

Fermented Dairy Products	References
Fermented Milks/Drinks	
Acidophilus milk drink	Itsaranuwat et al. (2003)
Synbiotic acidophilus milk	Amiri et al. (2008)
Acidophilus "sweet" drink	Speck (1978)
Whey-protein–based drinks	Lucas et al. (2004); Dalev et al. (2006)
Biogarde, mil–mil, and acidophilus milk with yeasts	Gomes and Malcata (1999)
Dairy fermented beverage	Almeida et al. (2000)
Fermented lactic beverages supplemented with oligofructose and cheese whey	de Castro et al. (2009)
Nonfermented goat's milk beverage	Neves (2000)
Fermented goat's milk	Martin-Diana et al. (2003)
High-pressure homogenized probiotic fermented milk	Patrignani et al. (2009)
Synbiotic fermented milk	Matijasic et al. (2016)
Whey-based synbiotic drink	Shah et al. (2016)

(Continued)

TABLE 10.1 (*Continued*)
Some Classified Probiotic Dairy Products Developed Worldwide

Fermented Dairy Products	References
Yogurts	
Regular full-fat yogurts	Aryana and Mcgrew (2007)
Low-fat yogurts	Penna et al. (2007)
Stirred fruit yogurts	Kailasapathy et al. (2008)
Dahi	Yadav et al. (2007)
Acidophilus butter and progurt	Gomes and Malcata (1999)
Peanut milk yogurt	Isanga and Zhang (2009)
Frozen yogurt	Davidson et al. (2000)
Mango soy fortified probiotic yogurt	Kaur et al. (2009)
Traditional Greek yogurt	Maragkoudakisa et al. (2006)
Corn milk yogurt	Supavititpatana et al. (2008)
Banana-based yogurt	Sousa et al. (2007)
Graviola and cupuassu-based yogurts	Silveira et al. (2007)
Acai yogurt	Almeida et al. (2008)
Synbiotic yogurt	Gabrial et al. (2010); Madhu et al. (2012)
Cheeses	
Cheddar cheese	Ong and Shah (2009)
Minas fresco cheese	Souza and Saad (2009)
Feta cheese	Kailasapathy and Masondole (2005)
Cheese from caprine milk	Kalavrouzioti et al. (2005)
Kazar cheese	Ozer et al. (2008)
Semihard reduced-fat cheese	Thage et al. (2005)
White-brined cheese	Yilmaztekin et al. (2004)
Cottage cheese	Blanchette et al. (1996)
Canestrato pugliese hard cheese	Corbo et al. (2001)
Argentine fresco cheese	Vinderola et al. (2000)
Goat semisolid cheese	Gomes and Malcata (1999)
Petit–suisse cheese supplemented with inulin and/or oligofructose	Cardarelli et al. (2008)
Crescenza cheese	Gobbetti et al. (1997)
Turkish Beyaz cheese	Kilic et al. (2009)
Whey Portuguese cheese	Madureira et al. (2005)
Minas fresh cheese	Buriti et al. (2005)
Ice Cream	
Synbiotic ice cream	Homayouni et al. (2008)
Probiotic ice cream	Kailasapathy and Sultana (2003); Akin et al. (2007)
Low-fat ice cream	Haynes and Playne (2002); Akalin and Erisir (2008)
Acidophilus milk-based ice cream	Andrighetto and Gomes (2003)
Frozen synbiotic dessert	Saad et al. (2008)

Source: Adapted from Granato, D. et al., *Comp. Rev. Food Sci. Food Saf.*, 9, 455–470, 2010.

BASIC CONCEPTS OF PROBIOTICS AND PREBIOTICS

Early in the twentieth century, Élie Metchnikoff first suggested the benefits of probiotic bacteria. He described the colonization ability of beneficial flora in the gut, and he postulated that yogurt consumption by the Bulgarian peasants meant that they lived longer (Brown and Valiere, 2004). Later, the definition of probiotics were given by FAO/WHO (2001), and updated by Hill et al. (2014): "Probiotics are live microorganisms that, when administered in adequate amounts, confer a health benefit on the host." Probiotic bacteria may be present in different food products like infant formula, medicinal foods, dietary supplements, fermented foods, and so on. The incorporation of probiotics in food can be in the form of microencapsulated or freeze-dried powder. The form depends on the supplementation medium that makes the probiotic bacteria live during consumption. On the other hand, prebiotics are defined as selectively fermented ingredients, whose fermentation results in specific changes in the composition and/or activity of the gastrointestinal microbiota, thus conferring benefit(s) upon host health (Gibson et al., 2011). The complex carbohydrates that are nondigestible by humans, such as fructo-oligosaccharides, galacto-oligosaccharides, inulin, and so on, are the best studied prebiotics.

PROBIOTICS

The worldwide accepted definition of probiotics is as follows: "live microorganisms which, when administered in adequate amounts, confer a health benefit on the host." Probiotic terms include the specific bacterial strains, represented by lactic acid bacteria (LABs) such as *Bifidobacterium* spp. and *Lactobacillus* spp. These two strains are extensively used in the preparation of fermented dairy and food products, such as yogurt, cheese, beverages, kefir, and lassi. Hence, fermented milk and milk products with pure, active, and live bacterial cultures are the best sources of probiotics (Balakrishnan and Floch, 2012). These types of milk products, prepared or fortified with probiotics, may be useful for a large number of gastrointestinal tract (GIT) conditions. They have also been shown to reduce symptoms for a number of gut diseases and conditions, including diarrhea, antibiotic-associated diarrhea, *Helicobacter pylori* infection, and irritable bowel syndrome. In general, probiotic dairy products enrich the GIT microbial community and have many beneficial health effects.

PROBIOTIC BACTERIAL STRAINS

Many LABs have been studied for their potential probiotic properties, but only a few strains meet the standards of the United Nations of being well documented clinically. The most studied probiotic bacteria are the *Bifidobacterium* and *Lactobacillus* species. The food industry employs these species in functional product developments, including *Bifidobacterium animalis*, *B. bifidum*, *B. brevis*, *B. infantis*, *B. longum*, *Lactobacillus acidophilus*, *L. casei*, *L. delbrueckii* ssp. *bulgaricus*, *L. reuteri*, and *L. rhamnosus* (Knorr, 1998). A more detailed list of probiotic bacteria is shown in Table 10.2.

TABLE 10.2
List of Some Studied Probiotic Bacteria

Bifidobacterium Species	Lactobacillus Species	Others
B. adolescentis	*L. acidophilus*	*Bacillus cereus*
B. animalis	*L. amylovorus*	*Clostridium botyricum*
B. bifidum	*L. brevis*	*Enterococcus faecalis*
B. breve	*L. casei*	*Enterococcus faecium*
B. infantis	*L. rhamnosus*	*Escherichia coli*
B. lactis	*L. crispatus*	*Lactococcus lactis* ssp. *cremoris*
B. longum	*L. delbrueckii* ssp. *bulgaricus*	*Lactococcus lactis* ssp. *lactis*
	L. fermentum	*Leuconostoc mesenteroides* ssp.
	L. gasseri	*dextranicum*
	L. helveticus	*Pediococcus acidilactici*
	L. johnsonii	*Propionibacterium freudenreichii*
	L. lactis	*Saccharomyces boulardii*
	L. paracasei	*Streptococcus salivarius* ssp.
	L. plantarum	*thermophilus*
	L. reuteri	*Sporolactobacillus inulinus*
	L. salivarius	
	L. gallinarum	

Source: Adapted from Prado, F. C. et al., *Food Res. Int.*, 41, 111–123, 2008; Leroy, F. et al., Latest developments in probiotics, in *Meat Biotechnology*, Toldra, F., (Ed.), Brussels, Belgium, Springer, pp. 217–229, 2008.

ROLE OF PROBIOTICS IN MAJOR MILK PRODUCTS

Numerous studies have shown that food matrixes play an incredibly vital role in providing health benefits to the host (Espirito Santo et al. 2011). Fermented dairy foods, mostly fermented milk products, are normally used as carriers for the probiotic bacteria. Among fermented dairy foods, dairy beverages have been adopted into the human diet in several countries because the fermentation technique is inexpensive, and it not only preserves the food materials safely but also improves the nutritional value and sensory properties of the products (Gadaga et al., 1999). Hence, demand for new and innovative probiotic products by consumers has encouraged the maximum production of dairy food matrixes for successful delivery of probiotic products such as cheese, yogurt, ice cream, lassi, infant milk powder, and so on. Davidson et al. (2000) determined the viability of the probiotic strains *Bifidobacterium longum*, *Lactobacillus acidophilus*, *Lactobacillus delbrueckii* ssp. *Bulgaricus*, and *Streptococcus salivarius* ssp. *Thermophilus*, which were used as culture in the low-fat ice cream. This study has shown evidence that culture bacterial populations did not decrease when they were stored under frozen conditions. In addition, no alterations in the sensory characteristics of ice cream were seen in the presence of probiotic bacteria. Therefore, it has been suggested that the ice cream matrix could provide an excellent way to deliver probiotic culture. Although probiotic ice cream contained comparatively high pH around (5.5–6.5), it did not show any significant reduction in the survival of lactic acid cultures during frozen storage. Products with lower acidity led to an increase in consumer acceptance, especially by those consumers who choose mild acidic products (Cruz et al. 2009). It has been noticed in the commercial bioyogurt industry that survival and growth of probiotic dairy yeast *Saccharomyces boulardii* along with yogurt bacteria were quite appreciable. Lourens-Hattingh and Viljoen (2001) reported that probiotic yeast has the ability to survive in dairy food matrixes, specifically in ultra-heat-treated (UHT) milk, UHT milk yogurt, and bioyogurt. A study involving a 4-week period under refrigeration conditions (4°C) was conducted using above-mentioned dairy foods and incorporating yeast, *S. boulardii*. This study revealed that the probiotic yeast species, *S. boulardii* has the ability of maximum survival (10^7 CFU/g) in bioyogurt. It was found that in the fruit-based yogurt, yeast populations were relatively higher because of high amount of fructose and sucrose found in the fruit. The probiotic dairy yeast *S. boulardii* was unable to utilize lactose, but this species efficiently utilized the other available nutrients such as galactose, glucose, and organic acid, which were obtained from lactose metabolism by bacterial species.

The stirred fruit yogurt, prepared with mixed berry, mango, strawberry, and passion fruit, was analyzed for the survivability of *Bifidobacterium animalis* ssp. *lactis* and *L. acidophilus* during storage (Godward et al., 2000; Kailasapathy et al., 2008). No effect on the counts of both probiotic strains on addition of any of the fruit extractions except the cell concentrations was found.

Increased numbers of *L. acidophilus* and *L. casei* were found in fermented milk fortified with lemon and orange fibers compared with the control set during cold storage. This number pattern was not seen in the *B. bifidum* because bifidobacteria species are very sensitive to acidic environments (Sendra et al., 2008).

Probiotic-Incorporated Cheeses

Among fermented dairy products, cheeses have been reported for the potential delivery of probiotic bacteria into the human gastrointestinal tract. The physiochemical properties of cheese favor the production of probiotic bacteria. The manufacturing process of cheeses depends on the type of cheese and its composition. Compositional factors of cheeses include higher buffering capacity and pH, higher fat and total solids content, nutrient availability, lower oxygen content, and titratable acidity. These factors contribute to making superior fermented dairy products, and they protect probiotic bacteria from the external adverse conditions and storage as well. However, the release of live and active probiotic bacteria is still possible for the host (Ong et al., 2006; Karimi et al., 2011).

In general, all probiotic bacteria have to be compatible during the food manufacturing processes without any changes having to be made to the technological aspect. Therefore, the cheesemaking process may have to be refined for the use of probiotic cultures in cheese products, and all the requirements needed for the particular probiotic strains must be employed. With respect to the preparation of probiotic cheeses, the probiotic strains to be used for inoculation must be high in number and uniform because the probiotic strains must proliferate in the processing conditions such as ripening and storage (Ross et al., 2002). Overall, there are not many differences in the attributes of probiotic cheese and conventional cheese. Moreover, biofunctional attributes of conventional cheese can be further enhanced by the incorporation of probiotic bacteria, which increases the value of the cheese simultaneously.

Probiotic-incorporated food products exhibit effectiveness in controlled clinical trials. Well-established probiotic characterization steps along with manufacturing steps should be validated to ensure that there is no alteration in the final probiotic product (Stanton et al. 2003). The viability of probiotic bacteria should remain in the final product so that consumers receive the benefits from the probiotic cheese. Hence, before addition of any probiotic bacteria in the cheese or any other food stuffs, it must be screened *in vitro*, and the safety of the probiotic strains must be ensured. The proper validation via *in vivo* clinical trials as well as human trials are also very important steps. However, the viability of probiotic bacteria must be ensured in the product at the time of consumption. The probiotic strain could be used directly to fortify cheeses and related products. A thorough study of an individual strain should be done for any clinical studies of multiple strains studied at the time. When any product contains multiple strains, each and every strain has to be well studied for its biofunctional properties. The symbiotic association of multiple strains must be analyzed for the effectiveness of the particular product (Aimutis, 2001). Many clinical trials on animals and humans have documented the health benefits of probiotic cheeses. During its ripening period, cheddar cheese was shown to be more effective for delivering *Enterococcus faecium* Fargo 688 live cells compared to yogurt. In pigs' feces, the numbers of viable cells were noted as 2.0×10^6 of the probitiotic cheddar cheese and 5.2×10^5 CFU/g of the probiotic yogurt. The same probiotic bacteria with different delivery system significantly differ and it was even better in terms of viability in the probiotic cheese (Gardiner et al. 1999).

A study reported that fresh probiotic cheese (Argentinean fresh cheese) containing culture *L. acidophilus* A9, *B. bifidum* A12, and *L. paracasei* A13 showed immunomodulating property in mice, with increased phagocytic activity in the small intestine of peritoneal macrophages, after 2, 5, and 7 days of its consumption. After 5 days of ingestion, there was also a significant increase in the number of IgA$^+$ producing cells in the large intestine. Probiotic bacteria as antigens interacted in the large intestine (lymphoid nodules) and in the small intestine (Peyer's patches) (Medici et al., 2004). The roles of phagocytic cells were also seen to protect the microbial infections. The humoral immunity was maintained by the mucosal IgA antibodies, which eliminated the adherence of pathogens to the gut mucosa (Gill, 1998).

Ahola et al. (2002) studied the effect of Edam cheese on the potential risk of dental caries. The probiotic bacteria *L. rhamnosus* GG ATCC53103 (LGG) and *Lactobacillus rhamnosus* LC705 were used as the cultures for preparation of probiotic Edam cheese. A high reduction in the number of the microorganism *S. mutans* was observed; that is, no elevation of *S. mutans* populations was found in the probiotic group subjects, whereas the concentration of *S. mutans* were found to be increased by 8% in the three subjects compared to the control. Throughout the 3-week post-study, a decreased concentration (21%) of *S. mutans* populations were found in the subjects who consumed probiotic cheese and only an 8% reduction in the control group subjects. The declined populations were observed in the probiotic group subjects who had high yeast populations. During cheesemaking, an increase in the lactobacilli population also increased salivary lactobacilli population, with continuous probiotic intervention. Henceforth, the consumption of probiotic cheese could reduce the risk of dental caries in general, although no significant differences in the salivary microbial populations were observed.

An investigation was done in elderly people to find the positive effects of probiotic cheese consumption on oral candidosis (Hatakka et al. 2007). A total of 92 subjects consumed cheese that contained a mixture of probiotic cultures such as *Propionibacterium freundenreichii* spp. *shermani* JS, *L. rhamnosus* LC705, and *L. rhamnosus* GG. Saliva samples were taken four times throughout the study, and oral yeasts analysis were done. Results showed that the high yeast populations declined by 75.0% in the probiotic treatment group. The analysis revealed the prevalence of high populations ($>10^4$ CFU/mL) after 8 and 16 weeks. This indicated that microbial populations were remarkably decreased to 25.0% and 20.7%, respectively. On the other hand, 31% of oral yeasts were increased in the control cheese group, meaning those who did not ingest probiotic cheese. This study suggested that consumption of probiotics is highly effective for the composition of saliva, salivary immunoglobulins, and mucins concentration. Finally, the authors suggested that probiotic cheese could be used as a prophylactic approach for the reduction of hyposalivation risk and dry mouth. Thus, probiotics could be considered as having factors that promote oral health.

Probiotic Yogurt

Yogurt is a semisolid food that is the product of lactic acid fermentation of milk, and it is consumed around the world. High-quality yogurt has pleasant sensory characteristics and can prevent numerous diseases. Thus, it can be called a "natural probiotic." It is extremely rich in protein, calcium, and B vitamins, it increases the number of beneficial microflora in the intestinal tract, and it facilitates direct consumption of live bacteria. Commercially, yogurts are prepared by fermentation of milk with mixture of lactic cultures consisting of *Streptococcus thermophilus* (ST) and *Lactobacillus delbrueckii* ssp. *bulgaricus* (LB). Emphasis has been placed on developing probiotic yogurt containing probiotic cultures, namely, *Lactobacillus acidophilus* and *Bifidobacterium bifidum*, for obtaining therapeutic benefits. The suggested minimum level of probiotics in yogurt is 10^5–10^6 viable cells per gram of product, and an adequate number of the probitotics must be alive to exert their positive effect on the host. This attribute is known as "viability." Hence, viability of these bacteria during storage and up to the moment of consumption is an important criterion.

Probiotic yogurt is widely available in the market as plain yogurt, low-fat yogurt, and flavored yogurt under different brands.

Probiotics play an important role in reducing diarrhea, especially infectious diarrhea and antibiotic-associated diarrhea. Many studies have reported that certain probiotic yogurt strains may be helpful in reducing ulcerative colitis, bloating, and gas in patients with irritable bowel syndrome (IBS). Certain strains of *L. casei* and

B. lactis have also been found to improve stool consistency and bowel movement frequency in people with constipation. For example, VSL#3, a probiotic medical food consisting of a combination of eight different probiotic strains, is very useful in managing ulcerative colitis and irritable bowel syndrome. It claims to deliver the highest available concentration of live beneficial bacteria than any other probiotic (Huynh et al., 2009; Miele et al. 2010; Ng et al., 2010). It has been reported that drinking fermented milk prepared with a particular strain of *Lactobacillus gasseri* for up to 12 weeks significantly reduced abdominal fat and body weight in comparison with people who drank control fermented milk (Kadooka et al., 2010). Thus, it has been proved that fermented milk has benefits for consumers.

Ejtahed et al. (2011) studied the antidiabetic effect of probiotics and reported that the effect of probiotic yogurt on the lipid profile of individuals with type 2 diabetes significantly improved total cholesterol and LDL cholesterol. Immune stimulatory responses (such as to flu vaccines) of probiotics have also been reported. Evidence suggests that friendly bacteria in the colon help to boost the immune system. Ganguli et al. (2013) studied and reported that probiotics prevent necrotizing enterocolitis by modulating enterocyte genes that regulate innate immune-mediated inflammation. Similarly, a prospective study was conducted to examine the effect of probiotic yogurt on 38 *Helicobacter pylori*–infected 38 children on systemic immunological response. This study revealed that regular consumption of probiotic yogurt stimulated the cellular and humoral immunity in children. The balance of intestinal microbiota was also maintained for these children (Yang and Sheu 2012). Two probiotic strains, *Bifidobacterium animalis* ssp. *lactis*, BB-12w and *Lactobacillus paracasei* ssp. *paracasei*, *L. casei* 431w, also showed immune benefits in the influenza vaccination model in a randomized, double-blind, placebo-controlled study (Rizzardini et al., 2012).

P. freudenreichii have been reported for its preventive effects on colon cancer cells during *in vitro* and *in vivo* experiments (Lan et al., 2008; Cousin et al., 2012). Similarly, yogurt containing *L. bulgaricus* and *S. thermophilus* exhibited the anti-cancer effect (Perdigon et al., 2002; Miele et al., 2010), whereas strain *L. helveticus* was also reported for the prevention of colon cancer (de Moreno and Perdigon, 2010).

Microflora populate the mouth as well. Probiotic yogurt has also been documented for better oral health such as the reduction of throat infections, periodontal disease, and bad breath. Probiotics associated with yogurt have been claimed to lower blood pressure; decreases oxidative stress; improve eczema; and treat ulcers, colon cancer, urinary tract infections (UTI), depression, and anxiety. Probiotic yogurt is also beneficial for lactose-intolerant individuals because the live bacteria digest some of the lactose (milk sugar).

PROBIOTIC MARKETS IN INDIA

Indian consumers are more concerned today about their health and about healthy foods, especially probiotics and nutraceutical and therapeutic food products. Thus, demand for probiotic products is increasing. According to data published by TechSci Research, the Indian probiotic market is expected to grow at around 20% by 2019. Many industries are producing probiotic food products in India, among the leading

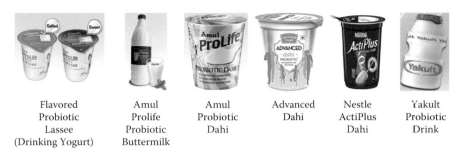

| Flavored Probiotic Lassee (Drinking Yogurt) | Amul Prolife Probiotic Buttermilk | Amul Probiotic Dahi | Advanced Dahi | Nestle ActiPlus Dahi | Yakult Probiotic Drink |

FIGURE 10.1   Available probiotic dairy products in Indian market.

producers are Amul, Nestle, Mother Dairy, and Danone. Functional foods, especially probiotic foods, dairy products, and beverages, make up an important revenue share in the Indian functional food and probiotic markets. It has been seen that North India dominates the Indian probiotic market compared to the southern and central regions of the country in terms of demand and sales revenue. According to TechSci Research, the future probiotic market in India will be segmented into probiotic beverages, functional foods, probiotic dietary supplements, probiotic drugs, and probiotic animal feeds. Figure 10.1 shows some of the currently available probiotic dairy foods in Indian markets.

PREBIOTICS

The human intestine is part of a system that is required for absorption of essential nutrients and minerals. The intestinal microflora comprises about 95% of total cells in the body. Intestinal microbes mainly include bacteria, although archaea and eukaryotes are also present. The colon is the most intensely populated area of the gastrointestinal tract. Therefore, on the basis of activities of resident microflora, the colon plays an essential part in host nutrition and health (Gibson and Roberfroid, 1999). *Lactobacilli* and *Bifidobacteria* are considered as the health-promoting constituents in the human colon. These genera are selectively grown and promoted by intake of available nonviable substances into the colon well known as prebiotics. Due to the presence of more bifidobacteria than lactobacilli, they exhibit a preference for oligosaccharides.

The term *prebiotics* was given by Gibson and Roberfroid (1995) to a nondigestible food ingredient that benefits the host health by stimulation of a number of probiotic bacteria in the colon. But it was noticed that this definition of prebiotics was found to overlap the term *dietary fibers*. So Cummings et al. (2001) explained that prebiotics are short chain length carbohydrates. Gibson et al. (2004) redefine *prebiotic* as "a selectively fermented substance that allows specific changes, both in the activity and composition in the GIT microflora that confers benefits upon host well-being and health." Since the introduction of the concept, prebiotics have attracted much attention and are involved in stimulating scientific as well as industrial interest. Most of the bacteria in the gastrointestinal tract are benign, but pathogenic species are also

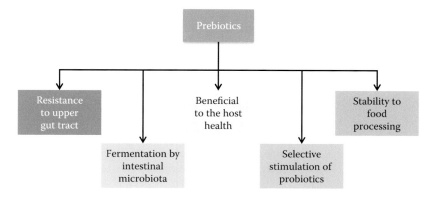

FIGURE 10.2 Criteria for classifying a food ingredient as a prebiotic.

present and can cause acute and chronic disorders. In nutritional sciences, there is much interest in dietary modulation of human gut microorganisms by prebiotics, which improve health by increasing the number of lactobacilli and bifidobacteria, which in turn can increase resistance to pathogenic species and also increase stimulation of immune response.

These are the classification criteria for dietary substances as prebiotics (Figure 10.2):

- The substance must not be hydrolyzed or absorbed in the stomach or small intestine.
- The substance must be selective for beneficial bacteria in the colon such as bifidobacteria and lactobacilli.
- Fermentation of such substances should induce beneficial effects within the host.

The prebiotic principle is based on ingesting a diet containing nondigestible oligosaccharides, also termed as short chain polysaccharides, which are fermented by indigenous beneficial microorganisms. Oligosaccharides are sugars containing 2–20 saccharide units. The oligosaccharides having prebiotic potential mainly are lactulose, galacto-oligosaccharides, fructo-oligosaccharides, lactosucrose, gluco-oligosaccharides, xylo-oligosaccharides, and soy oligosaccharides.

The probiotic approach has been defined as the consumption of live bacteria in appropriate cell numbers. In general, lactobacilli or bifidobacteria have been proven to strengthen the gut. However, probiotic bacteria must be live during the supplementation. Many probiotic strains have various health benefits like immune system stimulation. The availability of prebiotics containing hese probiotic strains enables the development of synbiotic with increased survivability in the gut. Prebiotics are noted for their ability to survive degrading by the host enzymes present in the GIT; therefore, probiotics reach the colon and are utilized by the beneficial probiotic bacteria, which may be either *Bifidobacterium* species or *Lactobacillus* species. Survivability of these bacteria in the intestine means greater potential health benefits to the host.

ESTABLISHED PREBIOTICS

Prebiotics are mainly classified as the inulin-derived fructans (fructo-oligosaccharides [FOSs]: inulin and oligofructose); galacto-oligosaccharides (GOSs) include sucrose-derived oligofructose and lactulose (Sarbini and Rastall, 2011). The possibility for generation of other prebiotics such as oligosaccharides can be done through synthesis or hydrolysis of the polysaccharide (Rastall, 2010).

Inulin Type Fructans

Glu $\alpha1-2[\beta$ Fru $1-2]n$, where $n > 10$ is the form of inulin polysaccharide (Crittenden and Playne, 1996). Inulin occurs naturally in Western foods such as onion, wheat, garlic, leek, and asparagus. The structurally similar fructo-oligosaccharides (a lower-molecular-weight version) are close relatives of inulin. FOSs are noted as the best oligosaccharides for the intestinal microflora bifidobacteria because they are very effective prebiotics for the growth of bifidobacteria. FOSs are Glu $\alpha1-2[\beta$ Fru $1-2]n$, in which $n = 2-9$. FOSs are either synthesized from sucrose or from the hydrolysis of inulin. Wang and Gibson (1993) reported that FOSs and inulin significantly increase the number of bifidobacteria, which indicates that these substrates are prebiotic in nature. However, both FOSs and inulin have been found to be less stable at low pH and at high temperatures than other prebiotic oligosaccharides. A study found that very acidic conditions partially hydrolyzed the $\beta(2-1)$ bonds of the fructose moiety (Bosscher, 2009). Moreover, a FOS solution heated at 145°C for only 10 seconds at pH 3.5 hydrolyzed it by approximately 10% (Voragen, 1998). A similar report was given by Petersen et al. (2010) on the FOS solution. The prebiotic activity was considerably reduced on exposure at high temperatures such as 85°C for 30 min. The FOS gets hydrolyzed during pasteurization and degraded up to 80% in the fruit juices (Klewicki, 2007). The hydrolysis pattern of FOS also depends upon the processing conditions.

Another significant technological feature of any specific prebiotic is its impact on the functional properties of any dairy or food product such as organoleptic and physicochemical properties. Various research studies have been done on the many prebiotics, but inulin is generally recognized as safe (GRAS) by the U.S. Food and Drug Administration (FDA). Franck (2008) studied the properties of inulin as a fat replacer and/or texture modifier in the food industry. Due to its moderate solubility (10% soluble at room temperature) in water, inulin is very easily incorporated into the liquid foods. Inulin is almost neutral in taste and is slightly sweet (less than 10% compared to sucrose). Based on such properties, inulin is a good choice as a fat replacer in many dairy products like yogurts, fermented milks, cheeses, ice creams, and dairy desserts (Kusuma et al., 2009; Meyer et al., 2011; Buriti et al., 2016). The gelling properties of inulin at high concentration (>25% in water for native inulin and >15% for long-chain inulin) makes it a good replacement for fat and also improves its mouthfeel. Dissolving inulin in water makes a white, creamy, spreadable gel. Its smooth, fatty mouthfeel means that it can completely replace fats in food materials. FOSs have been reported to be much more soluble than prebiotic inulin (up to 85% soluble at room temperature). FOSs are moderately sweet (30%–35% compared to sucrose) and their technical properties are almost similar to glucose and sucrose syrups; hence, their use can be as a sugar replacer (Bosscher, 2009).

Galacto-Oligosaccharides

Galacto-oligosaccharides are defined by Crittenden and Playne (1996) as Glu α1–4[β Gal 1–6]n, (n = 2–5). GOSs are traditionally manufactured from lactose. The enzyme β-galactosidase exhibits the transgalactosylase activity on the production of GOS. The substrate lactulose is used for the development of prebiotic GOS, and the resultant product oligosaccharides showed similar fermentation characteristics to the traditional GOS using *in vitro* testing with fecal batch cultures. This technique used for preparation of GOS may prove to be more effective per gram than the traditional techniques (Cardelle-Cobas et al., 2012). The stability of GOS is very high in acidic conditions and at high temperatures, which is why the addition of GOS is preferable to both acidic and heat-treated foods. For example, GOSs are added to pasteurized fruit juices, bakery products, fermented milks, yogurts, and buttermilks. The addition of GOSs to infant formula has the most prospects for profitability. Data indicate that infant formula contains 6.0–7.2 g/L GOS and 0.6–0.8 g/L FOS together with GOS (Sangwan et al., 2011).

Recently, interest has been focused on the application of gluco-oligosaccharides (GlOSs) for their prebiotic potential. Sarbini et al. (2013) reported that commercial GlOS products were very effective in the selective growth of bifidobacteria and the growth of bacteroides *Faecalibacterium prausnitzii* was decreased in fecal batch cultures during *in vitro* study. Increased concentration of bifidobacteria would be considered to have positive effects on health, while reduction in the *F. prausnitzii* cell numbers might not be desirable (Sarbini et al., 2013).

Prebiotic Lactulose

Synthetic disaccharide lactulose is present in the form of Gal β1–4 Fru. Lactulose has also received the attention due to its potential as a prebiotic. Saunders and Wiggins (1981) reported that initially lactulose was not hydrolyzed or absorbed in the small intestine because it was used as a laxative. The property of lactulose to increase the gut microflora bifidobacteria and lactobacilli and to reduce simultaneously the number of bacteroides in mixed continuous fecal culture was reported by Fadden and Owen (1992). Many human trials have reported on the prebiotic potentials of lactulose, which is why lactulose is a promising prebiotic candidate. However, lactulose is not yet widely distributed. It has an established presence in the food and medical sectors.

Prebiotics from Waste

Currently, food processing waste and agricultural waste biomass are also potential sources of prebiotics (Gullon et al., 2013). Plant oligosaccharides have been the traditional source for generation of oligosaccharides with application of an enzyme; however, the use of autohydrolysis has become more useful and interesting (Rivas et al., 2012). The treatment of polysaccharide-containing material involves elevated temperature and pressure for efficient production.

Mushrooms: A Potential Source of Prebiotics

A recent development in prebiotics involves the search for new sources of prebiotics. Mushrooms could be used as a potential source of prebiotics because they contain carbohydrates like chitin, hemicellulose, band a-glucans, mannans, xylans, and galactans. Linear and branched glucans with various types of glycosidic linkages such as $(1 \to 3)$, $(1 \to 6)$ β-glucans and $(1 \to 3)$ α-glucans are present in most mushrooms. However, few of the mushrooms that contain mannose, xylose, arabinose, galactose, fucose, glucuronic acids, and glucose are true heteroglycans, which contain the main side chain components. The carbohydrates present in mushrooms are nondigestible; thus, mushrooms can be considered as the potential prebiotic alternatives. The mushrooms extracts *Pleurotus ostreatus* and *P. eryngii* were capable of stimulating the growth of probiotics *Lactobacillus* ssp. and *Bifidobacterium* ssp. (Synytsya et al., 2009).

The selective stimulation of the growth of intestinal microbiota is one of the major criteria of prebiotics classification, and this criterion is generally associated with the promotion of health benefits (Gibson, 2004). Figure 10.3 represents the potential mechanism whereby dietary substrates present in the gut lumen. Wang (2009) reported that prebiotics enhance the growth and activities of the probiotic bacteria, especially lactobacilli and bifidobacteria. The suppressive effect of prebiotics has also been observed in bacteroides and clostridia. A comparative quantitative technique, the prebiotic index (PI) measurement, was given by Palframan et al. (2003) for assessing *in vitro* prebiotic effects. The main purpose of this equation is consideration of positive effects on the increasing number of lactobacilli and bifidobacteria,

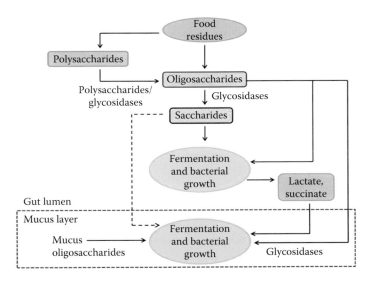

FIGURE 10.3 Potential mechanisms for dietary components available in mucosa-associated microbiota in large intestine.

while negative effects are indicated by the increase in the population of clostridia and bacteroides. The following equation can be used to calculate the PI:

$$\text{Prebiotic Index} = \frac{\text{Bif}}{\text{Total}} + \frac{\text{Bac}}{\text{Total}} + \frac{\text{Lac}}{\text{Total}} + \frac{\text{Clos}}{\text{Total}}$$
$$\text{(PI)}$$

where:
    Bif denotes bifidobacterial numbers
    Bac denotes bacteroides numbers
    Lac denotes lactobacilli numbers
    Clos denotes Clostridia numbers
    Total is the total bacterial numbers at sample time/numbers at inoculation

APPLICATIONS OF PREBIOTICS IN VARIOUS FOODS, PARTICULARLY DAIRY PRODUCTS

The main function of prebiotics is to improve the organoleptic characteristics of functional foods and also enhance the mouthfeel and characteristic taste. A good prebiotic must be chemically stable to various food-processing techniques, such as low pH, high temperature, Maillard reaction conditions, and low temperature. Therefore, the applications of prebiotics offer a double advantage: a well-balanced nutritional composition and enhanced organoleptic properties. Today, prebiotics are increasingly being used as food ingredients that promote the intestinal bacteria, particularly the probiotic bacteria. Some recent research that has been conducted in prebiotic food development is discussed in the following sectons.

Significance of Prebiotics in Cheese

Among all the food products, milk and milk products are considered the best media for supplementation of both prebiotics and probiotics. The composition of cheese and its matrix efficiently support the addition of probiotic bacteria due to its fat content and less acidic environment. Research was conducted *in vitro* in five petit–suisse cheese formulations to check the prebiotic potential of inulin, oligofructose, and honey. Human fecal slurry analysis revealed the highest fermentation rate in the cheese to which prebiotics were added. The fermentation rate was checked by analysis of lactic acid production. The addition of prebiotics in probiotic cheese also promoted the growth rate of lactobacilli and bifidobacteria. Many prebiotic-supplemented probiotic cheeses were studied for maintaining viability of probiotic bacteria in the product during long-term storage. Kinik et al. (2017) studied the effects of the use of the prebiotics oligofructose and inulin on symbiotic goat cheese during ripening and reported that the aromatic compounds were found to be increased in the probiotic cheese. The textural properties of cheese were also significantly changed on the cheese to which both prebiotics and probiotics were added.

Prebiotics in Fermented Milk

Rodrigues et al. (2012) evaluated the physiochemical composition and rheological properties of the prebiotic inulin added to microfiltered cow's milk. Addition of prebiotic increased the total solid content and acidity of the products. Moreover, addition of inulin increased the apparent viscosity of the product during storage temperatures of $6.0°C \pm 0.1°C$ and $4.0°C \pm 0.1°C$. Greater thixotropy and lowered hysteresis have also been observed in the prebiotic fermented milk.

Remarkable human health effects have been observed for fermented milks that incorporated prebiotics. The nutritional and technical properties of prebiotics make them superior components that can be added to many foodstuffs.

Prebiotics in Yogurts

Today, prebiotics are added more and more frequently to yogurt because of the use of probiotic bacteria in the yogurt. Many studies discuss the various aspects of synbiotic yogurts. Shakerian et al. (2014) reported that *L. acidophilus* and *B. animalis* have grown well in yogurt up to 10^6 CFU/mL. One percent inulin had no significant effect on organic acid production, but it was beneficial for promoting the growth of *B. animalis* and for reducing the degree of proteolysis. Grimoud et al. (2010) screened some LABs for their probiotic characteristics (resistance to intestinal conditions, inhibition of pathogenic bacteria). *Bifidobacterium* and *L. farciminis* were the most effective for inhibiting-pathogen growth, whereas bifidobacteria showed the most resistance to harsh gastrointestinal conditions. The prebiotics oligodextran and oligoalternan were selected on the basis of their ability to support the growth of the tested probiotics. It was observed that bifidobacteria most effectively metabolized the glucooligosaccharides, the strongest inhibitory effects against enteric pathogens were displayed by lactobacilli.

Allgeyer et al. (2010) prepared six different synbiotic drinkable yogurts containing the selected prebiotics chicory inulin, polydextrose, and soluble corn fiber added separately to the yogurts. The concentration of fiber was increased by adding 5 g of fiber/serving or 2.5 g of fiber/serving to claim an excellent source of fiber. Yogurt drinks were also prepared using a prebiotic concentration 5 g for each and individual prebiotics with the selected probiotic bacteria *L. acidophilus* LA-5 and *B. lactis* Bb-12. A control sample without prebiotics and probiotics was also prepared. Yogurt drinks with soluble corn fiber and inulin exhibited variable sweet versus sour attributes. The next yogurt drink with polydextrose was noted variability in the mouthfeel attributes. During 30 days storage the survivability of probiotics decreased from 2 to 3 log in all the yogurt treatments.

Guven et al. (2005) prepared set-type low-fat yogurt (0.1% fat and solid not fat (SNF) 14%) with inulin addition (1%, 2%, and 3%) as a fat replacer. Synbiotic yogurt (2.5% fat) was prepared with probiotic bacteria (*L. rhamnosus* and *L. reuteri*) and 1.5% prebiotics (inulin, lactulose, and oligofructose). The samples containing inulin showed the lowest syneresis and had the highest viscosity. *L. rhamnosus* and *L. reuteri* also showed the best viability in the samples containing inulin (Shaghaghi et al., 2013).

Chemical characteristics such as pH, titratable acidity, and the acetaldehyde of yogurt were not influenced by the inulin (Guven et al., 2005). Aryana et al. (2007) reported that yogurt containing prebiotic has a significantly lower pH than other yogurts.

Yogurts containing inulin have better body and texture and less syneresis than other prepared yogurts and the control yogurt (Aryana et al. 2007). Yogurt stickiness, airiness, and thickness contribute to the creamy mouthfeel. The addition of inulin significantly affects the thickness (Kip et al., 2006). Rheological properties were performed by shear, compression–extrusion, and dynamic assay, and results showed no significant changes in the rheological properties (Dello Staffolo et al., 2004). The viscoelastic behavior is not significantly affected by the addition of any of the fiber, although it increased the consistency of the yogurts (Sanz et al., 2008).

The addition of prebiotics affects sensory evaluations of yogurts. The yogurt containing 1% inulin was almost similar to the control yogurt, which was prepared with whole milk (Guven et al., 2005). It has been reported that inulin improves the creamy mouthfeel of low-fat yogurts (Kip et al. 2006). The flavor scores of yogurt containing inulin were similar to that of the control yogurts (Aryan and McGrew, 2007). When these yogurts were compared with the control yogurt, only the color difference in the apple fiber yogurt was observed. The rheological properties of the plain yogurt were modified by the use of fibers. The panelists suggested that the yogurts supplemented with fibers were found to be more acceptable (Dello Staffolo et al., 2004). The viability and activity of probiotic bacteria *L. casei* LC-01 could be improved by the addition of prebiotic inulin to the food products (Nazzaro et al., 2009; Paseephol and Sherkat, 2009). The adhesion property of *L. rhamnosus* was significantly increased, and the adhesion of harmful bacteria *Salmonella typhimurium* to Caco-2 cells was decreased in the inulin and kiwifruit-pectin–supplemented product. The ability of *Bifidobacterium bifidum* to adhere to Caco-2 cells was also significantly enhanced in the inulin and citrus-pectin–supplemented product (Parkar et al., 2010). The populations of *Lactobacillus-Enterococcus* group, *Atopobium* group, and *Bifidobacterium* genus significantly increased after the inulin and konjac glucomannan hydrolysate fermentation (Connolly et al., 2010).

Probiotics and Prebiotics (Synbiotics) in Human Health

Probiotics and prebiotics together or synbiotics modulate the gut microbiota and may perhaps promote the host's health. The health promotion may be due to the mechanism of synbiotics through the modulation of the immune system, the production of metabolites, and maintaining the viability and survivability of intestinal bacteria long enough to work effectively in the harsh environment of the GIT. Prebiotics are not generally digested in the GIT by the digestive enzymes, but some groups of bacteria, the so-called beneficial bacteria, combine with these non-digestible ingredients and enhance their activity in the colon by producing many short chain fatty acids. Prebiotics help in the improvement of intestinal health by increasing the absorption of minerals. In addition to their health benefits, prebiotics may increase the rheological and the sensory properties of yogurt and other dairy products (Al-Sheraji et al., 2013).

The format of delivery of probiotics is an important aspect for improving their efficacy, in other words, improving their physiology, viability, stability, and potential health benefits. For this, fermented milk products like yogurt could be the best choice. It has been suggested that symbiotic products are more effective than either probiotics or prebiotics alone (Sanders and Marco, 2010). Synbiotics change the gut microbiota and ecology via synergistic effects, including increasing mineral absorption and reducing the loss of bone mineral density, which was indicated by bone alkaline phosphatase (Scholz-Ahrens et al. 2016). Inulin has also been reported to improve calcium and magnesium absorption, reduce triglyceridemia and associated heart disease, and minimize the risk of diseases related to abnormality of the gastro-intestinal defense mechanisms (Roberfroid, 2005).

Shah et al. (2016) studied the antioxidant potential and the physiochemical and microbiological activity during storage of two synbiotic dairy products: synbiotic lassi, which was prepared with the *S. thermophilus* MTCC 5460 (MD2) and honey, and whey-based synbiotic drink made with inulin and orange juice using *L. helveticus* MTCC 5463 (V3). The physiochemical results showed that pH and titratable acidity of both types of synbiotic products decreased pH and increased titratable acidity under long-term refrigeration. There was no change in the viability of pro-biotic cultures was observed under storage conditions. The freshly prepared synbi-otic lassi with honey exhibited 28.43% of the DPPH (α,α-diphenyl-β-picrylhydrazyl) radical scavenging activity, whereas the activity was found to be decreased to 23.03% on the seventh day of storage. The hydroxyl radical scavenging activity of this prod-uct decreased significantly from 107.76% to 79.41% at the end of the storage condi-tions. The whey-based synbiotic drink showed hydroxyl radical scavenging activity up to 100.32% (day 0), but it declined sharply to 79.21% on the seventh day; however, it increased again on the fourteenth day (102.59%). The radical scavenging activity by the DPPH method decreased from 26.85% on the starting day to 17.12% on the seventh day, and after that it continued to decline.

Madhu et al. (2012) reported about yogurt prepared with yogurt cultures along with probiotic bacteria *L. fermentum* CFR 2192, *L. plantarum* CFR 2194, and pre-biotic FOS. The growth promotion of *L. plantarum* and *L. fermentum* was signifi-cantly ($p < 0.05$) affected by the FOS supplementation. DPPH radical scavenging activity was significantly ($p < 0.05$) higher in synbiotic yogurt (85%) containing *L. plantarum* and FOS compared to the control yogurt (72%). Ferric reducing power and total phenolics in the synbiotic yogurt were significantly higher compared to the other test samples for the entire storage period. Thus, incorporating prebiotic FOS and probiotics improved the functionality of the synbiotic yogurt.

Kleniewska et al. (2016) studied the antioxidant capacity of probiotic *L. casei* (4×10^8 CFU) combined with prebiotic inulin (400 mg). They demonstrated that this synbiotic was effective in protecting the human body from oxidative stress damage. The administration of synbiotics significantly increased the Ferric reducing anti-oxidant power (FRAP) value ($p = 0.00008$) and catalase (CAT) activity ($p = 0.02$). The level of glutathione peroxidase (GP_x) and superoxide dismutase (SOD) activ-ity were found to be insignificant in comparison with controls. They suggested that synbiotics might be considered as a food supplement suitable for the treatment and prevention of the oxidative stress injury. Riordan et al. (2007) studied short-term synbiotic treatment for liver function in patients with cirrhosis. They observed that a synbiotic regimen modulated the gut microbiota and significantly improved liver function in patients with cirrhosis. They concluded that the benefit of synbiotic treat-ment is unrelated to reduction in endotoxemia and may be mediated by treatment-related induction of IL-6 synthesis by TNF-α. Prebiotics are also suggested for their hypocholesterolemic effects. Beitane and Ciprovica (2012) studied the influence of lactulose as a prebiotic as well as inulin on the ability of *Bifidobacterium lactis* to reduce cholesterol in milk during fermentation. Prebiotics inulin-RAFTILINE®HP (ORAFTI, Belgium) and syrup of lactulose (Duphalac®, the Netherlands) were used in different concentrations: 0%, 1%, 2%, 3%, 4%, and 5%. They found a reduction in cholesterol level in fermented milk using *B. lactis* and that this cholesterol reduction was influenced by the addition of prebiotics. The lower cholesterol content was determined in fermented milk samples with 4% of lactulose (9.5 mg/100 g) and with 1% of inulin (10.4 mg/100 g). Kiessling et al. (2002) also demonstrated that consumption of synbiotic yogurt containing oligofructose and *B. longum* 913 and *L. acidophilus* 145 improved HDL cholesterol levels in women.

Matijasic et al. (2016) reported that the daily consumption of synbiotic fermented milk prepared with probiotic strains *L. acidophilus* La-5 ($\geq 6.5 \times 10^9$ cfu) and *B. animalis* ssp. BB-12 ($\geq 9 \times 10^9$ cfu) and with dietary fiber (90% inulin, 10% oligofructose) had a short-term effect on the proportion and amount of La-5 like strains and *B. animalis* ssp. *lactis* in the fecal microbiome of IBS patients. The safety evaluation study of probiotics and synbiotics in children aged 0–18 years was conducted by van den Nieuwboer et al. (2015); the study revealed that the probiotic and synbiotic products are safe for consumption by children because no adverse effect was observed. Fateh et al. (2011) studied the efficacy of commercially available mixtures of pre- and probiotics (synbiotic) in improving stool frequency and consistency.

Turkish-fermented cereal food formula synbiotic tarhana and synbiotic yogurt prepared as functional foods were studied for their effect on plasma lipid profiles. Synbiotic yogurt was prepared with prebiotic inulin and lactulose, each at 3%, and with different concentration of the probiotic culture: at 0.5%, 1.5%, 3.0%, and 4.5% DVS-ABT2 containing *B. bifidum*, *S. thermophilus*, and *L. acidophilus*. The result showed that dried tarhana significantly reduced low-density lipoproteins (LDL-C), total plasma cholesterol, and triglycerides, whereas high-density lipoprotein (HDL-C) was increased significantly (Gabrial et al., 2010).

CONCLUSION

Prebiotics and well-studied probiotic bacteria, along with probiotic yeasts, are gaining attention widely not only because of their positive physiological effects but also because of the nutritive value that they add to probiotic-containing food products. It is clear that the beneficial properties of particular probiotic bacteria are highly strain dependent; that is, during *in vivo* demonstrations, each strain used in the products exhibits specific effects on the targeted sites. Many studies have stated the various health benefits of probiotic bacteria for human health. Few of the proven beneficial effects in human trials include the application of *L. rhamnosus* GG in lactose intolerance, antibiotic-associated diarrhea, irritable bowel syndrome, and reduction of bad cholesterol. The most promising application of certain probiotics is the potential for boosting and strengthening the immune system at the mucosal level.

It has been recommended that fermented dairy foods containing selected probiotic strains are very useful in the treatment of inflammatory bowel diseases. Fermented dairy products like yogurt and acidophilus milks and cheeses are good for supplementing beneficial probiotic bacteria. The available findings on these documented health benefits need to be validated by long-term clinical studies and large randomized controlled trials with human subjects. In developing countries, more research needs to be done on the claimed health benefits of fermented probiotic dairy products, mainly for gastric cancer and lactose intolerance, because these are growing health concerns. Many reports on animal studies clearly suggest the positive health effects of synbiotic products, including their antioxidant, hypocholesterolemic, anti-allergic properties and the effects on asthma, and their use in preventing colorectal cancer and inflammatory diseases. But these beneficial aspects of synbiotic products must be confirmed and investigated at clinical and molecular levels.

Increased demand for probiotic fermented milk products encourages more and more development of these products. Designing new and innovative technology in this area of functional foods development is growing day by day. Innovation may come in the use of specific probiotic bacteria and in fortification of fermented milks with prebiotics and other biofunctional ingredients. In this regard, fermented milk products are a great option for their potential in improving gut health and overall well-being.

REFERENCES

Ahola, A. J., Yli-Knnuttila, H., Suomalainen, T., Poussa, T., Ahlstrom, A., et al. 2002. Short-term consumption of probiotic containing cheese and its effect on dental caries risk factors. *Arch. Oral Biol.* 47(11): 799–804.

Aimutis, W. R., 2001. Challenges in developing effective probiotic functional foods including scientific and regulatory considerations: Dairy nutrition for a healthy future. *Bulletin-IDF.* 363: 30–38.

Akalin, A. S. and Erisir, D., 2008. Effects of inulin and oligofructose on the rheological characteristics and probiotic culture survival in low-fat probiotic ice cream. *J. Food Sci.* 73(4): M184–M188.

Akin, M. B., Akin, M. S., and Kirmaci, Z., 2007. Effects of inulin and sugar levels on the viability of yogurt and probiotic bacteria and the physical and sensory characteristics in probiotic ice cream. *Food Chem.* 104(1): 93–99.

Allgeyer, L. C., Miller, M. J., and Lee, S.-Y., 2010. Sensory and microbiological quality of yogurt drinks with prebiotics and probiotics. *J. Dairy Sci.* 93(10): 4471–4479.

Almeida, K. E., Bonassi, I. A., and Gomes, M. I. F. V., 2000. Caracteristica microbiologica de bebida l'actea preparada com microrganismos probioticos. In: *Proceedings of XVII Congresso Brasileiro de Ciencia e Tecnologia de Alimentos*, Fortaleza, Brazil.

Almeida, M. H. B., Zoellner, S. S., Cruz, A. G., Moura, M. R. L., Carvalho, L. M. J., and Sant'ana, A. S., 2008. Potentially probiotic acai yogurt. *Int. J. Dairy Technol.* 61(2): 178–182.

Al-Sheraji, S. H., Ismail, A., Manap, M. Y., Mustafa, S., Yusof, R. M., and Hassan, F. A., 2013. Prebiotics as functional foods: A review. *J. Funct. Foods.* 5(4): 1542–1553.

Amiri, Z. R., Khandelwal, P., Aruna, B. R., and Sahebjamnia, N., 2008. Optimization of process parameters for preparation of synbiotic acidophilus milk via selected probiotics and prebiotics using artificial neural network. *J. Biotechnol.* 136: S460.

Andrighetto, C. and Gomes, M. I. F. V., 2003. Produção de picolés utilizando leite acidófilo. *Braz. J. Food Technol.* 6: 267–71.

Annamaria Staiano, A., 2009. Effect of a probiotic preparation (VSL#3) on induction and maintenance of remission in children with ulcerative colitis. *Am. J. Gastroenterol.* 104: 437–443.

Aryana, K. J. and McGrew, P., 2007. Quality attributes of yogurt with *Lactobacillus casei* and various prebiotics. *LWT- Food Sci. Technol.* 40: 1808–1814.

Aryana, K. J., Plauche, S., Rao, R. M., McGrew, P., and Shah, N. P., 2007. Fat-free plain yoghurt manufactured with inulins of various chain lengths and *Lactobacillus acidophilus*. *J. Food Sci.* 72: M79–M84.

Balakrishnan, M. and Floch, M. H., 2012. Prebiotics, probiotics and digestive health. *Curr. Opin. Clin. Nutr. Metab. Care.* 15: 580–585.

Beitane, I. and Ciprovica, I., 2012. The study of cholesterol content in synbiotic fermented dairy products. *J. Life Sci.* 6: 1077–1081.

Blanchette, L., Roy, D., Belanger, G., and Gauthier, S. F., 1996. Production of cottage cheese using dressing fermented by bifidobacteria. *J. Dairy Sci.* 79: 8–15.

Bosscher, D., 2009. Fructan prebiotics derived from inulin. In *Prebiotics and Probiotics Science and Technology*, (pp. 163–205). Springer, New York.

Brown, A. C. and Valiere, A., 2004. Probiotics and medical nutrition therapy. *Nutr. Clin. Care.* 7(2): 56–68.

Buriti, F. C. A., Rocha, J. S., and Saad, S. M. I., 2005. Incorporation of *Lactobacillus acidophilus* in Minas fresh cheese and its implications for textural and sensorial properties during storage. *Int. Dairy J.* 15(12): 1279–1288.

Buriti, F. C. A., Bedani, R., and Saad, S. M. I., 2015. Probiotic and prebiotic dairy desserts. In *Probiotics, Prebiotics, and Synbiotics: Bioactive Foods in Health Promotion.* pp. 345–360.

Cardarelli, H. R., Buriti, F. C. A., Castro, I. A., and Saad, S. M. I., 2008. Inulin and oligofructose improve sensory quality and increase the probiotic viable count in potentially synbiotic petit-suisse cheese. *LWT—Food Sci. Technol.* 41: 1037–1046.

Cardelle-Cobas, A., Olano, A., Corzo, N., Villamiel, M., Collins, M., et al. 2012. *In vitro* fermentation of lactulose-derived oligosaccharides by mixed fecal microbiota. *J. Agric. Food Chem.* 60(8): 2024–2032.

Connolly, M. L., Lovegrove, J. A., and Tuohy, K. M., 2010. Konjac glucomannan hydrolysate beneficially modulates bacterial composition and activity within the faecal microbiota. *J. Funct. Foods.* 2: 219–224.

Corbo, M. R., Albenzio, M., De Angelis, M., Sevi, A., and Gobbetti, M., 2001. Microbiological and biochemical properties of *Canestrato pugliese* hard cheese supplemented with bifidobacteria. *J. Dairy Sci.* 84: 551–561.

Cousin, F. J., Jouan-Lanhouet, S., Dimanche-Boitrel, M. T., Corcos, L., and Jan, G., 2012. Milk fermented by *Propionibacterium freudenreichii* induces apoptosis of HGT-1 human gastric cancer cells. *PLoS One.* 7(3): e31892.

Crittenden, R. G. and Playne, M., 1996. Production, properties and applications of food-grade oligosaccharides. *Trends Food Sci. Technol.* 7(11): 353–361.

Cruz, A. G., Antunes, A. E. C., Sousa, A. L. O. P., Faria, J. A. F., and Saad, S. M. I., 2009. Ice-cream as a probiotic food carrier. *Food Res. Int.* 42: 1233–1239.

Cummings, J. H., Macfarlane, G. T., and Englyst, H. N., 2001. Prebiotic digestion and fermentation. *Am. J. Clin. Nutr.* 73(2): 415s–420s.

Dalev, D., Bielecka, M., Troszynska, A., Ziajka, S., and Lamparski, G., 2006. Sensory quality of new probiotic beverages based on cheese whey and soy preparation. *Pol. J. Food Nutr. Sci.* 15(56): 71–77.

Davidson, R. H., Duncan, S. E., Hackney, C. R., Eigel, W. N., and Boling, J. W., 2000. Probiotic culture surival and implications in fermented frozen yogurt characteristics. *J. Dairy Sci.* 83: 666–673.

de Castro, F. P., Cunha, T. M., Ogliari, P. J., Teofilo, R. F., Ferreira, M. M. C., and Prudencio, E. S., 2009. Influence of different content of cheese whey and oligofructose on the properties of fermented lactic beverages: Study using response surface methodology. *LWT—Food Sci. Technol.* 42(5): 993–997.

de Moreno, L. A. and Perdigon, G., 2010. The application of probiotic fermented milks in cancer and intestinal inflammation. *Proc. Nutr. Soc.* 69: 421–428.

Dello Staffolo, M., Bertola, N., Martino, M., and Bevilacqua, A., 2004. Influence of dietary fibre addition on sensory and rheological properties of yoghurt. *Int. Dairy J.* 14: 263–268.

Ejtahed, H. S., Mohtadi-Nia, J., Homayouni-Rad, A., Niafar, M., Asghari-Jafarabadi, M., et al. 2011. Effect of probiotic yogurt containing *Lactobacillus acidophilus* and *Bifidobacterium lactis* on lipid profile in individuals with type 2 diabetes mellitus. *J. Dairy Sci.* 94: 3288–3294.

Espirito Santo, A. P., Perego, P., Converti, A., and Oliveira, M. N., 2011. Influence of food matrices on probiotic viability: A review focusing on the fruity bases. *Trends Food Sci. Technol.* 22: 377–385.

Fadden, K. and Owen, R. W., 1992. Faecal steroids and colorectal cancer: The effect of lactulose on faecal bacterial metabolism in a continuous culture model of the large intestine. *Eur. J. Cancer Prevent.* 1(2): 113–128.

Fateh, R., Iravani, S., Frootan, M., Rasouli, M. R., and Saadat, S., 2011. Synbiotic preparation in men suffering from functional constipation: A randomised controlled trial. *Swiss Med Wkly.* 141: w13239. 1–7.

Food and Agricultural Organization of the United Nations and World Health Organization. 2001. Health and nutritional properties of probiotics in food including powder milk with live lactic acid bacteria. World Health Organization.

Franck, A., 2008. *Food Applications of Prebiotics: Handbook of Prebiotics.* pp. 437–448. CRC Press, Boca Raton, Florida.

Gabrial, S. G. N., Zaghloul, A. H., Khalaf-Allah, A. E. M., El-Shimi, N. M., Mohamed, R. S., and Gabrial, G. N., 2010. Synbiotic Tarhana as a functional food. *J. Am. Sci.* 6(12): 847–857.

Gadaga, T. H., Mutukumira, A. N., Narvhus, J. A., and Feresu, S. B., 1999. A review of traditional fermented foods and beverages of Zimbabwe. *Int. J. Food Microbiol.* 53: 1–11.

Ganguli, K., Meng, D., Rautava, S., Lu, L., Walker, W. A., and Nanthakumar, N., 2013. Probiotics prevent necrotizing enterocolitis by modulating enterocytes genes that regulate innate immune-mediated inflammation. *Am. J. Physiol.-Gastro. Liver Physiol.* 304(2): G132–G141.

Gardiner, G., Stanton, C., Lynch, P. B., Collins, J. K., Fitzgerald, G., and Ross, R. P., 1999. Evaluation of cheddar cheese as a food carrier for delivery of a probiotic strain to the gastrointestinal tract. *J. Dairy Sci.* 82(7): 1379–1387.

Gibson, G. R., 2004. From probiotics to prebiotics and a healthy digestive system. *J. Food Sci.* 69(5): M141–M143.

Gibson, G. R., Probert, H. M., Van Loo, J., Rastall, R. A., and Roberfroid, M. B., 2004. Dietary modulation of the human colonic microbiota: Updating the concept of prebiotics. *Nutr. Res. Rev.* 17(02): 259–275.

Gibson, G. R. and Roberfroid, M. B., 1995. Dietary modulation of the human colonic microbiota: Introducing the concept of prebiotics. *J. Nutr.* 125(6): 1401–1412.

Gibson, G. R. and Roberfroid, M. B. (Eds.), 1999. *Colonic Microbiota, Nutrition and Health,* p. 44. Kluwer Academic, Dordrecht, the Netherlands.

Gibson, G. R., Scott, K. P., Rastall, R. A., Tuohy, K. M., Hotchkiss, A., et al., 2011. Dietary prebiotics: Current status and new definition. *IFIS Funct. Foods Bulletin.* 7: 1–19.

Gill, H. S., 1998. Stimulation of the immune system by lactic cultures. *Int. Dairy J.* 8(5–6): 535–544.

Gobbetti, M., Corsetti, A., Smacchi, E., Zocchetti, A., and De Angelis, M., 1997. Production of Crescenza cheese by incorporation of bifidobacteria. *J. Dairy Sci.* 81: 37–47.

Godward, G., Sultana, K., Kailasapathy, K., Peiris, P., Arumugaswamy, R., and Reynolds, N., 2000. The importance of strain selection on the viability and survival of probiotic bacteria in dairy foods. *Milchwissenschaft* 55: 441–445.

Gomes, A. M. P., and Malcata, F. X., 1999. *Bifidobacterium* spp. and *Lactobacillus acidophilus*: Biological, biochemical, technological and therapeutical properties relevant for use as probiotics. *Trends Food Sci. Technol.* 10: 139–157.

Granato, D., Branco, G. F., Cruz, A. G., Faria, J. de A. F., and Shah, N. P., 2010. Probiotic dairy products as functional foods. *Comp. Rev. Food Sci. Food Safety.* 9: 455–470.

Grimoud, J., Durand, H., Courtin, C., Monsan, P., Ouarne, F., et al. 2010. *In vitro* screening of probiotic lactic acid bacteria and prebiotic glucooligosaccharides to select effective synbiotics. *Anaerobe.* 16: 493–500.

Gullon, B., Gomez, B., Martinez-Sabajanes, M., Yanez, R., Parajo, J. C., and Alonso, J. L., 2013. Pectic oligosaccharides: Manufacture and functional properties. *Trends Food Sci. Technol.* 30(2): 153–161.

Guven, M., Yasar, K., Karaca, O. B., and Hayaloglu, A. A., 2005. The effect of inulin as a fat replacer on the quality of set-type low-fat yogurt manufacture. *Int. J. Dairy Technol.* 58(3): 180–184.

Hatakka, K., Ahola, A. J., Yli-Knuuttila, H., Richardson, M., Poussa, T., et al. 2007. Probiotics reduce the prevalence of oral Candida in the elderly — A randomized controlled trial. *J. Dental Res.* 86(2): 125–130.

Haynes, I. N. and Playne, M. J., 2002. Survival of probiotic cultures in low-fat ice cream. *Aust. J. Dairy Technol.* 57: 10–14.

Hill, C., Guarner, F., Reid, G., Gibson, G. R., Merenstein, D. J., et al., 2014. The International Scientific Association for Probiotics and Prebiotics consensus statement on the scope and appropriate use of the term probiotic. *Nature Rev. Gastroenterol. Hepatol.* 11(8): 506–514.

Homayouni, A., Azizi, A., Ehsani, M. R., Yarmand, M. S., and Razavi, S. H., 2008. Effect of microencapsulation and resistant starch on the probiotic survival and sensory properties of synbiotic ice cream. *Food Chem.* 111: 50–55.

Huynh, H. Q., Debruyn, J., Guan, L., Diaz, H., Li, M., et al. 2009. Probiotic preparation VSL#3 induces remission in children with mild to moderate acute ulcerative colitis: A pilot study. *Inflamm. Bowel. Dis.* 15: 760–768.

Isanga, J. and Zhang, G., 2009. Production and evaluation of some physicochemical parameters of peanut milk yogurt. *LWT—Food Sci. Technol.* 42: 1132–1138.

Itsaranuwat, P., Al-Haddad, K. S. H., and Robinson, R. K. 2003. The potential therapeutic benefits of consuming 'health-promoting' fermented dairy products: A brief update. *Int. J. Dairy Technol.* 56: 203–210.

Kadooka, Y., Sato, M., Imaizumi, K., Ogawa, A., Ikuyama, K., et al. 2010. Regulation of abdominal adiposity by probiotics (*Lactobacillus gasseri* SBT2055) in adults with obese tendencies in a randomized controlled trial. *Eur. J. Clin. Nutr.* 64(6): 636–643.

Kailasapathy, K., Harmstorf, I., and Phillips, M., 2008. Survival of *Lactobacillus acidophilus* and *Bifidobacterium animalis* spp. lactis in stirred fruit yogurts. *LWT—Food Sci. Technol.* 41: 1317–1322.

Kailasapathy, K. and Masondole, L., 2005. Survival of free and microencapsulated *Lactobacillus acidophilus* and *Bifidobacterium lactis* and their effect on texture of feta cheese. *Aus. J. Dairy Technol.* 60(3): 252–258.

Kailasapathy, K. and Sultana, K., 2003. Survival and β-D-galactosidase activity of encapsulated and free *Lactobacillus acidophilus* and *Bifidobacterium lactis* in ice cream. *Aus. J. Dairy Technol.* 58: 223–227.

Kalavrouzioti, I., Hatzikamari, M., Litopoulou-Tzanetaki, E., and Tzanetakis, N., 2005. Production of hard cheese from caprine milk by use of probiotic cultures as adjuncts. *Int. J. Dairy Technol.* 58: 30–38.

Karimi, R., Mortazavian, A. M., and Da Cruz, A. G., 2011. Viability of probiotic microorganisms in cheese during production and storage: A review. *Dairy Sci. Technol.* 91: 283–308.

Kaur, H., Mishra, H. N., and Umar, P., 2009. Textural properties of mango soy fortified probiotic yogurt: Optimisation of inoculum level of yogurt and probiotic culture. *Int. J. Food Sci. Technol.* 44: 415–424.

Kiessling, G., Schneider, J., and Jahreis, G., 2002. Long-term consumption of fermented dairy products over 6 months increases HDL cholesterol. *Eur. J. Clin. Nutr.* 56(9): 843–849.

Kilic, G. B., Kuleansan, H., Eralp, I., and Karahan, A. G., 2009. Manufacture of Turkish Beyaz cheese added with probiotic strains. *LWT—Food Sci. Technol.* 42(5): 1003–1008.

Kinik, O., Kesenkas, H., Ergonul, P. G., and Akan, E., 2017. The effect of using pro and prebiotics on the aromatic compounds, textural and sensorial properties of symbiotic goat cheese. *Mljekarstvo* 67 (1): 71–85.

Kip, P., Meyer, D., and Jellema, R. H., 2006. Inulins improve sensoric and textural properties of low-fat yoghurts. *Int. Dairy J.* 16: 1098–1103.

Kleniewska, P., Hoffmann, A., Pniewska, E., and Pawliczak, R., 2016. The influence of probiotic *Lactobacillus casei* in combination with prebiotic inulin on the antioxidant capacity of human plasma. *Oxid. Med. Cell. Longev.*, Article ID 1340903, 1–10.

Klewicki, R., 2007. The stability of gal-polyols and oligosaccharides during pasteurization at a low pH. *LWT-Food Sci. Technol.* 40(7): 1259–1265.

Knorr, D., 1998. Technology aspects related to microorganisms in functional foods. *Trends Food Sci. Technol.* 9: 295–306.

Kusuma, G. D., Paseephol, T., and Sherkat, F., 2009. Prebiotic and rheological effects of Jerusalem artichoke inulin in low-fat yogurt. *Aus. J. Dairy Technol.* 64(2): 159–163.

Lan, A., Bruneau, A., Bensaada, M., Philippe, C., Bellaud, P., et al. 2008. Increased induction of apoptosis by *Propionibacterium freudenreichii* TL133 in colonic mucosal crypts of human microbiota-associated rats treated with 1,2-dimethylhydrazine. *B. J. Nutr.* 100: 1251–1259.

Leroy, F., Falony, G., and Vuyst, L., 2008. Latest developments in probiotics. In: Toldra F, (Ed.). *Meat Biotechnology.* Springer, Brussels, Belgium, pp. 217–229.

Lourens-Hattingh, A. and Viljoen, B. C., 2001. Growth and survival of a probiotic yeast in dairy products. *Food Res. Int.* 34: 791–796.

Lucas, A., Sodini, I., Monnet, P., Jolivet, P., and Corrieu, G., 2004. Probiotic cell counts and acidification in fermented milks supplemented with milk protein hydrolysates. *Int. Dairy J.* 14(1): 47–53.

Madhu, A. N., Amrutha, N., and Prapulla, S. G., 2012. Characterization and antioxidant property of probiotic and synbiotic yogurts. *Probiotics Antimicrob. Proteins.* 4: 90–97.

Madureira, A. R., Pereira, C. I., Truszkowska, K., Gomes, A. M. P., Pintado, M. E., and Malcata, F. X., 2005. Survival of probiotic bacteria in a whey cheese vector submitted to environmental conditions prevailing in the gastrointestinal tract. *Int. Dairy J.* 15(6–9): 921–927.

Maragkoudakisa, P. A., Miarisa, C., Rojeza, P., Manalisb, N., Magkanarib, F., et al. 2006. Production of traditional Greek yogurt using *Lactobacillus* strains with probiotic potential as starter adjuncts. *Int. Dairy J.* 16(1): 52–60.

Martın-Diana, A. B., Janer, C., Pelaez, C., and Requena, T., 2003. Development of a fermented goat's milk containing probiotic bacteria. *Int. Dairy J.* 13: 827–833.

Matijasic, B. B., Obermajer, T., Lipoglavsek, L., Sernel, T., Locatelli, I., et al. 2016. Effects of synbiotic fermented milk containing *Lactobacillus acidophilus* La-5 and *Bifidobacterium animalis* ssp. *lactis* BB-12 on the fecal microbiota of adults with irritable bowel syndrome: A randomized double-blind, placebo-controlled trial. *J. Dairy Sci.* 99: 5008–5021.

Medici, M., Vinderola, C. G., and Perdigon, G., 2004. Gut mucosal immunomodulation by probiotic fresh cheese. *Int. Dairy J.* 14(7): 611–618.

Meyer, D., Bayarri, S., Tarrega, A., and Costell, E., 2011. Inulin as texture modifier in dairy products. *Food Hydrocoll.* 25(8): 1881–1890.

Miele, E., Pascarella, F., Giannetti, E., Quaglietta, L., Robert, N., et al., 2010. Inhibitory effect of yogurt on aberrant crypt foci formation in the rat colon and colorectal tumorigenesis in RasH2 mice. *Exp. Anim.* 59: 487–494.

Nazzaro, F., Fratianni, F., Coppola, R., Sada, A., and Orlando, P., 2009. Fermentative ability of alginate-prebiotic encapsulated *Lactobacillus acidophilus* and survival under simulated gastrointestinal conditions. *J. Funct. Foods.* 1: 319–323.

Neves, L. S., 2000. *Produção de um Derivado de leite de cabra, não fermentado, Com bactérias probióticas.* Londrina, Paraná, Brazil, Universidade Estadual de Londrina, 100.

Ng, S. C., Plamondon, S., Kamm, M. A., Hart, A. L., Al-Hassi, H. O., et al. 2010. Immunosuppressive effects via human intestinal dendritic cells of probiotic bacteria and steroids in the treatment of acute ulcerative colitis. *Inflamm. Bowel. Dis.* 16: 1286–1298.

Ong, L., Henriksson, A., and Shah, N. P., 2006. Development of probiotic Cheddar cheese containing *Lactobacillus acidophilus, Lb. casei, Lb. paracasei* and *Bifidobacterium* spp. and the influence of these bacteria on proteolytic patterns and production of organic acid. *Int. Dairy J.* 16: 446–456.

Ong, L. and Shah, N. P., 2009. Probiotic Cheddar cheese: Influence of ripening temperatures on survival of probiotic microorganisms, cheese composition and organic acid profiles. *LWT—Food Sci. Technol.* 42(7): 1260–1268.

Ozer, B., Uzun, Y. S., and Kirmaci, H. A., 2008. Effect of microencapsulation on viability of *Lactobacillus acidophilus* La-5 and *Bifidobacterium bifidum* Bb-12 during kasar cheese ripening. *Int. J. Dairy Technol.* 61: 237–244.

Palframan, R., Gibson, G. R., and Rastall, R. A., 2003. Development of a quantitative tool for the comparison of the prebiotic effect of dietary oligosaccharides. *Lett. Appl. Microbiol.* 37(4): 281–284.

Parkar, S. G., Redgate, E. L., Wibisono, R., Luo, X., Koh, E. T. H., and Schroder, R., 2010. Gut health benefits of kiwifruit pectins: Comparison with commercial functional polysaccharides. *J. Funct. Foods.* 2: 210–218.

Paseephol, T. and Sherkat, F., 2009. Probiotic stability of yoghurts containing Jerusalem artichoke inulins during refrigerated storage. *J. Funct. Foods.* 1: 311–318.

Patrignani, F., Burns, P., Serrazanetti, D., Vinderola, G., Reinheimer, J., et al. 2009. Suitability of high pressure-homogenized milk for the production of probiotic fermented milk containing *Lactobacillus paracasei* and *Lactobacillus acidophilus. J. Dairy Res.* 76: 74–82.

Penna, A. L. B., Gurram, S., and Barbosa-Canovas, G. V., 2007. High hydrostatic pressure processing on microstructure of probiotic low-fat yogurt. *Food Res. Int.* 40(4): 510–519.

Perdigon, G., De Moreno, D. L., Valdez, J., and Rachid, M., 2002. Role of yoghurt in the prevention of colon cancer. *Eur. J. Clin. Nutr.* 56(3): S65–S68.

Petersen, A., Bergstrom, A., Andersen, J., Hansen, M., Lahtinen, S., et al. 2010. Analysis of the intestinal microbiota of oligosaccharide fed mice exhibiting reduced resistance to *Salmonella* infection. *Beneficial Microbes* 1(3): 271–281.

Prado, F. C., Parada, J. L., Pandey, A., and Soccol, C. R., 2008. Trends in non-dairy probiotic beverages. *Food Res. Int.* 41: 111–123.

Rastall, R. A., 2010. Functional oligosaccharides: Application and manufacture. *Ann. Review Food Sci. Technol.* 1: 305–339.

Riordan, S. M., Skinner, N. A., Mciver, C. J., Liu, Q., Bengmark, S., et al. 2007. Synbiotic-associated improvement in liver function in cirrhotic patients: Relation to changes in circulating cytokine messenger RNA and protein levels. *Microb. Ecol. Health Dis.* 19: 7–16.

Rivas, S., Gullon, B., Gullon, P., Alonso, J. L., and Parajo, J. C., 2012. Manufacture and properties of bifidogenic saccharides derived from wood mannan. *J. Agric. Food Chem.* 60(17): 4296–4305.

Rizzardini, G., Eskesen, D., Calder, P. C., Capetti, A., Jespersen, L., and Clerici, M., 2012. Evaluation of the immune benefits of two probiotic strains *Bifidobacterium animalis* ssp. lactis, BB-12w and *Lactobacillus paracasei* ssp. *paracasei, L. casei* 431w in an influenza vaccination model: A randomised, double-blind, placebo-controlled study. *B. J. Nutr.* 107: 876–884.

Roberfroid, M. B., 2005. Introducing inulin-type fructans. *B. J. Nutr.* 93: 13–26.

Rodrigues, D., Rocha-Santos, T. A., Gomes, A. M., Goodfellow, B. J., and Freitas, A. C., 2012. Lipolysis in probiotic and synbiotic cheese: The influence of probiotic bacteria, prebiotic compounds and ripening time on free fatty acid profiles. *Food Chem.* 131(4): 1414–1421.

Ross, R. P., Fitzgerald, G., Collins, K., and Stanton, C., 2002. Cheese delivering biocultures: Probiotic cheese. *Aus. J. Dairy Technol.* 57(2): 71–78.

Saad, S. M. I., Castro, I. A., and Harami, J. B., 2008. Avaliação senaorial de uma nova sobremesa láctea congelada simbiótica. In: *Proceedings of XXI Congresso Brasileiro de Ciência e Tecnologia de Alimentos*, Belo Horizonte.

Sanders, M. E. and Marco, M. L., 2010. Food formats for effective delivery of probiotics. *Ann. Rev. Food Sci. Technol.* 1: 65–85.

Sangwan, V. and Tomar, S. K., 2011. Estimation of Microbial GOS by High Performance Liquid Chromatography. Chemical Analysis of Value Added Dairy Products and Their Quality Assurance, Compendium, p. 233.

Sanz, T. A., Salvador, A., Jimenez, A., and Fiszman, S. M., 2008. Yogurt enrichment with functional asparagus fibre. Effect of fibre extraction method on rheological properties, colour, and sensory acceptance. *Eur. Food Res. Technol.* 227: 1515–1521.

Sarbini, S. R., Kolida, S., Gibson, G. R., and Rastall, R. A., 2013. *In vitro* fermentation of commercial α-gluco-oligosaccharide by faecal microbiota from lean and obese human subjects. *B. J. Nutr.* 109(11): 1980–1989.

Sarbini, S. R. and Rastall, R. A., 2011. Prebiotics: Metabolism, structure, and function. *Funct. Food Rev.* 3(3): 93–106.

Saunders, D. R. and Wiggins, H. S. 1981. Conservation of mannitol, lactulose, and raffinose by the human colon. *Am. J. Physiol.-Gastro. Liver Physiol.* 241(5): G397–G402.

Scholz-Ahrens, K. E., Adolphi, B., Rochat, F., Barclay, D. V., de Vrese, M., et al. 2016. Effects of probiotics, prebiotics, and synbiotics on mineral metabolism in ovariectomized rats—Impact of bacterial mass, intestinal absorptive area and reduction of bone turnover. *NFS Journal.* 3: 41–50.

Sendra, E., Fayos, P., Lario, Y., Fernandez-Lopez, J., Sayas-Barbera, E., and Perez-Alvarez, J., 2008. Incorporation of citrus fibers in fermented milk containing probiotic bacteria. *Food Microbiol.* 25: 13–21.

Shaghaghi, M., Pourahmad, R., and Adeli, H. R. M., 2013. Synbiotic yogurt production by using prebiotic compounds and probiotic lactobacilli. *Int. Res. J. Appl. Basic. Sci.* 5(7): 839–846.

Shah, C., Mokashe, N., and Mishra, V., 2016. Preparation, characterization and in vitro antioxidative potential of synbiotic fermented dairy products. *J. Food Sci. Technol.*53(4):1984–1992.

Shakerian, M., Razavi, S. H., Khodaiyan, F., Ziai, S. A., Yarmand, M. S., and Moayedi, A., 2014. Effect of different levels of fat and inulin on the microbial growth and metabolites in probiotic yogurt containing nonviable bacteria. *Int. J. Food Sci. Technol.* 49(1): 261–268.

Silveira, G., Guergoletto, K. B., Pelissari, F. M., Pagamunici, L. M., Zampieri, D. F., et al. 2007. Avaliação sensory de iogurte de polpa de cupuaçu (*Theobroma grandiflorum* Schum.) e graviola (*Annona muricata* L.) com probióticos. In: *Proceedings of IX Encontro Regional Sul de Ciência e Tecnologia de Alimentos.* Curitiba, Brazil: Anais do IX ERSCTA, pp. 486–489.

Sousa, R. C. S., Lira, R. A., Oliveira, F. C., Santos, D. O., and Sierra, O. A. P., 2007. Desenvolvimento e aceitação sensory de iogurte probiótico light de banana. In: *Proceedings of IX Encontro Regional Sul de Ciência e Tecnologia de Alimentos.* Curitiba, Brazil: Anais do IX ERSCTA. pp. 549–553.

Souza, C. H. B. and Saad, S. M. I., 2009. Viability of *Lactobacillus acidophilus* La-5 added solely or in co-culture with a yogurt starter culture and implications on physicochemical and related properties of Minas fresh cheese during storage. *LWT—Food Sci. Technol.* 42(2): 633–640.

Speck, M. L., 1978. The development of sweet acidophilus milk. *Dairy Ice Cream Field J.* 70: A–D.

Stanton, C., Desmond, C., Coakley, M., Collins, J. K., Fitzgerald, G., and Ross, R. P., 2003. Challenges facing development of probioticcontaining functional foods. In Farnworth E. R. (Ed.), *Handbook of Fermented Functional Foods.* Boca Raton, FL: CRC Press. pp. 27–58.

Supavititpatana, P., Wirjantoro, T. I., Apichartsrangkoon, A., and Raviyan, P., 2008. Addition of gelatin enhanced gelation of corn–milk yogurt. *Food Chem.* 106: 211–216.

Synytsya, A., Mickova, K., Synytsya, A., Jablonsky, I., Spevacek, J., et al. 2009. Glucans from fruit bodies of cultivated mushrooms *Pleurotus ostreatus* and *Pleurotus eryngii*: Structure and potential prebiotic activity. *Carbohydrate Polymers.* 76(4): 548–556.

Thage, B. V., Broe, M. L., Petersen, M. H., Petersen, M. A., Bennedsen, M. A., and Ardo, Y., 2005. Aroma development in semi-hard reduced-fat cheese inoculated with *Lactobacillus paracasei* strains with different aminotransferase profiles. *Int. Dairy J.* 15: 795–805.

van den Nieuwboer, M., Brummer, R. J., Guarner, F., Morelli, L., Cabana, M., and Claassen, E., 2015. Safety of probiotics and synbiotics in children under 18 years of age. *Beneficial Microbes.* 6(5): 615–630.

Vinderola, C. G., Prosello, W., Ghiberto, T. D., and Reinheimer, J. A., 2000. Viability of probiotic (*Bifidobacterium*, *Lactobacillus acidophilus* and *Lactobacillus casei*) and nonprobiotic microflora in Argentinian fresco cheese. *J. Dairy Sci.* 83: 1905–1911.

Voragen, A. G., 1998. Technological aspects of functional food-related carbohydrates. *Trends Food Sci. Technol.* 9(8): 328–335.

Wang, X. and Gibson, G. R., 1993. Effects of the *in vitro* fermentation of oligofructose and inulin by bacteria growing in the human large intestine. *J. Appl. Bacteriol.* 75(4): 373–380.

Wang, Y., 2009. Prebiotics: Present and future in food science and technology. *Food Res. Int.* 42(1): 8–12.

Yadav, H., Jain, S., and Sinha, P. R., 2007. Production of free fatty acids and conjugated linoleic acid in probiotic dahi containing *Lactobacillus acidophilus* and *Lactobacillus casei* during fermentation and storage. *Int. Dairy J.* 17: 1006–1010.

Yang, Y. J. and Sheu, B. S., 2012. Probiotics-containing yogurts suppress *Helicobacter pylori* load and modify immune response and intestinal microbiota in the *Helicobacter pylori*-infected children. *Helicobacter.* 17(4): 297–304.

Yilmaztekin, M., Ozer, B. H., and Atasoy, F., 2004. Survival of *Lactobacillus acidophilus* La-5 and *Bifidobacterium bifidum* BB-02 in white-brined cheese. *Int. J. Food Sci. Nutr.* 55: 53–60.

11 Bacterial Endophytes as Cell Factories for Sustainable Agriculture

Pratibha Vyas

CONTENTS

INTRODUCTION

Environmentally sound and sustainable crop production is one of the main challenges for agriculture in the twenty-first century. Excessive use of fertilizers and pesticides for enhanced agricultural yield has placed an extensive burden on the environment. Plant disease control has also remained a major challenge for improving crop productivity. Novel solutions are required to improve productivity and sustainability in agriculture. Ecologically safe, efficient, and cheap biological alternatives are required to reduce the consumption of fertilizers and to improve agriculture productivity. Microorganisms have huge potential in offering an alternative to the use of inorganic fertilizers and chemical pesticides.

Microorganisms are ubiquitous in nature; they are vital components of all known ecosystems on earth and play an important role in the functioning of ecosystems through nutrient cycling, decomposition, and energy flow. Because plants grow in intimate association with microbial communities, these microorganisms play a critical role in promoting plant growth and productivity by providing an adequate supply of nutrients. Endophytes reside within plant tissues at some phases of their life cycle without causing any disease symptoms. Microbial endophytes have developed a mutualistic association with their plant hosts wherein the host plant supplies sufficient nutrients and habitation for endophytes. These endophytes can be exploited as cell factories for synthesizing a large number of agriculturally important compounds, including plant hormones, enzymes, organic acids, siderophores, hydrogen cyanide, antibiotics, and antifungal metabolites.

Phytohormones are signal molecules that regulate plant growth and development. Many bacterial endophytes have been reported to produce auxins, absicic acid, cytokinins, and gibberellins (GA). Auxins are important phytohormones that influence many cellular functions that in turn regulate plant growth and development. Indole-3-acetic acid (IAA) production is widespread among bacterial endophytes; it increases root growth and root length, enabling plants to gain more nutrients from the soil. Bacteria also stimulate legume–rhizobia symbiosis through various modes of action, the most common being the IAA-induced increase in root growth, which provides more sites for nodule formation. This stimulation can also be through the supply of phosphorus required for nodule formation and nitrogen fixation by rhizobia. Cytokinins, which control cell division and the cell cycle and stimulate developmental processes in plants, have been detected in the culture medium of several bacteria (Srivastava, 2002). GA secretion by bacterial endophytes has been reported by several researchers and shows their importance in plant growth and development, especially under nutrient-deficient conditions.

Phosphorus, an essential plant nutrient, affects cellular plant structure, stimulates growth, and hastens maturity. Phosphorus deficiency is a major limitation to crop production because applied phosphorus rapidly binds into fixed forms that are not available to plants. Bacterial endophytes produce a large number of organic acids, including gluconic acid; 2-ketogluconic acid; and acetic, formic, lactic, glycolic, oxalic, malonic, maleic, and succinic acids, that help to mobilize insoluble phosphates in the rhizosphere. Phytate, the most widespread organic phosphorus form in soil, represents about 10% to 50% of total organic phosphorus. Phytate is hydrolyzed to *myo*-inositol and phosphate by bacteria through the production of phytases.

The nitrogen cycle that is so important in maintaining soil fertility is dominated by four major microbial processes, including nitrogen fixation, nitrification, denitrification, and nitrogen mineralization (Jetten, 2008). *Azotobacter, Azospirillum, Beijernickia, Clostridium, Desulfovibrio, Frankia, Klebsiella, Paenibacillus*, and *Rhizobium* have been reported as nitrogen-fixing bacteria (Betancourt et al., 2008, Jin et al., 2011; Rahi et al., 2012). Biological N_2-fixation has huge importance for the reason of the unacceptable levels of water pollution caused by nitrogenous fertilizers.

Ethylene, a gaseous plant hormone, is involved in a number of biological processes in plants. Ethylene in low concentrations enhances root elongation, whereas higher concentrations inhibit root extension. Several bacterial endophytes are able to produce enzyme 1-amino cyclopropane-1-carboxylate (ACC) deaminase, cleaving plant ethylene precursor ACC to α-ketobutyrate and ammonia and thus lowering ethylene levels. Bacteria producing ACC-deaminase are also important because they provide plants with tolerance against salinity, desiccation, metals, organic contamination, and resistance to pathogens.

Iron is an essential micronutrient and serves as a cofactor of many enzymes. Soil iron is largely present in the insoluble form of ferric hydroxide, which acts as a limiting factor for plant growth. Siderophores are low-molecular-weight iron chelators produced by microorganisms to combat low-iron stress. Siderophores bind Fe^{3+} with high affinity and help in iron uptake. Siderophore-producing bacterial endophytes make iron unavailable for fungal growth, thereby enhancing plant growth indirectly by suppressing soil-borne plant pathogens. Pathogenic microorganisms affect plant health and are a main hazard to crop production. Plant-growth-promoting bacterial endophytes produce several antibiotics, enzymes, and metabolites reducing the growth or activity of phytopathogens. The production of hydrogen cyanide, gluconic acid, IAA, and ammonia has also been implicated in suppressing the growth of fungal pathogens.

In order to take advantage of bacterial endophytes for plant growth enhancement, it is necessary to inoculate target bacteria at a higher concentration than that found in soil. The positive effects of bacterial application depend on the plant variety, growth conditions, and bacterial strains (Nowak et al., 1998; Mehnaz and Lazarovits, 2006). Increased yields with the application of endophytic bacteria have been reported in many plants. However, variable field performance by the microbial inoculants, despite promising results in laboratory and greenhouse experiments, demands more effective approaches in selection of plant-associated beneficial microorganisms for greater consistency in their field performance.

BACTERIAL ENDOPHYTES

Bacterial endophytes can be divided into two groups based on their dependency on the host plant. "Obligate" endophytes depend on their host for growth and survival; "facultative" can exist outside the host plants. Bacterial phytopathogens, obligate or facultative, can also be included as endophytes because of their occurrence in avirulent forms in plants. For example, *Xylella fastidiosa* has been found as an endophyte and does not cause any harm to plants (Araújo et al., 2002).

The relationship between the bacterial endophyte and its host plant ranges from latent phytopathogenesis to mutualism (Strobel and Long, 1998). Several bacterial species are usually associated with a single plant and among them, at least one species show host specificity. From nearly 300,000 plant species, each one hosts several to hundreds of endophytes (Qin et al., 2011), creating an enormous biodiversity. Bacterial endophytes may enter the interior of the root through auxin-induced tumors, wounds, or lateral branching sites, or by hydrolyzing wall-bound cellulose (Hallmann et al., 1997; Siciliano et al., 1998).

Endophytes provide protection to plants because of their ability to produce large numbers of antimicrobial metabolites and compounds. Bacterial endophytes increase the emergence of seedlings, the establishment of plants under adverse conditions, and plant growth. In addition, endophytes also have the ability to degrade xenobiotics and organic compounds, and to resist heavy metals or antimicrobials, which may originate from their exposure to diverse compounds in the plants or soils. Bacterial endophytes have been demonstrated to enhance plant growth, provide resistance to drought stress, and to increase tolerance to inappropriate soil conditions (Swarthout et al., 2009; Taurian et al., 2010).

Endophytic bacteria have been isolated from various sources (Figure 11.1; Table 11.1). *Cellulomonas, Clavibacter, Curtobacterium,* and *Microbacterium* have been isolated from *Glycine max, Sorghum bicolor, Triticum aestivum,* and *Zea mays* (Zinniel et al., 2002). In a study carried out on endophytic bacteria isolated from common bean by Costa et al. (2012), it was found that, out of 158 endophytic bacterial isolates, the majority (36.7%) belonged to Proteobacteria followed by Firmicutes, Actinobacteria, and Bacteroidetes. Kaur et al. (2017) reported a fluorescent *Pseudomonas* sp. with plant-growth–promoting activities from *Tinospora* stem.

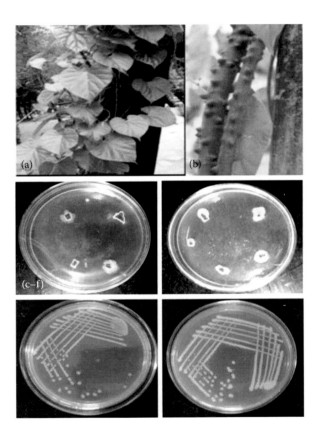

FIGURE 11.1 Isolation of endophytic bacteria from medicinal plant. (a) *Tinospora* stem and leaves, (b) bacteria growing in the vicinity of leaves and stem, and (c–f) pure cultures of endophytic bacteria on nutrient agar after 48 h incubation at 28°C.

TABLE 11.1
Isolation of Bacterial Endophytes from Plants

Bacterial Endophyte	Plant	References
Aureobacterium saperdae, Bacillus pumilus, Burkholderia solanacearum, Phyllobacterium rubiacearu, and Pseudomonas putida	Cotton	Chen et al. (1995)
Cellulomonas, Clavibacter, Curtobacterium, and Microbacterium	Glycine max, Sorghum bicolor, Triticum aestivum, Zea mays	Zinniel et al. (2002)
Different taxonomic groups	Alyssum bertolonii	Barzanti et al. (2007)
Achromobacter xiloxidans, Alcaligenes sp., pumilus	Sunflower	Forchetti et al. (2007)
Bacillus, Pseudomonas, Brevibacterium	Prosopis strombulifer	Sgroy et al. (2009)
Bacillus thuringiensis, B. amyloliquifaciens	Chelidonium majus	Goryluk et al. (2009)
Bacillus and Sphingopyxis	Strawberry	Dias et al. (2009)
Enterobacter sp.	Populus trichocarpa	Taghavi et al. (2010)
Actinobacteria, Proteobacteria, Bacteroidetes, and Firmicutes	Solanum nigrum L.	Luo et al. (2011)
Methylobacterium sp. and Curtobacterium sp.	Rice	Elbeltagy et al. (2012)
Bacillus, Delftia, Methylobacterium, Microbacterium, Paenibacillus, Staphylococcus, and Stenotrophomonas	Phaseolus vulgaris	Costa et al. (2012)
Acinetobacter calcoaceticus, Bacillus megaterium, Bacillus licheniformis, Bacillus pumilus, Micrococcus luteus, Paenibacillus sp., and Pseudomonas sp.	Plectranthus tenuiflorus	El-Deeb et al. (2013)
Pseudomonas sp.	Zingiber officinale	Jasim et al. (2014)
Alcaligenes, Bacillus, Curtobacterium, Pseudomonas, and Staphylococcus	Phyllostachys edulis	Yuan et al. (2015)
Exiguobacterium profundum	Amaranthus spinosus	Sharma and Roy (2015)
Alcaligenes faecalis	Withania somnifera	Abdallah et al. (2016)
Bacillus cereus, Bacillus pumilus, Pseudomonas putida, Clavibacter michiganensis	Curcuma longa	Kumar et al. (2016)
Pseudomonas sp.	Tinospora cordifolia	Kaur et al. (2017)

MECHANISMS OF PLANT GROWTH PROMOTION USED BY BACTERIAL ENDOPHYTES

Bacterial endophytes use a number of mechanisms to promote plant growth (Figure 11.2). They enhance plant growth directly by phosphate solubilization; nitrogen fixation; siderophore production; ACC-deaminase; and phytohormones such as auxins, cytokinins, and GA (Glick et al., 2007; Yang et al., 2009). Indirect

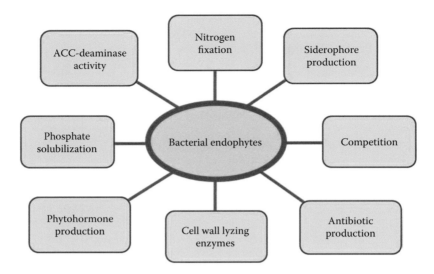

FIGURE 11.2   Mechanisms for plant growth promotion used by bacterial endophytes.

mechanisms are iron depletion, antibiotic production, fungal cell wall lyzing enzyme production, competition for sites, and induced systemic resistance (ISR) (Glick et al., 1999, 2007; Sayyed and Chincholkar, 2009).

PRODUCTION OF AUXINS

Auxins, an important class of phytohormones, regulate growth and development of plants. They help in orienting the growth of roots and shoots in response to light and gravity, differentiating vascular tissues, initiating root development, apical dominance, and stems and roots elongation (Patten and Glick, 2002; Cecchetti et al., 2008). IAA is involved in host–parasite interactions and has also been reported to have biocontrol activity against pathogenic fungi by inhibiting germination of spores and the growth of mycelium (Hamill, 1993). The auxin concentration is also very important for the physiological response by the plant.

Bacterial endophytes produce auxins and increase root growth and root length. IAA production has been reported for several endophytic bacteria (Table 11.2). Plant-growth-promoting bacterial endophytes isolated and characterized by Rashid et al. (2012) have been shown to produce IAA, in addition to performing phosphate solubilization, siderophore production, and nitrogen fixation. Recently, *Pseudomonas* sp. isolated from the stem of *Tinospora cordifolia* showed IAA production (Kaur et al., 2017).

TABLE 11.2
Plant-Growth–Promoting Attributes of Bacterial Endophytes

Bacterial Endophyte	Plant	Attribute	References
Pseudomonas spp. and *Serratia* spp.	*Brassica napus* and *Lycopersicon lycopersicum* L.	Antagonism against *Verticillium dahliae* Kleb and *Fusarium oxysporum* f. sp. *lycopersici* and plant growth promotion	Nejad and Johnson (2000)
Aureobacterium saperdae, *Bacillus pumilus*, *Burkholderia solanacearum* *Phyllobacterium rubiacearum, Pseudomonas putida,* and *P. putida*	Cotton	Antagonism against *Fusarium oxysporum* f. sp. *vasinfectum*	Chen et al. (1995)
Herbaspirillum	Rice	Nitrogen fixation	Elbeltagy et al. (2001)
Pantoea agglomerans	Rice	IAA, P-solubilization, nitrogen fixation, plant growth promotion	Verma et al. (2001)
Herbaspirillum seropedicae	Rice	Nitrogen fixation	James et al. (2002)
Acinetobacter, Enterobacter, Pantoea, Pseudomonas, and *Ralstonia*	Soybean	IAA, P-solubilization, nitrogen fixation	Kuklinsky-Sobral et al. (2004)
Methylobacterium extorquens, and *Pseudomonas synxantha*	Soybean	Adenine derivatives	Pirttilä et al. (2004)
Burkholderia sp.	*Vitis vinifera* L. cv. Chardonnay	Plant growth promotion	Compant et al. (2005)
Bacillus, Burkholderia, Erwinia, and *Pseudomonas*	*Paphiopedilum*	IAA	Tsavkelova et al. (2007)
Achromobacter xiloxidans, Alcaligenes sp. and *Bacillus pumilus*	Sunflower	Jasmonic acid, ABA	Forchetti et al. (2007)
Azospirillum spp.	Maize	IAA, nitrogen fixation	Roesch et al. (2007)
Burkholderia	Sugarcane	pyrrolnitrin	Mendes et al. (2007)
Bacteria	*Solanum nigrum*	ACC deaminase, IAA, phosphate solubilization	Long et al. (2008)
Acinetobacter, Agrobacterium, Bacillus, Burkholderia, Pantoea, and *Serratia*	Soybean	IAA, phosphate solubilization, nitrogen fixation	Li et al. (2008)
Serratia	Banana	Biocontrol against *Fusarium oxysporum*	Ting et al. (2008)
Burkholderia kururiensis	Rice	IAA	Mattos et al. (2008)
Pseudomonas, Acinetobacter, Pantoea, Agrobacterium, and *Aeromonas*	*Solanum nigrum*	ACC deaminase, IAA, phosphate solubilization	Long et al. (2008)

(*Continued*)

TABLE 11.2 (*Continued*)
Plant-Growth–Promoting Attributes of Bacterial Endophytes

Bacterial Endophyte	Plant	Attribute	References
Achromobacter xylosoxidans	Wheat	IAA, phosphate solubilization, nitrogen fixation	Jha and Kumar (2009)
Bacillus spp., *Klebsiella* spp., *Staphylococcus* spp.	*Pachycereus pringlei* (Cactus)	Rock phosphate solubilization, nitrogen fixation, volatile and nonvolatile organic acids	Puente et al. (2009)
Bacillus, *Pseudomonas*, and *Brevibacterium*	*Prosopis strombulifer*	IAA, zeatin, gibberallic acid, abscisic acid, protease, ACC deaminase, phosphate solubilization, and nitrogen fixation	Sgroy et al. (2009)
Bacillus and *Sphingopyxis*	Strawberry	IAA, phosphate solubilization, plant growth promotion	Dias et al. (2009)
Enterobacter sp., *Stenotrophomonas maltophilia*, *Pseudomonas putida,* and *Serratia proteamaculans*	*Populus* spp.	IAA, ACC deaminase production and plant growth promotion	Taghavi et al. (2009)
Coryneform bacteria	Winter rye	IAA	Merzaeva and Shirokikh (2010)
Bacillus megaterium, B. cereus, Micrococcus luteus, Lysinibacillus fusiformis	Ginseng	IAA, phosphate solubilization, nitrogen fixation, siderophores	Vendan et al (2010)
Pantoea	*Arachis hypogaea*	phosphate solubilization, siderophore, antagonism against fungal pathogens and plant growth promotion	Taurian et al. (2010)
Pseudomonas sp.	*Alyssum serpyllifolium*	Plant growth promotion, Ni uptake	Ma et al. (2011)
Bacillus megaterium, Enterobacter sakazakii, and *Pseudomonas putida*	*Mammillaria fraileana*	Phosphate solubilization, nitrogen fixation	Lopez et al. (2011)
Ralstonia sp., *Pantoea agglomerans,* and *Pseudomoans thivervalensis*	*Brassica napus*	ACC deaminase, phosphate solubilization, IAA, metal resistance, and siderophores	Zhang et al. (2011)
Methylobacterium sp., and *Curtobacterium* sp.	Rice	IAA, nitrogen fixation, cellulase	Elbeltagy et al. (2012)

(Continued)

TABLE 11.2 (*Continued*)
Plant-Growth–Promoting Attributes of Bacterial Endophytes

Bacterial Endophyte	Plant	Attribute	References
Achromobacter xylosoxidans, *Pseudomonas putida,* *Stenotrophomonas* *maltophilia*	*Amaranthus* *hybridus,* *Cucurbita* *maxima,* and *Solanum* *lycopersicum*	Phosphate solubilization, HCN, ammonia, antagonism against *Fusarium oxysporum*	Ngoma et al. (2013)
Bacillus	Avacado, black grapes	IAA, HCN, ammonia, protease, lipase	Prassad and Dagar (2014)
Azospirillum, Burkholderia, *Bradyrhizobium, Ideonella,* and *Pseudomonas acidovorax*	*Solanum* *tuberosum*	IAA, nitrogen fixation, antagonism against pathogens, plant growth promotion	Pageni et al. (2014)
Bacillus cereus, B. pumillus, *Pseudomonas putida,* and *Clavibacter michiganensis*	*Curcuma longa*	Phosphate solubilization, siderophores, antagonism against fungal pathogens *Fusarium solani,* and *Alternaria alternate*	Kumar et al. (2016)
Pseudomonas sp.	*Tinospora* *cordifolia*	IAA, phosphate solubilization, siderophores, HCN, antagonism against fungal pathogens *Fusarium moniliforme,* *F. verticillioides,* plant growth promotion	Kaur et al. (2017)

PRODUCTION OF ORGANIC ACIDS AND PHOSPHATE SOLUBILIZATION

Phosphorus, an essential plant nutrient, affects cellular structure, stimulates growth, and accelerates maturity. The symptoms of phosphorus deficiency in plants include stunted growth, wilting of leaves, delayed maturity, and reduced yield (Loria and Sawyer, 2005). Most of the Indian soils have been reported to be poor in available phosphorus: 43.9% of soil areas fall in the low category, 48.8% of soil areas in the medium category, and only 1.9% of soil areas in the high category (Hasan, 1994; Fernández et al., 2007). Inorganic phosphate fertilizers applied to soils are rapidly fixed into the insoluble forms, which are not available to plants depending on the pH and soil type. In the acidic soils, phosphorus is fixed by free oxides and hydroxides of aluminum and iron, while it gets fixed by calcium in alkaline soils (Halford, 1997). Endophytic microorganisms play an important role in making phosphorus available to plants. Endophytic bacteria including *Bacillus, Burkholderia, Pseudomonas,*

Enterobacter, Pantoea agglomerans, and *Ralstonia* sp. have been involved in solubilization of different phosphate substrates (Table 11.2).

Organic acid production by microorganisms leading to pH lowering of the medium is the main mechanism involved in phosphate solubilization (Patel et al., 2008; Park et al., 2009). Organic acids strongly chelate metal ions, originally bound to phosphate, thereby liberating orthophosphate ions.

$$\underset{\text{(Insoluble)}}{Ca_3(PO_4)_2} \xrightarrow[\text{Organic acids}]{\text{P-solubilizing microbes}} \underset{\text{(Orthophosphate,soluble)}}{Ca^{2+} + PO_4{}^{3-}}$$

$$\underset{\text{(Insoluble)}}{FePO_4} \xrightarrow[\text{Organic acids}]{\text{P-solubilizing microbes}} \underset{\text{(Orthophosphate,soluble)}}{Fe^{3+} + PO_4{}^{3-}}$$

$$\underset{\text{(Insoluble)}}{AlPO_4} \xrightarrow[\text{Organic acids}]{\text{P-solubilizing microbes}} \underset{\text{(Orthophosphate,soluble)}}{Al^{3+} + PO_4{}^{3-}}$$

Different organic acids have been reported to be produced by bacteria during phosphate solubilization (Vyas and Gulati, 2009; Gulati et al., 2010). Gluconic acid has been reported as the main organic acid produced by bacteria (Vyas and Gulati, 2009; Gulati et al., 2010). The endophytic bacteria *Bacillus* spp., *Klebsiella* spp., *Staphylococcus* spp., and *Pseudomonas* spp. are noted for volatile and nonvolatile organic acid production (Puente et al., 2009).

Phosphate solubilizing activity by microorganisms can be screened on Pikovskaya agar with insoluble phosphate substrate. A clear zone around the bacterial colonies is an indication of phosphate solubilization (Figure 11.3).

Nitrogen Fixation

Nitrogen is the most important nutrient required by plants. The nitrogen cycle involving different microorganisms plays an important role in improving the nitrogen status and fertility of soils. A large number of nitrogen-fixing microorganisms have been grouped into 38 bacterial genera, 20 cyanobacterial genera, and

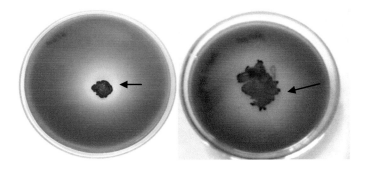

FIGURE 11.3 Endophytic bacterial colonies growing on modified Pikovskaya agar showing yellow zone of phosphate solubilization after 5 days of incubation at 28°C.

2 archaeal genera (Zahran et al., 1995). Several bacterial endophytes, including *Acinetobacter, Azospirillum, Agrobacterium, Bacillus, Bradyrhizobium Burkholderia, Brevibacterium, Ideonella, Herbaspirillum seropedicae, Pantoea agglomerans, Pseudomonas, Pseudacidovorax,* and *Serratia,* have been noted for nitrogen fixation (Table 11.2). In a study carried out by Kuklinsky-Sobral et al. (2004), nedophytic bacteria from soybean belonging to the families Burkholderiaceae, Enterobacteriaceae, and Pseudomonadaceae showed nitrogen fixation, in addition to the production of IAA and mineral phosphate solubilization. Roesch et al. (2007) found that 29 *Azospirillum* spp. strains and one *Herbaspirillum seropedicae* strain obtained from maize stems and roots showed nitrogen fixation ranging from 15.4 to 95.2 μg N/mg protein/day. The strains were also shown to have a *nifH* gene. In addition, these 30 strains could also show IAA production.

1-Amino Cyclopropane-1-Carboxylate-Deaminase Activity

The gaseous plant hormone ethylene is involved in a wide range of biological processes in plants. Low concentrations of ethylene enhance root extension, while higher concentrations inhibit root elongation (Glick et al., 2007). Several endophytic bacteria, including *Acinetobacter, Agrobacterium, Aeromonas, Bacillus, Brevibacterium, Pseudomonas,* and *Pantoea,* produce the enzyme ACC deaminase, which cleaves the plant ethylene precursor ACC to α-ketobutyrate and ammonia, thereby lowering the level of ethylene in the rhizosphere (Table 11.2). IAA produced by plant-growth-promoting bacteria can stimulate plant cell proliferation and plant cell elongation or induce the transcription of ACC synthase catalyzing the formation of ACC (Kim et al., 2001). The cleavage of ACC by ACC deaminase leads to more ACC exudation from inside the plant to maintain the equilibrium, thus reducing ACC and ethylene levels evolved by the plant. The plants grown in association with these bacteria have longer roots and shoots. ACC-deaminase-producing bacteria have also been found to provide resistance to plants against pathogens, and tolerance against salinity, drought, flooding, and metal and organic contamination (Glick et al., 2007; Sgroy et al., 2009; Karthikeyan et al., 2012).

Siderophore Production

Iron is an essential plant micronutrient; it serves as a cofactor of many enzymes with redox activity. A large portion of iron in the soil is in the highly insoluble form of ferric hydroxide, which acts as a limiting factor for plant growth even in iron-rich soils. Many bacteria produce low-molecular-weight iron-binding molecules, less than 1 kDa siderophores under low-iron conditions (Gulati et al., 2010; Vyas et al., 2010). Siderophores bind Fe^{3+} with high affinity and help in iron uptake (Glick et al., 1999). Studies on inoculation with siderophore-producing bacteria have provided evidence for the absorption of bacterial iron-siderophore complexes by the plants, especially in calcareous soils (Masalha et al., 2000). Siderophore-producing bacteria suppress fungal pathogens by making iron unavailable for fungal growth (Sayyed and Chincholkar, 2009). These bacteria also enhance availability of phosphorus to the plants through the solubilization of iron-bound phosphorus in the soil.

Siderophore-mediated competition for iron is also a major factor in determining the interaction among bacterial strains during rhizosphere competence and invasion of plant tissue by endophytes. Siderophores are classified into hydroxamate, catecholate, or carboxylate types based on functional groups (Glick et al., 1999). Catecholate-type siderophores have been reported for stronger binding to iron than hydroxamate-type siderophores (Sayyed and Chincholkar, 2009). Fluorescent *Pseudomonas* produce siderophores commonly referred to as pyochelins and pyoverdines. The water-soluble yellow–green pigments, called pyoverdins, give the fluorescent *Pseudomonas* their characteristic appearance and are involved in high-affinity transport of iron into the cell. Pyoverdines are comprised of a chromophore moiety, to which a peptide chain of variable composition and a carboxylic acid are bound, a catechol-type iron-binding site presented by the chromophore and two functional groups. One of the functional groups is hydroxamate-type, while the other may be a hydroxy acid such as hydroxyaspartic acid (Glick et al., 1999).

Several endophytic bacteria, including *Bacillus megaterium, Micrococcus luteus, B. cereus, Lysinibacillus fusiformis, Pseudomonas*, and *Brevibacterium*, have been shown to produce siderophores (Table 11.2). In addition to the production of IAA and antagonism against the fungal pathogens including *Verticillium dahliae, Rhizoctonia solani, Sclerotinia sclerotiorum*, and *Phytophthora cactorum*, the endophytic bacteria from potato tubers has also been reported for siderophore production (Sessitsch et al., 2004). Similarly, bacterial endophytes from canola have been shown to produce siderophores and to be characterized by IAA production, ACC-deaminase activity, phosphate solubilization, and salt tolerance (Rashid et al., 2012). Recently, *Pseudomonas* sp. isolated from *Tinospora* stem tissue has been shown to produce siderophores and to be characterized by IAA production, phosphate solubilization, and antagonism against fungal pathogens (Kaur et al., 2017).

BIOCONTROL AGENTS/PRODUCTION OF ENZYMES AND METABOLITES

Pathogenic microorganisms that affect plant health are a major threat to crop production. Biological control of plant pathogens using antagonistic bacteria is an effective and eco-friendly alternative to synthetic chemicals (Pageni et al., 2014). Endophytic bacteria produce several metabolites, including siderophores, antibiotics, hydrogen cyanide, pyoluteorin, and pyrrolnitrin, and cell-wall-degrading enzymes such as chitinases, cellulases, and proteases that reduce the growth or activity of phytopathogens (Table 11.2). Biological control may also result from direct interactions between bacteria and the host plants whereby the host disease defense response is stimulated, leading to ISR.

Bacterial endophytes are suitable biocontrol agents by virtue of their ability to colonize an ecological niche similar to that of phytopathogens and their ability to produce antibiotics and enzymes (Berg et al., 2005). Many studies have demonstrated the ability of bacterial endophytes to control fungal and bacterial phytopathogens, insects, and nematodes (Table 11.2). Sessitsch et al. (2004) studied the plant-growth-promoting activities of endophytic bacteria isolated from potato tubers. In dual plate, bacterial isolates showed antagonism against fungal pathogens *Verticillium dahliae*,

Rhizoctonia solani, *Sclerotinia sclerotiorum*, and *Phytophthora cactorum* and to the bacterial pathogens *Erwinia carotovora*, *Streptomyces scabies*, and *Xanthomonas campestris* by virtue of their ability to produce enzymes, antibiotics, siderophores, and plant growth hormone IAA.

PLANT GROWTH PROMOTION

Inoculations with a target microorganism at a much higher concentration than that found in the soil is necessary to take advantage of bacteria for plant growth and yield enhancement. The benefits of bacterial application depend on plant species/variety, growth conditions, and bacterial strains (Nowak et al., 1998; Mehnaz and Lazarovits, 2006). The overall performance and health of plants improve due to increased availability of limiting nutrients, increasing the ability of infected plants to defend themselves. Increased yields have been reported with the application of endophytic bacteria, including *Azospirillum, Azotobacter, Bacillus, Burkholderia, Pseudomonas, Rhizobium,* and *Serratia,* selected for various plant-growth-promoting activities (Table 11.2). In a study by Nejad and Johnson (2000), it was found that the seed bacterization of oilseed rape and tomato with endophytes significantly enhanced seed germination and growth, and reduced disease symptoms caused by the pathogens *Verticillium dahliae* Kleb and *Fusarium oxysporum* f. sp. *lycopersici* (Sacc.). Similarly, dry bean inoculated with bacterial endophytes increased biomasss of shoots up to 34% and total biomass up to 25% (Pageni et al., 2014). The bacterial isolates showed nitrogen fixation; production of IAA; and antagonism against potato pathogens *Pectobacterium atrosepticum, Fusarium sambucinum,* and *Clavibacter michiganensis* ssp. *epedonicus*. Recently, endophytic bacterium *Pseudomonas* sp. from the medicinal plant *Tinospora* has been reported to promote the growth of pea plants (Kaur et al., 2017). The bacterium showed phosphate solubilization, and production of IAA, siderophores, HCN, and ammonia.

CONCLUSIONS AND PERSPECTIVES

Bacterial endophytes are important components of sustainable agriculture and have gained importance in view of their ability to synthesize large number of important metabolites for agriculture. They can be considered as cell factories because they produce phytohormones, organic acids, ACC-deaminase, proteases, cellulases, siderophores, and fungal cell-wall–lyzing enzymes. Keeping in view the beneficial roles of bacterial endophytes, there has been a tremendous increase in studies on plant–bacterial associations and the use of bacterial endophytes as microbial inoculants.

The current knowledge about endophytes is not sufficient, and some gaps still exist in the studies carried out so far. Researchers are focusing on various genes to help particular bacteria to invade plant tissues and provide clues about their life cycle. In the future, researchers may be able to engineer endophytic bacteria to be used as cell factories and microbial inoculants after the functions of endophytic bacteria are fully understood.

REFERENCES

Abdallah, R. A. B., Trabelsi, B. M., Nefzi. A., Khiareddine, H. J., Remadi, M. D., 2016. Isolation of endophytic bacteria from *Withania somnifera* and assessment of their ability to suppress Fusarium wilt disease in tomato and to promote plant growth. *Journal of Plant Pathology and Microbiology*. 7:352.

Adesemoye, A. O., Obini, M., Ugoji, E. O., 2008. Comparison of plant growth-promotion with *Pseudomonas aeruginosa* and *Bacillus subtilis* in three vegetables. *Brazilian Journal of Microbiology*. 39(3):423–426.

Araújo, W. L., Marcon, J., Maccheroni, W., van Elsas, J. D., van Vuurde, J. W., Azevedo, J. L., 2002. Diversity of endophytic bacterial populations and their interaction with *Xylella fastidiosa* in citrus plants. *Applied and Environmental Microbiology*. 68(10):4906–4914.

Barzanti, R., Ozino, F., Bazzicalupo, M., Gabbrielli, R., Galardi, F., et al. 2007. Isolation and characterization of endophytic bacteria from the nickel hyperaccumulator plant *Alyssum bertolonii*. *Microbial Ecology*. 53(2):306–316.

Berg, G., Krechel, A., Ditz, M., Sikora, R. A., Ulrich, A., Hallmann, J., 2005. Endophytic and ectophytic potato-associated bacterial communities differ in structure and antagonistic function against plant pathogenic fungi. *FEMS Microbiology Ecology*. 51(2):215–229.

Betancourt, D. A., Loveless, T. M., Brown, J. W., Bishop, P. E., 2008. Characterization of diazotrophs containing Mo-independent nitrogenases, isolated from diverse natural environments. *Applied and Environmental Microbiology*. 74(11):3471–3480.

Cecchetti, V., Altamura, M. M., Falasca, G., Costantino, P., Cardarelli, M., 2008. Auxin regulates *Arabidopsis* anther dehiscence, pollen maturation, and filament elongation. *The Plant Cell*. 20(7):1760–1774.

Chen, C., Bauske, E. M., Musson, G., Rodriguezkabana, R., Kloepper, J. W., 1995. Biological control of Fusarium wilt on cotton by use of endophytic bacteria. *Biological Control*. 5(1):83–91.

Compant, S., Reiter, B., Sessitsch, A., Nowak, J., Clément, C., Barka, E. A., 2005. Endophytic colonization of *Vitis vinifera* L. by plant growth-promoting bacterium *Burkholderia* sp. strain PsJN. *Applied and Environmental Microbiology*. 71(4):1685–1693.

Costa, L. E., Queiroz, M. V., Borges, A. C., Moraes, C. A., Araújo, E. F., 2012. Isolation and characterization of endophytic bacteria isolated from the leaves of the common bean (*Phaseolus vulgaris*). *Brazilian Journal of Microbiology*. 43(4):1562–1575.

Dias, A. C., Costa, F. E., Andreote, F. D., Lacava, P. T., Teixeira, M. A., et al. 2009. Isolation of micropropagated strawberry endophytic bacteria and assessment of their potential for plant growth promotion. *World Journal of Microbiology and Biotechnology*. 25(2):189–195.

Elbeltagy, A., Nishioka, K., Sato, T., Suzuki, H., Ye, B., et al. 2001. Endophytic colonization and in planta nitrogen fixation by a *Herbaspirillum* sp. isolated from wild rice species. *Applied and Environmental Microbiology*. 67(11):5285–5293.

Elbeltagy, A., Nishioka, K., Suzuki, H., Sato, T., Sato, Y. I., et al. 2000. Isolation and characterization of endophytic bacteria from wild and traditionally cultivated rice varieties. *Soil Science and Plant Nutrition*. 46(3):617–629.

El-Deeb, B., Fayez, K., Gherbawy, Y., 2013. Isolation and characterization of endophytic bacteria from *Plectranthus tenuiflorus* medicinal plant in Saudi Arabia desert and their antimicrobial activities. *Journal of Plant Interactions*. 8(1):56–64.

Fernández, L. A., Zalba, P., Gómez, M. A., Sagardoy, M. A., 2007. Phosphate-solubilization activity of bacterial strains in soil and their effect on soybean growth under greenhouse conditions. *Biology and Fertility of Soils*. 43(6):805–809.

Forchetti, G., Masciarelli, O., Alemano, S., Alvarez, D., Abdala, G., 2007. Endophytic bacteria in sunflower (*Helianthus annuus* L.): Isolation, characterization, and production of jasmonates and abscisic acid in culture medium. *Applied Microbiology and Biotechnology*. 76(5):1145–1152.

Glick, B. R., Cheng, Z., Czarny, J., Duan, J., 2007. Promotion of plant growth by ACC deaminase-producing soil bacteria. *European Journal of Plant Pathology*. 119(3):329–339.

Glick, B. R., Patten, C. L., Holguin, G., Penrose, D. M., 1999. Biochemical and genetic mechanisms used by plant growth promoting bacteria. *World Scientific*. (1999):267.

Goryluk. A., Rekosz-Burlaga, H., Blaszczyk, M., 2009. Isolation and characterization of bacterial endophytes of *Chelidonium majus* L. L. *Pol J Microbiology*. 58(4):355–361.

Gulati, A., Sharma, N., Vyas, P., Sood, S., Rahi, P., et al. 2010. Organic acid production and plant growth promotion as a function of phosphate solubilization by *Acinetobacter rhizosphaerae* strain BIHB 723 isolated from the cold deserts of the trans-Himalayas. *Archives of Microbiology*. 192(11):975–983.

Hallmann, J., Quadt-Hallmann, A., Mahaffee, W. F., Kloepper, J. W., 1997. Bacterial endophytes in agricultural crops. *Canadian Journal of Microbiology*. 43(10):895–914.

Hamill, J. D., 1993. Alterations in auxin and cytokinin metabolism of higher plants due to expression of specific genes from pathogenic bacteria: A review. *Functional Plant Biology*. 20(5):405–423.

Hasan, R., 1994. Phosphorus fertility status of soils in India. *Phosphorus Researches in India* (Ed.)G. Dev). Potash & Phosphate Institute of Canada, India Programme, Gurgaon, India. 7–13.

Holford, I. C., 1997. Soil phosphorus: Its measurement, and its uptake by plants. *Soil Research*. 35(2):227–240.

James, E. K., Gyaneshwar, P., Mathan, N., Barraquio, W. L., Reddy, P. M., et al. 2002. Infection and colonization of rice seedlings by the plant growth-promoting bacterium *Herbaspirillum seropedicae* Z67. *Molecular Plant-Microbe Interactions*. 15(9):894–906.

Jasim, B., Joseph, A. A., John, C. J., Mathew, J., Radhakrishnan, E. K., 2014. Isolation and characterization of plant growth promoting endophytic bacteria from the rhizome of *Zingiber officinale*. *3 Biotechnology*. 4(2):197–204.

Jetten, M. S., 2008. The microbial nitrogen cycle. *Environmental Microbiology*. 10(11):2903–2909.

Jha, P., Kumar, A., 2009. Characterization of novel plant growth promoting endophytic bacterium *Achromobacter xylosoxidans* from wheat plant. *Microbial Ecology*. 58(1):179–188.

Jin, H. J., Lv, J., Chen, S. F., 2011. Paenibacillus sophorae sp. nov., a nitrogen-fixing species isolated from the rhizosphere of *Sophora japonica*. *International Journal of Systematic and Evolutionary Microbiology*. 61(4):767–771.

Karthikeyan, B., Joe, M. M., Islam, M. R., Sa, T., 2012. ACC deaminase containing diazotrophic endophytic bacteria ameliorate salt stress in *Catharanthus roseus* through reduced ethylene levels and induction of antioxidative defense systems. *Symbiosis*. 56(2):77–86.

Kaur, R., Mainam, A., Vyas, P., 2017. Endophytic *Pseudomonas* sp. TCA1 from *Tinospora cordifolia* stem with antagonistic and plant growth-promoting potential. *Research Journal of Pharmacy and Technology*. 10(2):456–460.

Kim, J. H., Kim, W. T., Kang, B. G., 2001. IAA and N6-benzyladenine inhibit ethylene-regulated expression of ACC oxidase and ACC synthase genes in mungbean hypocotyls. *Plant and Cell Physiology*. 42(10):1056–1061.

Kuklinsky-Sobral, J., Araújo, W. L., Mendes, R., Geraldi, I. O., Pizzirani-Kleiner, A. A., Azevedo, J. L., 2004. Isolation and characterization of soybean-associated bacteria and their potential for plant growth promotion. *Environmental Microbiology.* 6(12):1244–1251.

Kumar, A., Singh, R., Yadav, A., Giri, D. D., Singh, P. K., Pandey, K. D., 2016. Isolation and characterization of bacterial endophytes of *Curcuma longa* L. 3 *Biotechnology.* 6(1):1–8.

Li, J. H., Wang, E. T., Chen, W. F., Chen, W. X., 2008. Genetic diversity and potential for promotion of plant growth detected in nodule endophytic bacteria of soybean grown in Heilongjiang province of China. *Soil Biology and Biochemistry.* 40(1):238–246.

Long, H. H., Schmidt, D. D., Baldwin, I. T., 2008. Native bacterial endophytes promote host growth in a species-specific manner; phytohormone manipulations do not result in common growth responses. *PLoS One.* 3(7):e2702.

Lopez, B. R., Bashan, Y., Bacilio, M., 2011. Endophytic bacteria of *Mammillaria fraileana*, an endemic rock-colonizing cactus of the southern Sonoran Desert. *Archives of Microbiology.* 193(7):527–541.

Loria, E. R., Sawyer, J. E., 2005. Extractable soil phosphorus and inorganic nitrogen following application of raw and anaerobically digested swine manure. *Agronomy Journal.* 97(3):879–885.

Luo, S. L., Chen, L., Chen, J. L., Xiao, X., Xu, T. Y., et al. 2011. Analysis and characterization of cultivable heavy metal-resistant bacterial endophytes isolated from Cd-hyperaccumulator *Solanum nigrum* L. and their potential use for phytoremediation. *Chemosphere.* 85(7):1130–1138.

Ma, Y., Rajkumar, M., Luo, Y., Freitas, H., 2011. Inoculation of endophytic bacteria on host and non-host plants—Effects on plant growth and Ni uptake. *Journal of Hazardous Materials.* 195:230–237.

Masalha, J., Kosegarten, H., Elmaci, Ö., Mengel, K., 2000. The central role of microbial activity for iron acquisition in maize and sunflower. *Biology and Fertility of Soils.* 30(5):433–439.

Mattos, K. A., Pádua, V. L., Romeiro, A., Hallack, L. F., Neves, B. C., et al. 2008. Endophytic colonization of rice (*Oryza sativa* L.) by the diazotrophic bacterium *Burkholderia kururiensis* and its ability to enhance plant growth. *Anais da Academia Brasileira de Ciências.* 80(3):477–493. 3.

Mehnaz, S., Lazarovits, G., 2006. Inoculation effects of *Pseudomonas putida*, *Gluconacetobacter azotocaptans*, and *Azospirillum lipoferum* on corn plant growth under greenhouse conditions. *Microbial Ecology.* 51(3):326–335.

Mendes, R., Pizzirani-Kleiner, A. A., Araujo, W. L., Raaijmakers, J. M., 2007. Diversity of cultivated endophytic bacteria from sugarcane: Genetic and biochemical characterization of *Burkholderia cepacia* complex isolates. *Applied and Environmental Microbiology.* 73(22):7259–7267.

Merzaeva, O. V., Shirokikh, I. G., 2010. The production of auxins by the endophytic bacteria of winter rye. *Applied Biochemistry and Microbiology.* 46(1):44–50.

Nejad, P., Johnson, P. A., 2000. Endophytic bacteria induce growth promotion and wilt disease suppression in oilseed rape and tomato. *Biological Control.* 18(3):208–215.

Ngoma, L., Esau, B., Babalola, O. O., 2013. Isolation and characterization of beneficial indigenous endophytic bacteria for plant growth promoting activity in Molelwane Farm, Mafikeng, South Africa. *African Journal of Biotechnology.* 12(26):4105–4114.

Nowak. J., Asiedu, S. K., Bensalim, S., Richards, J., Stewart, A., et al. 1998. From laboratory to applications: Challenges and progress with in vitro dual cultures of potato and beneficial bacteria. *Plant Cell, Tissue and Organ Culture.* 52(1–2):97–103.

Pageni, B. B., Lupwayi, N. Z., Akter, Z., Larney, F. J., Kawchuk, L. M., Gan, Y., 2014. Plant growth-promoting and phytopathogen-antagonistic properties of bacterial endophytes from potato (*Solanum tuberosum* L.) cropping systems. *Canadian Journal of Plant Science*. 94(5):835–844.

Park, K. H., Lee, C. Y., Son, H. J., 2009. Mechanism of insoluble phosphate solubilization by *Pseudomonas fluorescens* RAF15 isolated from ginseng rhizosphere and its plant growth-promoting activities. *Letters in Applied Microbiology*. 49(2):222–228.

Patel, D. K., Archana, G., Kumar, G. N., 2008. Variation in the nature of organic acid secretion and mineral phosphate solubilization by Citrobacter sp. DHRSS in the presence of different sugars. *Current Microbiology*. 56(2):168–174.

Patten, C. L., Glick, B. R., 2002. Role of *Pseudomonas putida* indoleacetic acid in development of the host plant root system. *Applied and Environmental Microbiology*. 68(8):3795–3801.

Pirttilä, A. M., Joensuu, P., Pospiech, H., Jalonen, J., Hohtola, A., 2004. Bud endophytes of Scots pine produce adenine derivatives and other compounds that affect morphology and mitigate browning of callus cultures. *Physiologia Plantarum*. 121(2):305–312.

Prassad, M., Dagar, S., 2014. Identification and characterization of Endophytic bacteria from fruits like Avacado and Black grapes. *International Journal Microbiology and Applied Sciences*. 3(8):937–947.

Puente, M. E., Li, C. Y., Bashan, Y., 2009. Rock-degrading endophytic bacteria in cacti. *Environmental and Experimental Botany*. 66(3):389–401.

Qin, S., Xing, K., Jiang, J. H., Xu, L. H., Li, W. J., 2011. Biodiversity, bioactive natural products and biotechnological potential of plant-associated endophytic actinobacteria. *Applied Microbiology and Biotechnology*. 89(3):457–473.

Rahi, P., Kapoor, R., Young, J. P., Gulati, A., 2012. A genetic discontinuity in root-nodulating bacteria of cultivated pea in the Indian trans-Himalayas. *Molecular Ecology*. 21(1):145–159.

Rajkumar, M., Ae, N., Freitas, H., 2009. Endophytic bacteria and their potential to enhance heavy metal phytoextraction. *Chemosphere*. 77(2):153–160.

Rashid, S., Charles, T. C., Glick, B. R., 2012. Isolation and characterization of new plant growth-promoting bacterial endophytes. *Applied Soil Ecology*. 61:217–224.

Roesch, L. F., de Quadros, P. D., Camargo, F. A., Triplett, E. W., 2007. Screening of diazotrophic bacteria *Azopirillum* spp. for nitrogen fixation and auxin production in multiple field sites in southern Brazil. *World Journal of Microbiology and Biotechnology*. 23(10):1377–1383.

Sayyed, R. Z., Chincholkar, S. B., 2009 Siderophore-producing *Alcaligenes feacalis* exhibited more biocontrol potential vis-à-vis chemical fungicide. *Current Microbiology*. 58(1):47–51.

Sessitsch, A., Reiter, B., Berg, G., 2004. Endophytic bacterial communities of field-grown potato plants and their plant-growth-promoting and antagonistic abilities. *Canadian Journal of Microbiology*. 50(4):239–249.

Sgroy, V., Cassán, F., Masciarelli, O., Del Papa, M. F., Lagares, A., Luna, V., 2009. Isolation and characterization of endophytic plant growth-promoting (PGPB) or stress homeostasis-regulating (PSHB) bacteria associated to the halophyte *Prosopis strombulifera*. *Applied Microbiology and Biotechnology*. 85(2):371–381.

Sharma, S., Roy, S. 2015. Isolation and identification of a novel endophyte from a plant *Amaranthus spinosus*. *International Journal of Current Microbiology and Applied Science*. 4(2):785–798.

Siciliano, S. D., Theoret, C. M., De Freitas, J. R., Hucl, P. J., Germida, J. J., 1998. Differences in the microbial communities associated with the roots of different cultivars of canola and wheat. *Canadian Journal of Microbiology*. 44(9):844–851.

Srivastava, L. M., 2002. *Plant Growth and Development: Hormones and Environment.* Oxford, UK: Academic Press.

Strobel, G. A., Long, D. M., 1998. Endophytic microbes embody pharmaceutical potential. *ASM News-American Society for Microbiology.* 64(5):263–268.

Sun, Y., Cheng, Z., Glick, B. R., 2009. The presence of a 1-aminocyclopropane-1-carboxylate (ACC) deaminase deletion mutation alters the physiology of the endophytic plant growth-promoting bacterium *Burkholderia phytofirmans* PsJN. *FEMS Microbiology Letters.* 296(1):131–136.

Swarthout, D., Harper, E., Judd, S., Gonthier, D., Shyne, R., et al. 2009. Measures of leaf-level water-use efficiency in drought stressed endophyte infected and non-infected tall fescue grasses. *Environmental and Experimental Botany.* 66(1):88–93.

Taghavi, S., Garafola, C., Monchy, S., Newman, L., Hoffman, A., et al. 2009. Genome survey and characterization of endophytic bacteria exhibiting a beneficial effect on growth and development of poplar trees. *Applied and Environmental Microbiology.* 75(3):748–757.

Taghavi, S., van Der Lelie, D., Hoffman, A., Zhang, Y. B., Walla, M. D., et al. 2010. Genome sequence of the plant growth promoting endophytic bacterium *Enterobacter* sp. 638. *PLoS Genet.* 6(5):e1000943.

Taurian, T., Anzuay, M. S., Angelini, J. G., Tonelli, M. L., Ludueña, L., et al. 2010. Phosphate-solubilizing peanut associated bacteria: Screening for plant growth-promoting activities. *Plant and Soil.* 329(1–2):421–431.

Ting, A. S., Meon, S., Kadir, J., Radu, S., Singh, G., 2008. Endophytic microorganisms as potential growth promoters of banana. *BioControl.* 53(3):541–553.

Tsavkelova, E. A., Cherdyntseva, T. A., Botina, S. G., Netrusov, A. I., 2007. Bacteria associated with orchid roots and microbial production of auxin. *Microbiological Research.* 162(1):69–76.

Vendan, R. T., Yu, Y. J., Lee, S. H., Rhee, Y. H., 2010. Diversity of endophytic bacteria in ginseng and their potential for plant growth promotion. *The Journal of Microbiology.* 48(5):559–565.

Verma, S. C., Ladha, J. K., Tripathi, A. K., 2001. Evaluation of plant growth promoting and colonization ability of endophytic diazotrophs from deep water rice. *Journal of Biotechnology.* 91(2):127–141.

Vyas, P., Gulati, A., 2009. Organic acid production in vitro and plant growth promotion in maize under controlled environment by phosphate-solubilizing fluorescent *Pseudomonas. BMC Microbiology.* 9(1):174.

Vyas, P., Joshi, R., Sharma, K. C., Rahi, P., Gulati, A., Gulati, A., 2010. Cold-adapted and rhizosphere-competent strain of *Rahnella* sp. with broad-spectrum plant growth-promotion potential. *Journal of Microbiology and Biotechnology* 20(12):1724–1734.

Yang, J., Kloepper, J. W., Ryu, C. M., 2009. Rhizosphere bacteria help plants tolerate abiotic stress. *Trends in Plant Science.* 14(1):1–4.

Yuan, Z. S., Liu, F., Zhang, G. F., 2015. Isolation of culturable endophytic bacteria from *Moso bamboo* (*Phyllostachys edulis*) and 16S rDNA diversity analysis. *Archives of Biological Sciences.* 67(3):1001–1008.

Zahran, H. H., Ahmad, M. S., Afkar, E. A., 1995. Isolation and characterization of nitrogen-fixing moderate halophilic bacteria from saline soils of Egypt. *Journal of Basic Microbiology.* 35(4):269–275.

Zehr, J. P., Jenkins, B. D., Short, S. M., Steward, G. F., 2003. Nitrogenase gene diversity and microbial community structure: A cross-system comparison. *Environmental Microbiology.* 5(7):539–554.

Zhang, Y. F., He, L. Y., Chen, Z. J., Wang, Q. Y., Qian, M., Sheng, X. F., 2011. Characterization of ACC deaminase-producing endophytic bacteria isolated from copper-tolerant plants and their potential in promoting the growth and copper accumulation of *Brassica napus*. *Chemosphere*. 83(1):57–62.

Zinniel, D. K., Lambrecht, P., Harris, N. B., Feng, Z., Kuczmarski, D., et al. 2002. Isolation and characterization of endophytic colonizing bacteria from agronomic crops and prairie plants. *Applied and Environmental Microbiology*. 68(5):2198–2208.

12 Role of Exopolysaccharides in Cancer Prevention

Nahid Akhtar and Navneet Kumar

CONTENTS

Carbohydrates are some of the most important molecules on earth, and they have many roles, including structural, storage, signaling, and so on. They can be divided into three categories: monosaccharides, oligosaccharides, and polysaccharides. Monosaccharides are the hydroxyl alcohols and have carbons numbering from three to seven. They are further categorized into aldoses and ketoses. Oligosaccharides and polysaccharides are formed by repeating units of monosaccharides linked by glycosidic bonds. In oligosaccharides, disaccharides are the most common. Polysaccharides can be either homopolysaccharides (HoPs), which are composed of a single type of monomeric unit, or heteropolysaccharides (HePs), which are composed of different types of monomeric units. Polysaccharides can have a very high molecular weight, and they are very diverse because of the enormous number of possible combinations of the monosaccharide units.

Microbes are the smallest entities on earth and cannot be seen with the naked eyes, but they show biological as well as nonbiological effects in terms of causing disease, curd production, fermentation, bioremediation, and so on. They can act as minifactories and can produce a large variety of biomolecules that can be very useful for humanity. They use materials in cells and convert them into various products. Bacteria produce a large variety of biopolymers by using simple to complex substrates. These biopolymers can have a variety of chemical properties. One of these polymers, polysaccharides, are produced by bacteria such as lactic acid bacteria (LABs). These extracellular polysaccharides, called exopolysaccharides (EPSs) are either associated with cell-surface-like capsular polysaccharides or are produced outside the cell (Sutherland, 1972). The first extracellular polysaccharide was reported by Louis Pasteur in 1861 as a "viscous fermentation." The bacteria were identified as *Leuconostoc mesenteroides* by Van Tieghem (Robyt, 1998).

The use of polysaccharides for the prevention of disease is an emerging field. Polysaccharides are seen as alternatives with fewer side effects for the purpose of treating diseases with fewer side effects compared to modern medicines. One such disease is cancer, for which the scope of the use of polysaccharides is under investigation.

Cancer is the second leading cause of death after cardiovascular disease. It is a generic term for a group of diseases that are caused by uncontrolled growth of previously healthy cells. Any normal cell can become cancerous and can invade other parts of the body. According to the World Health Organization (WHO), approximately 14 million new cases were reported worldwide in 2012, and the number of cases is expected to increase by 70% in the next two decades. Around 8.8 million deaths were reported due to cancer in 2015, which is equivalent to 1 in 6 deaths due to cancer globally. Deaths due to cancer are listed here in decreasing order of frequency: cancer of the lung (1.69 million deaths), liver (788,000 deaths), colorectal (774,000 deaths), stomach (754,000 deaths), and breast (571,000 deaths). Among men, lung, prostate, colorectal, stomach, and liver cancer are the most common, while in women, breast, colorectal, lung, cervical, and stomach cancer are the most common. The economic impact for the treatment of cancer is gigantic, and it is increasing day by day. It was expected that the total cost for the treatment of cancer in 2010 was around $1.16 trillion (World Health Organization, 2017).

The anticancer potential of EPS is receiving high interest due to the increasing mortality of cancer patients. Anticancer drugs currently in use are effective, but their safety and side effects, such as vomiting, fatigue, and nausea, lessen the quality of life for many patients (Adamsen et al., 2006; Wagner et al., 2006). Therefore, the search for alternative strategies for the prevention and treatment of cancer is essential. EPSs produced by microbes for the treatment of cancer could be an effective strategy (Table 12.1; Figure 12.1). Several studies for finding EPSs to treat cancer are underway. This chapter focuses on all possible strategies for using EPSs to treat cancer.

TABLE 12.1
Bacterial Species Used for Treatment of Cancer

Form of Cancer	Source of Exopolysaccharide	References
Stomach cancer	*Fomes fomentarius, Lactobacillus species, Bifidobacterium bifidum*	Chen et al. (2008); Chen et al. (2009); Li et al. (2014); Wang et al. (2014); Zhang et al. (2014b).
Lung cancer	*L. acidophilus, L. plantarum, L. lactis, Clitocybe maxima, Rhizopus nigricans, Cordyceps sinensis, Prunella vulgaris*	Deepak et al. (2016); Feng et al. (2010); Hu et al. (2015); Yang et al. (2005).
Bone cancer	*Alteromonas infernus*	Heymann et al. (2016).
Breast cancer	*Trichoderma pseudokoningii, Halomonas maura, Lasiodilpodia theobromae, Sphingomonas elodea, Thraustochytriidae microalgae, L. lactis, Paecilomyces hepialid*	Alves da Cunhan et al. (2012); Park et al. (2017); Raveendran et al. (2013); Sivakumar et al. (2014); Wang et al. (2016); Wu et al. (2014).
Cervical cancer	*Aphanothece halaphytica, Paecilomyces hepiali*	Ou et al. (2014); Wu et al. (2014).
Skin cancer	*C. sinensis, Tolypocladium,*	Leung et al. (2006); Wong et al. (2011).
Colon cancer	*L. acidophilus, L. helveticus, L. casei*	Deepak et al. (2016); Li et al. (2005); Li et al. (2015); Liu et al. (2011).
Leukemia	*Halomonas stenophila*	Ruiz-Ruiz et al. (2011).
Liver cancer	*Bionectria ochroleuca, Rhizobium sp.* N613, *C. sinensis*	Li et al. (2016); Yang et al. (2005); Zhang et al. (2008); Zhao et al. (2010).

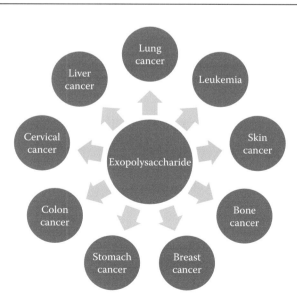

FIGURE 12.1   List of cancers studied for their treatment by use of exopolysaccharides.

LUNG CANCER

Lung cancer is a malignant disease characterized by uncontrolled growth of the lung cells. If it is not treated, this growth can spread beyond the lung to nearby tissues or other parts of the body by the process of metastasis. Most cancers that start in the lung, known as primary lung cancers, are carcinomas that derive from epithelial cells. The primary types of lung cancer are small-cell lung carcinoma and non-small-cell carcinoma. Small-cell lung cancer is a highly malignant tumor derived from cells exhibiting neuroendocrine characteristics; it accounts for 15% of lung cancer cases (Dela Cruz et al., 2011). Non-small-cell lung cancer, which accounts for the remaining 85% of cases, is further divided into three major pathologic subtypes: (1) adenocarcinoma, (2) squamous cell carcinoma, and (3) large-cell carcinoma (Dela Cruz et al., 2011).

Lung cancer is the leading cause of cancer death in the United States and around the world. Almost as many Americans die from lung cancer every year than of prostate, breast, and colon cancer combined (Dela Cruz et al., 2011). Globally, it is the largest contributor to new cancer diagnoses (1,350,000 new cases and 12.4% of total new cancer cases) and death from cancer (1,180,000 deaths and 17.6% of total cancer deaths). There has been a substantial relative increase in the numbers of cases of lung cancer in developing countries. Approximately half (49.9%) of the cases now occur in developing countries; in 1980, 69% of cases were in developed countries (Dela Cruz et al., 2011). The estimated number of lung cancer cases worldwide has increased by 51% since 1985 (a 44% increase in men and a 76% increase in women) (Parkin et al., 1994). In the United States, cancer of the lung and bronchus ranks second in both genders, with an estimated 117,920 new cases in men (14% of all new cancers) and 106,470 in women (13% of all new cancers) (Siegel et al., 2016).

As cancer cells proliferate and metabolize hastily, the level of reactive oxygen species in such cells is elevated. Reactive oxygen species (ROS) oxidize DNA, which causes various mutations that eventually cause cancer. Also, ROS plays an important role in the expression of numerous genes that aid in the proliferation and survival of tumors. An elevated level of ROS is associated with expression of transcription factors that affect tumor suppressor genes and help in metastasis (Gupta et al., 2012). EPSs from different bacteria like *Lactobacillus acidophilus*, *L. plantarum,* and *L. lactis* have shown the ability to scavenge free radicals, protect DNA from oxidation, decrease the expression of p53 gene, and suppress tumor growth by producing different antioxidant enzymes (Deepak et al., 2016). Thus, it is suggested that EPSs can be very useful in the treatment of lung cancer. Various studies have shown that EPSs possess the ability to prevent lung cancer. EPSs obtained from *Clitocybe maxima* mushroom have been found to lower the proliferation of pulmonary sarcoma (Hu et al., 2015). Hu et al. demonstrated that when mice with artificially induced pulmonary tumors were fed a diet containing EPSs, the proliferation of pulmonary sarcoma was reduced and the number of T-cells and macrophages increased (Hu et al., 2015). Medicinal mushrooms can also be used as a promising candidate for effectively curbing the problems caused by lung cancer. EPSs extracted from *Cordyceps sinensis*, a parasitic fungus commonly used in Chinese medicine, has shown antitumor activity. *C. sinensis* EPS has inhibited the growth of lung tumors in tumor-induced mice (Yang et al., 2005). Also, EPS from *C. sinensis* has also reduced the expression of c-MYC, c-Fos, Bcl-2, and vascular endothelial growth factor (VEGF) (Yang et al., 2005; Zhang et al., 2005). Overexpression of C-myc is believed to be associated with turning normal cells into transformed cells (Miller et al., 2012). The abnormal expression of c-Fos, a protooncogene, is associated with cancer development and progression (Wang et al., 2016). Bcl-2 is an anti-apoptotic protein. VEGF is necessary for cancer cells for angiogenesis, their growth and metastasis. A polysaccharide consisting of rhamnose, arabinose, xylose, mannose, glucose, and galactose obtained from *Prunella vulgaris* has shown anti-lung cancer activity in a C57BL/6 mouse–Lewis lung carcinoma model (Feng et al., 2010). *P. vulgaris* is traditionally used in Chinese medicine to treat tumors (Feng et al., 2010).

EPS from *C. sinensis* and *P. vulgaris* have shown antitumor activity and reduced the expression of various genes that play a role in development and progression of cancer. Thus, EPS can be considered an effective agent for the therapy of lung cancer.

STOMACH CANCER

The stomach looks like a sac and helps in the digestion of the ingested food. It consists of cardia, fundus, corpus, antrum, and pylorus. It secretes gastric juice having an acidic pH and enzymes such as pepsin that help in the killing of the pathogens (thus provides innate immunity). It also secretes intrinsic factor, which helps in the absorption of the vitamin B12. The stomach has five layers: (1) the innermost layer mucosa, (2) submucosa, (3) muscularis propria, (4) subserosa, and (5) serosa. Stomach cancer can develop in any section of the stomach, but most cancers develop in the mucosa, which is the inner lining of the stomach.

The progression of stomach cancer is a slow process and remains undetected for a long time because of the lack of symptoms. The different types include adenocarcinoma, lymphoma, gastrointestinal stromal tumor, carcinoid tumor, and so on. Adenocarcinoma is the most common and occurs in 90%–95% of stomach cancers. It develops from the mucosal layer.

According to Globocan (2012), stomach cancer is a fifth most common cancer in the world. It is estimated that 952,000 cases were diagnosed in 2012, which is 6.8% of total cancers diagnosed. Around 70% of cases occurred in developing countries, especially in eastern Asia. It is almost twice more common in men than in women. It is the third leading cause of cancer death in males as well as females and accounts for 8.8% of total cancer deaths. Males in the Republic of Korea represent the most number of cases, followed by Mongolia and Japan. Females in the Republic of Korea, followed by Guatemala and Mongolia, represent the most number of cases of stomach cancer (Globocan, 2012).

Stomach cancer occurrence is affected by gender, age, ethnicity, geography, *Helicobacter pylori* infection, stomach lymphoma, diet, tobacco use, obesity, inherited characteristics, and so on. *H. pylori* infection is one of the leading causes of stomach cancer. Long-term infection leads to inflammation, and precancerous changes start in the mucosal layer of the stomach. Large consumption of smoked foods, salted fish and meat, and pickled vegetables increase the risk of stomach cancer. Nitrates and nitrites present in cured meat are converted by certain bacteria, such as *H. pylori*, into cancer-causing compounds (American Cancer Society 2017). Treatments for stomach cancer include surgery, chemotherapy, targeted therapy, and radiation therapy. Use of phytochemicals for the treatment of stomach cancer is still an emerging field, and phytochemicals are not currently used in such treatment.

Use of EPSs could be promising in avoiding stomach cancer and reducing the suffering of patients with the disease. Among EPSs medicinal mushrooms might be most promising. Medicinal mushrooms are used in China, Japan, and other Asian countries as a tonic food and herbal remedy. They are the source of polysaccharides with immune-stimulating and antitumor properties (Wasser, 2002). One of the useful mushrooms is *Fomes fomentarius*, which belongs to Basidiomycete and has anti-inflammatory, antidiabetic, and anti-tumor properties. It has been used for centuries in traditional Chinese medicine for the treatment of inflammation, oral ulcer, hepatocirrhosis, gastroenteric disorders, and various cancers (Ito et al., 1976; Park et al., 2004; Lee, 2005). Mushroom polysaccharides have been found to possess antiproliferative properties against cancer cells (Li et al., 2004; Cui et al., 2007). Chen et al. (2008) found that EPS from *F. fomentarius* reduced the cell viability of human gastric cancer cells SGC-7901. At a higher concentration of EPS, cell proliferation was reported to almost cease (Chen et al., 2008). Polysaccharides at a low dose can be useful in promoting doxorubicin (DOX)-induced growth inhibition and apoptosis of few cancer cells (Collins et al., 2006). Chen et al. used EPS from *F. fomentarius* along with DOX and found the effect of DOX was significantly increased compared to DOX used alone against SGC-7901 cells. Thus, polysaccharides could be used to enhance the efficacy of drugs already in use.

Lactobacillus (LAB) species could be another important microorganism in this category. Most of the EPS-producing LAB strains release EPS (r-EPS), but some of them also produce cell-bound EPS (c-EPS), along with r-EPS. The EPS produced by LABs can be HoPs as well as HePs (Badel et al., 2011). The EPS produced by LABs has repeating units composed of seven monosaccharides, the principal ones being galactose, mannose, glucose, and rhamnose (Jolly et al., 2002; Ruas-Madiedo et al., 2002; Badel et al., 2011). The EPS released by LABs are an attractive source of food additives and useful drugs. Many of them have been found to have antioxidant and anticancer effects, which are significant health benefits (Li et al., 2014a; Wang et al., 2014; Zhang et al., 2014b). Li et al. (2015a) used the *L. helveticus* MB2-1 strain in their study and found that it produces a lot of EPS. This strain was isolated from traditional Sayram ropy fermented milk in the Xinjiang region of China (Li et al., 2012b). Their study found that c-EPS and three fractions of r-EPS (i.e., r-LHEPS-1, r-LHEPS-2, and r-LHEPS-3) showed antioxidant activity by strongly scavenging free radicals (Li et al., 2012a, 2014b). In 2014, they found that fractions of r-EPS, especially r-LHEPS-2, were found to have anticancer activity against BCG-823 human gastric cells (Li et al., 2014c). c-EPS is a HePs of mannose, glucose, rhamnose, arabinose, and galactose. The treatment of BCG-823 cells with c-EPS from *L. helveticus* MB2-1 showed a protective effect with an increase in concentration for treatment (Li et al., 2015a).

Levan is a fructose polymer produced primarily from microorganisms such as *Bacillus* species, *Xanthomonas* species, *Pseudomonas* species, and *Streptococcus* species (Rosell and Birkhed, 1974; Whiting and Coggins, 1967). Levan has β-(2,6)-glycosidic bonds, with some β-(2,1)-linked branch chains. Yoo et al. (2004) produced levan from the cultures of four different microorganisms: *Microbacterium laevaniformans, Gluconoacetobacter xylinus, Zymomonas mobilis,* and *Rahnella aquatilis.* They investigated the antitumor activity of levan against several cell lines, including gastric cancer cell line SNU-1. In this preliminary study, they found the suppression activity of levan against the SNU-1 cell line.

Liu et al. (2012) used levan-type EPS from *Paenibacillus polymyxa* EJS-3 and synthesized its derivatives via acetylation, phosphorylation, and benzylation. They found significant scavenging activity against superoxide and hydroxyl radicals, and higher reducing power. Free radical scavengers generally have anti-tumor effects also, so they used them against gastric cell line BGC-823. All the derivatives of levan were found to have inhibitory effects against the BGC-823 cell line, but the effect was dose-dependent. The inhibitory effect of levan derivatives was found to be more significant than natural levan (Liu et al., 2012).

EPS extracted from *Bifidobacterium bifidum* (B.EPS) has been found to possess protective effects against gastric cancer. The protective effects were shown on the gastric cancer cell line BGC-823. B.EPS treatment showed inhibition of the growth of BGC-823 cells in a dose- and time-dependent manner. Treatment led to a reduction in the expression of hTERT mRNA and an increase in the concentration of calcium ions, which could be the reason for the protective effects of B.EPS (Chen et al., 2009).

COLON CANCER

The colon, or the large intestine, is the last part of the gastrointestinal tract, where water, some nutrients, and salts are retained from the solid waste before it is defecated through the anus. Colon cancer is the abnormal growth of the cells of the colon. Colon cancer is one of the major causes of deaths related to cancer in general. In 2016, 95,270 new cases of colon cancer were diagnosed, and 49,190 individuals lost their lives to colon cancer in the United States alone (Siegel et al., 2016). Colon cancer is a serious global threat. Most cases of colon cancer arise from polyps on the wall of the large intestine and can metastasize to other parts of body. Individuals with a family history of colon cancer, obesity, diabetes and Crohn's disease, consumption of alcohol and red meat, and smoking are at increased risk of colon cancer (National Cancer Institute 2017a). Irritable bowel syndrome, pain in the abdomen, blood in the stool, weight loss, and weakness are signs of colon cancer. Colectomy; laparoscopic surgery; chemotherapy; radiotherapy; and drugs like fluorouracil, bevacizumab, and irinotecan hydrochloride are used for treating colon cancer. But the side effects of these therapies have made scientists explore other avenues for treating colon cancer. EPSs could be one of the promising avenues to treat colon cancer.

EPS from *L. acidophilus* (L.EPS) has shown the ability to inhibit colon cancer angiogenesis and proliferation (Deepak et al., 2016). L.EPS has shown antioxidant activity and cytotoxicity against colon cancer cell lines (Deepak et al., 2016). The EPS-treated colon cell lines had discontinuous and rough cell membranes as well as an increased leakage of lactate dehydrogenase from those cells, thus implying that EPSs affect the integrity of the colon cancer cell membrane. VEGF is found to be overexpressed in colon cancer. Treatment of colon cancer cell lines with L.EPS has been found to downregulate the expression of VEGF in colon cancer cell lines under both normal and hypoxic conditions (Deepak et al., 2016). Tissue inhibitor of metalloproteinases-3 (TIMP-3) expression was increased in HCT15 and CaCo$_2$ colon cancer cell lines (Deepak et al., 2016). TIMP-3 inhibits binding of VEGF to its receptor, inhibiting the matrix metalloproteinase necessary for cell migration and proliferation of cancer cells. Hypoxia-inducible factor (HIF) is suggested to be associated with colon cancer (Li et al., 2005; Dang et al., 2007). Tumor size and volume were reported to be decreased in mice where the expression of HIF-1 was downregulated (Li et al., 2015b). Treatment of colon cancer cells with EPS has downregulated expression of HIF1. Another HIF, HIF2 has the ability to suppress tumor growth, and in the study by Deepak et al. there was upregulation of the expression of HIF2. Expression of homoxygenase-1 (HO-1), which protects the cell from ultraviolet (UV) irradiation and ROS, was increased in colon cancer cell lines treated with EPS under both hypoxic and normal conditions (Deepak et al., 2016). Thus, upregulation of HIF2, HO-1, and TIMP 3 and downregulation of VEGF and HIF-1 in EPS-treated colon cancer cell lines suggest that EPS can play an important role in the proliferation, metastasis, and growth of colon cancer. EPS obtained from *L. helveticus*, which has a decasaccharide repeating unit, inhibited the proliferation of Caco-2 cancer cell lines (Li et al., 2015a). EPS from *L. casie* has also shown the ability to prevent the proliferation of HT 29 colon cancer cell lines (Liu et al., 2011).

BONE CANCER

Bone cancer is the growth of malignant or benign tumor(s) in the cells of bones. Benign tumors are more common than malignant tumors. There are two types of bone cancer: primary and secondary. Primary bone cancer arises in the cells of bone; secondary bone cancer occurs when tumors from other body parts metastasize to the bones. Individuals with Paget's disease who have undergone radiation therapy and who have hereditary retinoblastoma are at higher risk of bone cancer (National Cancer Institute). An estimated 3,300 new cases of bone cancer and 1490 deaths from the cancer occur in the United States each year (Siegel et al., 2016).

Osteosarcoma, a rare form of bone tumor, mostly affects teenagers. Osteosarcoma is the third most common form of cancer among teenagers in the United States; it is characterized primarily by lung metastases. Lung metastases are the primary cause of death in patients with osteosarcoma. Heparin is commonly used to prevent metastasis, its use is restricted because it can cause adverse bleeding and because of the risk of cross-species contamination (heparin is of animal origin) (Heymann et al., 2016). EPSs have shown the potential to treat bone cancer. Oversulfated EPSs extracted from the marine bacteria *Alteromonas infernus* inhibited the migration, invasion (by 90%), and proliferation of cells in human and murine osteosarcoma cell lines (Heymann et al., 2016). Mouse models of osteosarcoma developed by retro-orbital injection of POS1 cells showed inhibition of lung metastasis (Heymann et al., 2016). The oversulfated EPS of *A. infernus*, with a molecular weight of 15 kDa and with the ability to mimic glycoaminoglycans like heparin sulfate and heparin, has inhibited the metastasis of bone tumors to the lung without any adverse side effects (Heymann et al., 2016). Thus, EPS can be considered a promising candidate for the treatment of bone cancer.

BREAST CANCER

Breast cancer is the malignancy of cells in glands producing milk, called lobules, and the cells of milk ducts that transfer milk to the nipples. It is the most common form of cancer in women worldwide. It was estimated that there were 249,260 new cases of breast cancer in the United States and that 40,890 patients died because of breast cancer in 2016 (Siegel et al., 2016). Breast cancer affects both males and females, but breast cancer in males is rare (2,600 cases in men out of a total of 249,260 cases) (Siegel et al., 2016). Formation of a lump in the breast is the first symptom of breast cancer, and it can be detected by mammogram. Other symptoms include a change in the shape of nipple, nipple inversion, unequal size of the breasts, pain in the breast, redness of breast skin, and bloody or clear discharge from nipples (National Cancer Institute). Breast cancer cells can metastasize to other body parts like the lungs and the brain. Being female is the main risk factor associated with breast cancer. Obesity, the absence of breastfeeding, age at menopause, estrogen levels, smoking, alcohol consumption, radiation, exposure to environmental and workplace chemicals, and mutations in BRCA1 and BRCA2 genes are other risk factors associated with breast cancer (American Cancer Society). Tamoxifen; Herceptin; Fulvestrant; Pertuzumab; Herceptin, which is an inhibitor of human epidermal growth factor 2 (HER 2); and aromatase inhibitors like Letrozole, anastrazole, and raloxifene are used to treat breast cancer (Lukong, 2017).

EPSs from different sources like bacteria, fungi, and microalgae have demonstrated the potential to cure breast cancer. EPS obtained from *Trichoderma pseudokoningii* inhibited the proliferation of the human breast cancer Mcf-7 cell line. This EPS also arrested the Mcf-7 cells at S-phase and led to the apoptosis of these cells. *T. pseudokonigini* is also associated with altered nuclear morphology. ROS accumulation and disruption of the mitochondrial membrane potential eventually lead to the apoptosis of Mcf-7 breast cancer cell lines. The mechanism behind the prevention of breast cancer by EPSs is the activation of the mitochondrial apoptotic pathway (Wang et al., 2016a). Mauran is an EPS obtained from the halophilic bacterium *Halomonas maura*. Mauran is a high uronic acid-captaining sulfated EPS (Sivakumar et al., 2014). Mauran has high molecular weight; viscoelasticity; pseudoplasticity; thixotropic properties; and resistance to high pH, temperature, and salt content (Sivakumar et al., 2014). The high sulfate content provides mauran with antiproliferative properties, making mauran a good candidate for preventing growth and progression of breast cancer. Mauran base magnetic nanoparticles have been found to kill about 80% of a human breast adenocarcinoma cell line synergistically when loaded with 5-fluorouracil drug (Sivakumar et al., 2014). These EPS-based magnetic nanoparticles were biocompatible, decreased the viability of cancer cells, and had low cytotoxicity (Sivakumar et al., 2014). Mauran nanoparticles synthesized along with chitosan showed prolonged delivery of 5-FU and were more efficient in killing breast adenocarcinoma cells in a controlled manner (Raveendran et al., 2013). Thus, mauran can be used effectively in chemotherapy and drug delivery. Another EPS lasiodiplodan produced by *Lasiodilpodia theobromae* also inhibited the proliferation of MCF-7 breast cancer cells (Alves da Cunha et al., 2012). EPS gellan gum was also found to be promising in treating breast cancer. Gellan gum is an anionic EPS secreted by *Sphingomonas elodea*. It is used commercially as a thickening and stabilizing agent in various cosmetic and pharmaceutical products. Gellan gum–based magnetic nanoparticles carrying 5-FU have been shown to inhibit the viability of breast cancer cells (Sivakumar et al., 2014). EPS extracted from *Thraustochytriidae microalgae* inhibited the growth of MCF-7 breast cancer cell line (Park et al., 2017). These EPSs also reduced the progression of breast cancer cells by reducing the expression of cell cycle progression genes like cyclin D1 and E (Park et al., 2017). EPS from *L. lactis* increased the level of tumor necrosis factor alpha and NO synthase in MCF-7 cell line, thus helping to suppress breast cancer (Wu et al., 2016). EPS obtained from *Paecilomyces hepiali* HN1 has shown antiproliferative activity against breast cancer cells (Wu et al., 2014). EPS could be used to treat breast cancer effectively because some have been found to induce apoptosis, inhibit proliferation of breast cancer cell lines, hinder cell cycle progression, and increase the level of various factors that suppress breast cancer.

CERVICAL CANCER

The cervix is the lowermost part of the uterus. Cervical cancer is the malignancy of cells of the lining of the cervix or cells producing mucus in the cervix. Cancer of the cells of the lining of the cervix is called squamous cell cervical carcinoma; cancer of the mucus-secreting cells is called adenocarcinoma. The human papillomavirus (HPV) is associated with the majority of cervical cancer cases, and the Papanicolaou test (also called the PAP smear) is done to screen for abnormal cervical cells. HPV vaccines are used to prevent cervical cancer. Drugs like avastin topotecan hydrochloride and bleomycin are approved by the U.S. Food and Drug Administration (FDA) to treat cervical cancer. In the United States, 12,990 new cases were reported, and 4,120 females were estimated to die of cervical cancer in 2016 (Siegel et al., 2016).

EPS extract from *Aphanothece halaphytica* has induced apoptosis in a cervical cancer cell line (Ou et al., 2014). The anticancer property of EPS was due to its effect on Grp 78 protein. Grp 78 is an unfolded protein response regulator that activates mitochondria-mediated apoptosis. EPS derived from the fungus *Paecilomyces hepiali* has inhibited proliferation of cervical cancer cells in vitro (Wu et al., 2014). The mechanism by which these different fungal species show antitumor activity can be attributed to the induction of apoptosis, cell cycle arrest, and necrosis and antiangiogenesis by fungus EPSs (Wu et al., 2014).

SKIN CANCER

Skin is the outer covering of animals and is considered the largest organ of the body. Skin cancer is the malignancy of melanocytes (cells that produce melanin) or cells in the epidermal layer of the skin. Cancer of the melanocytes is called melanoma.

Malignancy of epidermal skin cells is called nonmelanoma skin cancer; it can be further categorized as basal cell skin carcinoma, squamous cell skin cancer, Merkel cell carcinoma, and Kaposi sarcoma. Melanomas metastasize more commonly and are more deadly than nonmelanoma skin cancer, which is easier to cure. Most skin cancer is caused by exposure to UV light. Damage to the earth's ozone layer has increased the amount of UV light entering the atmosphere. Exposure to the sun's UV light can cause skin cancer. UV light forms pyrimidine dimers in the DNA; these eventually cause mutations by interfering with DNA replication. Not all these mutations are harmful, but some mutations can cause skin cancer. Other causes of skin cancer include exposure to environmental and work-related carcinogens and ionizing radiation, smoking tobacco, taking immunosuppressive drugs like cyclosporin A, HPV infection, HIV infection, nonhealing wounds, and inflammation of the skin (Saladi and Persaud, 2005; Kuschal et al., 2012). Skin cancer is one of the most common forms of cancer worldwide. In 2016, there were 83,510 new cases of skin cancer, and 13,650 individuals died from skin cancer in the United States (Siegel et al., 2016). Chemotherapy, radiation therapy, cryotherapy, interferon therapy, Ipilimumab and drugs that inhibit B-raf (vemurafenib and dabrafenib), and a mitogen-activated protein kinase (trametinib) are used to treat skin cancer (Maverakis et al., 2015).

The role of polysaccharides in the prevention of skin cancer has also been observed. The role of fungus belonging to the genus *Tolypocladium* has been studied. The *Tolypocladium* species are anamorphic and parasites of other fungi, insect pathogens, and so on. Leung et al. (2006) isolated *Tolypocladium* species Cs-HK1 fungus from wild fungus *Cordyceps sinensis* and studied its antitumor effects. They used an extract of Cs-HK1, which was found to be rich with saccharides along with polysaccharides. Their study showed the reduction in the cell proliferation of melanoma B16 cells by treatment with mycelium extract. More than one dose of treatment did not show any further increase in the reduction of the cell proliferation, which showed its limited effect. When the same mycelium extract was used in vivo, they found that inhibition of tumor weight and tumor volume was much more significant than when it was used in vitro testing. It could be because of some other mechanisms in animal study (Leung et al., 2006).

EPS from *Cordyceps sinensis* has also shown the ability to prevent skin cancer (Wong et al., 2011). As previously mentioned, *C. sinensis* is a parasitic fungus infecting the moth *Hepialis armoricanus*. Wong et al. (2011) treated human fibroblast cells with EPS from *C. sinensis* and then irradiated these cells with UVB light. The cells pretreated with EPS showed less DNA damage and had 34% reduction in the formation of pyrimidine dimers than those cells that were not treated with EPS.

LIVER CANCER

Liver cancer involves tumor growth of liver cells (primary liver cancer), or it may be caused by metastasis of tumor(s) from other body parts to the liver (secondary liver cancer). Symptoms include weight loss, swollen abdomen, jaundice, abdominal pain, enlarged liver, and fever. Risk factors include cirrhosis of the liver, alcohol consumption, smoking, obesity, hepatitis B infection, steroid consumption, and family history of liver cancer. In 2016, 39,230 new cases of liver cancer were reported and 27,170 individuals died of liver cancer in the United States (Siegel et al., 2016). Radiation therapy, liver transplant, chemotherapy, segmentectomy, and drugs like cisplastin and doxorubicin are used to treat liver cancer.

EPS produced by the endophytic fungus *Bionectria ochroleuca* inhibited the proliferation of HepG2 liver cancer cell lines without cytotoxicity to human liver cells (Li et al., 2016). Beta-glucan EPS obtained from *Rhizobium sp.* N613, with a molecular weight of 35 kDa, was able to decrease the formation of tumors in mice bearing hepatoma 22 in a study by Zhao et al. (2010). EPS from *C. sinensis* was able to inhibit tumor growth in H22 tumor (hepatoma)–bearing mice by increasing activity of TNF-alpha and IFN-gamma phagocytosis ability of macrophages (Zhang et al., 2008). In the liver of tumor-bearing mice, the levels of c-Myc, c-Fos, and VEGF were lower when the mice were treated with EPS obtained from *C. sinensis*, thus exhibiting its antitumor activity in the liver (Yang et al., 2005). Thus, the outcomes of these studies corroborate the ability of EPS to treat liver cancer.

LEUKEMIA

Leukemia is cancer of the white blood cells that originate in bone marrow. Although the exact cause of leukemia is unknown, family history of leukemia, ionizing radiation, Down syndrome, previous treatment with chemotherapy, and exposure to certain carcinogens are risk factors. Swollen lymph nodes, enlarged liver and/or spleen, fatigue, development of petechiae, frequent infections, and anemia are symptoms of leukemia. In 2016, 60,140 new cases of leukemia were diagnosed and 24,400 people died of leukemia in the United States (Siegel et al., 2016). Bone marrow transplant, chemotherapy, and radiation therapy are used to treat leukemia. Methotrexate, nelarabine, vincristine sulfate, cyclophosphamide, and dexamethasone are some of the drugs for treating different forms of leukemia alone or in combination with other drugs (National Cancer Institute).

Bacterial and fungal polysaccharides are getting attention for their ability to cure leukemia. Sulfated EPS extracted from the halophilic bacteria *Halomonas stenophila* has antitumor properties for acute lymphoblastic leukemia. The EPS-induced, caspase-dependent apoptosis of the tumoral T cell line, and primary T cells were resistant to apoptosis (Ruiz-Ruiz et al., 2011). This study suggests that further research about using *H. stenophila* and other halophilic EPS for developing an effective treatment for different forms of leukemia must be done.

REFERENCES

Adamsen, L., Quist, M., Midtgaard, J., Andersen, C., Moller, T., et al., 2006. The effect of a multidimensional exercise intervention on physical capacity, well-being and quality of life in cancer patients undergoing chemotherapy. *Support. Care Cancer* 14: 116–127.

Alves da Cunha, M. A., Turmina, J. A., Ivanov, R. C., Barroso, R. R., Marques, P. T., et al., 2012. Lasiodiplodan, an exocellular (1-6)- B-D: Glucan from *Lasiodilpdia theobromaae* MMPI: Production on glucose, fermentation kinetics, rheology and antiproliferative activity. *J. Ind. Microbiol. Biotechnol.* 39(8): 1179–1188.

American Cancer Society. Stomach cancer. 2017b. Atlanta, Georgia. https://www.cancer.org/cancer/stomach-cancer.html. (Accessed March 2.)

American Cancer Society. 2017b. Atlanta, Georgia. https://www.cancer.org/cancer/breast-cancer.html. (Accessed March 17.)

Badel, S., Bernardi, T., Michaud, P., 2011. New perspectives for Lactobacilli EPSs. *Biotechnol. Adv.* 29: 54–66.

Chen, W., Zhao, Z., Chen, S. F., Li, Y. Q., 2008. Optimization for the production of EPS from *Fomes fomentarius* in submerged culture and its antitumor effect in vitro. *Bioresour Technol.* 99(8): 3187–3194.

Chen, X., Jiang, H., Yang, Y., Liu, N., 2009. Effect of EPS from *Bifidobacterium bifidum* on cell of gastric cancer and human telomerase reverse transcriptase. *Wei Sheng Wu Xue Bao* 49(1): 117–122.

Collins, L., Zhu, T., Guo, J., Xiao, Z. J., Chen, C. Y., 2006. *Phellinus linteus* sensitises apoptosis induced by doxorubicin in prostate cancer. *Br. J. Cancer.* 95: 282–288.

Cui, F. J., Tao, W. Y., Xu, Z. H., Guo, W. J., Xu, H. Y., et al., 2007. Structural analysis of antitumor heteropolysaccharide GFPS1b from the cultured mycelia of *Grifola frondosa* GF9801. *Bioresour. Technol.* 98: 395–401.

Dang, D. T., Chen, F., Gardner, L. B., Cummins, J. M., Rago, C., et al., 2006. Hypoxia-inducible factor-1α promotes nonhypoxia-mediated proliferation in colon cancer cells and xenografts. *Cancer Res.* 66(3): 1684–1693.

Deepak, V., Ramachandran, S., Balahmar, R. M., Pandian, S. R., Sivasubramaniam, S. D., Nellaiah, H., Sundar, K., 2016. In vitro evaluation of anticancer properties of EPSs from *Lactobacillus acidophilus* in colon cancer cell lines. *In Vitro Cell Dev Biol -Animal.* 52(2): 163–173.

Dela Cruz, C. S., Tanoue, L. T., Matthay, R. A., 2011. Lung cancer: Epidemiology, etiology, and prevention. *Clin Chest Med* 32(4): 605–644.

Feng, L., Jia, X. B., Shi, F., Chen, Y., 2010. Identification of two polysaccharides from *Prunella vulgaris* L. and evaluation on their anti-lung adenocarcinoma activity. *Molecules* 15(8): 5093–5103.

Globocon. 2012. Estimated Incidence, Mortality and Prevalence Worldwide in 2012. http://globocan.iarc.fr/Pages/fact_sheets_cancer.aspx. (Accessed March 2.)

Gupta, S. C., Hevia, D., Patchva, S., Park, B., Koh, W., Aggarwal, B. B., 2012. Upsides and downsides of reactive oxygen species for cancer: The roles of reactive oxygen species in tumorigenesis, prevention and therapy. *Antioxid. Redox Signal.* 16(11): 1295–322.

Heymann, D., Ruiz-Velasco, C., Chesneau, J., Ratiskol, J., Sinquin, C., Colliec-Jouault, S., 2016. Anti-metastatic properties of a marine bacterial EPS-based derivative designed to mimic glycosaminoglycans. *Molecules* 21(3): 309.

Hu, S. H., Cheung, P. C., Hung, R. P., Chen, Y. K., Chang, S. J., 2015. Antitumor and immunomodulating activities of EPS produced by big cup culinary medicinal mushroom *Clitocybe maxima* (Higher Basidiomycetes) in liquid submerged culture. *Int. J. Mushrooms* 17(9): 891–901.

Ito, H., Sugiura, M., Miyazaki, T., 1976. Antitumor polysaccharide fraction from the culture filtrate of *Fomes fomentarius*. *Chem. Pharm. Bull.* 24: 2575.

Jolly, L., Vincent, S. J. F., Duboc, P., Neeser, J., 2002. Exploiting EPSs from lactic acid bacteria. *Antonie van Leeuwenhoek.* 82: 367–374.

Kohler, B., Ward, E., McCarthy, B., Schymura, M. J., Ries, L. A., et al., 2011. Annual report to the nation on the status of cancer, 1975–2007, featuring tumors of the brain and other nervous system. *J. Natl. Cancer Inst.* 103: 1–23.

Kuschal, C., Thoms, K. M., Schubert, S., Schäfer, A., Boeckmann, L., et al., 2012. Skin cancer in organ transplant recipients: Effects of immunosuppressive medications on DNA repair. *Exp. Dermatol.* 21(1): 2–6.

Lee, J. S., 2005. Effects of *Fomes fomentarius* supplementation on antioxidant enzyme activities, blood glucose, and lipid profile in streptozotocin-induced diabetic rats. *Nutr. Res.* 25: 187–195.

Leung, P. H., Zhang, Q. X., Wu, J. Y. 2006. Mycelium cultivation, chemical composition and antitumour activity of a *Tolypocladium* sp. fungus isolated from wild *Cordyceps sinensis*. *J. Appl. Microbiol.* 101(2): 275–283.

Li, C., Li, W., Chen, X., Feng, M., Rui, X., et al., 2014a. Microbiological, physicochemical and rheological properties of fermented soymilk produced with EPS (EPS) producing lactic acid bacteria strains. *LWT–Food Sci. Technol.* 57: 477–485.

Li, G., Kim, D. H., Kim, T. D., Park, B. J., Park, H. D., et al., 2004. Protein-bound polysaccharide from *Phellinus linteus* induces G2/M phase arrest and apoptosis in SW480 human colon cancer cells. *Cancer Lett.* 216: 175–181.

Li, L., Lin, X., Staver, M., Shoemaker, A., Semizarov, D., et al., 2005. Evaluating hypoxia-inducible factor-1α as a cancer therapeutic target via inducible RNA interference in vivo. *Cancer Res.* 65(16): 7249–7258.

Li, W., Ji, J., Chen, X., Jiang, M., Rui, X., Dong, M., 2014b. Structural elucidation and antioxidant activities of EPSs from *Lactobacillus helveticus* MB2-1. *Carbohyd. Polym.* 102: 351–359.

Li, W., Ji, J., Tang, W., Rui, X., Chen, X., et al., 2014c. Characterization of an antiproliferative EPS (LHEPS-2) from *Lactobacillus helveticus* MB2-1. *Carbohydr. Polym.* 105: 334–340.

Li, W., Ji, J., Xu, X., Hu, B., Wang, K., et al., 2012a. Extraction and antioxidant activity in vitro of capsular polysaccharide from *Lactobacillus helveticus* MB2-1 in Sayram yogurt from Xinjiang. *Food Sci.* 33: 34–38.

Li, W., Mutuvulla, M., Chen, X., Jiang, M., Dong, M., 2012b. Isolation and identification of high viscosity-producing lactic acid bacteria from a traditional fermented milk in Xinjiang and its role in fermentation process. *Eur. Food Res. Technol.* 235: 497–505.

Li, W., Tang, W., Ji, J., Xia, X., Rui, X., et al., 2015b. Characterization of a novel polysaccharide with anti-colon cancer activity from *Lactobacillus helveticus* MB2-1. *Carbohydr. Res.* 411: 6–14.

Li, W., Xia, X., Tang, W., Ji, J., Rui, X., et al., 2015a. Structural characterization and anticancer activity of cell-bound EPS from *Lactobacillus helveticus* MB2-1. *J. Agric. Food Chem.* 63(13):3454–63.

Li, Y., Guo, S., Zhu, H., 2016. Statistical optimization of culture medium for production of exopolysaccharide from endophytic fungus Bionectria ochroleuca and its antitumor effect in vitro. *EXCLI J.* 15: 211–220.

Liu, C. T., Chu, F. J., Chou, C. C., Yu, R. C., 2011. Antiproliferative and anticytotoxic effects of cell fractions and EPSs from Lactobacillus casei 01. *Mutat. Res.* 721(2): 157–162.

Liu, J., Luo, J., Ye, H., Zeng, X., 2012. Preparation, antioxidant and antitumor activities in vitro of different derivatives of levan from endophytic bacterium *Paenibacillus polymyxa* EJS-3. *Food Chem. Toxicol.* 50(3–4): 767–772.

Lukong, K. E., 2017. Understanding breast cancer-the long and unwinding road. *BBA Clinical* 7: 64–77.

Maverakis, E., Cornelius, L. A., Bowen, G. M., Phan, T., Patel, F. B., et al., 2015. Metastatic melanoma - a review of current and future treatment options. *Acta Derm Venereol.* 95(5): 516–524.

Miller, D. M., Thomas, S. D., Islam, A., Muench, D., Sedoris, K., 2012. c-Myc and cancer metabolism. *Clin. Cancer Res.* 18(20): 5546–5553.

National Cancer Institute. 2017a. National Institute of Health, Bethesda, Maryland. https://www.cancer.gov/types/bone/bone-fact-sheet. (Accessed March 17, 2017).

National Cancer Institute. 2017b. National Institute of Health, Bethesda, Maryland. https://www.cancer.gov/types/breast. (Accessed March 17, 2017).

National Cancer Institute. 2017c. National Institute of Health, Bethesda, Maryland. https://www.cancer.gov/types/leukemia. (Accessed March 17, 2017).

Ou, Y., Xu, S., Zhu, D., Yang, X., 2014. Molecular mechanism of exopolyasaccharide from *Aphanothece halaphytica* (EPSAH) induced apoptosis in HeLa cells. *PLoS One* 9(1): e87223.

Park, G. T., Go, R. E., Lee, H. M., Lee, G. A., Kim, C. W., et al., 2017. Potential anti-proliferative and immunomodulatory effects of marine microalgal EPS on various human cancer cells and lymphocytes in vitro. *Mar. Biotechnol. (NY)* 19(2): 136–146.

Park, Y. M., Kim, I. T., Park, H. J., Choi, J. W., Park, K. Y., et al., 2004. Anti-inflammatory and anti-nociceptive effects of the methanol extract of *Fomes fomentarius*. *Biol. Pharm. Bull.* 27: 1588–1593.

Parkin, D. M., Pisani, P., Lopez, A. D., Masuyer, E., 1994. At least one in seven cases of cancer is caused by smoking. Global estimates for 1985. *Int. J. Cancer.* 59(4): 494–504.

Raveendran, S., Poulose, A. C., Yoshida, Y., Maekawa, T., Kumar, D. S., 2013. Bacteria EPS based nanoparticles for sustained drug delivery, cancer chemotherapy and bioimaging. *Carbohydr. Polym.* 91(1): 22–32.

Robyt J. F., 1998. *Essentials of Carbohydrate Chemistry*. Spinger-Verlag, New York.

Rosell, K. G., Birkhed, D., 1974. An insulin-like fructan produced by *Streptococcus* mutans, strain JC2. *Acta Chem. Scand. B.* 28(5): 589.

Ruas-Madiedo, P., Hugenholtz, J., Zoon, P., 2002. An overview of the functionality of EPSs produced by lactic acid bacteria. *Int. Dairy J.* 12: 163–171.

Ruiz-Ruiz, C., Srivastava, G. K., Carranza, D., Mata, J. A., Llamas, I., et al., 2011. An EPS produced by the novel halophilic bacterium *Halomonas stenophila* strain B100 selectively induces apoptosis in human T leukaemia cells. *Appl. Microbiol. Biotechnol.* 89(2): 345–355.

Saladi, R N., Persaud, A. N., 2005. The causes of skin cancer: A comprehensive review. *Drugs Today (Barc).* 41(1): 37–53.

Siegel, R. L., Miller, K. D., Jemal, A., 2016. Cancer statistics, 2016. *CA Cancer J. Clin.* 66: 7–30.

Sivakumar, B., Aswathy, R. G., Sreejith, R., Nagaoka, Y., Iwai, S., Suzuki, M., Fukuda, T., et al., 2014. Bacterial EPS based magnetic nanoparticles: A versatile nanotool for cancer cell imaging, targeted drug delivery and synergistic effect of drug and hyperthermia mediated cancer therapy. *J. Biomed. Nanotechnol.* 10(6): 885–899.

Sutherland, I. W., 1972. Bacterial EPSs. *Adv. Microb. Physiol.* 8: 143–212.

Wagner, AD., Grothe, W., Haerting, J., Kleber, G., Grothey, A., Fleig, W. E. 2006. Chemotherapy in advanced gastric cancer: A systematic review and meta-analysis based on aggregate data. *J. Clin. Oncol.* 24(18): 2903–2909.

Wang, G., Liu, C., Liu, J., Liu, B., Li, P., et al., 2016a. EPS from *Trichoderma pseudokonningii* induces the apoptosis of Mcf-7 cells through an intrinsic mitochondrial pathway. *Carbohydr. Polym.* 136: 1065–1073.

Wang, K., Li, W., Rui, X., Chen, X., Jiang, M., Dong, M., 2014. Structural characterization and bioactivity of released EPSs from *Lactobacillus plantarum* 70810. *Int. J. Biol. Macromol.* 67: 71–78.

Wang, S., Xu, X., Xu, F., Men, Y., Sun, C., et al., 2016b. Combined expression of c-jun, c-fos, and p53 improves estimation of prognosis in oral squamous cell carcinoma. *Cancer Invest.* 34(8): 393–400.

Wasser, S. P., 2002. Medicinal mushrooms as a source of antitumor and immunomodulating polysaccharides. *Appl. Microbiol. Biotechnol.* 60: 258–274.

Whiting, G., Coggins, R., 1967. Levan formation by acetomonas. *J. Inst. Brew.* 73: 422.

Wong, W. C., Wu, J. Y., Benzie, I. F., 2011. Photoprotective potential of *Cordyceps polysaccharides* against ultraviolet B radiation-induced DNA damage to human skin cells. *Br. J. Dermatol.* 164(5): 980–986.

World Health Organization, 2017. http://www.who.int/cancer/en/ (Accessed March 14, 2017).

Wu, Z., Lu, J., Wang, X., Hu, B., Ye, H., et al., 2014. Optimization for production of exoplysaccharides with antitumor activity in vitro from *Paecilomyces hepialid. Carbohydr. Polym.* 99: 226–234.

Wu, Z., Wang, G., Pan, D., Guo, Y., Zeng, X., et al., 2016. Inflammation related pro- apoptotic activity of exoplysaccharides isolated from *Lactococcus lactis* subsp. *lactis. Benef. Microbes.* 7(5): 761–768.

Yang, J., Zhang, W., Shi, P., Chen, J., Han, X., Wang, Y., 2005. Effects of exoplysaccharide fraction (EPSF) from a cultivated *Cordyceps sinensis* fungus on c-Myc, c-Pos and VEGF expression in B16 melanoma bearing mice. *Pathol. Res. Pract.* 201(11): 745–750.

Yoo, S. H., Yoon, E. J., Cha, J., Lee, H. G., 2004. Antitumor activity of levan polysaccharides from selected microorganisms. *Int. J. Biol. Macromol.* 34(1–2): 37–41; 2004. *Erratum in: Int. J. Biol. Macromol.* 34(1–2): 149.

Zhang, S., Nie, S., Huang, D., Feng, Y., Xie, M., 2014a. A novel polysaccharide from *Ganoderma atrum* exerts antitumor activity by activating mitochondria-mediated apoptotic pathway and boosting the immune system. *J. Agric. Food Chem.* 62: 1581–1589.

Zhang, S., Nie, S., Huang, D., Huang, J., Feng, Y., Xie, M., 2014b. A polysaccharide from *Ganoderma atrum* inhibits tumor growth by induction of apoptosis and activation of immune response in CT26- bearing mice. *J. Agric. Food Chem.* 62: 9296–9304.

Zhang, W., Li, J., Qiu, S., Chen, J., Zheng, Y., 2008. Effects of exopolysaccharide fraction (EPSF) from a cultivated Cordyceps sinensis on immunocytes of H22 tumor bearing mice. *Fitoterapia* 79(3): 168–173.

Zhang, W., Yang, J., Chen, J., Huo, Y., Han, X., 2005. Immunomodulatory and antitumor effects of an EPS fraction from cultivated *Cordyceps sinensis* (Chinese caterpillar fungus) on tumor bearing mice. *Biotechnol. Appl. Biochem.* 42(1): 9–15.

Zhao, L., Chen, Y., Ren, S., Han, Y., Cheng, H., 2010. Studies on the chemical structure and antitumor activity of an exopolysaccharide from *Rhizobium* sp. N613. *Carbohydr. Res.* 345(5): 637–643.

13 Probiotics and Its Efficacy Assessment in Diabetic Intervention

Amarish Kumar Sharma and Anjana Rana Sharma

CONTENTS

INTRODUCTION

A group of experts assembled together by the Food and Agriculture Organization (FAO) of the United Nations defined the term "probiotics" in 2001 and updated its definition in 2014. Probiotics are live microorganisms that provide a great health benefit when delivered in the living host system in an adequate amount [1]. Probiotics are mostly isolated from the intestinal tracts of humans and animals. End products of bacteria, dead bacteria, or any by-products derived from the bacterial system are

TABLE 13.1

Essential Genera and Species of Microbial System Investigated and Used as Probiotics

Genus	Species
Lactobacillus	*johnsonii*
	paracasei
	plantarum
	reuteri
	rhamnosus
	salivarius
Saccharomyces	*cerevisiae*
Bacillus	*coagulans*
	clausii
Escherichia	*coli*
Enterococcus	*faecium*
Streptococcus	*thermophilus*
	salivarius
Bifidobacterium	*breve*
	infantis
	longum
	adolescentis
	animalisb
	bifidum

Source: Sanders, M.E. et al., Probiotics: Their potential to impact human health, Council for Agricultural Science and Technology Issue Paper 36, 1–20, 2007.

not considered to be probiotics because they are not alive when they are delivered or administered to the host body. A range of potent probiotics are investigated for both human and animal applications [1]. Essential microbial species are listed in Table 13.1 (see also Figure 13.1).

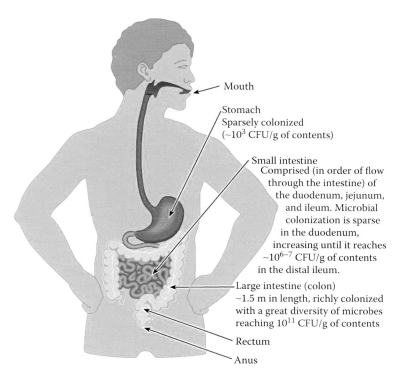

Mouth

Stomach
Sparsely colonized
($\sim 10^3$ CFU/g of contents)

Small intestine
Comprised (in order of flow
through the intestine) of
the duodenum, jejunum,
and ileum. Microbial
colonization is sparse
in the duodenum,
increasing until it reaches
$\sim 10^{6-7}$ CFU/g of contents
in the distal ileum.

Large intestine (colon)
~ 1.5 m in length, richly colonized
with a great diversity of microbes
reaching 10^{11} CFU/g of contents

Rectum

Anus

FIGURE 13.1 The human gastrointestinal tract depicting microbial colonization. (From Sanders, M.E. et al., Probiotics: Their potential to impact human health, Council for Agricultural Science and Technology Issue Paper 36, 1–20, 2007.)

A very diverse and extensive array of probiotic products is on the market. Yogurt is the most widely consumed probiotic product worldwide. Cheese could be the second most widely used probiotic food consumed worldwide. Many fermented and nonfermented milks and nutritional diet formulas are based on different probiotic formulations. Apart from food consumables, probiotics are also sold as dietary supplements, medical food, and drugs. Most often these products are concentrated, dried forms of microbes packed into capsules, tablets, or sachets, which make it convenient for their delivery in large numbers [2].

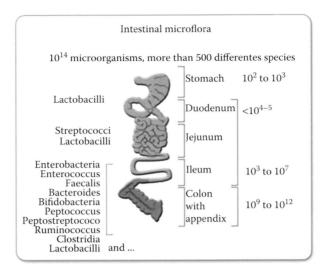

Intestinal microflora

10^{14} microorganisms, more than 500 differentes species

Lactobacilli	Stomach 10^2 to 10^3
	Duodenum $<10^{4-5}$
Streptococci Lactobacilli	Jejunum
Enterobacteria Enterococcus Faecalis	Ileum 10^3 to 10^7
Bacteroides Bifidobacteria Peptococcus Peptostreptococo Ruminococcus Clostridia Lactobacilli and ...	Colon with appendix 10^9 to 10^{12}

From Priyadarsini, N. et al., *Int. J. Pharm. Sci. Rev. Res.*, 34(1), 276–280, 2015; Kumar, N. et al., *J. Gastroenterol. Hepatol.*, 23, 1834–1839, 2008.

REQUIREMENTS FOR A MICROBE TO BE CONSIDERED A PROBIOTIC

A microbe must meet a simple set of requirements to be considered a probiotic. During administration into the host system, the microorganism must be alive, it must provide health benefits, and it must be administered at appropriate levels to confer those benefits [5].

As per "Guidelines for the Evaluation of Probiotics in Food," a probiotic must undergo the following minimum qualifying assessment:

1. Using accurate molecular and physiological techniques, probiotics should be identified at the genus, species, and strain levels.
2. The probiotic strain should be submitted to an internationally recognized culture repository center where scientists can replicate the research and get it published on the strain so that it can serve as a reference strain.
3. For better understanding of the physiological attributes of the probiotic strain, appropriate *in vitro* and animal assessment must be conducted. The choice of assessment should be based on the functions of the probiotic in the target host.
4. The safety of the microbe used a source of the probiotics should be fully evaluated.

5. All the properly conducted controlled studies justifying the health benefits of the probiotics in the target host should be documented.
6. The viable final product must contain the efficacious dose of the viable probiotics through the end of the product's shelf life.

This list of requirements does not include properties such as adherence to the intestinal mucosa, bile and acid resistance, bacteriocin production, antipathogenic activity, and human origin and sustenance through intestinal transit. The array of potential health targets, host systems, and probiotics' specific delivery methods are so diverse that any characteristics beyond those mentioned in the list become important for only a subset of probiotics, and it may be unclear if these evaluations are truly predictive as far as *in vivo* efficacy is concerned [6].

It is often claimed that the probiotics must remain viable during intestinal transit to be effective, although the potential ability of the probiotics to grow and metabolize as they travel through the intestinal tract can contribute extensively to health benefits. At a minimum, a probiotic should be safe and effective, and its functional efficacy should remain intact through the end of the product shelf life. The probiotic's product label must identify the microbial strains and physiological conditions of storage so that consumers can be confident that the probiotic will stay alive until the end of its shelf life [7].

Considerations [2]	Review Comments
Probiotics should be described adequately and identified to the strain level.	Biochemical, morphological, physiological, and DNA-based techniques can contribute to the description of commercial probiotic strains. Total genomic DNA sequencing is becoming more common on fully characterized probiotic strains [8].
Each probiotic strain should be able to be identified and enumerated from the product label.	This can be a challenge because culture microbiology methods often are not enumerated on the product label to differentiate among different species of the same genus. DNA-based approaches can often solve this problem.
Product formulation should be evidence-based.	Decisions on product format (type of food or supplement), dose, and choice of strain(s) should be consistent with those used in clinical studies.
Product labeling should be truthful and not misleading.	Product labels and any supplementary communications should provide clear, accurate information on the types and levels of probiotics; any documented health benefits; and the amount of product that must be consumed for an effect.
Probiotic strains and products should be supported by a dossier substantiating efficacy.	A dossier should be developed that is composed at least in part of peer-reviewed publications documenting the ability of the probiotics to have a positive impact on human health and supporting any claims made.

Benefits of Probiotics [9]

Health Target	References
Lipid profiles of blood	[10]
Dental caries	[11]
Blood pressure	[12]
Tumors of intestinal colon	[13]
Stunted growth form malnourishment at a young age	[14]
Cold and cough	[15]
Intestinal microbiota alteration	[16]
Allergic symptoms and their development	[17,18]
Digestion of lactose	[19]
H. pylori colonization of the stomach	[20]
Irritable bowel syndrome	[21,22]
Delivery of cloned components active in gut (IL10, vaccines, antiviral agents, toxin receptors)	[23]
Harmful intestinal microbe activities	[24]
Absence from work, daycare	[25,26]
Vaginal infections	[27]
Diarrhea (rotavirus, travelers', antibiotic-associated, C. difficile)	[28–30]

PROBIOTICS' CONTRIBUTION TO THE HEALTH INDUSTRY

Scientists and researchers have suggested that probiotic bacteria can improve digestive function; minimize diarrhea associated with antibiotic therapy; reduce crying time in newborn babies with severe abdominal pain, often caused by spasm, obstruction, or distention of intestines; improve lactose intolerance, and improve immune function [31].

Several papers cite the characterization of and potential health benefits of probiotics, and the rate of future publications on this area of study is expected to increase tremendously. Many clinical studies now under way are designed to evaluate the positive influence of probiotic cultures in a variety of health conditions. It is very important to recognize and understand the different strains, species, and genera of the bacteria that are under consideration for their health benefits to the target host [32].

HYPERLIPIDEMIA, OR HYPERCHOLESTEROLEMIA

Cholesterol is a waxy, fat-like substance that is found in all cells of the body. It makes hormones, vitamin D, and other essential substances that help digest foods by the digestive system. Cholesterol moves through the bloodstream in small packages called lipoproteins [33]. Two kinds of lipoproteins carry cholesterol throughout the body: low-density lipoproteins (LDLs) and high-density lipoproteins (HDLs). A balance of both types is essential for normal body functioning. HDL cholesterol is called "good" cholesterol; it carries cholesterol from other parts of the body back to the liver. The liver removes the cholesterol from the entire body system. LDL cholesterol sometimes is called "bad" cholesterol, and high levels of it can lead to a buildup of cholesterol in the arteries, which leads to serious disease outcome like coronary heart disease [34].

Clinical studies have shown that use of probiotic cultures has played an important role in lowering blood serum cholesterol. Studies proved that consuming probiotic dairy products has led to lower low-density lipid levels in humans [10].

OBESITY AND METABOLIC SYNDROME

This is one of the exciting and fascinating areas of metabolic research where the role of probiotics has been highly acknowledged. Research in this area examines how the gut-colonizing microbiota affect the onset of obesity and diabetes or metabolic syndrome. A deranged pattern of microbiota colonization is associated with the onset of diabetes and/or obesity, but it is unclear whether regularizing these deranged patterns could cure the disease or prevent obesity. Due to microbial metabolism of food in the gut, microbes can directly affect energy production, but microbes and their metabolic products may act as cellular metabolic regulators through interacting with host cellular targets [35].

In humans, a probiotic strain of *Lactobacillus gasseri* was subjected to experimental animal models of obesity. The study, has shown an extensive decrease in body mass index (BMI) and fat mass in visceral and subcutaneous regions. In another study, a specific probiotic strain improved insulin sensitivity. The results from these studies have encouraged more clinical studies in the area of metabolic syndrome and obesity [36].

LACTOSE INTOLERANCE

People with lactose intolerance cannot digest lactose, a sugar found in milk products. People suffering from this condition may have symptoms that include abdominal pain, bloating, diarrhea, gas, and nausea. Lactose intolerance occurs due to insufficient secretion of the lactase enzyme in the small intestine to digest lactose sugar down to glucose and galactose [37].

The inability to consume milk and its different food products potentially can mean that some people do not take in enough calcium, which leads to serious bone health and its associated malfunctions. It has been well accepted worldwide that consuming yogurt aids digestion of lactose because lactic acid bacteria used to make yogurt deliver lactase enzyme to the small intestine, where it breaks down lactose to glucose and galactose before it reaches the intestinal colon for absorption into body fluids. *Lactobaccilus acidophilus*, *Lactobaccilus bulgaricus*, *Streptococcus thermophilus*, and *bifidobacteria* have been proven to be potent yogurt probiotic bacteria that improve digestion of lactose [34].

WORKING MECHANISM OF PROBIOTICS

The health effects of probiotics result from several mechanisms interacting synergistically. The interaction mechanisms differ for different strains, as do their specific sites and modes of action. The mechanism may include competitive binding sites to the intestinal mucosal wall, nutrient specific competition, production of antimicrobial metabolites, stimulation of mucin production, intestinal barrier stabilization, gut transit facilitation, metabolism of essential nutrients to fatty acids metabolites, and modulation of the immune system. Some of the above mechanisms have not been substantiated in humans and have been seen only in laboratory trials [38].

Transient effects have been observed on populations of intestinal microbes in the presence of probiotics in the target host system because the native microbiota are acclimatized and well adapted to the environment. The naturally stable synergistic association of gut microbes effectively resists physiological changes compared to probiotics, which explains the transient effects. It is possible that probiotics take over the situation efficiently and disrupt the normal microbial balance (such as during antibiotic therapy), thus normalizing the microbial balance in the intestinal environment and improving intestinal biochemistry [39].

Figure 13.2 depicts the working mechanism of probiotic bacteria to inhibit the enteric bacteria colonization and enhance the function of the mucosal barrier. Probiotic bacteria perform antibacterial activity by (1) producing defensin/bacteriocin, (2) inhibiting pathogenic bacteria through competitive inhibition, (3) inhibiting bacterial adherence and transboundary movement of enteric bacteria, and (4) enhancing

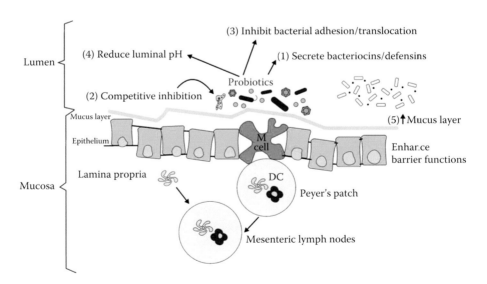

FIGURE 13.2 The working mechanism of probiotic bacteria to inhibit the enteric bacteria colonization and functional enhancement of mucosal barrier. From Otutumi, L.K. et al., *Variations on the Efficacy of Probiotics in Poultry*, Rigobelo, E.C. (Ed.), InTech Open Access Publisher, Rijeka, Croatia, 2012.

the acidity of the intestinal lumen. (5) Extensive production of mucus by probiotic bacteria is also one of the mechanisms for increasing the intestinal barrier function (Ng et al., 2009) [41].

Diabetes Mellitus: A Sweet Poison and a Silent Killer

Diabetes is a metabolic syndrome characterized by altered biological metabolism and significantly high blood sugar (hyperglycemia) resulting due to either insufficient release or low level of insulin hormone in the blood or its abnormal resistance to blood glucose [42]. Diabetes mellitus is a metabolic disorder that sets the stage for several chronic diseases, and it is an epidemic of the twenty-first century. It poses a major threat to a large part of the global population, especially in India, and to economic development. A recent study conducted by the International Diabetes Federation, the current number of people affected by diabetes is expected to rise to 551 million by 2030. The sharp rise in the number of people with diabetes is occurring in two-thirds of the entire world, and more than 60% of people affected with diabetes come from middle-income countries. Upper-middle-income countries have a higher proportion of the population affected (10.1%) compared to lower-middle-income countries. Sedentary life style, high level of work stress, population, and urbanization are stated as the major contributing factors for the onset of diabetes. India and China are the two major developing countries with a high prevalence of Type 2 diabetes (T2D). Both Type 1 and Type 2 diabetes are responsible for the onset of obesity and cardiovascular disease (CVD), one of the main causes of death in India. The prevalence of diabetes and related mortality rises with the prosperity of the country. Prosperity translates into more sophistication and sedentary lifestyles, junk food habits, and extensive dependence on electronic gadgets [43].

Nearly 1 million casualties are due to diabetes or its associated diseases. Keeping in view the alarming increase in diabetes and its associated risk to the global human population, the World Health Organization (WHO) has called India the "Diabetic Capital of the World." The most probable reasons for Indians being highly affected with this disease are high psychological stress, wide disparities in income levels, changes to a sedentary lifestyle, poor immune system, and obesity. Research data, observed trends, and the risk factors for the onset of diabetes has pushed the world community to develop natural and eco-friendly drugs to achieve minimum side effects and long-term efficacy. Probiotics have the maximum potential to fulfill these requirements and could carve a path for future medicine [44].

Role of Probiotics in Type 2 Diabetes

T2D is an altered metabolic condition in which the body cells becomes resistant to the presence of blood glucose, leading to its hyperaccumulation. It in turn can lead to many serious diseases. In T2D, insulin, secreted by the beta cells of the pancreas, becomes desensitized toward blood glucose, thereby creating a situation in which extra blood glucose is stored in the form of fats. Storage of fats in adipose tissues above threshold limits leads to serious outcomes such as obesity and CVD.

The prevalence of Type 2 diabetes mellitus (T2DM) has increased to a serious level in the past decade and is associated with the onset of many serious disease outcomes. It works as a sweet poison by making a person lethargic. It can lead to dementia and kidney failure, and can ultimately decreases life expectancy for many people worldwide [45].

In 2011, 61.3 million people in India were estimated to have been affected with T2DM, out of which 31.2 million were undiagnosed, according to the study conducted by the International Diabetes Federation (IDF) [2]. A similar study conducted by Indian Council of Medical Research-India Diabetes study (ICMR-INDIAB) projected that 62.4 million people are suffering with diabetes and 77.2 million people have prediabetes.

Recent research and clinical studies on probiotics have concluded that gut microbiota play an important and decisive role in controlling the effects of metabolic disorders such as Type 2 diabetes mellitus (T2DM) [46]. Accumulating evidence from research data generated through metagenomic and metabolomics studies using high throughput technologies such as nuclear magnetic resonance (NMR) spectrometry supports the new hypothesis that metabolic disorder like diabetes, and its associated abnormalities like obesity and CVD, occurs due to low-grade systemic inflammation caused by a high-fat and fructose diet, which progressively leads to a disruption of normal gut microflora colonization. The gut microbiome and their associated health phenotypes are extensively modulated through the kinds of nutrients consumed. A poor diet can replace the healthy microflora with unhealthy ones, leading to chronic disease. Hence, the microbiota of the human intestinal system could serve as a template for the resource material to explore strategies for developing novel dietary probiotic supplements in the management of specific gut-related diseases. The intestinal microbiota of human adults affected with Type 2 diabetes studied by high throughput, tag-encoded amplicon pyrosequencing of the V4 region of the 16S rRNA gene showed decreased population of clostridia and firmicutes and an increased population of betaproteobacteria. An increased ratio of phylum firmicutes and bacteroides prevotella to clostridium coccoides in correlation with plasma glucose concentration is also observed (Figure 13.3). Bacteroidetes related taxa either remain neutral or sometimes increase in people with diabetes [47] (Figure 13.4).

Recent studies of bifidobacteria lactobacilli showed that compositional changes do occur during the onset of insulin resistance in mice fed a high-fat diet. The intestinal microbiota profile estimated the reduction in population of *Bifidobacterium* species and *Lactobacillus* species, which resulted in an increased level of lipopolysaccharides in the blood, which in turn might have resulted in NFkB activation (which leads to insulin resistance and ultimately Type 2 diabetes mellitus). In mice fed a high-fat diet and that were profiled for gut microbial alterations, permeability in the human gut system, and metabolic endotoxemia, it was clearly observed that lactobacillus colonization in drastically reduced in gut microbial profile; this leads to transepithelial resistance and increased metabolic endotoxemia, which has a direct link to obesity and CVD [43]. Several investigations have claimed that there is altered endocrine signaling because of changes in gut microbiota population, which ultimately leads to an altered level of secretion of gut hormones to the central nervous system. Such alterations have a direct connection to food intake and to the secretion and

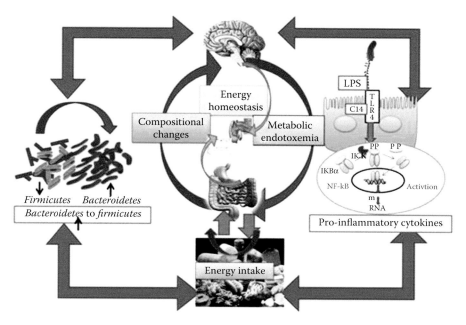

FIGURE 13.3 Role of gut microbiota in the development and control of Type 2 diabetes. (From Panwar, H. et al., *Diabetes Metab. Res. Rev.,* 29, 103–112, 2013.)

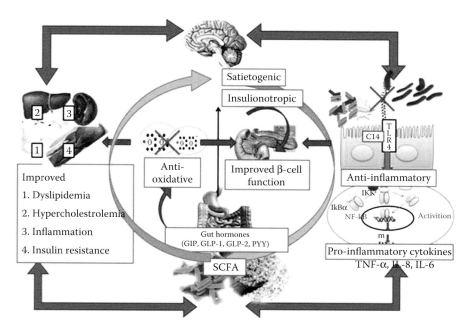

FIGURE 13.4 Probable mechanisms of probiotics action in the management of Type 2 diabetes. (From Panwar, H. et al., *Diabetes Metab. Res. Rev.,* 29, 103–112, 2013.)

expression of gut hormones such as glucagon-like peptide-1 (GLP-1) and glucagon-like peptide-2 (GLP-2), glucose-dependent insulinotropic peptide, which regulates energy balance through insulintropipc, satietogenic properties that affect pancreatic cell mass and its function, insulin secretion, nutrient absorption, and energy storage [44–46,48].

The scientific study of the set of metabolites present within the human gut system shows a considerable contribution of gut microbial metabolites in the homeostasis of glucose in the vasculature. Some studies have proved the metabolic role of gut microbial secretions in decreasing the inflammation-associated biomarkers and activation of free fatty acid receptors to control the upstream regulation of gut hormones [47,48]. Study outcomes through Liquid chromatography-mass spectrometry (LCMS) and validated by metabolomics analysis of clinical serum and urine samples claim that hyperactivation of glucose tolerance in the gut microenvironment may be due to the presence of gut flora–associated metabolites such as hippuric acid, methyluria, and methyl xanthin [49].

Healthy individuals can be differentiated easily from diabetic ones by determining the presence of secondary metabolites of bile acids in the bloodstream. The presence of the secondary metabolite deoxycholate is more prominent in diabetic individuals, whereas cholate was profiled in healthy individuals. This outcome clearly signifies the alteration in the bile acid pool due to unregulated biosynthetic pathway in diabetic patients [44,50]. Type 2 diabetes can be effectively controlled by modulating the intestinal microbiota through dietary control of specific nutrients, which will ultimately control the inflammatory metabolic disorder.

PHARMACOLOGICAL EFFICACY OF PROBIOTICS IN *IN VITRO* SCREENING FOR DIABETES

Putative probiotics of a therapeutic nature are highly strain-specific, and a judicious preselection of specific strains is based on the expression of their specific functional biomarkers. Authentication for a particular kind of medical condition is extremely crucial to demonstrate functional efficacy. The antihyperglycemic efficacy of probiotics has been investigated extensively in different *in vitro* studies on animal cell line models, and in *in vivo* research studies on live animal models were then validated by double-blind, placebo-controlled, randomized clinical trials in humans [51].

Various cell line models have recently been investigated to profile antihyperglycemic or hypoglycemic, inflammatory, and antioxidative effects for the management of Type 2 diabetes and to prove the potential therapeutic efficacy of probiotics. Ma et al. [52] investigated the expression of nerve growth factor (NGF) and anti-inflammatory metabolites by challenging the live and killed strains of *Lactobacillus reuteri* in *in vitro* conditions. The probiotic *lactobacillus reuteru* cells upregulate the expression of NGF and subsequently subsided the cellular expression of IL-8, induced by TNF-a [44].

HeLa cells were used in several research investigations as a potential *in vitro* model to investigate the expression of NFkB signaling, which is a potent inducer of inflammation. In another similar type of study, HeLa cells were incubated with *Lactobacillus reuteri* for one to two hours; it was observed that the IkB degradation was inhibited through NFkB regulation, simultaneously preventing the expression of various proinflammatory cytokines. Neish et al. [54] reported that NFkB activity can be suppressed or attenuated by heat inactivation in animal culture media, which could be due to inactivation of a blood immune component, thereby indicating that the bacterial epithelial cell contact was required to bring about the positive effect [52].

Genetically engineered *E. coli* was studied as one of the potent probiotic microbiota to regulate glucose homeostasis in animal cell lines in *in vitro* conditions. GLP-1 and transcriptional activator PDX-1 expression was profiled for the role of gut hormones in the regulation of glucose and energy homeostasis through their insulinotropic mechanism, in the Caco-2 intestinal cell line. The study results clearly show that the engineered *E. coli* strain stimulated the secretion of insulin from 164 pmol/mL to 164 nmol/mL, which proves the potential role of probiotics for the treatment of diabetes [42]. A study conducted by Paszti-Gere et al. [44,53] proved the antioxidative role of probiotics. The study, conducted in the IPEC-J2 cell line, reported that there is a progressive decrease in oxidative stress by inhibiting the expression of IL-8 and TNF-a, on islets of Langerhans cells of the pancreatic system, by metabolites of *Lactobacillus plantarum* 2142.

EVALUATION OF PROBIOTICS FOR COMBATING DIABETES IN THE ANIMAL MODEL SYSTEM

Per reported studies, probiotics have regulated glucose and energy homeostasis exceptionally well. Many reports claim that the probiotics exert their antidiabetic effects by sensitizing the insulin for glucose by increasing the expression of natural killer T-cells. Inflammation-mediated insulin resistance, for which the liver is thought to be the responsible target organ, regulates inflammation through NKT cells by producing more pro-inflammatory and anti-inflammatory cytokines. The depletion of NKT cells in the liver could lead to overexpression of inflammatory cytokines, which could disturb the metabolic condition and insulin resistance. It has been observed that the oral administration of VSL3 probiotic preparation for almost 4 weeks to mice kept on a high-fat diet improved insulin resistance, reduced weight loss, and significantly reduced inflammatory cytokine expression [54].

A study conducted by Amar et al. [42] inferred that the knockout mouse model lacking microbial recognition receptors Nod1 or CD14 could significantly reduce bacterial translocation and glucose metabolism, but they were subsequently increased in knockout Myd88 mice and ob/ob mice under the same conditions. Pro-inflammatory cytokine expression of TNF-a, IL-1b, IL-6, and PAI-1 was significantly reduced in mesenteric adipose tissue, muscles, and liver, respectively, and significantly reduced insulin resistivity [42] (Table 13.2).

TABLE 13.2
Antidiabetic Effectiveness of Probiotic Treatment in Animal Models

Probiotic Microbiota	Animal Model	Result
Lactobacillus plantarum DSM 15313	HFD C57BL/6 J mice	Increased NKT cells, improved insulin resistance, reduced inflammation
Lactobacillus reuteri GMNL-263	STZ-induced diabetic rats	Reduced glycated haemoglobin and blood glucose
Lactobacillus casei, Lactobacillus reuteri, Lactobacillus plantarum	DCs from NOD mice stimulated with probiotic lactobacilli for 24 hours	Lactobacillus casei induced DC to produce high level of IL-10, delay in diabetes incidence
Bifidobacterium longum (BIF CGMCC NO. 2107)	HFD rats	Reduced metabolic endotoxin (LPS) concentrations and intestinal inflammation and increased the expression of intestinal Reg I as a regulator of growth factor
Bifidobacterium animalis subsp. lactis 420	C57bl6, ob/ob, CD14⁻/⁻, ob/obxCD14⁻/⁻, Myd88⁻/⁻, Nod1⁻/⁻, Nod2⁻/⁻ with normal chow diet and HFD	Reversed bacterial translocation process, improved animals inflammatory and metabolic status
Lactobacillus casei	NOD mice	Improved blood glucose and host immune response
Lactobacillus casei	Alloxan treated BALB/c mice	Inhibited the disappearance of insulin-secreting beta-cells
Lactobacillus casei	T2D-KK-Ay mice	Lowered plasma glucose level and modified the host immune responses
Lactobacillus rhamnosus GG	Neonatal STZ-induced diabetic rats	Lowered blood HbA1c, suppressed oxidative stress, improved glucose tolerance and enhanced insulin secretion
Lactobacillus acidophilus NCDC14 and *Lactobacillus casei* NCDC19	Fructose-induced diabetic rats	Significantly lowered the blood glucose and HbA1c levels and free fatty acids and triglycerides
Lactobacillus acidophilus NCDC14 and *Lactobacillus casei* NCDC19	STZ-induced diabetic rats	Improved diabetic dyslipidemia, inhibited lipid peroxidation and nitrite formation
Probiotic mixture *Lactobacillus acidophilus*	Alloxan-induced diabetic rats	Reduced blood glucose by improving gliclazide bioavailability in diabetic rats

Source: Panwar, H. et al., *Diabetes Metab. Res. Rev.,* 29, 103–112, 2013.

CONCLUSION

Intestinal microbiota could serve as effective probiotic tools to bioremediate metabolic disorders by maintaining human metabolism and homeostasis. The gut microbiota have the potential to counteract the adverse effects of a high-fat diet, maintain the intestinal microenvironment, and control inflammation by regulating endotoxemia.

From the above documented research study and clinical trials conducted by several research groups around the world, we are in a position to justify the potential effects of probiotics in recovering the human health from several chronic metabolic disorders and their associated diseases. From the above study, it is well proved that probiotics can be used as natural tools to treat metabolic syndromes through controlling the release of proinflammatory cytokines under the influence of insulin resistance and adiposity.

FUTURE PERSPECTIVES

Very few research studies have been conducted in the area of probiotics, so it is impossible to come to a decisive conclusion about the effectiveness of probiotics in the treatment of metabolic disorders and their associated diseases. Leads generated through research data up to now point to the potential effect of antidiabetic probiotics.

Type 2 diabetes has a multigenic etiology associated with multiple risk factors, and the exact mechanism showing how a probiotic performs a target-based action of its antihyperglycemic effect at the molecular and genomic levels remains for future study. Rapid advancement during the last decade in the fields of genomics, proteomics, transcriptomics, metabolomics, and nutrigenomics could pave the way to discovering the pathophysiological and pharmacological effects. Future clinical trials will pave the way for development in the field of antidiabetic probiotics.

Future probiotic drug trials to evaluate the functional efficacy of probiotics in the target human host system is very important and challenging because most of the clinical trials for probiotic study have been conducted under controlled and defined conditions. Many compounding factors such as use of antibiotics, endotoxins, and dietary nutrients may affect intestinal gut microbiota, subsequently affecting their energy balance, and glucose metabolism and corresponding insulin secretions and other useful hormones. Hence, understanding the factors in the probiotic mechanism of action in the target host is of extreme importance and should be the future scope of study for the discovery of novel probiotic products in the field of antidiabetics.

REFERENCES

1. Hill, C., F. Guarner, G. Reid, G. R. Gibson, D. J. Merenstein, B. et al. Expert consensus document: The International Scientific Association for Probiotics and Prebiotics consensus statement on the scope and appropriate use of the term probiotic. *Nature Reviews Gastroenterology & Hepatology* 11(8) (2014): 506–514.
2. Sanders, M. E., G. R. Gibson, H. S. Gill, and F. Guarner. Probiotics: Their potential to impact human health. Council for Agricultural Science and Technology Issue Paper 36 (2007): 1–20.

3. Priyadarsini, N., T. Mishra, M. Behera, D. Mohapatra, and P. Panda. Role of Probiotics in Type 2 Diabetes Mellitus. *International Journal of Pharmaceutical Sciences Review and Research* 34(1) (2015): 276–280.

4. Kumar, N., S. Navalpur, R. Balamurugan, K. Jayakanthan, A. Pulimood, et al. Probiotic administration alters the gut flora and attenuates colitis in mice administered dextran sodium sulfate. *Journal of Gastroenterology and Hepatology* 23(12) (2008): 1834–1839.

5. Morelli, L, and E. Bessi. From research in microbiology to guidelines. In *Ending the War Metaphor: The Changing Agenda for Unravelling the Host-Microbe Relationship-Workshop Summary*, p. 237. National Academies Press, Washington, DC, June 9, 2006.

6. Klaenhammer, T. R., and M. J. Kullen. Selection and design of probiotics. *International Journal of Food Microbiology* 50(1) (1999): 45–57.

7. Turnbaugh, P. J., R. E. Ley, M. A. Mahowald, V. Magrini, E. R. Mardis, and J. I. Gordon. An obesity-associated gut microbiome with increased capacity for energy harvest. *Nature* 444(7122) (2006): 1027–1131.

8. Altermann, E., W. M. Russell, M. A. Azcarate-Peril, R. Barrangou, B. L. Buck, et al. Complete genome sequence of the probiotic lactic acid bacterium Lactobacillus acidophilus NCFM. *Proceedings of the National Academy of Sciences of the United States of America* 102(11) (2005):3906–3912.

9. Vyas, U., and N. Ranganathan. Probiotics, prebiotics, and synbiotics: Gut and beyond. *Gastroenterology Research and Practice* 2012 (2012): 872716.

10. Hlivak, P., J. Odraska, M. Ferencik, L. Ebringer, E. Jahnova, and Z. Mikes. One-year application of probiotic strain Enterococcus faecium M-74 decreases serum cholesterol levels *Bratisl Lek Listy* 106(2) 2005:67–72.

11. Nikawa, H., S. Makihira, H. Fukushima, H. Nishimura, Y. Ozaki, et al. Lactobacillus reuteri in bovine milk fermented decreases the oral carriage of mutans streptococci. *International Journal of Food Microbiology* 95(2) (2004):219–223.

12. Miguel, M., M. M. Contreras, I. Recio, and A. Aleixandre. ACE-inhibitory and antihypertensive properties of a bovine casein hydrolysate. *Food Chemistry* 112(1) (2009):211–214.

13. Ishikawa, H., I. Akedo, T. Otani, T. Suzuki, T. Nakamura, et al. Randomized trial of dietary fiber and Lactobacillus casei administration for prevention of colorectal tumors. *International Journal of Cancer* 116(5) (2005):762–767.

14. Saran, S., S. Gopalan, and T. P. Krishna. Use of fermented foods to combat stunting and failure to thrive. *Nutrition* 18(5) (2002):393–356.

15. Winkler, P., M. De Vrese, C. Laue, and J. Schrezenmeir. Effect of a dietary supplement containing probiotic bacteria plus vitamins and minerals on common cold infections and cellular immune parameters. International *Journal of Clinical Pharmacology & Therapeutics* 43(7) (2005).

16. Turck, D. Safety aspects in preparation and handling of infant food. *Annals of Nutrition and Metabolism* 60(3) 2012:211–214.

17. Wills-Karp, M., J. Santeliz, and C. L. Karp. The germless theory of allergic disease: revisiting the hygiene hypothesis. *Nature Reviews Immunology* 1(1) (2001):69–75.

18. Viljanen, M., E. Savilahti, T. Haahtela, K. Juntunen-Backman, R. Korpela, et al. Probiotics in the treatment of atopic eczema/dermatitis syndrome in infants: a double-blind placebo-controlled trial. *Allergy* 60(4) (2005):494–500.

19. Marteau, P., P. Pochart, B. Flourie, P. Pellier, L. Santos, et al. Effect of chronic ingestion of a fermented dairy product containing Lactobacillus acidophilus and Bifidobacterium bifidum on metabolic activities of the colonic flora in humans. *The American Journal of Clinical Nutrition* 52(4) (1990):685–688.

20. Sheu, B. S., H. C. Cheng, A. W. Kao, S. T. Wang, Y. J. Yang, et al. Pretreatment with Lactobacillus-and Bifidobacterium-containing yogurt can improve the efficacy of quadruple therapy in eradicating residual Helicobacter pylori infection after failed triple therapy. *The American Journal of Clinical Nutrition* 83(4) (2006):864–869.
21. Gionchetti, P., F. Rizzello, A. Venturi, and M. Campieri. Probiotics in infective diarrhoea and inflammatory bowel diseases. *Journal of Gastroenterology and Hepatology* 15(5) (2000):489–493.
22. Kruis, W. Antibiotics and probiotics in inflammatory bowel disease. *Alimentary Pharmacology & Therapeutics* 20(s4) (2004):75–78.
23. Berlec, A., M. Ravnikar, and B. Štrukelj. Lactic acid bacteria as oral delivery systems for biomolecules. *Die Pharmazie-An International Journal of Pharmaceutical Sciences* 67(11) (2012):891–898.
24. Poul, M., G. Jarry, M. O. Elhkim, and J. M. Poul. Lack of genotoxic effect of food dyes amaranth, sunset yellow and tartrazine and their metabolites in the gut micronucleus assay in mice. *Food and Chemical Toxicology* 47(2) (2009):443–448.
25. Tubelius, P., V. Stan, and A. Zachrisson. Increasing work-place healthiness with the probiotic Lactobacillus reuteri: A randomised, double-blind placebo-controlled study. *Environmental Health* 4(1) (2005):25.
26. Weizman, Z., G. Asli, and A. Alsheikh. Effect of a probiotic infant formula on infections in child care centers: Comparison of two probiotic agents. *Pediatrics* 115(1) (2005):5–9.
27. Anukam, K. C., E. O. Osazuwa, I. Ahonkhai, and G. Reid. Lactobacillus vaginal microbiota of women attending a reproductive health care service in Benin city, Nigeria. *Sexually Transmitted Diseases* 33(1) (2006):59–62.
28. Szajewska, H., M. Ruszczyński, and A. Radzikowski. Probiotics in the prevention of antibiotic-associated diarrhea in children: A meta-analysis of randomized controlled trials. *The Journal of Pediatrics* 149(3) (2006):367–372.
29. Sazawal, S., G. Hiremath, U. Dhingra, P. Malik, S. Deb, and R. E. Black. Efficacy of probiotics in prevention of acute diarrhoea: A meta-analysis of masked, randomised, placebo-controlled trials. *The Lancet Infectious Diseases* 6(6) (2006):374–382.
30. McFarland, L. V., G. W. Elmer, and M. McFarland. Meta-analysis of probiotics for the prevention and treatment of acute pediatric diarrhea. *International Journal of Probiotics and Prebiotics* 1(1) (2006):63.
31. U. S. Probiotics. org (California Dairy Research Foundation and Dairy and Food Culture Technologies) Probiotics Basics, 2006.
32. Zoetendal, E. G., M. Rajilić-Stojanović, and W. M. De Vos. High-throughput diversity and functionality analysis of the gastrointestinal tract microbiota. *Gut* 57(11) (2008): 1605–1615.
33. Moroti, C., L. F. S. Magri, M. de Rezende Costa, D. C. U. Cavallini, and K. Sivieri. Effect of the consumption of a new symbiotic shake on glycemia and cholesterol levels in elderly people with type 2 diabetes mellitus. *Lipids in Health and Disease* 11(1) (2012): 29.
34. Ejtahed, H. S., J. Mohtadi-Nia, A. Homayouni-Rad, M. Niafar, M. Asghari-Jafarabadi, and V. Mofid. Probiotic yogurt improves antioxidant status in type 2 diabetic patients. *Nutrition* 28(5) (2012): 539–543.
35. Duncan, S. H., G. E. Lobley, G. Holtrop, J. Ince, A. M. Johnstone, et al. Human colonic microbiota associated with diet, obesity and weight loss. *International Journal of Obesity* 32(11) (2008): 1720–1724.
36. de Vrese, M., P. Winkler, P. Rautenberg, T. Harder, C. Noah, et al. Effect of Lactobacillus gasseri PA 16/8, Bifidobacterium longum SP 07/3, B. bifidum MF 20/5 on common cold episodes: A double blind, randomized, controlled trial. *Clinical Nutrition* 24(4) (2005): 481–491.

37. Kolars, J. C., M. D. Levitt, M. Aouji, and D. A. Savaiano. Yogurt—An autodigesting source of lactose. *New England Journal of Medicine* 310(1) (1984): 1–3.
38. Holzapfel, W. H., P. Haberer, J. Snel, U. Schillinger, and J. H. J. Huis in't Veld. Overview of gut flora and probiotics. *International Journal of Food Microbiology* 41(2) (1998): 85–101.
39. Marteau, P., P. Seksik, and R. Jian. Probiotics and intestinal health effects: A clinical perspective. *British Journal of Nutrition* 88(S1) (2002): s51–s57.
40. Otutumi, L. K., E. R. de Moraes Garcia, M. B. Góis, and M. M. Loddi. *Variations on the Efficacy of Probiotics in Poultry.* E. C. Rigobelo (Ed.). InTech Open Access Publisher, Rijeka, Croatia, 2012.
41. Harzallah, D., and H. Belhadj. Lactic acid bacteria as probiotics: Characteristics, selection criteria and role in immunomodulation of human GI muccosal barrier. In *Lactic Acid Bacteria—R&D for Food, Health and Livestock Purposes*, Kongo, M. (Ed.). InTech, Rijeka, Croatia, 2013.
42. Amar, J., C. Chabo, A. Waget, P. Klopp, C. Vachoux, et al. Intestinal mucosal adherence and translocation of commensal bacteria at the early onset of type 2 diabetes: Molecular mechanisms and probiotic treatment. *EMBO Molecular Medicine* 3(9) (2011): 559–572.
43. Mengual, L., P. Roura, M. Serra, M. Montasell, G. Prieto, and S. Bonet. Multifactorial control and treatment intensity of type-2 diabetes in primary care settings in Catalonia. *Cardiovascular Diabetology* 9(1) (2010): 14.
44. Panwar, H., H. M. Rashmi, V. K. Batish, and S. Grover. Probiotics as potential biotherapeutics in the management of type 2 diabetes–prospects and perspectives. *Diabetes/ Metabolism Research and Reviews* 29(2) (2013): 103–112.
45. Larsen, N., F. K. Vogensen, F. W. J. van den Berg, D. S. Nielsen, A. S. Andreasen, et al. Gut microbiota in human adults with type 2 diabetes differs from non-diabetic adults. *PloS one* 5(2) (2010): e9085.
46. Whiting, D., L. Guariguata, C. Weil, and J. Shaw. IDF Diabetes Atlas. Global estimates of the prevalence of diabetes for 2011 and 2030. *Diabetes Research and Clinical Practice* 94(3) (2011): 311–321.
47. Martin, F.-P., S. Collino, S. Rezzi, and S. Kochhar. Metabolomic applications to decipher gut microbial metabolic influence in health and disease. *Frontiers in Physiology* 3 (2012): 113.
48. Cani, P. D., E. Lecourt, E. M. Dewulf, F. M. Sohet, B. D. Pachikian, et al. Gut microbiota fermentation of prebiotics increases satietogenic and incretin gut peptide production with consequences for appetite sensation and glucose response after a meal. *The American Journal of Clinical Nutrition* 90(5) (2009): 1236–1243.
49. Freeland, K. R., C. Wilson, and T. M. S. Wolever. Adaptation of colonic fermentation and glucagon-like peptide-1 secretion with increased wheat fibre intake for 1 year in hyperinsulinaemic human subjects. *British Journal of Nutrition* 103(1) (2010): 82–90.
50. Suhre, K., C. Meisinger, A. Döring, E. Altmaier, P. Belcredi, et al. Metabolic footprint of diabetes: A multiplatform metabolomics study in an epidemiological setting. *PloS One* 5(11) (2010): e13953.
51. Zhao, X., J. Fritsche, J. Wang, J. Chen, K. Rittig, et al. Metabonomic fingerprints of fasting plasma and spot urine reveal human pre-diabetic metabolic traits. *Metabolomics* 6(3) (2010): 362–374.
52. Ma, D., P. Forsythe, and J. Bienenstock. Live Lactobacillus reuteri is essential for the inhibitory effect on tumor necrosis factor alpha-induced interleukin-8 expression. *Infection and Immunity* September 1, 2004. 72(9):5308–5314.

53. Paszti-Gere, E., K. Szeker, E. Csibrik-Nemeth, R. Csizinszky, A. Marosi, et al. Metabolites of Lactobacillus plantarum 2142 prevent oxidative stress-induced overexpression of proinflammatory cytokines in IPEC-J2 cell line. *Inflammation* 35(4) (2012): 1487–1499.

54. Collins, T., M. A. Read, A. S. Neish, M. Z. Whitley, D. Thanos, and T. Maniatis. Transcriptional regulation of endothelial cell adhesion molecules: NF-kappa B and cytokine-inducible enhancers. *The FASEB Journal* July 1, 1995. 9(10):899–909.

14 Bacterial Metabolites in Food Preservation

Robinka Khajuria and Shalini Singh

CONTENTS

INTRODUCTION

Despite modern advances in food manufacturing and processing operations, preservation of food is still a debated issue. According to the Centers for Disease Control and Prevention (CDC) report (Scallan, et al., 2011), approximately 48 million food poisoning cases are reported annually in the United States alone, out of which 128,000 require hospitalization and 3,000 result in fatality. CDC recognizes 31 pathogens that are known to cause food-borne illness, including *Escherichia coli*, *Listeria monocytogenes*, *Salmonella* spp., *Bacillus cereus*, *Staphylococcus aureus*, *Clostridium perfringens*, *Clostridium botulinum*, *Yersinia enterocolytica*, and *Campylobacter jejuni*. In addition to these known pathogens, other agents that have not yet been identified as causing food-borne illness but are known to affect health with symptoms such as acute gastroenteritis are also recognized as threats by the

CDC (Scallan et al., 2011). Except for the United States, statistical data on the occurrence of food-borne diseases worldwide is extremely fragmented. As a result, the true measure of food-borne illness on a global scale is not clear.

In addition to microbial contamination posing a threat to human health, it also affects greatly the food industry in terms of food spoilage. Even with current good manufacturing practices and preservation methods adopted by the food industry, around 25% of the total food produced annually is lost due to microbial damage (Sillankorva et al., 2012). Controlling economic losses due to food spoilage, reducing food processing costs, and providing contamination-free food products to consumers are the major challenges faced by the food industry. In spite of adopting acceptable cleaning procedures, microbes are found in foods and food contact surfaces. Food products can be contaminated at different stages, from cultivation, production, and final consumption. The inherent ability of pathogens to form biofilms that allow them to attach to living and inert surfaces also contributes to the prevalence of pathogens in foods and food contact surfaces (Holah et al., 2002). Therefore, it has become necessary that new food preservation techniques are continually developed to ensure consumer safety.

Conventionally, chemical preservatives such as nitrates/nitrites, sulfites, sodium benzoate, propyl gallate, and potassium sorbate have been used in food products to prevent microbial spoilage. However, the past few decades have seen a massive decline in the use of these chemicals due to their reported side effects (Sharma, 2015). For instance, nitrites and nitrates have been linked to leukemia and to colon, bladder, and stomach cancer. Sorbate and sorbic acid have been reported to cause urticaria and contact dermatitis. Benzoates have been suspected to cause allergies, asthma, and skin rashes, thereby leading to a decline in their use as food preservatives (Lee and Paik, 2016).

Consumer awareness about food additives and about the health benefits of natural, traditional, and minimally processed foods with no added chemical preservatives are continuing to grow. Consumer demand for better quality and natural food products and strict government requirements for guarantees of food safety has forced the food industry to adopt alternate methods of food preservation. This has led to an increased interest in the use of natural preservatives to prevent food spoilage. Biopreservation deals with extending food shelf life and enhancing food safety using plants, animals, microorganisms, and/or their metabolites as preservatives (Fangio and Fritz, 2014).

The empirical use of microorganisms and/or their natural products for the preservation of foods has become a more common practice (Gálvez et al., 2007). Some microorganisms can inhibit the growth of microorganisms directly by producing toxic or antimicrobial components such as bacteriocins, antibiotics, and so on. Or they can inhibit this growth indirectly by changing the pH, osmotic pressure, or surface tension. This situation is called antagonistic relation. These antagonistic interactions among microorganisms have often been used in biologic attribution of food. Many microorganisms such as lactic acid bacteria (LABs), yeast, fungi, and bacteriophages are known to have antagonistic characteristics, thus making them natural choices for use as natural preservatives in food products (Erginkaya et al., 2011). This chapter focuses on the use of these microorganisms and their metabolites for preservation of food products.

LACTIC ACID BACTERIA

LABs are gram-positive, typically nonsporulating rod- or coccus-shaped microbes that are known to produce either a mixture of lactic acid, carbon dioxide, acetic acid and/ or ethanol, or lactic acid only. LABs include the genera *Lactococcus, Lactobacillus, Streptococcus, Pediococcus, Enterococcus, Leuconostoc, Aerococcus, Carnobacterium, Tetragenococcus, Oenococcus, Vagococcus,* and *Weisella* (Ananou et al., 2007). LABs present attractive physiological properties and technological applications such as resistance to bacteriophages' proteolytic activity, high resistance to freezing and lyophilization, capacity for adhesion and colonization of the digestive mucosa, and production of antimicrobial substances (Wigley, 1999). In general, LABs are generally recognized as safe (GRAS) and play an essential role in food fermentation given that a wide variety of strains are employed as starter or protective cultures in the manufacture of dairy, meat, and vegetable products. The most important contribution of these microorganisms is the preservation of the nutritional qualities of the raw material through extended shelf life and the inhibition of spoilage and pathogenic bacteria (Ray, 1992).

The idea of using LABs to prevent food spoilage through in situ acid production dates back to the 1950s. LABs were initially used to prevent the growth of *Clostridium botulinum* in food products. This technology relied on the inability of *C. botulinum* to grow at pH 4.6. LABs and a fermentable carbohydrate are added to the food. The LABs produce acid, thereby creating an unfavorable environment for the growth of *C. botulinum*. Saleh and Ordal (1955) also reported the use of *Lactobacillus bulgaricus* or *Lactococcus lactis* containing a fermentable carbohydrate inoculated with spores of *C. botulinum* to prevent toxin production in chicken. When incubated at 30°C in the presence of the *Lactobacillus* culture, samples did not become toxic, which can be attributed to reduction in pH due to acid production. Microgard is a Food and Drug Administration (FDA) approved cultured milk product added to cottage cheese as a safe food preservative. It is made by fermenting milk using *Propionibacterium shermanii* to produce acetate, propionic acid, and low-molecular-weight proteins. Although Microgard contains a bacteriocin, propionic acid plays a major role in its activity (Ananou et al., 2007). Table 14.1 lists some of the commercially produced LAB preparations used for food preservation. The major antimicrobial substances produced by LABs include organic acids, diacetyl, hydrogen peroxide, reuterin, reutericyclin, and bacteriocins (Gálvez et al., 2007). The following sections discuss these antimicrobial agents in detail.

ORGANIC ACIDS

LABs species such as *Lactobacillus, Lactococcus, Leuconostoc, Pediococcus,* and *Streptococcus* are used extensively as preservatives in fermented foods. While the homofermentative LABs are known to produce lactic acid only, the heterofermentative LABs can synthesize acetic acid and lactic acid (Erginkaya et al., 2011). Both lactic acid and acetic acid are reported to exhibit antimicrobial activities against a wide spectrum of fungi, yeasts, and bacteria (Schnürer and Magnusson, 2005). The antimicrobial effect of these organic acids lies in their ability to reduce pH and in their undissociated forms. Low external pH leads to acidification of the cell

TABLE 14.1
Commercially Available LAB-Based Preservatives

Microorganisms	Application	Protective Action	Manufacturer
Lactic acid bacteria (e.g., *L. sakei, L. curvatus, L. plantarum*)	Fermented meat products, dairy products	Inhibition of *Listeria monocytogenes*	Chr. Hansen (Denmark), DuPont (United States)
Carnobacterium sp.	Fish and seafood Sacco	Inhibition of *Listeria monocytogenes*	Italy
Lactococcus lactis	Cheese	Inhibition of *Clostridia tyrobutyricum*	CSK (the Netherlands)
Lactobacillus sp.	Fresh dairy products	Inhibition of mold and yeasts	Chr. Hansen (Denmark)
L. rhamnosus, L. paracasei, Propionobacterium sp.	Fresh dairy products	Inhibition of mold and yeasts	DuPont (United States)

Source: Gravesen, D.E. and Gravesen, A.E., *Advances in Biochemical Engineering/Biotechnology*, 143, 29–49, 2014.

cytoplasm, whereas the undissociated lipophilic acid diffuses passively across the membrane. The undissociated acid acts by disrupting the electrochemical proton gradient or by altering the cell membrane permeability, which in turn leads to disruption of substrate transport systems (Davidson et al., 2005).

Lactic and acetic acid hold GRAS status, and their concentration in food is regulated by sensory parameters (Peláez et al., 2012). Although acetic acid is considered to be more toxic to microorganisms than lactic acid, the use of acetic acid in foods is limited due to its pungent odor and taste. Lactic acid, on the other hand, has a very mild taste, which allows it to be applied in substantial concentrations in fermented dairy products, meat, sauces, pickled vegetables, and salad dressings. Lactic acid has been used for a very long time for the preservation of vegetables because this method is low cost, has low energy requirements, and yields highly acceptable and diversified flavors. In order to strike a balance between low-acid content in foods and microbial stability of food products, however, manufacturers prefer to use acetic acid–lactic acid mixtures instead of high acetic acid concentrations. Furthermore, acetic acid and lactic acid have been reported to exhibit synergistic inhibitory effects (Dang et al., 2009). Lactic acid has been reported to exhibit antimicrobial effects on a number of different microorganisms such as *Mycobacterium tuberculosis, Listeria monocytogenes, Yersinia enterocolitica, Aeromonas hydrophila, Bacillus coagulans, Clostridium botulinum, Clostridium sporogenes, Enterobacteriaceae, Lactobacillaceae, Pseudomonas fragi, Vibrio vulnificus, Helicobacter pylori, Escherichia coli O157:H7, Pseudomonas* sp., and *Salmonella typhimurium* (Naidu, 2000). Besides antibacterial activity, lactic acid and lactate compounds such as sodium lactate demonstrate antifungal activities. They have been reported to inhibit the growth of aflatoxin-producing *Aspergillus* sp. Because of these attributes, lactic acid and lactates are widely used for decontamination of beef, pork, and poultry during processing and packaging.

Acetic acid in the form of vinegar has been used as a preservative for a very long time because of its antimicrobial effect, thus ensuring food quality and safety. Acetic acid exhibits antimicrobial activities against *Salmonella typhimurium, Salmonella bareilly, Salmonella enteritidis, Listeria monocytogenes, Helicobacter pylori, Yersinia enterocolitica, E. coli* O157:H7, *Bacillus spp., Campylobacter jejuni, Staphylococcus aureus*, and *Enterobacteriaceae.* Acetic acid is more toxic compared to other organic acids such as lactic acid, formic acid, citric acid, and sulfuric acids (Naidu, 2000). Therefore, several derivatives of acetic acid are currently in use as antimicrobial agents, especially in meat and meat products. However, the salt forms of acetic acid, unlike lactates, require different handling and utilization. For instance, sodium acetate is used in combination with potassium sorbate (10%) and phosphates (10%) to extend the shelf life of pork chops. A surface application of sodium diacetate extends the shelf life of chicken by about 4 days when stored at 2°C (Lucera et al., 2012).

Hydrogen Peroxide

Hydrogen peroxide (H_2O_2) is produced during aerobic growth of LABs. In the presence of oxygen, LABs produce hydrogen peroxide through electron transport via the action of flavoprotein oxidases or nicotinamide adenine hydroxy dinucleotide (NADH) peroxidase. The presence of H_2O_2 leads to the formation of destructive hydroxyl radicals from superoxide anions. This process in turn leads to peroxidation of membrane lipids and increased membrane permeability. The resulting bactericidal effect of these oxygen metabolites is due to the oxidation of sulfhydryl groups leading to the denaturing of a number of proteins. H_2O_2 also acts a precursor for the synthesis of free radicals such as superoxide (O^{2-}) and hydroxyl ($OH·$) radicals that can cause DNA damage (Naidu, 2000).

Hydrogen peroxide production by *Lactobacillus* and *Lactococcus* strains has been reported to inhibit the growth of *Staphylococcus aureus, Pseudomonas* sp., and various psychotrophic microorganisms in food products. In raw milk, H_2O_2 is known to activate the lactoperoxidase system, thereby leading to the production of hypothiocyanate ($OSCN^-$), oxyacids (O_2SCN^- and O_3SCN^-), and intermediate oxidation products that inhibit a wide array of gram-positive and gram-negative bacteria (Yang, 2000). Application of small quantities of hydrogen peroxide to apple skin can serve as an alternative to fungicides used to inhibit *P. expansum*. The rate of spore germination of *F. graminearum* was affected by hydrogen peroxide due the strong oxidizing effect on the bacterial cell and destruction of basic molecular structures of cellular proteins. The inhibition of food-borne pathogens by LABs has been ascribed at least in part to the activity of H_2O_2 (Magnusson et al., 2003; Muhialdin et al., 2011).

Diacetyl

Diacetyl is a product of citrate metabolism and is produced by LAB strains of *Leuconostoc, Lactococcus, Pediococcus*, and *Lactobacillus*. Homofermentative LABs produce more diacetyl than heterofermentative LABs (Erginkaya et al., 2011). The antimicrobial effect of diacetyl has been known since the 1930s.

It inhibits the growth of gram-negative bacteria by reacting with the arginine-binding protein and thus affecting arginine utilization. Diacetyl is more toxic to gram-negative bacteria, yeasts, and molds. However, diacetyl is rarely present in food fermentations at sufficient levels to make a major contribution to antibacterial activity (Yang, 2000); therefore, high concentrations of diacetyl are required to achieve inhibition of spoilage bacteria. But higher concentration of diacetyl affects the sensory properties of the food, thus limiting the use of diacetyl-producing cultures for protective purposes to foods where sensory attributes are not essential (Gálvez et al., 2014).

Nevertheless, its selective antimicrobial activity and nontoxicity against humans and animals makes diacetyl a potential candidate for microbial food preservatives. The antimicrobial activity of diacetyl has been reported since 1927. Diacetyl has been reported to exhibit antibacterial activity against *Listeria, Salmonella, Escherichia coli* O157:H7, *Salmonella typhimurium, Yersinia,* and *Aeromonas* (Gálvez et al., 2014). Lanciotti et al. (2003) reported the inhibitory effect of diacetyl against *S. typhimurium* and *E. coli* O157:H7 during meat fermentation. Because of its low yield during lactic fermentation and ability to affect the sensory experience unfavorably, its commercial use as a food preservative is restricted. However, diacetyl can be used at low concentrations because it has been reported to act synergistically with other antimicrobial agents and contribute to combined preservation systems in fermented foods (Yang, 2000).

ACETALDEHYDE

Acetaldehyde is a reactive, low-molecular-weight compound used to impart flavor to a variety of products such as yogurt, cheese, wine, beer, and so on. Acetaldehyde is produced during the metabolism of carbohydrates in heterofermentative LABs and is converted to ethanol by reoxidation of pyridine nucleotides by alcohol dehydrogenase. *L. delbrueckii* subsp. *bulgaricus* produces acetaldehyde by cleaving threonine into acetaldehyde and glycine, a reaction catalyzed by threonine aldolase. *L. delbrueckii* subsp. *bulgaricus* cannot metabolize acetaldehyde, leading to its accumulation in the product. This accumulation inhibits *Staphylococcus aureus, Salmonella typhimurium,* and *E. coli* growth in dairy products (Yang, 2000). The antimicrobial effect of acetaldehyde is attributed to the ability of added acetaldehyde to replace intracellular acetaldehyde that is lost from the cell when the permeability of the plasma membrane is disturbed by ethanol (Barber et al., 2002). Pure acetaldehyde was shown to be inhibitory to *L. monocytogenes* and *S. typhimurium.*

REUTERIN

Reuterin (3-hydroxypropionaldehyde) is a low-molecular-weight compound with antimicrobial properties that is produced by *Lactobacillus reuteri.* It is produced as an intermediate during the metabolism of glycerol to 1,3-propanediol under anaerobic conditions (Talarico et al., 1988; Talarico and Dobrogosz, 1989). The antimicrobial activity of reuterin is due to its ability to inhibit the synthesis of DNA (Talarico and Dobrogosz, 1989). Reuterin has been reported to inhibit the growth of fungi, and gram-positive and gram-negative bacteria. It has been reported to exhibit bacteriostatic activity against *L. monocytogenes* and bactericidal activities against *Staphylococcus aureus*, *E. coli* O157:H7, *Campylobacter jejuni, Yersinia enterocolitica, Aeromonas hydrophila* subsp. *hydrophila, and Salmonella choleraesuis* (Arqués et al., 2004). Reuterin producer *L. reuteri* has GRAS organism status, thus making it easier for authorities to accept reuterin as a food preservative (Lacroix, 2011).

REUTERICYCLIN

Reutericyclin is a negatively charged, hydrophobic tetramic acid that acts as a proton ionophore, resulting in dissipation of the proton motive force. It has been shown to exhibit antimicrobial activities against *Lactobacillus* spp., *Bacillus cereus, Bacillus subtilis, S. aureus, Enterococcus faecalis,* and *Listeria innocua*. As seen in the case of many other antimicrobial agents, the inhibition of gram-negative bacteria is seen under the conditions that promote disruption of outer membranes; such conditions include truncated lipopolysaccharides, high salt concentrations, and low pH. Reutericyclin is produced in high concentrations during growth of *Lactobacillus reuteri* in sourdough. Reutericyclin, like reuterin, may be a potential candidate for biopreservation of foods (Gänzle, 2004; Gálvez et al., 2014).

BIOFILMS

A biofilm is a multicellular layer of adherent bacteria surrounded by a matrix of extracellular polysaccharides with growth and survival advantages over planktonic cells because it has a documented increased resistance to antimicrobial compounds and thermal stress. Bacteria, with the help of biofilms, attach to the surfaces of equipment used for food processing and remain viable even after disinfection, thus compromising food quality. Most of the work done on biofilms is related to their role in food spoilage. However, in recent years, it has been reported that the biofilms produced by LABs have antibacterial effects on certain pathogens found in meat and dairy products. Biofilms have also been reported to inhibit the growth of fungi. Wu et al. (2010) reported the antibacterial activity of exopolysaccharide (EPS), a component of biofilms, against *E. coli, S. typhimurium, P. aeruginosa, V. parahaemolyticus, S. aureus, B. subtilis*, and *B. cereus*. However, a comprehensive and focused study is needed on use of LAB biofilms as biocontrol agents.

BACTERIOCINS

Bacteriocins are extracellular bioactive peptides or peptide complexes synthesized by ribosomes and exhibit bactericidal or bacteriostatic activity. Bacteriocins are produced by a wide array of bacteria, including many LABs. The bacteriocins produced from LABs are known as lantibiotics (Jeevaratnam et al., 2005). Many of the LAB bacteriocins have been reported to be effective against food-borne pathogens and microorganisms associated with spoilage. As a result, bacteriocins have attracted considerable interest in recent years for their use as natural food preservatives (Table 14.2).

TABLE 14.2
Bacteriocins Produced by LABs and Their Target Pathogens

Bacteriocin	Producer Organisms	Effective Against
Nisin	*Lactococcus lactis*	*Listeria monocytogenes, Brochothrix thermosphacta*
Nisin Z	*Lactococcus lactis lactis*	*S. aureus*
Lacticin 481	*Lactococcus lactis*	Gram-positive bacteria
Lactacin B	*Lactococcus acidophilus*	*Lactobacillus leichmannii, L. helveticus, L. bulgaricus, L. lactis*
Lactocin	*Lactobacillus helveticus*	*L. acidophilus*
Leucocin B	*Leuconostoc mesenteroides*	*Lactobacillus* spp.
AcH Pediocin	*Lactobacillus plantarum*	*L. monocytogenes*
Pediocin PA-1/AcH	*Pediococcus acidilactic*	Gram-positive bacteria, *Listeria monocytogenes*
Helveticin J	*Lactobacillus helveticus* 481	*L. bulgaricus, L. lactis*
Lactocin S, Sakacin P, Sakadin A	*Lactobacillus sake*	*Lactobacillus* spp., *Leuconostoc* spp. *Pediococcus* spp., *Carnobacterium* spp., *Carnobacterium piscicola, Enterococcus* spp.,*Listeria monocytogenes*
Bavaricin A	*Lactobacillus bavaricus*	*Lactobacillus* spp., *Lactococcus* spp., *Pediococcus* spp. *Enterococcus* spp., *Listeria monocytogenes*
Curvacin A	*Lactobacillus curvatus*	*Lactobacillus* spp. *Carnobacterium* spp. *Listeria monocytogenes*
Enterocin	*Enterococcus faecium, Enterococcus faecalis*	*L. monocytogenes, Staphylococcusaureus*
Mundticin	*Enterococcus mundtii*	*Listeria monocytogenes, Clostridium botulinum, Lactobacillus spp*
Enterocin A	*Enterococcus faecium*	*Listeria monocytogenes*
Enterolysin A	*Enterococcus faecalis* LMG 2333	Enterococci, Pediococci, Lactococci, and Lactobacilli

Source: Erginkaya, et al. Microbial Metabolites as Biological Control Agents in Food Safety. *Food Processing: Strategies for Quality Assessment, Food Engineering Series.* p. 225. Springer Science+Business Media, New York. 2014; Ivey, M. et al., *Annual Review of Food Science and Technology,* 4, 41–62, 2013.

The bacteriocins produced by LAB are classified into four major groups:

1. Lantibiotics (<5 kDa) are a class of bacteriocins that contain the unusual thio-ether amino acids lanthionine and β-methyl lanthionine, in addition to other modified amino acids such as dehydrated serine and threonine (Jung, 1991). The most studied bacteriocin in this group is nisin, which is produced by *Lactococcus lactis* subsp. *lactis.* Class I bacteriocins are further subdivided into two subclasses: Ia and Ib. Class Ia bacteriocins consist of cationic and hydrophobic peptides that form pores in the target membranes. Class Ib bacteriocins are globular in nature and have no net negative charge

(Altena et al., 2000). They have comparatively more rigid structures than Class Ia bacteriocins.

2. Small thermostable peptides (nonlantibiotics) are bioactive peptides (<10 kDa) that do not contain any modified amino acid residues. They are further subdivided into two classes. Class IIa includes pediocin-like bacteriocin having anti-listerial activity with a conserved *N*-terminal sequence Tyr–Gly–Asn–Gly–Val and two cysteines forming an S–S bridge in the *N*-terminal half of the peptide. Class IIb bacteriocins are composed of two different peptides with different primary amino acid sequences (Jeevaratnam et al., 2005).

3. High-molecular-weight bacteriocins are large (>30 kDa), heat-labile protein bacteriocins such as helveticin J.

4. Large peptides form large complexes with carbohydrates or lipids. Currently, no such bacteriocin has been purified. It is argued that these are artifacts that result in the formation of complexes with other macromolecules due to their cationic and hydrophobic properties. This phenomenon has been demonstrated in the case of plantaricin S (Stoyanova et al., 2012; Balciunas et al., 2013).

The majority of bacteriocins used as biopreservatives belong to Classes I and II bacteriocins. Among the Class I bacteriocins, nisin is the best known bacteriocin with GRAS status for use as a direct human food ingredient and has a broad inhibitory spectrum against gram-positive bacteria, including many pathogens, and can prevent outgrowth of *Bacillus* and *Clostridium* spores. However, it is not effective against gram-negative bacteria, yeasts, and molds. Among the Class II bacteriocins, the pediocin-like bacteriocins having anti-listerial activity are the most common. Pediocins are produced by *Pediococcus* spp. and are known to inhibit *Listeria monocytogenes* effectively compared to nisin. Bacteriocins have an advantage over classical antimicrobials because they are destroyed by digestive enzymes (Cleveland et al., 2001; Šušković et al., 2010).

Bacteriocins can be used in food preservation in different ways. The most commonly adopted strategies for the application of bacteriocins include the following:

1. Inoculation with bacteriocin-producing LAB cultures in the product (*in situ*).
2. Direct addition of bacteriocin in purified or semipurified form.
3. Using a product that has previously been fermented with a bacteriocin-producing strain.

The selection of an approach for bacteriocin application depends on the product type and the process parameters maintained during processing, storage, and distribution. Bacteriocin production *in situ* by starter cultures will be preferred in the preservation of fermented foods. For nonfermented refrigerated products such as prepackaged salads, purified bacteriocins are added directly. An example of the former would be the use of *P. pentosaceus* and *P. acidilactici* strains as starter cultures in the natural fermentation of meat, vegetables, and dairy products. Use of psychrotrophic LAB has been reported to reduce the risk of *Salmonellae* and other vegetative pathogen growth during sausage fermentation. It has also been reported to inhibit *L. monocytogenes* growth in perishable meat products (Jeevaratnam et al., 2005). The following sections discuss some of the major bacteriocins with probable application as food preservatives.

Nisin

Nisin is a polypeptide bacteriocin belonging to the lantibiotic family that is produced by strains of *Lactococcus lactis* subsp. *lactis*. Nisin has been used as a food preservative because of its antimicrobial activity and low toxicity for humans. Nisin was first discovered in England in 1928 and was used to prevent clostridial spoilage of Gruyere cheese. Aplin and Barrett commercialized nisin concentrate as Nisaplin, which is now produced by Danisco and used as a preservative in milk and dairy products, canned foods, cured meats, and other segments of the fermentation industry. Other nisin preparations available commercially include Delvoplus® (DSM, Holland), Chrisin® (Chr. Hansens, Denmark), and Silver Elephant Nisin (Zheijiang Silver Elephant Bio-Engineering, China). Most of these preparations contain approximately 1,000,000 international units (IUs) per gram. Nisin is the only bacteriocin that has been approved in Europe as a food additive and has been granted GRAS status in the United States (Schillinger et al., 2001; Lacroix, 2011).

Although various natural nisin variants have been discovered, only two natural variants, nisin A and nisin Z, are used in commercial preparations. A particular *lactococcus* producer strain produces a specific nisin variant. Nisin is cationic in nature due to the presence of three lysine and one or more histidine residues (varies in nisin variants) together (Naidu, 2000). Nisin is active against gram-positive bacteria but has no effect against gram-negative bacteria, yeasts, and molds. This could be due to the large size of nisin (1.8–4.6 kDa), which restricts its movement across the outer membrane of gram-negative bacteria (Kuwano et al., 2005). Among gram-positive bacteria *Bacillus*, *Clostridium*, *Alicyclobacillus*, *Desulfomaculum*, *Geobacillus*, and *Themoanaerobacterium* are susceptible to Nisin (Lacroix, 2011). Nisin has also been reported to inhibit the growth of *Listeria monocytogenesm* (Schillinger et al., 2001).

The activity of Nisin in a food matrix depends on the following factors:

1. Binding of nisin to food components (e.g., meat phospholipids).
2. Inactivation of nisin by food ingredients.
3. Changes in nisin solubility and charge.
4. Changes in the cell envelope of the target organisms in response to environmental factors.

Nisin is used in a variety of foods, from liquids to solids, canned to packaged, chill to warm ambient storage (Naidu, 2000). Nisin is normally added in aqueous solution form to the liquid portion of a product during processing. It can also be used, howeve, in powder form. It is essential in both cases to ensure uniform dispersal of nisin throughout the food matrix. Nisin can also be used at higher concentrations as a spray or dip for surface decontamination. The concentration of nisin depends on the food type, pH, temperature storage conditions, and the required shelf life. Nisin is often used in acidic foods, but it is more effective in products across a range of pH, varying from 3.5 to 8.0. It has also been utilized to inhibit undesirable LAB growth in beer and wine (Daeschel et al., 1991).

Pediocin

Pediocins are a type of Class II bacteriocins produced by the genus *Pediococcus*. Strains of *P. pentosaceous* and *P. acidilactici*, have been used extensively as starter cultures in the production of fermented plants, meat, fish, cereals, and dairy-based products (Yang and Ray, 1994). *Pediococcus acidilactici* is known to synthesisze a 44 amino acid Class IIa bacteriocin called Pediocin PA-1 (Renye et al., 2011). Pediocin PA-1 has been reported to exhibit strong activity against *Listeria monocytogenes,* a pathogen whose presence in dairy and meat products is responsible for certain food-borne illnesses (Beaulieu et al., 2005). Pediocin has been reported to exhibit higher activity and specificity against *L. monocytogenes* compared to nisin (Woraprayote et al., 2013). Pediocin PA-1–producing cultures and have found numerous applications in the food industry in terms of controlling microbial succession during fermentation and inhibiting the growth of microorganisms associated with spoilage during storage (Díez et al., 2012).

Several bacteriocins such as pediocin A, produced by *Pediococcus pentosaceus;* pediocin AcH (pediocin H), pediocin PA-1, pediocin JD1, and pediocin SJ-1, produced by *Pediococcus acidilactici*; and pediocin PD-1, produced by *Pediococcus damnosus* NCFB 1832, have been reported for pediococci. Compared to other bacteriocins in the pediocin family and some lantibiotics, pediocin A of *P. pentosaceus* FBB61 and pediocins from *P. acidilactici* strains have a wider bactericidal spectrum against gram-positive bacteria. Pediocin A inhibits growth of several strains of *P. acidilactici, P. pentosaceus, S. aureus, Lactobacillus* spp., *C. Perfringens, C. botulinum,* and *C. sporogenes.* Thus, the use of these bacteriocins to control these bacteria in foods can be suggested for further study (Naidu, 2000).

Among pediocins, Pediocin PA-1/AcH is the most studied bacteriocin of the LABs. Pediocin PA-1/AcH effectively reduces populations of *Listeria* strains in ice cream mix, sausage mix, fresh and ground beef, and whole milk. It has been found to be effective against many strains of gram-positive and gram-negative spoilage and pathogenic bacteria. Incorporation of pediocins as preservatives in foods can help in killing the pathogens associated with spoilage to ensure longer product shelf life and greater consumer safety. Many vacuum-packaged, refrigerated, processed food products such as meat, dairy, fish, and vegetables normally contain bacteria from the genera *Leuconostoc, Lactobacillus, Carnobacterium, Brochothrix,* and *Clostridium.* These microbes can multiply even under refrigeration and thus cause spoilage. By introducing pediocin PA-1/AcH during the formulation of these food products, spoilage in the final product could be avoided or reduced (Bennik, 1997; Ennahar et al., 1998). Many studies have reported the safety of pediocins in food products. When consumed, they are hydrolyzed by the proteolytic enzymes in the digestive tract, and the degradation products do not contain any unusual components such as unusual amino acids. In spite of greater interest, pediocin has yet not been legally approved by regulatory agencies in the United States and Europe for use as a preservative (Erginkaya et al., 2011).

LACTICIN

Lacticin 3147 is a plasmid-encoded bacteriocin produced by *Lactococcus lactis* subsp. *lactis* DPC3147. Lacticin 3147 is a two-component antibiotic that exhibits an antimicrobial spectrum similar to that of nisin A (Silkin et al. 2008). Lacticin 3147 exhibits antimicrobial activity against *Listeria, Clostridium, Staphylococcus, Streptococcus* species, *Propionibacterium acne, Streptococcus mutans*, methicillin-resistant *Staphylococcus aureus* (MRSA), vancomycin-resistant *Enterococcus faecalis* (VRE), and penicillin-resistant *Pneumococcus* (PRP). With its broad bactericidal action, lacticin 3147 offers considerable potential for improving food safety (Martínez-Cuesta et al., 2010).

Lacticin 481 is another bacitracin that was first isolated from *L. lactis* subsp. *lactis* CNRZ 481. *L. lactis* strains enjoy GRAS status; therefore, lacticin 481 may be regarded as a food-grade additive and the use of lacticin 481 produced *ex situ* or *in situ* for food preservation may not pose any legislative issues. Lacticin 481 exhibits bactericidal effect on all species of *Lactococcus*, *Lactobacilli*, and *Leuconostoc*. Lacitin 481 can be used specifically against *Clostridium tyrobutyricum* to prevent spoilage in Emmental-type cheese. Lacticin 481 has also been reported to control the growth of *L. monocytogenes* (Lacroix, 2011).

Sakacin

Sakacins are Class IIa bacteriocins produced by certain strains of *Lactobacillus sakei*. These bacteriocins are cationic and hydrophobic peptides that show strong antilisterial activity (Lacroix, 2011). Sakacin C2 is a bacteriocin secreted by *Lactobacillus sake* C2 that displays strong antibacterial activity against *Staphylococcus aureus, Streptococcus thermophilus, Listeria innocua, Bacillus cereus, Salmonella typhimurium*, and *E. coli*. Sakacin P produced by *Lactobacillus sakei* is a potent antimicrobial agent against food pathogen (*L. monocytogenes* and *E. faecalis*) and spoilage (*Carnobacterium* spp.). Anti-listerial activity and a narrow inhibitory spectrum make sakacin P one of the most promising bacteriocins for preservation of *Listeria*-contaminated foods (Trinetta et al., 2008; Gao et al., 2013).

Enterocins

Enterocin EJ97, a low-molecular-weight cationic peptide, is produced by *E. faecalis* EJ97. It exhibits antimicrobial activity against bacteria involved in food spoilage such as *B. coagulans, B. stearothermophilus*, and those responsible for food poisoning such as *Listeria monocytogenes* and *Staphylococcus aureus* (García et al., 2003, 2004). Enterocin AS-48 is another cationic cyclic antimicrobial peptide produced by *E. faecalis* S-48 and *E. faecium* (Gómez et al. 2013). It has broad bactericidal activity against most gram-positive bacteria, including several pathogens such as *Listeria monocytogenes, Staphylococcus aureus, Mycobacterium spp., Bacillus cereus,* and some gram-negative bacteria (Banos et al., 2012).

BACTERIOCIN FROM OTHER MICROORGANISMS

Besides LABs, several other bacteria also produce bacteriocins, although LAB bacteriocins have been studied extensively for their use as natural biopreservatives. Bacteria belonging to *Staphylococcus* spp., *Bacillus* spp., and *Listeria* spp. also produce bacteriocin with antimicrobial activity (Deegan et al., 2006; Balciunas et al., 2013). Like LABs, the genus *Bacillus* also includes a variety of industrially important species that have been given GRAS status by the U.S. FDA. The production of bacteriocins has been reported extensively for *B. subtilis, Bacillus cereus, B. coagulans, B. megaterium*, and *B. thuringiensis*, although the most studied bacteriocins include subtilin and coagulin (Compaoré et al., 2013; Kaewklom et al., 2013). Staphylococcins are another type of bacteriocin that are produced by bacteria belonging to the genus *Staphylococcus*. Staphylococcins include bacteriocins such as epidermin, epilancin K7, nukacin ISK-1 staphylococcin C55/BacR1 aureocin A70, and aureocin A53 (Nascimento et al., 2002). *Staphylococcus aureus* also synthesizes prominent bacteriocins such as the lantibiotic staphylococcin C55 and staphylococci BacR1. These bacteriocins show bactericidal activity against a broad range of LABs and *L. monocytogenes* (Ceotto et al., 2009).

Variacin is a lanthionine-containing bacteriocin produced by *Kocuria varians*. It has been used to inhibit the growth of *B. cereus* in chilled dairy products, vanilla, and chocolate desserts. Variacin is resistant to a wide range of temperatures and pH levels (2–10), and exhibits antimicrobial activity against *listeriae, staphylococci*, and the vegetative cells and spores of *clostridia* and *bacilli* (Balciunas et al., 2013).

KILLER YEASTS

The yeasts are a large group of microbes characterized by their ability to survive in different conditions. The traits of yeasts that act against other microorganisms have attracted increasing attention for their application as bioprotective agents in the food industry. Table 14.3 lists commercially used yeasts and their applications. The antagonistic characteristics of yeast have been attributed mainly to the following mechanisms:

1. Competition for nutrients.
2. Changes in the medium pH due to growth-coupled ion exchange or organic acid production.
3. Tolerance to high concentrations of ethanol.
4. Secretion of antimicrobial compounds, such as killer toxins or mycocins (Schmitt and Breinig 2006).

The competition for nutrients is considered to be the main mode of action against postharvest fungal pathogens (Janisiewicz, 1994). Yeast quickly depletes glucose, fructose, or sucrose, thereby preventing the growth of undesirable microbes. This action of yeast has been exploited in food and beverage fermentation for the species *Saccharomyces cerevisiae*. The production of iron-scavenging molecules, called siderophores, is another major antimicrobial mechanism. Iron sequestration by yeast has been exploited in systems used for biological control of postharvest pathogens sensitive to iron deprivation (Zhang et al., 2007).

Yeast killer toxins, also known as mycocins, were initially defined as extracellular proteins that disrupt the cell membrane function in susceptible yeast bearing receptors for the compound (Kulakovskaya et al., 2003, 2004). The first mycocins were identified in association with *S. cerevisiae* in the brewing industry (Muccilli et al., 2011). Several others have since been isolated. Killer toxin production has been reported among many yeast genera, including *Saccharomyces, Candida, Debaryomyces, Cryptococcus, Kluyveromyces, Torulopsis, Pichia, Williopsis*, and *Zygosaccharomyces* (Schmitt and Breinig, 2002; Golubev et al., 2006; Muccilli et al., 2013).

TABLE 14.3
Use of Antagonistic Yeasts as a Preservative in Food Products

Species	Application
Saccharomyces cerevisiae	In winemaking against spoilage by yeast strains such as *Brettanomyces bruxellensis*, *Dekkera anomala*, *Pichia membranifacien*; in sake fermentation; in table olive fermentation against *C. boidinii*.
Debaryomyces hansenii	In olive fermentation against *C. boidinii*, *S. exiguous*, and *K. lactis*; in yogurt and on cheese against *Aspergillus*, *Byssochlamys*, and *Eurotium*
Kluyveromyces wickerhamii	In wine against *Dekkera* and *Brettanomyces*
Filobasidium floriforme	In apple against *B. cinerea*
Ustilago maydis	In grape juice against. *B. bruxellensis* strains
Williopsis mrakii	In yogurt and maize silage against *Candida krusei* D1241 and *Saccharomyces cerevisiae* D1247
Williopsis saturnus var. saturnus	In cheese biopreservation against *S. cerevisiae* and *K. marxianus*; in yogurt against *C. kefir*, *K. marxianus*, *S. cerevisiae*, *S. bayanus*, *Byssochlamys*, *Eurotium*, and *Penicillium*.
Williopsis anomalus	In airtight storage of wheat against *Penicillium roqueforti* and *Enterobacteriaceae*; on apples and grape vines against *B. cinerea*
Candida intermedia	In sorghum and maize against *Colletotrichum sublineolum* and *Colletotrichum graminicola*
Candida famata	On papaya against *Colletotrichum gloeosporioides*
Candida friedrichii	On grape berries against *A. carbonarius* and ochratoxin A (OTA) contamination in wine and grape juice
Candida zeylanoides	In ham against *P. nordicum* growth
Meyerozyma guilliermondii	On papaya against *C. gloeosporioides*
Tetrapisispora phaffii	In winemaking against *Hanseniaspora/Kloeckera*
Torulaspora globosa	In sorghum and maize against *C. sublineolum* and C. *graminicola*
Aureobasidium pullulans	On grape berries against *B. cinerea*; on plums and peaches against *M. laxa*

Source: Muccilli, S., and Restuccia, C., *Microorganisms*, 3, 588–611, 2015.

The first positive indications of the antagonistic activity of yeast were reported against *Escherichia coli* and *Staphylococci* (Viljoen, 2006). Fatichenti et al. (1983) showed the antibacterial activity of *Debaryomyces hansenii* against *Clostridium tyrobutyricum* and *Clostridium butyricum*. Antibacterial activity was also detected in *Kloeckera apiculata* and *Kluyveromyces thermotolerans* against beer-spoilage bacteria (Bilinski et al., 1985). *Geotrichum candidum* was reported to inhibit the growth of listeria (Dieuleveux et al., 1998). Hatoum et al. (2013) characterized anti-listerial hydrophobic peptides, extracted from four dairy yeast cultures, identified as *D. hansenii*, *Pichia fermentans*, *Candida tropicalis*, and *Wickerhamomyces anomalus*.

Several studies over the past few decades focused on the application of antagonistic yeast in various food and beverage processes for improving sensory qualities and inhibition of pathogenic and spoilage organisms. Killer yeasts are used extensively to prevent the growth of spoilage yeast and bacteria in wine fermentations.

S. cerevisiae strains producing K2 and Klus toxins have been found to prevent the growth of spoilage yeast strains (Maqueda et al. 2012). Numerous non-*Saccharomyces* yeasts have also been reported to produce killer toxins. The killer toxin secreted by *Tetrapisispora phaffii*, has extensive anti-*Hanseniaspora/–Kloeckera* activity under winemaking conditions (Comitini and Ciaani, 2010). Killer toxins secreted by *W. anomalus* and *Kluyveromyces wickerhamii* exhibit antimicrobial activity gainst *Dekkera* and *Brettanomyces* spoilage yeast that cause unpleasant odors in wine during fermentation, aging, and storage. De Ullivarri et al. (2014) reported the killer activity of *W. anomalus* against *Brettanomyces bruxellensis*, *Dekkera anomala*, *Pichia membranifaciens*, and *Meyerozyma guilliermondii*. Killer toxins from the *Candida pyralidae* exhibited killer activity against several *B. bruxellensis* strains. Killer toxins produced by *S. cerevisiae* and *W. anomalus* have been reported to inhibit the growth of *Lactobacillus hilgardii* in wine (De Ullivarri et al., 2014).

A number of yeast-based biocontrol products are available commercially, especially to prevent deterioration of fruits after harvest. Aspire is a U.S. FDA-approved product containing *Candida oleophila* for preventing spoilage in fruits such as citrus, apples, and pears during storage. Yield Plus, which contains *Cryptococcus albidus*, is used for biocontrol of *Botrytis, Penicillium*, and *Mucor*. Shemer is another biocontrol product based on *Metschnikowia fructicola* approved in 2001 in Israel; it is used on fruits such as grapes and strawberries and on sweet potatoes (Charalampopoulos et al. 2002; İzgü et al. 2004). *Debaryomyces* species is used to prevent spoilage of fruit and dairy products during storage. These yeasts have been used commercially for inhibition of fungi such as *Byssochlamys fulva, Byssochlamys nivea, Cladosporium* sp., *Penicillium candidum*, and *Penicillium roqueforti* (Liu and Tsao, 2009; Taqarort et al., 2008).

FUNGAL PIGMENTS

Several natural biocolorants show antagonistic activity to certain bacteria, viruses, and fungi thus can be used to prevent microbial spoilage in food products. Pigments produced by *Monascus* sp. are one of the most widely food colorants. They have been used in the Far East for many years as a colorant in wine, fish, cheese, beverages, and even sausages. In addition to imparting color, the antibacterial effects of these pigments have also been reported. The antimicrobial effect of *Monacus* pigment varies according to the type of target microorganism and pigment (Kim et al., 2006a). Yellow pigments produced by *M. purpureus* have been reported to inhibit the growth of *Bacillus subtilis* orange pigments (rubropunctatin and monascorubrin); *M. purpureus* also exhibit antimicrobial activities against *Bacillus subtilis* and *Escherichia coli* (Martinkova and Vesely, 1995). Kim et al. (2006b) reported antimicrobial activity of the red pigment produced by *Monascus* against the filamentous fungi *Aspergillus niger, Penicillium citrinum*, and *Candida albicans*. Cinnabarin, an orange pigment produced by *Pycnoporus sanguineus*, was reported to exhibit antimicrobial activity against food pathogens such as *Bacillus cereus, Escherichia coli, Enterococcus faecalis, Enterococcus faecium, Klebsiella pneumoniae, Leuconostoc mesenteroides, Leuconostoc plantarum, Staphylococcus aureus,*

Salmonella sp., *Salmonella typhimurium*, and *Pseudomonas aeruginosa* (Smania et al., 1998). *Streptomyces hygroscopicus* subsp. *ossamyceticus* has been reported to produce a yellowish antibiotic pigment that inhibited the growth of *Escherichia coli, Klebsiella* sp., and *Pseudomonas aeruginosa* (Selvameenal et al., 2009). Carotenoids obtained from *Dunaliella spp., Phafia rhodozyma*, and *Rhodotorula* spp. have also been reported to inhibit food-borne pathogens such as *Salmonella typhimurium, S. Enteritidis, Staphlococcus aureus, Escherichia coli*, and *Bacillus subtilis* (Mimee et al., 2005; Kim et al., 2006b). Carotenoids have also been reported to inhibit the synthesis of aflatoxin by *Aspergillus flavus* (90%) and by most of the *A. parasiticus* (30%) strains (Strack et al., 2003).

BACTERIOPHAGES

The natural biotherapeutic potential of bacteriophages is well recognized around the world. Bacteriophages are viruses whose only hosts are bacteria. Lytic bacteriophages have a cycle of cell infection and death that starts when they attach to sensitive bacterial cells and release endolysins. These endolysins degrade the cell wall from the outside to allow the phage DNA (or RNA) to enter the bacterium. If the phage DNA escapes the restriction/modification (R/M) system of the bacterium, it seizes the growing cell's metabolic machinery to produce phage components. The phage components self-assemble and are released during a lytic burst that kills the bacterial host. The released bacteriophages adsorb to additional bacteria to continue the lytic cycle. If high concentrations of bacteriophages attach to the cells, they may release enough endolysin to lyse the cell independently of the lytic cycle. This is called lysis from without (García et al., 2009).

In 2006, a major milestone was achieved with the approval of the first phage-based product (ListShield™) to control *Listeria monocytogenes* in meat and poultry products (Bren, 2007). Since then, other phage products have also been approved for use as biotherapeutics in food (Sulakvelidze, 2011). These advances in phage biocontrol highlight their potential in controlling additional food pathogens and spoilage organisms and also confirm that the use of phages is acceptable to the food industry. Many studies have been conducted in both preharvest (farm animals) and postharvest (meat, fresh and packaged foods) environments. Bacteriophages can be used in the food industry for several applications, such as for the prevention of colonization and diseases in livestock, decontamination of raw products such as fresh fruit and vegetables, disinfection of equipment and contact surfaces, and extension of shelf life of perishable manufactured foods (Sillankorv et al., 2012). This section discusses the use of phages as natural preservatives.

Atterbury et al. (2003) reported 95%–99% inactivation of *C. jejuni* isolated from chicken skin by bacteriophages. Another study reported the inhibition of *Listeria monocytogenes* by phages in infected melon and soft cheeses. Similarly, *Salmonella enteritidis* inhibition was reported after the application of phage therapy in raw and pasteurized milk. In a different study, *S. aureus* growth in dairy products was inhibited by using a lytic bacteriophage cocktail isolated from raw milk (O'Flynn et al., 2004; Milci et al., 2005; Scott, 2008). Phages have been incorporated into milk contaminated with *Salmonella* in cheddar production to reduce viable cells after storage (Modi et al., 2001). Similarly, *S. aureus* growth in milk during curd manufacture was inhibited by phages (García et al., 2009). Other examples of phage-based biopreservation approaches include inhibition of *Enterobacter sakazakii* in reconstituted infant milk formula and *Salmonella typhimurium* on chicken frankfurters (Whichard et al., 2003; Kim et al., 2007).

Hungaro et al. (2013) reported the use of a mixture of bacteriophages and chemical agents (dichloroisocyanurate, peroxyacetic acid, lactic acid) for reduction of *S. Enteritidis* on chicken skin. Anti-*Salmonella* phages were also evaluated on pig skin by Hooton et al. (2011). In this case, a phage mixture against *S. typhimurium* was shown to reduce cell numbers to undetectable levels. Immobilization of phages onto a modified cellulose membrane was shown to be effective against *L. monocytogenes* and *E. coli* O157:H7 in ready-to-eat (RTE) and raw meat (Anany et al., 2011). The immobilization method is based on charge, allowing the phage heads (net negative charge) to bind to the cellulose membranes (net positive charge) and thus leaving the tails free to capture and kill the contaminating bacteria. Viazis et al. (2011) reported the antimicrobial ability of a bacteriophage mixture alone and in combination with an essential *trans*-cinnamaldehyde oil on different *E. coli* O157:H7 strains contaminating lettuce and spinach leaves. Boyacioglu et al. (2013) reported the improved effect of an anti-*E. coli* O157:H7 bacteriophage mixture when used with modified atmosphere packaging of fresh-cut leafy greens. Guenther et al. (2012) reported complete eradication of *S. typhimurium* in a variety of RTE foods in the presence of phage F01-E2. In addition, Bigot et al. (2011) demonstrated the ability of a single bacteriophage, FWLLm1, to limit the growth of *L. monocytogenes* in RTE poultry. Zhang et al. (2012) demonstrated the efficacy of single phages and phage cocktails against *S. flexneri* 2a, *S. dysenteriae*, and *S. sonnei* that were artificially contaminated in RTE spiced chicken. Endersen et al. (2013) assessed the antibacterial potential of six mycobacteriophages, both individually and as a phage mixture, to inhibit the growth of *Mycobacterium smegmatis* in reconstituted skim milk.

The U.S. FDA approved the first bacteriophage preparation for commercial use on August 18, 2006. This preparation, called List-Shield™ (LMP-102), contained a mixture of phages against *Listeria monocytogenes*. It was comprised of a mixture of equal proportions of six individually purified LM-specific bacteriophages that belong to the family Siphoviridae. LMP-102 was prepared to be used on RTE meat and poultry products as an antimicrobial agent against *L. monocytogenes*. This was followed by another phage preparation developed by a U.S. company that received approval for a spray application in meat and poultry processing plants. The approved phage cocktail has antimicrobial activity against 170 strains of *L. monocytogenes*. Though initially it was designed for meat and poultry products, it was later found that the phage cocktail is also effective on fresh fruits, like apple and melon, especially in combination with the bacteriocin nisin. Another phage preparation, Listex P100, was developed by a Netherlands-based company against *L. monocytogenes*. It was granted approval under the U.S. FDA's GRAS procedure for use on cheese (O'Flynn et al., 2004; García et al., 2007; Hagens and Loessner, 2007; Parisien et al., 2008). Bacteriophages specific for *Salmonella* serotypes have also been used on various food substrates such as sprouted seeds and animal skins and carcasses. The commercial preparation SalmoFresh contains a cocktail of naturally occurring lytic bacteriophages that selectively and specifically kill *Salmonella*, including strains belonging to the most common/highly pathogenic serotypes: *Typhimurium, Enteritidis, Heidelberg, Newport, Hadar, Kentucky,* and *Thompson* (Gálvez et al., 2014). The commercial preparation EcoShield™ contains a cocktail of three lytic phages specific for *E. coli* O157:H7.

Bacteriophages are also being used for reducing the carriage of zoonotic agents in livestock and poultry. Bacteriophage preparations have been used to prevent *Salmonella* and *E. coli* infections in chickens, calves, and pigs, and in control of the food-borne pathogens *Salmonella* and *C. jejuni* in chickens and *E. coli* O157:H7 in cattle (Sulakvelidze, 2013). Selective application of bacteriophages could improve animal health and animal production and reduce the risks of transmission of zoonotic agents to humans.

One of the advantages of phages is their restricted host range, which could ensure that only pathogenic microbes could be killed without destroying desirable fermentative bacteria or resident human microbiota. However, this also means that different strains of bacteriophage would be required to kill different pathogens in a single food product. Multiple phage strains may be required against different serotypes of the same pathogen. For instance, 30 different phage serotypes would be required to lyse the majority of enteropathogenic and enterotoxigenic *E. coli* (Brüsson, 2005). Another concern about the use of bacteriophages on food products is that changes in surface receptors of the food-borne pathogens can lead to development of bacteriophage resistance, undermining the efficacy of bacteriophage biocontrol. Resistance can be controlled through the use of multiple-strain cocktails, rotation of the bacteriophage in the cocktails, or multiple hurdles to decrease the generation of phage-resistant pathogens (Montville and Chikindas, 2007). Bacteriophages can still serve as suitable candidates for biopreservation of food products. A main limiting factor for the commercial use of bacteriophages in foods has been the high production costs. This issue will presumably be solved soon because several companies are investing in development and production facilities.

REFERENCES

Altena, K., Guder, A., Cramer, C., and Bierbaum, G., 2000. Biosynthesis of the lantibiotic mersacidin: Organization of a type B lantibiotic gene cluster. *Applied and Environmental Microbiology* 66(6):2565–2571.

Ananou, S., Maqueda, M., Martínez-Bueno, M., and Valdivia, E., 2007. Biopreservation, an ecological approach to improve the safety and shelf-life of foods. *Communicating Current Research and Educational Topics and Trends in Applied Microbiology* 1:475.

Anany, H., Chen, W., Pelton, R., and Griffiths, M. W., 2011. Biocontrol of *Listeria monocytogenes* and *Escherichia coli* O157:H7 in meat by using phages immobilized on modified cellulose membranes. *Applied and Environmental Microbiology* 77(18):6379–6387.

Arqués, J. L., Fernández, J., Gaya, P., Nuñez, M., Rodríguez, E., and Medina, M., 2004. Antimicrobial activity of reuterin in combination with nisin against food-borne pathogens. *International Journal of Food Microbiology* 95(2):225–229.

Atterbury, R. J., Connerton, P. L., Dodd, C. E., Rees, C. E., and Connerton, I. F., 2003. Application of host-specific bacteriophages to the surface of chicken skin leads to a reduction in recovery of *Campylobacter jejuni. Applied and Environmental Microbiology* 69(10):6302–6306.

Balciunas, E. M., Martinez, F. A. C., Todorov, S. D., de Melo Franco, B. D. G., Converti, A., and de Souza Oliveira, R. P., 2013. Novel biotechnological applications of bacteriocins: A review. *Food Control* 32(1):134–142.

Banos, A., Ananou, S., Martínez-Bueno, M., Gálvez, A., Maqueda, M., and Valdivia, E., 2012. Prevention of spoilage by enterocin AS-48 combined with chemical preservatives, under vacuum, or modified atmosphere in a cooked ham model. *Food Control* 24(1):15–22.

Barber, A. R., Vriesekoop, F., and Pamment, N. B., 2002. Effects of acetaldehyde on *Saccharomyces cerevisiae* exposed to a range of chemical and environmental stresses. *Enzyme and Microbial Technology* 30(2):240–250.

Beaulieu, L., Groleau, D., Miguez, C. B., Jetté, J. F., Aomari, H., and Subirade, M., 2005. Production of pediocin PA-1 in the methylotrophic yeast *Pichia pastoris* reveals unexpected inhibition of its biological activity due to the presence of collagen-like material. *Protein Expression and Purification* 43(2):111–125.

Bennik, M., Smid, E. J., and Gorris, L., 1997. Vegetable-associated *Pediococcus parvulus* produces pediocin PA-1. *Applied and Environmental Microbiology* 63(5):2074–2076.

Bigot, B., Lee, W. J., McIntyre, L., Wilson, T., Hudson, et al., 2011. Control of Listeria monocytogenes growth in a ready-to-eat poultry product using a bacteriophage. *Food Microbiology* 28(8):1448–1452.

Bilinski, C. A., Innamorato, G., and Stewart, G. G., 1985. Identification and characterization of antimicrobial activity in two yeast genera. *Applied and Environmental Microbiology* 50(5):1330–1332.

Boyacioglu, O., Sharma, M., Sulakvelidze, A., and Goktepe, I., 2013. Biocontrol of *Escherichia coli* O157: H7 on fresh-cut leafy greens. *Bacteriophage* 3(1):e24620.

Bren, L., 2007. Bacteria-eating virus approved as food additive. *FDA Consum* 41(1):20–22.

Brüsson, H., 2005. Phage therapy: The *Escherichia coli* experience. *Microbiology* 151:2133–2140.

Ceotto, H., dos Santos Nascimento, J., de Paiva Brito, M. A. V., and de Freire Bastos, M. D. C., 2009. Bacteriocin production by *Staphylococcus aureus* involved in bovine mastitis in Brazil. *Research in Microbiology* 160(8):592–599.

Charalampopoulos, D., Wang, R., Pandiella, S. S., and Webb, C., 2002. Application of cereals and cereal components in functional foods: A review. *International Journal of Food Microbiology* 79(1):131–141.

Cleveland, J., Montville, T. J., Nes, I. F., and Chikindas, M. L., 2001. Bacteriocins: safe, natural antimicrobials for food preservation. *International Journal of Food Microbiology* 71(1):1–20.

Comitini, F., and Ciani, M., 2010. The zymocidal activity of *Tetrapisispora phaffii* in the control of *Hanseniaspora uvarum* during the early stages of winemaking. *Letters in Applied Microbiology* 50(1):50–56.

Compaoré, C. S., Nielsen, D. S., Ouoba, L. I., Berner, T. S., Nielsen, et al., 2013. Co-production of surfactin and a novel bacteriocin by *Bacillus subtilis* subsp. *subtilis* H4 isolated from Bikalga, an African alkaline *Hibiscus sabdariffa* seed fermented condiment. *International Journal of Food Microbiology* 162(3):297–307.

Daeschel, M. A., Jung, D. S., and Watson, B. T., 1991. Controlling wine malolactic fermentation with nisin and nisin-resistant strains of *Leuconostoc oenos*. *Applied and Environmental Microbiology* 57(2):601–603.

Dang, T. D. T., Vermeulen, A., Ragaert, P., and Devlieghere, F., 2009. A peculiar stimulatory effect of acetic and lactic acid on growth and fermentative metabolism of Zygosaccharomyces bailii. *Food Microbiology* 26(3):320–327.

Davidson, P. M., Sofos, J. N., and Branen, A. L. Eds., 2005. *Antimicrobials in Food*. Boca Raton, FL: CRC Press.

De Ullivarri, M. F., Mendoza, L. M., and Raya, R. R., 2014. Killer yeasts as biocontrol agents of spoilage yeasts and bacteria isolated from wine. In *BIO Web of Conferences* (Vol. 3). EDP Sciences.

Deegan, L. H., Cotter, P. D., Hill, C., and Ross, P., 2006. Bacteriocins: Biological tools for bio-preservation and shelf-life extension. *International Dairy Journal 16*(9):1058–1071.

Dieuleveux, V., Van Der Pyl, D., Chataud, J., and Gueguen, M., 1998. Purification and characterization of anti-Listeria compounds produced by *Geotrichum candidum*. *Applied and Environmental Microbiology 64*(2):800–803.

Díez, L., Rojo-Bezares, B., Zarazaga, M., Rodríguez, J. M., Torres, C., and Ruiz-Larrea, F., 2012. Antimicrobial activity of pediocin PA-1 against *Oenococcus oeni* and other wine bacteria. *Food Microbiology 31*(2):167–172.

Endersen, L., Coffey, A., Neve, H., McAuliffe, O., Ross, R. P., and O'Mahony, J. M., 2013. Isolation and characterisation of six novel mycobacteriophages and investigation of their antimicrobial potential in milk. *International Dairy Journal 28*(1):8–14.

Ennahar, S., Assobhei, O., and Hasselmann, C., 1998. Inhibition of Listeria monocytogenes in a smear-surface soft cheese by Lactobacillus plantarum WHE 92, a pediocin AcH producer. *Journal of Food Protection 61*(2):186–191.

Erginkaya, Z., Unal, E., and Kalkan, S., 2011. Importance of microbial antagonisms about food attribution. *Science Against Microbial Pathogens: Communicating Current Research and Technological Advances.* 3rd ed. Formatex Research center. Spain, 2,1342.

Erginkaya, Z., Ünal, E., and Kalkan, S., 2014. Microbial Metabolites as Biological Control Agents in Food Safety. *Food Processing: Strategies for Quality Assessment, Food Engineering Series* pp. 225. Springer Science+Business Media, New York.

Fangio, M. F., and Fritz, R., 2014. Potential use of a bacteriocin-like substance in meat and vegetable food biopreservation. *International Food Research Journal 21*:677–683.

Fatichenti, F., Bergere, J. L., Deiana, P., and Farris, G. A., 1983. Antagonistic activity of *Debaryomyces hansenii* towards *Clostridium tyrobutyricum* and *Cl. butyricum*. *Journal of Dairy Research 50*(04):449–457.

Gálvez, A, López, H. A. R. L., and Omar N. B., 2007. Bacteriocin-based strategies for food biopreservation. *International Journal of Food Microbiology* 120:51–70.

Gálvez, A., López, R. L., Pulido, R. P., and Burgos, M. J. G., 2014. Natural antimicrobials for food biopreservation. In *Food Biopreservation*. New York, NY: Springer, 3.

Gänzle, M. G., 2004. Reutericyclin: Biological activity, mode of action, and potential applications. *Applied Microbiology and Biotechnology 64*(3):326–332.

Gao, Y., Li, D., and Liu, X., 2013. Evaluation of the factors affecting the activity of sakacin C2 against *E. coli* in milk. *Food Control 30*(2):453–458.

García, M. T., Omar, N. B., Lucas, R., Pérez-Pulido, R., Castro, et al., 2003. Antimicrobial activity of enterocin EJ97 *on Bacillus coagulans* CECT 12. *Food Microbiology 20*(5):533–536.

García, P., Madera, C., Martínez, B., and Rodríguez, A., 2007. Biocontrol of *Staphylococcus aureus* in curd manufacturing processes using bacteriophages. *International Dairy Journal 17*(10):1232–1239.

García, P., Madera, C., Martínez, B., Rodríguez, A., and Suárez, J. E., 2009. Prevalence of bacteriophages infecting Staphylococcus aureus in dairy samples and their potential as biocontrol agents. *Journal of Dairy Science* 92:3019–3026.

García, T., Martí, M., Lucas, R., Omar, N. B., Pulido, R. P., and Gálvez, A., 2004. Inhibition of *Listeria monocytogenes* by enterocin EJ97 produced by *Enterococcus faecalis* EJ97. *International Journal of Food Microbiology 90*(2):161–170.

Golubev, W. I., Pfeiffer, I,. and Golubeva, E. W., 2006. Mycocin production in *Pseudozyma tsukubaensis*. *Mycopathologia 162*(4):313–316.

Gómez, N. C., Abriouel, H., Ennahar, S., and Gálvez, A., 2013. Comparative proteomic analysis of Listeria monocytogenes exposed to enterocin AS-48 in planktonic and sessile states. *International Journal of Food Microbiology 167*(2):202–207.

Gravesen, D. E., and Gravesen, A. E., 2014. Biopreservatives. *Advances in Biochemical Engineering/Biotechnology* 143:29–49. doi:10.1007/10_2013_234.

Guenther, S., Herzig, O., Fieseler, L., Klumpp, J., and Loessner, M. J., 2012. Biocontrol of *Salmonella typhimurium* in RTE foods with the virulent bacteriophage FO1-E2. *International Journal of Food Microbiology* 154(1):66–72.

Hagens, S., and Loessner, M. J., 2007. Application of bacteriophages for detection and control of foodborne pathogens. *Applied Microbiology and Biotechnology* 76(3):513–519.

Hatoum, R., Labrie, S., and Fliss, I., 2013. Identification and partial characterization of anti-listerial compounds produced by dairy yeasts. *Probiotics and Antimicrobial Proteins* 5(1):8–17.

Holah, J. T., Taylor, J. H., Dawson, D. J., and Hall, K. E., 2002. Biocide use in the food industry and the disinfectant resistance of persistent strains of *Listeria monocytogenes* and *Escherichia coli*. *Journal of Applied Microbiology* 92:111S–120S.

Hooton, S. P., Atterbury, R. J., and Connerton, I. F., 2011. Application of a bacteriophage cocktail to reduce *Salmonella typhimurium* U288 contamination on pig skin. *International Journal of Food Microbiology* 151(2):157–163.

Hungaro, H. M., Mendonça, R. C. S., Gouvêa, D. M., Vanetti, M. C. D., and de Oliveira Pinto, C. L., 2013. Use of bacteriophages to reduce Salmonella in chicken skin in comparison with chemical agents. *Food Research International* 52(1):75–81.

Ivey, M., Massel, M., and Phister, T. G., 2013. Microbial interactions in food fermentations. *Annual Review of Food Science and Technology* 4(1):41–62.

İzgü, F., Altınbay, D., and Derinel, Y., 2004. Immunization of the industrial fermentation starter culture strain of *Saccharomyces cerevisiae* to a contaminating killer toxin-producing *Candida tropicalis*. *Food Microbiology* 21(6):635–640.

Janisiewicz, W. J., 1994. Enhancement of biocontrol of blue mold with the nutrient analog 2-deoxy-D-glucose on apples and pears. *Applied and Environmental Microbiology* 60(8):2671–2676.

Jeevaratnam, K., Jamuna, M., and Bawa, A. S., 2005. Biological preservation of foods–Bacteriocins of lactic acid bacteria. *Indian Journal of Biotechnology* 4:446–454.

Jung, G., 1991. Lantibiotics—Ribosomally synthesized biologically active polypeptides containing sulfide bridges and α,β-didehydroamino acids. *Angewandte Chemie* 30(9):1051–1068.

Kaewklom, S., Lumlert, S., Kraikul, W., and Aunpad, R., 2013. Control of *Listeria monocytogenes* on sliced bologna sausage using a novel bacteriocin, amysin, produced by *Bacillus amyloliquefaciens* isolated from Thai shrimp paste (Kapi). *Food Control* 32(2):552–557.

Kim, C., Jung, H., Kim, J. H., and Shin, C. S., 2006a. Effect of monascus pigment derivatives on the electrophoretic mobility of bacteria, and the cell adsorption and antibacterial activities of pigments. *Colloids and Surfaces B: Biointerfaces* 47(2):153–159.

Kim, C., Jung, H., Kim, Y. O., and Shin, C. S., 2006b. Antimicrobial activities of amino acid derivatives of Monascus pigments. *FEMS Microbiology Letters* 264(1):117–124. doi:10.1111/j.1574-6968.2006.00451.x.

Kim, K. P., Klumpp, J., and Loessner, M. J., 2007. *Enterobacter sakazakii* bacteriophages can prevent bacterial growth in reconstituted infant formula. *International Journal of Food Microbiology* 115:195–203.

Kulakovskaya, T. V., Kulakovskaya, E. V., and Golubev, W. I., 2003. ATP leakage from yeast cells treated by extracellular glycolipids of *Pseudozyma fusiformata*. *FEMS Yeast Research* 3(4):401–404.

Kulakovskaya, T. V., Shashkov, A. S., Kulakovskaya, E. V., and Golubev, W. I., 2004. Characterization of an antifungal glycolipid secreted by the yeast Sympodiomycopsis paphiopedili. *FEMS Yeast Research* 5(3):247–252.

Kuwano, K., Tanaka, N., Shimizu, T., Nagatoshi, K., Nou, S., and Sonomoto, K., 2005. Dual antibacterial mechanisms of nisin Z against Gram-positive and Gram-negative bacteria. *International Journal of Antimicrobial Agents* 26(5):396–402.

Lacroix, C., 2011. Protective cultures, antimicrobial metabolites and bacteriophages for food and beverage biopreservation. vol 201, *Woodhead Publishing Series in Food Science, Technology and Nutrition*. Oxford, UK: Woodhead Publishing Limited.

Lanciotti, R., Patrignani, F., Bagnolini, F., Guerzoni, M. E., and Gardini, F., 2003. Evaluation of diacetyl antimicrobial activity against Escherichia coli, Listeria monocytogenes and Staphylococcus aureus. *Food Microbiology* 20(5):537–543.

Lee, N. K., and Paik, H. D., 2016. Status, antimicrobial mechanism, and regulation of natural preservatives in livestock food systems. *Korean Journal for Food Science of Animal Resources* 36(4):547–557.

Liu, S. Q., and Tsao, M., 2009. Biocontrol of dairy moulds by antagonistic dairy yeast *Debaryomyces hansenii* in yoghurt and cheese at elevated temperatures. *Food Control* 20(9):852–855.

Lucera, A., Costa, C., Conte, A., and Del Nobile, M. A., 2012. Food applications of natural antimicrobial compounds. *Frontiers in Microbiology* 3:287. doi:10.3389/fmicb.2012.00287.

Magnusson, J., Ström, K., Roos, S., Sjögren, J., and Schnürer, J., 2003. Broad and complex antifungal activity among environmental isolates of lactic acid bacteria. *FEMS Microbiology Letters* 219(1):129–135.

Maqueda, M., Zamora, E., Álvarez, M. L., and Ramírez, M., 2012. Characterization, ecological distribution, and population dynamics of *Saccharomyces sensu* stricto killer yeasts in the spontaneous grape must fermentations of southwestern Spain. *Applied and Environmental Microbiology* 78(3):735–743.

Martínez-Cuesta, M. C., Bengoechea, J., Bustos, I., Rodríguez, B., Requena, T., and Peláez, C., 2010. Control of late blowing in cheese by adding lacticin 3147-producing Lactococcus lactis IFPL 3593 to the starter. *International Dairy Journal* 20(1):18–24.

Martinkova, L., and Veselý, D., 1995. Biological activity of polyketide pigments produced by the fungus Monascus. *Journal of Applied Bacteriology* 79(6):609–616.

Milci, S., Goncu, A., Alpkent, Z., and Yaygin, H., 2005. Chemical, microbiological and sensory characterization of Halloumi cheese produced from ovine, caprine and bovine milk. *International Dairy Journal* 15(6):625–630.

Mimee, B., Labbé, C., Pelletier, R., and Bélanger, R. R., 2005. Antifungal activity of flocculosin, a novel glycolipid isolated from Pseudozyma flocculosa. *Antimicrobial Agents and Chemotherapy* 49(4):1597–1599.

Modi, R., Hirvi, Y., Hill, A., and Griffiths, M. W., 2001. Effect of phage on survival of *Salmonella enteritidis* during manufacture and storage of Cheddar cheese made from raw and pasteurized milk. *Journal of Food Protection* 64:927–933.

Montville, T. J., and Chikindas, M. L., 2007. Biopreservation of Foods. *Food Microbiology: Fundamentals and Frontiers*, 3rd ed. M.P. Doyle and L.R. Beuchat (Eds.). Washington, DC: ASM Press.

Muccilli, S., Caggia, C., Randazzo, C. L., and Restuccia, C., 2011. Yeast dynamics during the fermentation of brined green olives treated in the field with kaolin and Bordeaux mixture to control the olive fruit fly. *International Journal of Food Microbiology* 148(1):15–22.

Muccilli, S., and Restuccia, C., 2015. Bioprotective role of yeasts. *Microorganisms* 3: 588–611. doi:10.3390/microorganisms3040588.

Muccilli, S., Wemhoff, S., Restuccia, C., and Meinhardt, F., 2013. Exoglucanase-encoding genes from three *Wickerhamomyces anomalus* killer strains isolated from olive brine. *Yeast* 30(1):33–43.

Muhialdin, B. J., Hassan, Z., and Sadon, S. K., 2011. Biopreservation of food by lactic acid bacteria against spoilage fungi. *Annals Food Science and Technology* *12*(1):45–57.

Naidu, A. S. Ed., 2000. *Natural Food Antimicrobial Systems*. Boca Raton, FL: CRC Press.

Nascimento, J. S., dos Santos, K. R. N., Gentilini, E., Sordelli, D., and de Freire Bastos, M. D. C., 2002. Phenotypic and genetic characterisation of bacteriocin-producing strains of *Staphylococcus aureus* involved in bovine mastitis. *Veterinary Microbiology* *85*(2):133–144.

O'Flynn, G., Ross, R. P., Fitzgerald, G. F., and Coffey, A., 2004. Evaluation of a cocktail of three bacteriophages for biocontrol of Escherichia coli O157: H7. *Applied and Environmental Microbiology 70*(6):3417–3424.

Parisien, A., Allain, B., Zhang, J., Mandeville, R., and Lan, C. Q., 2008. Novel alternatives to antibiotics: Bacteriophages, bacterial cell wall hydrolases, and antimicrobial peptides. *Journal of Applied Microbiology 104*(1):1–13.

Peláez, A. L., Cataño, C. S., Yepes, E. Q., Villarroel, R. G., De Antoni, G. L., and Giannuzzi, L., 2012. Inhibitory activity of lactic and acetic acid on Aspergillus flavus growth for food preservation. *Food Control 24*(1):177–183.

Ray, B., 1992. *Food Biopreservatives of Microbial Origin*, In: Ray, B. and Daeschel, M. (Eds). Boca Raton, FL: CRC Press.

Renye, J. A., Somkuti, G. A., Garabal, J. I., and Du, L., 2011. Heterologous production of pediocin for the control of Listeria monocytogenes in dairy foods. *Food Control 22*(12): 1887–1892.

Saleh, M. A., and Ordal, Z., 1955. Studies on growth and toxin production of Clostridium botulinum in a precooked frozen food. *Journal of Food Science 20*(4):340–350.

Scallan, E., Hoekstra, R. M., Angulo, F. J., Tauxe, R. V., Widdowson, et al., 2011. Foodborne illness acquired in the United States—Major pathogens. *Emerging Infectious Diseases 17*(1):7–15. doi:10.3201/eid1701.P11101.

Schillinger, U., Becker, B., Vignolo, G., and Holzapfel, W. H., 2001. Efficacy of nisin in combination with protective cultures against Listeria monocytogenes Scott A in tofu. *International Journal of Food Microbiology, 71*(2):159–168.

Schmitt, M. J., and Breinig, F., 2002. The viral killer system in yeast: From molecular biology to application. *FEMS Microbiology Reviews 26*(3):257–276.

Schmitt, M. J., and Breinig, F., 2006. Yeast viral killer toxins: Lethality and self-protection. *Nature Reviews Microbiology 4*(3):212–221.

Schnürer, J., and Magnusson, J., 2005. Antifungal lactic acid bacteria as biopreservatives. *Trends in Food Science & Technology 16*(1):70–78.

Scott, D. L., 2008. UHT processing and aseptic filling of dairy foods. Master of Science, Food Science Graduate Program College of Agriculture, Kansas State.

Selvameenal, L., Radhakrishnan, M., and Balagurunathan, R., 2009. Antibiotic pigment from desert soil actinomycetes; biological activity, purification and chemical screening. *Indian Journal of Pharmaceutical Sciences 71*(5):499. doi:10.4103/0250-474X.58174.

Sharma, S., 2015. Food preservatives and their harmful effects. *International Journal of Scientific and Research Publications* 5:1–2.

Silkin, L., Hamza, S., Kaufman, S., Cobb, S. L., and Vederas, J. C., 2008. Spermicidal bacteriocins: Lacticin 3147 and subtilosin A. *Bioorganic & Medicinal Chemistry Letters 18*(10):3103–3106.

Sillankorva, S. M., Oliveira, H., and Azeredo, J., 2012. Bacteriophages and their role in food safety. *International Journal of Microbiology*. doi:10.1155/2012/863945.

Smania, E. D. F. A., Smânia Júnior, A., and Loguercio-Leite, C., 1998. Cinnabarin synthesis by *Pycnoporus sanguineus* strains and antimicrobial activity against bacteria from food products. *Revista de microbiologia 29*(4):317–320. doi:10.1590/S0001-37141998000400017.

Stoyanova, L. G., Ustyugova, E. A., and Netrusov, A. I., 2012. Antibacterial metabolites of lactic acid bacteria: their diversity and properties. *Applied Biochemistry and Microbiology 48*(3):229–243.

Strack, D., Vogt, T., and Schliemann, W., 2003. Recent advances in betalain research. *Phytochemistry 62*(3):247–269.

Sulakvelidze, A., 2011. Safety by nature: Potential bacteriophage applications. *Microbe* 6:122–126.

Sulakvelidze, A., 2013. Using lytic bacteriophages to eliminate or significantly reduce contamination of food by foodborne bacterial pathogens. *Journal of the Science of Food and Agriculture 93*(13):3137–3146.

Šušković, J., Blazenka, K., Beganović, J., Pavunc, A. L., Habjanič, K., and Matosic, S., 2010. Antimicrobial activity—the most important property of probiotic and starter lactic acid bacteria. *Food Technology and Biotechnology 48*(3):296–307.

Talarico, T. L., Casas, I. A., Chung, T. C., and Dobrogosz, W. J., 1988. Production and isolation of reuterin, a growth inhibitor produced by Lactobacillus reuteri. *Antimicrobial Agents and Chemotherapy 32*(12):1854–1858.

Talarico, T. L., and Dobrogosz, W. J., 1989. Chemical characterization of an antimicrobial substance produced by Lactobacillus reuteri. *Antimicrobial Agents and Chemotherapy 33*(5):674–679.

Taqarort, N., Echairi, A., Chaussod, R., Nouaim, R., Boubaker, et al., 2008. Screening and identification of epiphytic yeasts with potential for biological control of green mold of citrus fruits. *World Journal of Microbiology and Biotechnology 24*(12):3031–3038.

Trinetta, V., Rollini, M., and Manzoni, M., 2008. Development of a low-cost culture medium for sakacin A production by L. sakei. *Process Biochemistry 43*(11):1275–1280.

Viazis, S., Akhtar, M., Feirtag, J., and Diez-Gonzalez, F., 2011. Reduction of *Escherichia coli* O157: H7 viability on leafy green vegetables by treatment with a bacteriophage mixture and trans-cinnamaldehyde. *Food Microbiology 28*(1):149–157.

Viljoen, B. C., 2006. Yeast ecological interactions. Yeast–yeast, yeast–bacteria, yeast–fungi interactions and yeasts as biocontrol agents. In *Yeasts in Food and Beverages*. Berlin, Germany: Springer, p. 83.

Whichard, J. M., Sriranganathan, N., and Pierson, F. W., 2003. Suppression of Salmonella growth by wild-type and large-plaque variants of bacteriophage Felix O1 in liquid culture and on chicken frankfurters. *Journal of Food Protection* 66:220–225.

Wigley, R. C., 1999. Encyclopedia of Food Microbiology. In: Robinson, R. K., Batt, C. A., and Patel, P. D. (Eds). Oxford, UK: Academic Press, p. 2084.

Woraprayote, W., Kingcha, Y., Amonphanpokin, P., Kruenate, J., Zendo, T., et al., 2013. Anti-listeria activity of poly (lactic acid)/sawdust particle biocomposite film impregnated with pediocin PA-1/AcH and its use in raw sliced pork. *International Journal of Food Microbiology 167*(2):229–235.

Wu, M. H., Pan, T. M., Wu, Y. J., Chang, S. J., Chang, M. S., and Hu, C. Y., 2010. Exopolysaccharide activities from probiotic *bifidobacterium*: Immunomodulatory effects (on J774A. 1 macrophages) and antimicrobial properties. *International Journal of Food Microbiology 144*(1):104–110.

Yang, R., and Ray, B. 1994. Factors influencing production of bacteriocins by lactic acid bacteria. *Food Microbiology 11*(4):281–291.

Yang, Z., 2000. Antimicrobial compounds and extracellular polysaccharides produced by lactic acid bacteria: Structures and properties. Auditorium XII of the University Main Building, Aleksanterinkatu 5, Department of Food Technology, University of Helsinki.

Zhang, H., Bao, H., Billington, C., Hudson, J. A., and Wang, R. 2012. Isolation and lytic activity of the Listeria bacteriophage endolysin LysZ5 against *Listeria monocytogenes* in soya milk. *Food Microbiology 31*(1):133–136.

Zhang, H., Zheng, X., and Yu, T., 2007. Biological control of postharvest diseases of peach with *Cryptococcus laurentii. Food Control 18*:287–291.

15 *Trichoderma* spp. in Bioremediation
Current Status and Scope

Shalini Singh and Robinka Khajuria

CONTENTS

TRICHODERMA SPP.

Trichoderma spp. are common, soil-inhabiting, free-living fungi that interact with root, soil, and foliar environments, triggering various responses in plants (Kredics et al., 2014). *Trichoderma* species belong to Ascomycetes of the Order Hypocreales. They show great genetic diversity and hence exhibit a number of different capabilities (Wei, 1979; Harman et al., 2004a,b; Tripathi et al., 2013). These strains are known for controlling plant diseases and helping in improving plant growth, especially through root development. They are also found to help plants resist abiotic stresses, and they assist in nutrient uptake (Benítez et al., 2004; Harman et al., 2004a; Körmöczi et al., 2013b). *Trichoderma* spp. are also found to play a significant part in bioremediation and phytobioremediation; its strains are involved in the breakdown of pesticides, herbicides, insecticides, heavy metals, polycyclic aromatic hydrocarbons (PAHs), and so on (Ravelet et al., 2000; Saraswathy and Hallberg, 2002; Verdin et al., 2004; Machín-Ramírez et al., 2010; Afify and El-Beltagi, 2011; Tripathi et al., 2013; Petrović, 2014; Woo et al., 2014). Laccase-producing strains like *T. atroviride*, *T. harzianum*, and *T. assperellum* (Körmöczi et al., 2013c) play a role in bioremediation processes and in agricultural and industrial applications (Schuster and Schmoll, 2010; Tripathi et al., 2013; Błaszczyk et al., 2014). Because of its ability to produce significant quantities of ligninases, the genus *Trichoderma* is widely used in industrial applications (Miettinen-Oinen, 2004).

Metal Bioremediation

Heavy metal remediation in wastewater is an acute environmental issue because rapid industrialization has led to toxic compounds, including heavy metals, in the environment that can potentially cause serious harm to life. Excess concentration of these heavy metals disrupts natural ecosystems, including plants as well as animals (Blaylock and Huang, 2000; Meagher, 2000). Fungi are known to tolerate heavy metals (Kapoor and Viraraghavan, 1995; Leyval et al., 1997; Baldrian, 2003; Gavrilesca, 2004; Ezzouhri et al., 2009; Aisha and Al-Rajhi, 2013), even under extreme environmental conditions. Their cell walls exhibit great metal-binding properties (Gupta et al., 2000; Anand et al., 2006). Microorganisms have been found to transform metal ions by reductive processes. They are also used as indicators of metal pollution and toxicity levels and as various mechanisms for metal bioremediation (Nies, 1999; Gadd, 2000; Hall, 2002; Rosen, 2002).

Trichoderma harzianum has been found to accumulate heavy metals like zinc (Zn), cadmium (Cd), and mercury (Hg) (Ledin et al., 1996; Singh and Sharma, 2012). In fact, many *Trichoderma* species have a natural ability to uptake and provide metal ions to plants for the plants' growth. Hence, studies (Aisha and Al-Rajhi, 2013) elaborate on the role of *Trichoderma* spp. in the growth and development of plants in the presence of copper and zinc. Lopez and Vazquez (2003) studied the tolerance of *Trichoderma atroviride* isolated from sludge. Other researchers also support the use of *Trichoderma* in metal bioremediation (Errasquin and Vazquez, 2003; Howell, 2003; Ting and Choong, 2009).

Anthropogenic activities have led to an alarming increase in the environmental concentration of Zn (Yap et al., 2002). This has serious implications because human diseases like nephritis and anuria have been linked to Zn contact. Zn does not degrade easily in aquatic ecosystems; hence, it needs to be removed from such ecosystems because it is capable of disrupting aquatic life. Conventional chemical methods (Lopez and Vazquez, 2003) are enormously costly, especially when a low concentration of heavy metals is present in large quantities of wastewater (Wang and Chen, 2006), and are also linked to their nonspecific reactions (Price et al., 2001). Bioremediation (Volesky, 1994), particularly by fungi, offers a better alternative solution for these processes (Savvaidis, 1998). Yazdani et al. (2010b) reported that *Trichoderma atroviride* exhibited a significant capacity to uptake Zn, and had a great tolerance to Zn in the presence of a basal medium of potato dextrose broth and hence is a powerful bioremediator for Zn pollution. They showed that *T. atroviride* could effectively uptake 18.1–26.7 mg/g of Zn from liquid fermentation media, even at high concentrations. The isolate showed 47.6%–64% adsorption and 30.4%–45.1% absorption for Zn. The study confirmed the ability of *T. atroviride* as a potential bioremediator of Zn. Similar observations have been made by other researchers as well (Anand et al., 2006). Adams et al. (2007), compared different fungal strains

(*Trichoderma harzianum, Trichoderma reesei, and Coriolus versicolor*) for their influence on metal desorption. They reported that the fungal strains desorbed Zn significantly more (about three times more) than any of the controls used. They also studied the mechanism of metal desorption, elaborating upon the constitutive expression of chelation in *Trichoderma harzianum* and *Coriolus versicolor*, with the same induced by Zn in *Trichoderma reesei*. Zn was also found to reduce the production of chelators in *C. versicolor*. Only *C. versicolor* was found to produce oxalic acid (a strong metal chelator). *T. harzianum* was found to be the best in Zn desorption among the fungal strains tested. A *Trichoderma harzianum* strain was found to effectively solubilize phosphates and compounds containing manganese and zinc by Altomare et al. (1999).

Chromium (VI, or CrVI) is a highly toxic carcinogen and has been considered an environmental pollutant (Rangasamy et al., 2013). Wastewater from leather industries is the biggest contributor to chromium (VI) discharge in water bodies. Chromium (VI) rapidly penetrates into cell membranes, unlike chromium (III), which is a beneficial form of chromium, and has been found to be hazardous by all exposure routes. Skin ulceration, allergic contact dermatitis, and ulcers of the nasal septum have been reported due to exposure to Cr(VI). Eye exposure may cause permanent damage. Thus, chromium poses serious threats to life and ecosystems in general. A number of fungal strains have been found to play a role in chromium remediation but according to Vankar and Bajpai (2008), *Trichoderma* sp. (nonpathogenic) can remove chromium with an almost 100% uptake rate. The investigators also emphasized the role of polysaccharides in *Trichodermal* cells in the uptake of metal. Nida'a et al. (2016) also supported the ability of *Trichoderma harizianum* to remove total and hexavalent chromium as well as total chromium from tannery wastewater. Under variable conditions, the highest chromium removal was found to be 70.18% for total chromium and 99.67% for hexavalent chromium, where the fungal biomass significantly increased in the presence of chromium. In the presence of organic poultry manure and microbial strains *Pseudomonas* and *Trichoderma*, 90% Cr(VI) reduction was seen with *Pseudomonas fluorescens*. Cr(VI) was found to reduce to Cr(III) from soils containing chromium (Rangasamy et al., 2013). Absorption of Cr(VI) *Trichodermal* cells under aerobic conditions was evaluated by Vankar and Bajpai (2007), where the maximum efficiency of 97.39% was obtained at pH 5.5, but acidic pH further decreases the biosorption efficiency of fungus. Other researchers also evaluated *Trichoderma harizianum* for bioremediation of Cr(VI) and other heavy metals from industrial effluents) (Bishnoi et al., 2007). As a result, *Trichoderma harizianum* is considered important for removing environmental pollutants (Zafar et al., 2006; Nurliana et al., 2011).

A few studies report the use of *Trichoderma* for biosorption of copper (Cu). *Trichoderma viride* has also been found to absorb and immobilize copper found in wastewater. Townsley et al. (1986) studied its effect on copper remediation in simulated effluent. An isolate of *T. atroviride*, obtained from a river, was investigated for its ability to uptake and tolerate Cu, and it was observed the isolate was able to uptake up to 11.20 mg/g of Cu in liquid nutrient medium over variable Cu concentration (25–300 mg L^{-1}), suggesting the potential of *T. atroviride* in the bioremediation of Cu (Yazdani et al., 2010a). Anand et al. (2006) reported 17 mg L^{-1} Cu removal with

100 mg L^{-1} initial Cu concentration by *T. viride* at 30°C in 72 h. Factors such as incubation period, concentration of biomass, temperature, and pH have been found to affect the sorption of metals (Yan and Viraraghavan, 2003) and hence need to be carefully controlled. At the same time, metal tolerance varies according to tolerance strategies and/or mechanisms adopted by fungal strains (Zafar et al., 2006). Petrović et al. (2014), evaluated *Trichoderma* strains isolated from different ecosystems for their sustainability in the presence of variable concentration (0.25–10 mmol L^{-1}) of Cu(II), and some of the isolates exhibited great tolerance to high copper concentrations. Ambiental (2010) experimentally evaluated *Trichoderma* spp. in the soil of isolated copper and gold mines for its persistence in these contaminated sites. The results were encouraging because the fungal species tested successfully survived during the analysis. The tolerance of *Trichoderma* sp. for Cu has been tested by others too (Kredics et al., 2001a,b; Anand et al., 2006; Ting and Choong, 2009; Yazdani et al., 2009). Different fungal strains were isolated from agricultural soils with arsenic contamination, from West Bengal, India, and it was reported that *Trichoderma* sp. was the most successful in eliminating arsenic (As) (Srivastava et al., 2011). Su et al. (2011) investigated *Trichoderma asperellum* SM-12F1, along with *Penicillium janthinellum* SM-12F4 and *Fusarium oxysporum* CZ-8F1, for biotransformation of As, when exposed to various concentration of As(V). After 15 days of incubation, a significant reduction in As(V) was seen. Similar studies have been done previously too (Su et al., 2011).

Cd is recognized as one of the most noxious constituents of industrial waste. It shows mutagenic, carcinogenic, phytotoxic, and ecotoxic effects on all biological systems, including humans, making Cd a serious environmental threat (Bhattacharyya et al., 2000; Pepper, 2000; Järup, 2002; Satoh et al., 2002; Waisberg et al., 2003; Deckert, 2005). Fungi can effectively remove Cd from the environment. Fungal strains such as *Aspergillus terreus, Aspergillus flavus, Cladosporium cladosporioides, Fusarium oxysporum, Gioclaudium roseum, Penicillium* spp., *Mucor rouxii, Helminthosporium* sp., *Talaromyces helicus, Trichoderma koningii, Trichoderma harzianum*, and *Saccharomyces cerevisiae* have all shown effective removal of Cd (Kapoor and Viraraghavan, 1995). Lima et al. (2011) evaluated *Trichoderma harzianum* for its ability to tolerate various amounts of Cd, and it was found that the fungal strain showed good growth even in the presence of high concentrations of Cd; it also accumulated polyphosphate in controls. The findings supported the use of the *Trichoderma* sp. for remediation of Cd in polluted ecosystems. Lopez and Vazquez (2003), while evaluating Cd uptake by *Trichoderma atroviride*, demonstrated that the presence of Cd repressed fungal growth up to 50%, to concentrations lower than 1 mM. *Trichoderma asperellum, Trichoderma harzianum*, and *Trichoderma tomentosum*, were found to decrease Cd quantitatively, at variable concentrations (1, 100, and 200 ppm) and at different pH levels (5.0, 7.0, and 9.0) (Mohsenzadeh and Shahrokhi, 2014). *T. asperellum* exhibited the highest removal ability (76.17%), at alkaline levels of pH. Lima et al. (2011) used *Trichoderma harzianum* for Cd elimination, where the influence of polyphosphate was also studied for its effect on Cd removal. Similarly, *Trichoderma virens, T. asperellum, T. atroviride, T. longibrachiatum*, and *T. harzianum* isolated from paddy fields irrigated with industrial effluents, were inoculated in basal potato dextrose broth medium supplemented with potassium dichromate (as hexavalent chromium source), mercuric chloride (as source of mercury), and cadmium chloride ($CdCl_2$) (as Cd source) at different concentrations, that is, 0.4, 0.6, 0.8, and 1 mM (Bhavya et al., 2015). All five isolates that were tested exhibited the potential to uptake the metals tested, with this ability differing for different fungal species. The work supports that *Trichoderma* biomass is an effective biosorbent for the removal of metal ions. Teng et al. (2015) explored *Trichoderma reesei* FS10-C for phytoremediation ability of soil polluted with Cd, associated with *Sedum plumbizincicola*. It was found that the fungal strain could uptake up to 300 mg L^{-1} of Cd a direct influence on plant shoot growth, in comparison to the control. Studies of a similar nature have been carried out to substantiate the use of *Trichoderma* sp for bioremediation of Cd (Lima et al., 2011; Sahu et al., 2012; Babu et al., 2014a–c).

The behavior of fourteen *Trichoderma* strains were checked on nickel (Ni) and Cd (Nongmaithem et al., 2016), where three isolates showed high levels of Ni tolerance, followed by a few, average performers. Fungal biomass was found to improve in the presence of up to 60 ppm of Ni in all strains, with the best fungal strain found stable in the presence of up to 150 ppm of Ni. Among the selected isolates, the best one exhibited good biomass production and a maximum MIC50 value in Cd stress. Sarkar et al. (2010) reported *Trichoderma harzianum* to be moderately tolerant to up to 60 ppm of Ni; at that concentration fungal growth was inhibited by more than 30%. Lima et al. (2011) also observed the effects of Cd on the growth of *T. harzianum*.

When studied for remediation of iron and lead in polluted water, *Trichoderma* was found to reduce the concentration of heavy metals in bore well and car wash water with immobilized cells (Raj, 2014). Cd, Cr, Cu, lead (Pb), Zn, and Ni were tested in soil, soil leachate, and plant tissues for two strains of *Trichoderma*. The researchers reported an increase in both translocation index and metal bioconcentration factors for inoculated plants, except for Pb and *Salix* spp. The highest values of *Ti*—339% (Cr), 190% (Ni), and 110% (Cu)—were achieved when *Miscanteus giganteus* and *Trichoderma* sp. were combined, indicating the positive influence of the fungus on plant growth as well on solubility of heavy metals in soil (Kacprzak et al., 2014). Similarly, *Trichoderma aureoviride, T. harzianum,* and *T. virens* showed great tolerance for Ni^{3+} and Pb^{2+} at high metal concentrations. Other metals tested include, Cu^{2+} and Zn^{2+} (Siddiquee et al., 2013); Zn^{2+}, Ba^{2+}, and Fe^{2+} (Kacprzak et al., 2005); and Cd and Ni (Cao et al., 2008).

HERBICIDE REMEDIATION

Atrazine, a selective herbicide of the family of striazines, is often used (Chan and Chu, 2005) for weed control (Ribeiro et al., 2005). It is difficult to degrade, and it contaminates surface water and groundwater (Chan and Chu, 2005). Its breakdown has been seen with various fungal strains, including species of *Aspergillus, Rhizopus, Fusarium, Penicillium,* and *Trichoderma*, with different forms of degradation (Kaufman and Blake, 1970; Sene et al., 2010) products. Degradation of atrazine under in vitro conditions in polluted soils was done using indigenously isolated fungal strains (Pelcastre et al., 2013), and *Trichoderma* sp. was found to resist very high atrazine concentrations (10,000 mg L^{-1}).

Another study by Tang et al. (2009) showed that, through molecular breeding of the *Trichoderma atroviride* strain T23 in liquid medium, degradation levels between 81% and 96% of 600 g mL^{-1} of pesticides such as dichlorides, compared with 72% achieved by the original strain without improvement, can be obtained. Organochlorine pesticides such as DDT, dieldrin, and endosulfan have also been degraded by *Trichoderma* species (Llado et al., 2009).

Linuron is also used worldwide for weed control and is moderately persistent in soils. It is easily found in surface water, drinking water, and foodstuffs, with great toxicity for different organisms. Danilovic et al. (2015) demonstrated an effective decrease in linuron content when *Trichoderma asperellum* and *Phanerochaete chrysosporium* were applied to soil contaminated with different concentrations of linuron. The fungal strains individually, as well as in combination, were effective against the herbicide.

Some (Ahlawat et al., 2010) checked the biodegradation ability of button mushroom spent substrate and associated microflora for carbendazim and mancozeb, commonly used agricultural fungicides: 17.45% of carbendazim was found to be degraded by a bacterial strain isolated from the spent substrate, while *Trichoderma* sp. degraded mancozeb by 18.05%. All the isolates were found to produce extracellular lignolytic enzymes on solid media substrate (SMS). *Trichoderma* sp., along with *Aeromonas* sp., *Aspergillus* sp., *Penicillium* sp., and *Bacillus* sp., have been reported to degrade alachlor within 7 days of incubation (Huang et al., 1995, 1996). Takagi et al. (2011) reported degradation of endosulfan, isolated from polluted soil, using more than 30 strains of *Trichoderma* spp. *Trichoderma* sp. strain 93155 was capable of degrading dieldrin by 19.7% after 14 days.

PESTICIDE REMEDIATION

Extensive use of pesticides causes serious environmental concerns for both soil and water and endanger the existing biosystems via their multifaceted toxicity (Bouziani, 2007). Biodegradation is widely used for the treatment of pesticides in soil because it is a cost-effective and eco-friendly method (Ritmann et al., 1988; Enrica, 1994) compared to conventional approaches like land filling and incineration (Sayler et al., 1990). Among microorganisms, fungi, especially *Trichoderma* sp., have been found to show great potential in pesticide bioremediation (Maheshwari et al., 2014, Sivaramanan, 2014).

Organophosphates and carbamates are potential toxic compounds that have been found to be toxic to aquatic life. These insecticides lead to the accumulation of acetylcholine in the synaptic terminals and thus disrupt normal functions of the nervous system (WHO, 1986). Oxamyl and carbofuran has been used extensively in agriculture to control insect pests of crops (Chapalamadugu and Chaudhry, 1992). Bumpus et al. (1993) and Harish et al. (2013) have emphasized the significance of fungi in the degradation of organophosphorus pesticides. *Trichoderma harzianum* can effectively degrade carbofuran (Wootton et al., 1983); organochlorines through an oxidative system (Katayama and Matsumura, 2009); and even dichlorodiphenyltrichloroethane (DDT), dieldrin, endosulfan, pentachlororonitrobenzene, and pentachlorophenol (PCP) (Katayama and Matsumura, 1993). *T. harzianum*, *T. viride*, and

T. knoingii, when mutated with radiations, exhibited production of high amounts of exo-enzymes (Haggag and Mohamed, 2002; Javaid et al., 2016). Afify et al. (2013) irradiated *Trichoderma* spp., for improved production of hydrolases to use them in the degradation of oxaml pesticides. Interestingly enough, *Trichoderma* spp. used oxamyl for growth while degrading it by 72.5%. Kumar et al. (2011), also reported effective biodegradation of methyl parathion and endosulfan using *Trichoderma viridae*, along with *Pseudomonas aeruginosa* (Bumpus et al., 1993). Körmöczi et al. (2013a) isolated *Trichoderma* strains from vegetable rhizosphere samples for the production of laccase to act against common plant pathogens. Isolates simultaneously reduced the negative effects of the herbicide linuron. Zhang et al. (2015) studied the genetics involved in the degradation of dichlorvos by *Trichoderma atroviride*, for possible exploration in bioremediation processes. Pentachlorophenol (PCP) is used extensively as a fungicide and a pesticide. It can damage the nervous system, liver, and kidneys, and it can also cause cancer. Sing et al. (2014) successfully isolated four PCP-tolerant fungal isolates from sawdust, and these four grew efficiently even in areas with high PCP concentration. *Trichoderma* sp. were among the PCP degraders, with *T. virgatum* reducing toxicity of PCP by up to 95% (Cserjesi and Johnson, 1972). Similar reports were made by Duncan and Deverall (1964). *T. viride* and *T. harzianum* have also been found to successfully remediate pollution caused by pirimicarb (Romeh, 2001).

Isolation of *Trichoderma* sp., which has the ability to produce laccase, was accomplished (Divya et al., 2013) in the estuaries of Kerala, India. The tolerance of *T. viride* Pers. NFCCI-2745 to salinity and various phenolics was the most promising. Eshak et al. (2012) used effluent discharge samples from a sugarcane bagasse mill in Egypt, with phenolics as the main pollutants. The collected wastewater was used as a medium for growing the fungal strains *A. oryzea* plus *T. reesei*, and the strains were found to grow efficiently on the medium prepared, indicating degradation of phenolic compounds present in the medium. *T. viride* and *T. harzianum* have high potential to degrade pirimicarb (Romeh, 2001), while *Trichoderma viride* has also been found to degrade methyl parathion and endosulfan (Kumar et al., 2011). *T. virens* and *T. reesei* were found to tolerate aromatic amines, a major class of polluting and toxic pesticides, and it was concluded that *T. virens* and, *T. reesei* successfully detoxified the amines (Cocaign et al., 2013).

Dye Remediation

Dyes are widely used for coloring diverse materials (Walmik et al., 1998), especially in dyeing and printing industries. Synthetic azo dyes are used in various industries, and a significant part of them is lost in the effluents (Zollinger, 1985). These chemical compounds cause contact dermatitis, are metabolized in the human intestine and liver (Chung and Stevens, 1993), and have been associated with carcinogenicity. Also, their presence in water is not esthetically appealing and increases water turbidity (Banat, et al., 2006; Raju et al., 2007). Biological decolorization can be achieved by microorganisms, and fungi are the most potent decolorizers (Yazdi et al., 1990; Yuthu and Viraraghavan, 2001). Itavara et al. (1999) reported that a mixture of *Trichoderma reesei* culture filtrate, purified endoglucanase, and β-glucosidase of *Aspergillus niger* degraded 70% of cellulose material to carbon dioxide. Baskar and

Baskaran (2012) investigated the dye decolorization capability of different fungal species. The study showed that ramazol black and ramazol red were found to be decolorized by *Trichoderma* sp. by 84.3% and 87.1%, respectively, in 21 days of incubation, indicating significant dye decolorization ability of the strains used. Shahid et al. (2013) also studied the ability of *Trichoderma lignorum* along with *Aspergillus niger* and *Fusarium oxysporum* to degrade textile dyes.

Balcázar-López et al. (2016) tested the transgenic strain of *T. atroviride*, with a laccase from *T. sanguineus*, for degradation of bisphenol A (BPA), phenolic compounds in wastewater, and benzopyrene and phenanthrene and industrial dyes. The technique proved to be successful, with transgenic *Trichodermal* strain showing increased bioremediation abilities. Similar constructs for *Trichoderma* species have been prepared and successfully evaluated for bioremediation by others too (Schuster and Schmoll, 2010; Ortega et al., 2011; Hamzah et al., 2012).

CYANIDE DEGRADATION

Cyanide is used extensively in industry and has been found to contaminate wastewater through release from metal finishing, electroplating, and coal coking (Dash et al., 2009). Unfortunately, it is associated with high toxicity, carcinogenicity, and mutagenicity (Maniyam et al., 2011). Species like *Trichoderma* spp. and *Fusarium* spp. have previously been demonstrated to degrade metallocyanides through the release of extracellular cyanide hydratase and dihydratase enzymes (Ezzi and Lynch, 2002, 2005). Lynch (2002) reported the ability of rhizospheric *Trichoderma* sp. to degrade phytotoxic concentrations (10 mM) of cyanide. Studies reported by Harman et al. (2004a) mention that the *Trichoderma* sp. strain T22, with genetic modification, was able to withstand concentrations up to 2,000 mg of cyanide per gram of soil, exceeding the limits set by the U.S. Environmental Protection Agency (EPA, 2015). This level of tolerance is quite remarkable, and the activity of *Trichoderma* sp. strain T22 is associated with the cellular system of intoxication based on the production of the enzyme permeases.

REMEDIATION OF POLYAROMATIC HYDROCARBONS AND PETROLEUM PRODUCTS

PAHs are commonly found in leaves and in wood (lignin), but they are also the products of burning of wood and fossil fuels (Samanta et al., 2002). They are toxic: they can cause mutations and cancers and thus are priority pollutants (Mueller et al., 1996; Labana et al., 2007). They can be present at alarming concentrations in soils polluted with industrial wastes (Bossert and Bartha, 1989; Andelman and Snodgrass, 1974; Daisey et al., 1997), and hence removal of PAHs from soil is a priority. Although PAHs are toxic and recalcitrant, lignin-degrading organisms, including bacteria and fungi (Mester and Tien, 2000), can help in the degradation of PAHs because these organisms can use PAHs for growth (Boonchan, et al., 2000; Cerniglia and Sutherland 2010). Fungi offer greater degradative abilities for PAHs because they can colonize solid substrates easily and effectively (Chulalaksananukul et al., 2006). Undugoda et al. (2013) reported the ability of various phyllosphere fungi, for example, *Penicillium* spp., *Aspergillus* spp., and *Trichoderma* spp. to degrade phenanthrene, naphthalene, toluene, and xylene. They reported that initial experiments indicated that the highest degradation of aromatic hydrocarbons occurred after seven days. Gomez et al. (2009), while studying the bioremediation ability of various bacterial and fungal cultures, reported *Trichoderma viride* to be the most important microorganism in alleviating pollution caused by PAHs. The degradation of PAHs in affected soils by *Trichoderma reesei*, with simultaneous breakdown of benzopyrene, has been tested by Yao et al. (2015), where the isolate removed about 54% of benzopyrene after 12 days. Similar results have been reported by others too (Verdin, et al., 2004). Fungal strains in isolated PAH-contaminated soils were evaluated for their different enzyme activities as well as for the degradation of PAHs (Balaji et al., 2014). *Trichoderma,* along with the 20 other selected strains, was efficient in degrading PAHs. The fungal consortia show promise for bioremediation of PAH-contaminated environments. Delira et al. (2012) also evaluated the ability of different *Trichoderma* strains to degrade hydrocarbons, including crude oil, naphthalene, phenanthrene, and benzopyrene.

Andrea et al. (2001) used *Trichoderma* and *Phanerochaete* in hydrocarbon degradation of oil-polluted soils. Also, many others (Llanos and Kjoller, 1976; Bartha and Atlas, 1977; April, 2006, Obire et al., 2008; Hamzah et al., 2012) have shown the ability of *Aspergillus* species and *Trichoderma* species to break hydrocarbons. The presence of *Trichoderma reesei* and *Trichoderma harzianum* in water-soluble fraction of crude oil supports the potential of these fungal strains in the possible remediation of crude oil–polluted water (Edema and Okungbowa, 2012).

Species of *Trichoderma*, along with *Gliocladium, Mucor,* and *Scopulariopsis*, were shown to grow on diesel-supplemented medium (Kristin et al., 2003). Hashem (1996) isolated fungal and bacterial strains from petroleum-contaminated and uncontaminated soils. They observed that *Trichoderma harzianum* was the most predominant fungal species to grow in these conditions. Bokhary and Parvez (1995) reported *Trichoderma* and *Ulocladium* to degraded oil. *Trichoderma* sp. showed enhanced growth with increasing crude oil concentrations (Hashem and Harbi, 2000). Makut et al. (2014) studied different fungal species (*Cladosporium* spp., *Cuvularia lunata, Penicillium brevicompactum,* and *Trichoderma viride*) for their efficiency in the use of petroleum products for growth by adding gasoline, kerosene, diesel, brake fluid, and engine oil to a nutrient medium. Out of the strains evaluated, *Trichoderma viride* was found to be most versatile in its ability to degrade. Sanyaolu et al. (2012) also demonstrated the ability of various fungal cultures, including *Trichoderma* spp. to hydrolyze premium motor spirit (PMS). Uzoamaka et al. (2009) isolated *Aspergillus versicolor, Aspergillus niger, Aspergillus flavus, Syncephalastrum* spp., *Trichoderma* spp., *Neurospora sitophila, Rhizopus arrhizus,* and *Mucor* spp. from oil-polluted soil and demonstrated the potential of each for hydrocarbon degradation. Adams et al. (2014) investigated the bioremediation of spent oil-contaminated soil, where *Trichoderma* spp., along with other microorganisms tested, drastically reduced total petroleum hydrocarbon in spent oil–contaminated soil. Carvalho et al. (2009) studied PCP degradation using *Trichoderma longibrachiatum* DSM 16517 in experiments involving mycelium growth and percentage of PCP decay, under co-metabolic conditions with PCP concentrations between 5 and 15 mg L^{-1}. *T. longibrachiatum* DSM 16517 was able to degrade PCP; at a concentration of 15 mg L^{-1}, the strains failed to biotransform PCP. Rigot and Matsumura (2002), using *Trichoderma harzianum* 2023, evaluated PCP degradation at 10 ppm as an initial concentration. After nine days of incubation, the PCP was entirely metabolized (it was quickly and stechiometrically converted to PCA). Hadibarata and Tachibana (2009) degraded n-eicosane (C20) using *Trichoderma* sp., where the fungi converted it into nonadecanoic acid. Similar observations for *Trichoderma* strains have been made by others too (Llanos and Kjoller, 1976; Davies and Westlake, 1979; Dragun, 1988, Korda et al., 1997, Obire et al., 2008; Obire and Anyanwu, 2009; Hamzah et al., 2012; Dhar et al., 2014).

DETERGENT DEGRADATION

The possible use of *Trichoderma harzianum* Rifai, isolated from wastewater samples of the Rasina River in the vicinity of the industrial wastewaters of a plant in Henkel, Serbia, was tested for biodegradation of commercial detergent. The fungus was found to decrease successfully the concentration of the detergent formulation tested, with more than 70% degradation of the detergent under trial, after 16 days of incubation (Jakovljevic et al., 2015).

AGRICULTURAL WASTE REMEDIATION

Trichoderma harzianum is a well-known producer of cellulases, with numerous applications in textile and paper industries for the breakdown and hydrolysis of cellulose (Bondkly et al., 2010). Rathore et al. (2013) reported that *Trichoderma viridae* was found to be the best degrader of organic waste collected from various sources. *Trichoderma viridie, Beauveria bassiana, Verticillium lecanii,* and *Metarhizium anisopliae* were evaluated for degrading various agricultural wastes like that of vegetables and fruits, and *T. viridie* especially has proven to be a good remediating agent (Esposito and da Silva, 1998).

DEGRADED PAPER REMEDIATION

Various fungal isolates were obtained from soil polluted with degraded papers. The major isolates included different species of *Aspergillus, Penicillium,* and *Trichoderma* and yeast (Raju et al., 2007; Sharma et al., 2013). These fungi play an important role in degrading paper waste, which would otherwise accumulate in ecosystems, especially water bodies, with seriously harmful effects on life.

CONCLUSION

The polysaccharides in *Trichoderma* cells can significantly enhance metal uptake. Many studies have investigated this "wonder" fungi, but we still have to achieve a higher degree of success for the fungi to be used on a commercial scale. Improved techniques using mutation and/or genetic engineering to further enhance the ability of *Trichoderma* sp. in bioremediation processes is still needed. *Trichoderma* sp. may prove to be a promising, cheap, and natural sorbent for the treatment of industrial waste.

REFERENCES

Adams, G. O., Tawari-Fufeyin P., and Ehinomen, I., 2014. Bioremediation of spent oil contaminated soils using poultry litter. *Res J Eng Appl Sci.* 3(2):118–124.

Adams, P., Lynch, J. M., and De Leij, F. A. A. M., 2007. Desorption of zinc by extracellularly produced metabolites of *Trichoderma harzianum, Trichoderma reesei* and *Coriolus versicolor. J Appl Microbiol.* 103:2240–2247.

Afify, A. E. M. M. R., Seoud, M. A. A, Ibrahim, G. M., and Kassem, B. W., 2013. Stimulating of biodegradation of oxamyl pesticide by low dose gamma irradiated fungi. *Plant Pathol Microbiol.* 4(9):1–5.

Afify, A. M. R., and El-Beltagi, H. S., 2011. Effect of the insecticide cyanophos on liver function in adult male rats. *Fresenius Environ Bull.* 20:1084–1088.

Ahlawat, O. P. Gupta, P., Kumar, S., Sharma, D. K., and Ahlawat, K., 2010. Bioremediation of fungicides by spent mushroom substrate and its associated microflora. *Indian J Microbiol.* 50(4):390–395.

Al-Rajhi, A. M. (2013). Impact of biofertilizer Trichoderma harzianum Rifai and the biomarker changes in Eruca sativa L. plant grown in metal-polluted soils. *World Appl Sci J.* 22(2): 171–180.

Altomare, C., Norvell, W. A., Bjorkman, T., and Harman, G. E., 1999. Solubilization of phosphates and micronutrients by the plant-growth-promoting and biocontrol fungus *Trichoderma harzianum Rifai* 1295-22. *Appl Environ Microbiol.* 65:2926–2933.

Ambiental, E. Y. G., 2010. *Trichoderma* spp. and its potential in soil bioremediation. United Nations Convention to Combat Desertification. European Commission.

Anand, P., Isar, J., Saran, S., and Saxena, R. K., 2006.Bioaccumulation of copper by *Trichoderma viride. Bioresour Technol.* 97(8):1018–1025.

Andelman, J. B., and Snodgrass, J. E., 1974. Incidence and significance of polynuclear aromatic hydrocarbons in the water environment. *Crit Rev Environ Control.* 5:69–83.

Andrea, R., Tania, A., and Lucia, R., 2001. Biodegradation of polycyclic aromatic hydrocarbons by soil fungi. *Braz J Microbiol.* 32(4):1–11.

April, T., Foght, J., and Currah, R., 2006. Hydrocarbon degrading filamentous fungus isolated from flare pit soil in Northern and Western Canada. *Can J Microbiol.* 46(1):38–49.

Babu, A. G., Shea, P. J., and Oh, B.-T., 2014a. *Trichoderma* sp. PDR1-7 promotes *Pinus sylvestris* reforestation of lead-contaminated mine tailing sites. *Sci. Total Environ.* 476–477:561–567.

Babu, A. G., Shim, J., Bang, K.-S., Shea, P. J., and Oh, B.-T., 2014b. *Trichoderma virens* PDR-28: A heavy metal-tolerant and plant growth-promoting fungus for remediation and bioenergy crop production on mine tailing soil. *J. Environ. Manage.* 132:129–134.

Babu, A. G., Shim, J., Shea, P. J., and Oh, B.-T., 2014c. *Penicillium aculeatum* PDR-4 and *Trichoderma* sp. PDR-16 promote phytoremediation of mine tailing soil and bioenergy production with sorghum-sudangrass. *Ecol. Eng.* 69:186–191.

Balaji, V., Arulazhagan, P., and Ebenezer, P., 2014. Enzymatic bioremediation of polyaromatic hydrocarbons by fungal consortia enriched from petroleum contaminated soil and oil seeds. *J Environ Biol.* 35: 1–9.

Balcázar-López, E., Méndez-Lorenzo, L. H., Batista- García, R. A., Esquivel-Naranjo, U., Ayala, M., et al., 2016. Xenobiotic compounds degradation by heterologous expression of a Trametes sanguineus laccase in *Trichoderma atroviride. Plos One* 1: 13. doi:10.1371/journal.pone.0147997.

Baldrian, P., 2003. Interactions of heavy metals white rot fungi. *Eznym. Microb. Technol.* 32:78–91.

Banat. I. M., Nigam, P., Singh, D., and Marchant, R., 2006. Microbial decolorization of textile-dyecontaining effluents. *Biosour Technol.* 58: 217–227.

Bartha, R., and Atlas, M., 1977. The microbiology of aquatic oil spills. *Adv Appl Microbiol.* 22:225–226.

Baskar, B. B., and Baskaran, C. (2012). Bioremediation of Azo Dyes Using Fungi. *International Journal of Research in Pharmacy & Science*, 2(4).

Benítez, T., Rincón, A. M., Limón, M. C., and Codón, A. C., 2004. Biocontrol mechanisms of *Trichoderma* strains. *Int Microbiol.* 7:249–260.

Bhattacharyya, M. H., Wilson, A. K., Rajan, S. S., Jonah, M., 2000. Biochemical pathways in cadmium toxicity. In *Molecular Biology and Toxicology of Metals.* Zalups, R.K., Koropatnick, E.J., Eds.; Taylor & Francis Group: London, UK. 34–74.

Bhavya, G., Sunil, K. C. R., Nandini, B., Swati, K., Prakash, H. S., and Geetha, N., 2015. In search of industrial clean-up clients; Evaluation of heavy metal tolerability of Rhizospheric Trichoderma. *IJIRSET.* 2(5):948–952.

Bishnoi, N. R., Kumar, R., and Bishnoi, K. 2007. Biosorption of Cr (VI) with Trichoderma viride immobilized fungal biomass and cell free Ca-alginate beads.

Błaszczyk, L., Siwulski, M., Sobieralski, K., Lisiecka, J., and Jędryczka, M., 2014. *Trichoderma* spp.–application and prospects for use in organic farming and industry. *J Plant Prot Res.* 54(4):309–317.

Blaylock, M. J., and Huang, J. W., 2000. Phytoextraction of Metals, In: I. Raskin and B.D. Ensley (Ed.). *Phytoremediation of Toxic Metals: Using Plants to Clean up the Environment.* Toronto, Canada: John Wiley & Sons, pp. 303.

Bokhary, H. A., and Parvez, S. 1995. Fungi inhabiting household environments in Riyadh, Saudi Arabia. *Mycopathologia*, 130(2): 79–87.

Boonchan, S., Britz, M. L., and Stanley, G. A., 2000. Degradation and mineralization of high-molecular-weight polycyclic aromatic hydrocarbons by defined fungal-bacterial cocultures. *Appl. Environ. Microbiol.* 66:1007–1019.

Bossert, I., and Bartha, R., 1989. The fate of petroleum in soil ecosystems. In: Atlas, R.M., Ed. *Petroleum Microbiology.* New York: MacMillan. 435–473.

Bouziani, M., 2007. L'usage immodéré des pesticides. De graves conséquences sanitaires. *Le Guide de la Médecine et de la Santé.* Santémaghreb, Albin Michel.

Bumpus, J. A., Kakar, S. N., and Coleman, R. D., 1993. Fungal degradation of organophosphorous insecticides. *Appl Biochem Biotechnol.* 39(2):715–726.

Cao, L., Jiang, M., Zeng, Z., Du, A., Tan, H., and Liu, Y., 2008. *Trichoderma atroviride* F6 improves phytoextraction efficiency of mustard (*Brassica juncea* (L.) Coss. var. foliosa Bailey) in Cd, Ni contaminated soils. *Chemosphere* 71(9):1769–1773.

Carvalho, M. B., Martins, I., Leitão, M. C., Garcia, H., Rodrigues, C., et al., 2009. Screening pentachlorophenol degradation ability by environmental fungal strains belonging to the phyla Ascomycota and Zygomycota. *J Ind Microbiol Biotechnol.* 36:1249–1256.

Cerniglia, C. E., and J. B. Sutherland., 2010. Degradation of polycyclic aromatic hydrocarbons by fungi. In: K. Timmis (Ed.) *Handbook of hydrocarbon and lipid microbiology.* Berlin, Germany: Springer. pp. 2079–2110.

Chan, K. H., and Chu, W., 2005. Atrazine removal by catalytic oxidation processes with or without UV irradiation: Part II: An analysis of the reaction mechanisms using LC/ESI-tandem mass spectrometry. *Appl Catalysis B: Environ.* 58:165–174.

Chapalamadugu, S., and Chaudhry, G. R., 1992. Microbiological and biotechnological aspects of metabolism of carbamates and organophosphates. *Crit Rev Biotechnol.* 12:357–389.

Chávez-Gómez, B., Quintero, R., Esparza-García, F., Howard, A. M., Díaz de la Serna FJ, Z., et al., 2009. Removal of phenanthrene from soil by co-cultures of bacteria and fungi pregrown on sugarcane bagasse pith. *Bioresour Technol.* 89(2):177–186.

Chulalaksananukul, S., Gadd, G. M., Sangvanich, P., Sihanonth, P., Piapukiew, J., and Vangnai A. S., 2006. Biodegradation of benzo(a) pyrene by a newly isolated Fusarium sp. *FEMS Microbiol Lett.* 262:99–106.

Chung, K. T., and Stevens, S. E., 1993. Degradation of Azo dyes by environmental Microorganism and helminthes. *Environ Toxicol Chem.* 12: 2121–2132.

Cocaign, A., Bui, L. C., Silar, P., Tong L. C. H., Busi, F., et al., 2013. Biotransformation of *Trichoderma* spp. and their tolerance to aromatic amines, a major class of pollutants. *Appl Environ Microbiol.* 79(15):4719–4726.

Cserjesi, A. J., and Johnson, E. L., 1972. Methylation of pentachlorophenol by *Trichoderma virgatum. Can J Microbiol.*18:45–49.

Daisey, J. M., Leyko, M. A., and Kneip, T. J., 1997. Source identification and allocation of polynuclear aromatic hydrocarbon compounds in the New York City aerosol. In: Jones P.W, Leber P. (Eds.). *Polynuclear Aromatic Hydrocarbons.* Ann Arbor, MI: Ann Arbor Science Publishers, pp. 201–215.

Danilovic, G. M., Curcic, N. Z., Pucarevic, M. M., Jovanovic, L. B., Vagvolgyi, C., et al., 2015. Degradation of Linuron in soil by two fungal strains. *Matica Srpska J Nat Sci Novi Sad.* 129:45–54.

Dash, R. R., Gaur, A., and Balomajumder, C., 2009. Cyanide in industrial wastewater and its removal: A review on biotreatment. *J Hazard Mater.* 163: 1–11.

Davies, J. S., and Westlake, D. W. S., 1979. Crude oil utilization by fungi. *Can J Microbiol.* 25: 146–156.

Deckert, J., 2005. Cadmium toxicity in plants: Is there any analogy to its carcinogenic effect in mammalian cells? *Biometals* 18:475–481.

Delira, R. A., Alarco, A. Cerrato, R. F., Almaraz, J. J., and Cabriales, J. J. P., 2012. Tolerance and growth of 11 Trichoderma strains to crude oil, naphthalene, phenanthrene and benzo[a]pyrene. *J Environ Manage.* 95: S291–S299.

Dhar, K., Dutta, S., and Anwar, M. N., 2014. Biodegradation of Petroleum Hydrocarbon by indigenous Fungi isolated from Ship breaking yards of Bangladesh. *Int Res J Biol Sci.* 3(9):22–30.

Divya, L. M., Prasanth, G. K., and Sadasivan, C., 2013. Potential of the salt-tolerant laccase-producing strain *Trichoderma viride* Pers. NFCCI-2745 from an estuary in the bioremediation of phenol-polluted environments. *J Basic Microbiol.* 00: 1–6.

Dragun, J., 1988. Microbial degradation of petroleum products in soil. In: Calabrese, E. J. and Kostecki, P. T. (Eds.), *Soils Contaminated by Petroleum: Environmental and Public Health Effects.* New York, NY: Wiley-Interscience, pp. 289–300.

Duncan, C. G., and Deverall, F. J., 1964. Degradation of wood preservatives by fungi. *App. Environ Microbiol.* 12:57–62.

Edema, N. E., and Okungbowa, F. I., 2012. Bioremediation prospects of fungi isolated from water soluble fraction of crude oil samples. *Ife J Sci.* 14 (2):385–389.

El-Bondkly, A. M., Aboshosha, A. A. M., Radwan, N. H., and Dora, S. A., 2010. Successive construction of ß-glucosidase hyperproducers of *Trichoderma Harzianum* using microbial biotechnology techniques. *J Microbial Biochem Technol.* 2:070–073.

Enrica, G., 1994. The role of Microorganisms in environmental decontamination. In A. Renzoni, (Ed.). *Contaminants in the Environment: A Multidisciplinary Assessment of Risks to Man and Other Organisms* 25:235–246. Boca Raton, FL: Lewis Publishers.

EPA. 2015, April. "What Is a Pesticide?," http://www.epa.gov.

Errasquin, L. E., and Vazquez, C., 2003. Tolerance and uptake of heavy metals by *Trichoderma atroviride* isolated from sludge. *Chemosphere* 50: 137–143.

Eshak, M. G., Hassanane, M. M., Farag I. M., and Fadel, M., 2012. Bioremediation of polluted diets with industrial wastewater using marine and earth fungi: Molecular genetic, biochemical and histopathological studies in mice. *World Appl Sci J.* 20(2):290–304.

Esposito, E., and da Silva, M., 1998. Systematics and environmental application of the genus *Trichoderma. Crit Rev Microbiol.* 24: 89–98.

Ezzi, M. I., and Lynch, J. M. 2005. Biodegradation of cyanide by Trichoderma spp. and Fusarium spp. *Enzyme and Microbial Technol.,* 36(7): 849–854.

Ezzouhri, L., Castro, E., Moya, M., Espinola F., and Lairini, K., 2009. Heavy metal tolerance of filamentous fungi isolated from polluted sites in Tangier, Morocco. *Afr J Microbiol Res.* 3(2):35–48.

Gadd, G. M., 2000. Bioremedial potential of microbial mechanisms of metal mobilization and immobilization. *Curr Opin Biotechnol.* 11:271–279.

Gavrilesca, M., 2004. Removal of heavy metals fromthe environment by biosorption. *Eng Life Sci.* 4(3):219–232.

Gupta, R., Ahuja, P., Khan, S., Saxena, R. K., and Mohapatra, H., 2000. Microbial biosorbents: Meeting challenges of heavy metal pollution in aqueous solutions. *Curr Sci.* 78(8):967–973.

Hadibarata, T., and Tachibana, S., 2009. Microbial degradation of *n*-eicosane by filamentous fungi. In Y. Obayashi, T. Isobe, A. Subramanian, S. Suzuki, S. Tanabe (Eds.), *Interdisciplinary Studies on Environmental Chemistry Environmental Research in Asia.* Terrapub, Tokyo. 322–329.

Haggag, W. M., and Mohamed, H. A. A., 2002. Enhancement of antifungal metabolites production from gamma-rays induced mutants of some *Trichodema* sp. for control onion white rot disease. *Plant Pathol Bull.* 11:45–56.

Hall, J. L., 2002. Cellular mechanisms for heavy metal detoxification and tolerance. *J Exp Bot.* 53:1–11.

Hamzah, A., Zarin, M., Hamid, A., Othman, A., and Sahidan, S., 2012. Optimal physical and nutrient parameters for growth of Trichoderma virens UKMP-1M for heavy crude oil degradation. *Sains Malays.* 41: 71–79.

Harish, R., Supreeth, M., and Chauhan, J. B., 2013. Biodegradation of organophosphate pesticide by soil fungi. *Adv Bio Tech.* 12 (9):4–8.

Harman, G. E., Howell, C. R., Viterbo, A., Chet, I., and Lorito, M., 2004b. *Trichoderma* species–opportunistic, avirulent plant symbionts. *Nat Rev Microbiol.* 2:43–56.

Harman, G. E., Lorito, M., and Lynch, J. M., 2004a. Uses of *Trichoderma* spp. to alleviate or remediate soil and water pollution. *Adv Appl Microbiol.* 56:330–331

Hashem, A. R., 1996. Influence of crude oil contamination on the chemical and microbiological aspects of Saudi Arabian soil. *J King Saud Univ.* 8 (1):11–18.

Hashem, A. R. and Al-Harbi, S. A., 2000. Biodegradation of crude oil. In Mohamed, A. M. O. and Al-Hosani, K. I. (Eds.), *Geoengineering in Arid Lands.* Rotterdam, the Netherlands: Balkema Publication, pp. 567–569.

Howell, C. R., 2003. Mechanisms employed by *Trichoderma* species in the biological control of plant disease; the history and evolution of current concept. *Plant Dis.* 87:4–10.

Huang, J. W., Hu, C. K., and Shih, S. D., 1996. The role of soil microorganism in alleviations of root injury of garden pea seedlings by alachlor with spent golden mushroom compost. *Plant Pathol Bull.* 5(3):137–145.

Huang, J. W., Hu, C. K., Tzeng, D. D. S., and Ng, K. H., 1995. Effect of soil amended with spent golden mushroom compost on alleviating phytotoxicity of alachlor to seedling of garden pea. *Plant Pathol Bull* 4(2):76–82.

Iskandar, N. L., Zainudin, N. A., and Tan, S. G., 2011. Tolerance and biosorption of copper (Cu) and Lead (Pb) by filamentous fungi isolated from a fresh water ecosystem. *J Environ Sci.* 23:824–830.

Itavara, M., Siika-aho, M., and Vilkari, L., 1999. Enzymatic degradation of cellulose based materials. *J Environ Poly Deg.* 7:67–73.

Jakovljevic, V. D., Stojanovic, J. D., and Vrvic, M. M., 2015. The potential application of fungus, *Trichoderma harzianum* Rifai in biodegradation of detergent and industry. *Chem Ind Chem Eng Q.* 21 (1) 131–139.

Järup, L., 2002. Cadmium overload and toxicity. *Nephrol Dial Transplant.* 17:35–39.

Javaid, M. K., Ashiq, M., and Tahir, M., 2016. Potential of biological agents in decontamination of agricultural soil, *Scientifica*, Vol. 2016, Article ID 1598325, 9 pages, doi:10.1155/2016/1598325.

Kacprzak, M., and Malina, G., 2005. The tolerance and Zn^{2+}, Ba^{2+} and Fe^{3+} accumulation by *Trichoderma atroviride* and *Mortierella exigua* isolated from contaminated soil. *Can J Soil Sci.* 85(2):283–290.

Kacprzak, M. J., Rosikon, K., Fijalkowski, K., and Grobelak, A., 2014. The Effect of *Trichoderma* on Heavy Metal Mobility and Uptake by *Miscanthus giganteus*, *Salix* sp., *Phalaris arundinacea*, and *Panicum virgatum*. *Appl Environ Soil Sci.* 2014(Article ID 506142):10 pages.

Kapoor, A., and Viraraghavan, T., 1995. Fungi biosorption: An alternative treatment option for heavy metal bearing wastewaters: A review. *Bioresour Technol.* 53:195–206.

Katayama, A., and Matsumura, F., 1993. Degradation of organochlorine pesticides, particularly endosulfan, by *Trichoderma harzianum*. *Environ Toxicol Chem.* 12:1059–1065.

Katayama, A., and Matsumura, F., 2009. Degradation of organochlorine pesticides, particularly endosulfan, by *Trichoderma harzianum*. *Environl Toxicol Chem.* 12:1059–1065.

Kaufman, D. D., and Blake, J., 1970. Degradation of atrazine by soil fungi. *Soil Biol Biochem.* 2:73–80.

Korda, A., Santas, P., Tenente, A., and Santas, R., 1997. Petroleum hydrocarbon bioremediation: sampling and analytical techniques, in situ treatments and commercial microorganisms currently used. *Appl Microbiol Biotechnol.* 48: 677–686.

Körmöczi, P, Kredics, L., Danilovic, G., Jovanonic, L., Manczinger, L., et al. 2013a. Possibilities of bioremediation, biocontrol and plant growth promotion with Trichoderma strains isolated from vegetable rhizosphere samples. *Acta Microbiologica et Immunologica Hungarica.* 60(Suppl.): 163–164.

Körmöczi, P., Danilović, G., Manczinger, L., Jovanović, L., Panković, D., et al., and Kredics, L., 2013b. Species composition of *Trichoderma* isolates from the rhizosphere of vegetables grown in Hungarian soils. *Fresen Environ Bull.* 22:1736–1741.

Körmöczi, P., Manczinger, L., Sajben-Nagy, E., Vágvölgyi, C., Danilović, G., et al., 2013c. Screening of *Trichoderma* strains isolated from rhizosphere samples for laccase production. *Rev Agric Rural Develop.* 2:325–330.

Kredics, L., Antal, Z., Manczinger, L., and Nagy, E., 2001a. Breeding of mycoparasitic *Trichoderma* strains for heavy metals resistance. *Lett Appl Microbiol.* 33:112–116.

Kredics, L., Doczi, I., Antal, Z., and Manczinger, L., 2001b. Effect of heavy metals on growth and extracellular enzyme activities of mycoparasitic *Trichoderma* strains. *Bull Environ Contam Toxicol.* 66:249–254.

Kredics, L., Hatvani, L., Naeimi, S., Körmöczi, P., Manczinger, L., et al., 2014. Biodiversity of the genus Hypocrea/Trichoderma in different habitats. In: Gupta, V. K., Schmoll, M., Herrera-Estrella, A., Upadhyay, R. S., Druzhinina, I., Tuohy, M. (Eds.), *Biotechnology and Biology of Trichoderma*. Amsterdam, the Netherlands: Elsevier Science BV, pp. 3–24.

Kumar, S. Anthonisamy, A., and Arunkumar, S., 2011. Biodegradation of methyl parathion and endosulfan using: *Pseudomonas aeruginosa* and Trichoderma viridae. *J Environ Sci Eng.* 53(1):115–122.

Labana, S., Kapur, M., Malik, D., Prakash, D., and Jain, R. K., 2007. Diversity, biodegradation and bioremediation of polycyclic aromatic hydrocarbons. In S. Singh and R. Tripathi (Eds.), *Environmental Bioremediation Technologies*. Berlin, Germany: Springer, pp. 409–443.

Ledin, M., Krantz-Rulcker, C., and Allard, B., 1996. Zn, Cd and Hg accumulation by microorganisms, organic and inorganic soil components in multi-compartment systems. *Soil Biol. Biochem.* 28:791–799.

Leyval, C., Turnau, K., and Haselweter, K., 1997. Effect of heavy metal pollution on mycorrhizal colonization and function: Physiological, ecological and applied aspects. *Mycorrhiza* 7:139–153.

Lima De F. A., De Moura, G. F., De Lima, M. A. B., De Souza, P. M., Alves Da Silva, C. A., et al., 2011. Role of the morphology and polyphosphate in Trichoderma harzianum related to cadmium removal. *Molecules* 16:2486–2500.

Llado, S., Jiménez, N., Viñas, M., and Solanas A. M., 2009. Microbial populations related to PAH biodegradation in an aged biostimulated creosote-contaminated soil. *Biodegradation* 20:593–601.

Llanos, C., and Kjoller, A., 1976. Change in the flora of soil fungi following oil waste application. *Oikos* 27: 377–382.

Lopez, E., and Vazquez, C., 2003. Tolerance and uptake of heavy metals by *Trichoderma atroviride* isolated from sludge. *Chemosphere* 50:137–143.

Lynch, J. M., 2002. Resilience of the rhizosphere to anthropogenic disturbance. *Biodegradation* 13:21–27.

Machın-Ramırez, C., Morales, D., Martınez-Morales, F., Okoh, A. I., and Trejo-Hernandez, M. R., 2010. Benzo[a]pyrene removal by axenic- and co-cultures of some bacterial and fungal strains. *Int Biodeterior Biodegrad.* 64:538–544.

Maheshwari, R., Singh, U., Singh, P., Singh, N., Jat, B. L., and Rani, B., 2014. To decontaminate wastewater employing bioremediation technologies. *J Adv Sci Res.* 5(2):07–15.

Makut, M. D., Ogbonna, A. I., Ogbonna, C. I. C., and Olwuna, M. H., 2014. Utilization of petroleum products by fungi isolated from the soil environment of Keffi Metropolis, Nasarawa State, Nigeria. *IJSN.* 5(2):222–225.

Maniyam, M. N., Sjahrir, F., and Ibrahim, A. L., 2011. Biodegradation of cyanide by rhodococcus strains isolated in Malaysia, 2011 *International Conference on Food Engineering and Biotechnology*, IPCBEE vol. 9: IACSIT Press, Singapore.

Meagher, R. B., 2000. Phytoremediation of toxicelemental and organic pollutants. *Curr Opin Plant Biol.* 3:153–162.

Mester, T., and Tien, M., 2000. Oxidation mechanism of lignolytic enzymes involved in the degradation of environmental pollutants. *Int Biodet Biodegrad.* 46:51–59.

Miettinen-Oinonen, A., 2004. Trichoderma reesei strains for production of cellulases for the textile industry. http://www.vtt.fi/inf/pdf/.

Mohsenzadeh, F., and Shahrokhi, F., 2014. Biological removing of Cadmium from contaminated media by fungal biomass of *Trichoderma* species, *JEHSE.* 12:102:1–7.

Mueller, J. G., Cerniglia, C. E., and Pritchard, P. H., 1996. Bioremediation of environments contaminated by polycyclic araomatic hydrocarbons. In Crawford R. L., Crawford D. L. (Eds.), *Biotechnology Research Series*, (6):125–194.

Nida'a, S., Hamad Mayson, M., and Al-kidsawey, A. T. E. R., 2016. Mycoremedation of total and hexavlent chromium from tannery wastewater using fungus *Trichoderma harizianum. Mesopotamia Environ J.* 2(3):34–41.

Nies, D. H., 1999. Microbial heavy-metal resistance. *Appl Microb Biotechnol.* 51:730–750.

Nongmaithem, N., Roy, A., and Bhattacharya, P. M., 2016. Screening of Trichoderma isolates for their potential of biosorption of nickel and cadmium. *Brazilian J Microb.* 47: 305–313.

Obire, O., and Anyanwu, E., 2009. Impact of various concentrations of crude oil on fungal populations of soil. *Int J Environ Sci Technol.* 6: 211–218.

Obire, O., Anyanwu, E. C., and Okigbo, R. N., 2008. Saprophytic and crude oil-degrading fungi from cow dung and poultry droppings as bioremediating agents. *Int Agric Technol.* 4(2):81–89.

Ortega, S. N., Nitschke, M., Mouad, A. M., Landgraf, M. D., Rezende, M. O., et al., 2011. Isolation of Brazilian marine fungi capable of growing on DDD pesticide. *Biodegradation* 22: 43–50.

Pelcastre, M. I. Ibarra, J. R. V., Navarrete, A. M., Rosas, J. C., Ramirez, C. A. G., and Andoval, O. A. A., 2013. Bioremediation perspectives using autochthonous species of Trichoderma sp. for degradation of atrazine in agricultural soil from the Tulancingo valley, Hidalgo, Mexico. *Trop. Subtrop. Agro.* 16(2): 265–276.

Pepper, I. L., 2000. Microbial responses to environmentally toxic cadmium. *Microb Ecol.* 38:358–364.

Petrović, J. J. Danilovic, G., Ćurcic, N., Milinkovic, M., Stosic, N, et al., 2014. Copper tolerance of Trichoderma Species. *Arch Biol Sci.* Belgrade, 66(1):137–142.

Price, M. S., Classen, J. J., and Payne, G. A., 2001. *Aspergillus niger* absorbs copper and zinc from swine wastewater. *Bioresour Technol.* 77(1):41–49.

Raj, K. S., 2014. In-vitro screening of *Trichoderma* in rock phosphate solubilization and myco remediation of heavy metal contaminated water. *PIJR.* 3(1):24–29.

Raju, N. S., Venkataramana, G. V., Girish, S. T., Raghavendra, V. B., and Shivashankar, P., 2007. Isolation and evaluation of indigenous Soil fungi for decolourization of Textile dyes. *J Appl Sci.* 7(2):298–301.

Rangasamy, S. Alagirisamy, B., and Santiago, M., 2013. Poultry manure induce biotransformation of hexavalent chromium in soil. *IOSR-JESTFT.* 5(6):27–32.

Rathore, S., Gaur, R. C., Suwalka, D., and Mehta, J., 2013. Bioremediation of various agro waste using microorganism in Hadoti region of Rajasthan. *Int J Rec Biotechnol.* 1 (1):39–42.

Ravelet, C., Krivobok, S., Sage, L., and Steiman, R., 2000. Biodegradation of pyrene by sediment fungi. *Chemosphere* 40:557–563.

Ribeiro, A. B., Rodríguez-Maroto, J. M., Mateus, E. P., and Gomes, H., 2005. Removal of organic contaminants from soils by an electrokinetic process: The case of atrazine. Experimental and modeling.*Chemosphere* 59(9): 1229–1239.

Rigot, J., and Matsumura, F., 2002. Assessment of the rhizosphere competency and pentachlorophenol-metabolizing activity of a pesticide-degrading strain of *Trichoderma harzianum* introduced into the root zone of corn seedlings. *J Environ Sci Health.* 37: 201–210.

Ritmann, B. E., Jacson, D. E., and Storck, S. L., 1988. Potential for treatment of hazardous organic chemicals with biological Process. *Biotr. Sys.* 3:15–64.

Romeh, A. A., 2001. Biodegradation of carbosulfan, pirimicarb and diniconazole pesticides by Trichoderma spp. *J Environ Res.* 3: 162–172.

Rosen, B. P., 2002. Transport e detoxification systems for transition metals, heavy metals and metalloids in eukaryotic and prokaryotic microbes. *Comp Biochem Physiol.* 133:689–693.

Sahu, A., Mandal, A., Thakur, J., Manna, M. C., and Rao, A. S., 2012. Exploring bioaccumulation efficacy of *Trichoderma viride*: An alternative bioremediation of cadmium and lead. *Natl Acad Sci Lett.* 35:299–302. doi:10.1007/s40009-012-0056-4.

Samanta, S. K., Singh, O. V., and Jain, R. K., 2002. Polycyclic aromatic hydrocarbons: Environmental pollution and bioremediation. *Trends Biotechnol.*20:243–248.

Sanyaolu, A. A. A., Sanyaolu, V. T., Kolawole-Joseph, O. S., and Jawando, S., 2012. Biodegradation of premium motor spirit by fungal species. *Int J Sci Nat.* 3(2):276–285.

Saraswathy, A., and Hallberg. R., 2002. Degradation of pyrene by indigenous fungi from a former gasworks site. *FEMS Microbiol Lett.* 210:227–232.

Sarkar, S., Satheshkumar, A., Jayanthi, R., and Premkumar R., 2010. Biosorption of nickel by live biomass of *Trichodermaharzianum*. *Res J Agric Sci.* 1(2):69–74.

Satoh, M., Koyama, H., Kaji, T., Kito, H., and Tohyama, C., 2002. Perspectives on cadmium toxicity research. *Tohoku J Exp Med.* 196:23–32.

Savvaidis, I., 1998. Recovery of gold from thiourea solutions using microorganisms. *Biometals* 11:145–151.

Sayler, G. S., Hooper, S. W., Layton, A. C., and King, J. M. H., 1990. Catabolic plasmids of environmental and ecological significance. *Microbial Ecology.*19 (1):1–20.

Schuster, A., and Schmoll, M., 2010. Biology and biotechnology of *Trichoderma. Appl Microbiol Biotechnol.* 87:787–799.

Sene, L., Converti, A., Secchi, G. A. R., and Simão, R.de C. G., 2010. New aspects on atrazine biodegradation. *Braz Arch Biol Technol.* 53(2):487–496.

Shahid, A., Singh, J., Bisht, S., Teotia, P., and Kumar, V., 2013. Biodegradation of textile dyes by fungi isolated from North Indian field soil. *Environ Asia.* 6(2):51–57.

Sharma, R., Chandra, S., and Singh, A., 2013. Isolation of microorganism from soil contaminated with degraded paper in Jharna village. *J Soil Sci Environ Manage.* 4(2):23–27.

Siddiquee, S., Aishah, S. N., Azad, S. A., Shafawati, S. N., and Naher, L., 2013. Tolerance and biosorption capacity of Zn^{2+}, Pb^{2+}, Ni^{3+} and Cu^{2+} by filamentous fungi (*Trichoderma harzianum, T. aureoviride* and *T. virens*). *Adv Biosci Biotechnol.* 4:570–583.

Sing, N. N., Zulkharnain, A., Roslan, H. A., Assim, Z., and Husaini, A., 2014. Bioremediation of PCP by *Trichoderma* and *Cunninghamella* strains isolated from sawdust. *Braz Arch Biol Technol.* 57(6):811–820.

Singh, M., and Sharma, O. P., 2012. *Trichoderma*–A savior microbe in the era of climate change. *IJABR.* 2(4):784–786.

Sivaramanan, S., 2014. Biodegradation of Saw in Plant Fertilizer. *Res J Agri Forestry Sci.* 2(2):13–19.

Srivastava, P. K., Vaish, A., Dwivedi, S., Chakrabarty, D., Singh, N., and Tripathi, R. D., 2011. Biological removal of arsenic pollution by soil fungi. *Earth Environ Sci.* 409:2430–2442.

Su, S. Zeng, X., Bai, L. Li, L., and Duan, R., 2011. Arsenic biotransformation by arsenic-resistant fungi *Trichoderma asperellum* SM-12F1, *Penicillium janthinellum* SM-12F4, and *Fusarium oxysporum* CZ-8F1. *Sci Total Environ.* 409:5057–5062.

Takagi, K., Kataoka, R., and Yamazaki, K., 2011. Recent technology on bio-remediation of POPs and persistent pesticides. *JARQ.* 45(2):129–136.

Tang, J., Liu, L., Hu, S., Chen, Y., and Chen, J., 2009. Improved degradation of organophosphate dichoruos by Trichoderma atroviride transformats generated by restriction enzyme-mediated interaction (REMI). *Bioresour Technol.* 100:480–483.

Teng, Y., Luo, Y., Ma, W., Zhu, L., Ren, W., et al., 2015. Trichoderma reesei FS10-C enhances phytoremediation of Cd-contaminated soil by Sedum plumbizincicola and associated soil microbial activities, Vol.6: Article 438.

Ting, A. S. Y., and Choong, C. C., 2009. Bioaccumulation and biosorption efficacy of *Trichoderma* isolates SP2F1 in removing Copper (Cu II) from aqueous solutions. *World J Microbiol Biotechnol.* 25:1431–1437.

Townsley, C. C., Ross, I. S., and Atkins, A. S., 1986. Copper removal from a simulated leach effluent using filamentous fungus *Trichoderma viridie*. In H. Eccles and S. Hunt (Eds.), *Immobilization of Ions by Biosorption*. Chichester, UK: Ellis Horwood, pp. 159–170.

Tripathi, P., Singh, P., Mishra, A., Chauhan, P., Dwivedi, S., et al., 2013. Trichoderma: A potential bioremediator for environmental cleanup. *Clean Technol Environ Policy.* 15:541–550. doi:10.1007/s10098-012-0553-7.

Undugoda, L. J. S., Kannangara, S., and Sirisena, D. M., 2013. Aromatic hydrocarbon degrading phyllosphere fungi. *Proceedings of the International Forestry and Environment Symposium of the Department of Forestry, and Environmental Science*. University of Sri Jayewardenepura, Sri Lanka.

Uzoamaka, G. O., Floretta, T., and Florence, M. O., 2009. Hydrocarbon degradation potentials of indigenous fungal isolates from petroleum contaminated soils. *J Phys Nat Sci.* 3(1):1–6.

Van Gestela, K., Mergaertb, J., Swingsb, J., Coosemansa, J., and Ryckeboer, J., 2003. Bioremediation of diesel oil-contaminated soil by composting with biowaste. *Environ Pollut.* 125 (2003) 361–368.

Vankar, P. S., and Bajpai, D., 2007. Phytoremediation of chrome (VI) of tannary effluent by *Trichoderma* species. *Conference on Dasilination and the Environment.* Sponsored by the European Desalination Society and Center for Research and Technology, Hellas (CERATH), Sani Resort, Halkidiki, Greece.

Vankar, P. S., and Bajpai, D. 2008., Phyto-remediation of chrome-VI of tannery effluent by *Trichoderma* species. *Desalination* 222:255–262.

Verdin, A., Sahraoui, A. L.-H., and Durand, R., 2004. Degradation of benzo [a]pyrene by mitosporic fungi and extracellular oxidative enzymes. *Int Biodeterior Biodegrad.* 53:65–70.

Volesky, B., 1994. Advances in biosorption of metals: Selection of biomass types. *FEMS Microbiol.* 14: 291–302.

Waisberg, M., Joseph, P., Hale, B. E., and Beyersmann, D., 2003. Molecular and cellular mechanisms of cadmium carcinogenesis. *Toxicology* 192:95–117.

Walmik, A., Sani, R. K., and Banerjee, V. C., 1998. Biodegradation of textile azo dyes by P.chrysosporium. *Enzyme Microb Technol.* 22: 185.

Wang, J., and Chen, C., 2006. Biosorption of heavy metals by *Saccharomyces cerevisiae*: A review, *Biotechnol Adv.* 24:427–451.

Wei, J. C., 1979. *Handbook of Fungi Identification.* Shanghai, China: Technology Press.

WHO (World Health Organization). 1986. Organophosphorus Insecticides: A General Introduction. *Environmental Health Criteria.* Geneva, Switzerland.

Woo, S. L., Ruocco, M., Vinale, F., Nigro, M., Marra, R., et al., 2014. *Trichoderma*-based products and their widespread use in agriculture. *Open Mycol J.* 8(Suppl-1, M4):71–126.

Wootton, M. A., Kremer, R. J., and Keaster, A. J., 1993. Effects of carbofuran and the corn rhizosphere on growth of soil microorganisms. *Bull Environ Contain Toxicol.* 50:49–56.

Yan, G., and Viraraghavan, T., 2003. Heavy-metal removal from aqueous solution by fungus. Mucor rouxii. *Water Res.* 37:4486–4496.

Yao, L., Teng, Y., Luo, Y., Christie, P., Ma, W., et al., 2015. Biodegradation of Polycyclic Aromatic Hydrocarbons (PAHs) by Trichoderma reesei FS10-C and Effect of Bioaugmentation on an Aged PAH-Contaminated Soil. *Biorem J.* 19:9–17.

Yap, C. K., Ismail, A., Tan, S. G., and Omar, H., 2002. Correlation between speciation of Cd, Cu, Pb and Zn in sediment and their concentrations in total soft tissue of green-lipped mussel *Perna viridis* from the west coastal of Peninslar Malaysia. *Environ Int.* 28:117–126.

Yazdani, M., Yap, C. K., and Abdullah, F., 2010a. Adsorption and absorption of Cu in *Trichoderma atroviride. Pertanika J. Trop. Agric. Sci.* 33(1):71–77.

Yazdani, M., Yap, C. K., Abdullah, F., and Tan, S. G., 2009. *Trichoderma atroviride* as a bioremediator of Cu pollution: An in vitro study. *Toxicological and Environmental Chemistry.* 91(7):1305–1314.

Yazdani, M., Yap, C. K., Abdullah, F., and Tan, S. G., 2010b. An *in vitro* study on the adsorption, absorption and uptake capacity of Zn by the bioremediator *Trichoderma atroviride. Environment Asia.* 3(1):53–59.

Yazdi, M. T., Woodward, G., and Radford, A., 1990. Cellulase production by Neurospora crassa: The enzymes of the complex and their regulation. *Enzyme Microb Technol.* 12:116–119.

Yuthu, F., and Viraraghavan, T., 2001. Fungal decolorization of dye wastewaters. *Bio Tech*.79: 251–262.

Zafar, S., Aqil, F., and Ahmad, I., 2006. Metal tolerance and biosorption potential of filamentous fungi isolated from metal contaminated agricultural soil. *Bioresource Technology Journal*. 96:2557–2561.

Zhang, T., Tang, J. Sun, J., Yu, C., Liu, Z., and Chen, J., 2015. Hex1-related transcriptome of *Trichoderma atroviride* reveals expression patterns of ABC transporters associated with tolerance to dichlorvos. *Biotechnol Lett*. 37:1421–1429, doi:10.1007/s10529-015-1806-4.

Zollinger, H., 1985. Colour chemistry synthesis: Properties and applications of organic dyes and pigments. New York, NY: VCH Publishers.

16 Probiotics and Their Applications in Aquaculture

Arun Chauhan and Rahul Singh

CONTENTS

Alteration of the body or one of its organs that disturbs normal physiological function is known as disease. The disease can be infectious due to the action of microorganisms or noninfectious due to nonliving causes (environmental, other). The disease can be treatable or nontreatable depending on the nature of the alterations and their intensity. The main causative agent of disease is stress because animals must then expend more energy to maintain homeostasis and less energy to combat disease.

321

Some disease agents are always present in the environment and try to enter a suitable home when the opportunity presents itself. Infectious disease only occurs when three factors present simultaneously:

Mortality curves:

When infectious agents move into the population, proliferate cause disease but then after time fail to show no longer effects in population bell-shaped mortality curves create in which transmission is horizontal with width of curve proportional to incubation time and period of communicability shows. (Pic. 1)

Sigmoidal curve of mortality form when slight deviation occurs in lac period of bell-shaped curve which shows non-communicable period of diseases in the case of typical bacterial infection. (Pic. 2)

Point source mortality curve in population can be seen at high virulent infectious type disease and all susceptible members affected conditions such as chemical and viral infection. (Pic. 3)

Plateau and multiple spiked curves form by non-infectious diseases. (Pic. 4 and 5)

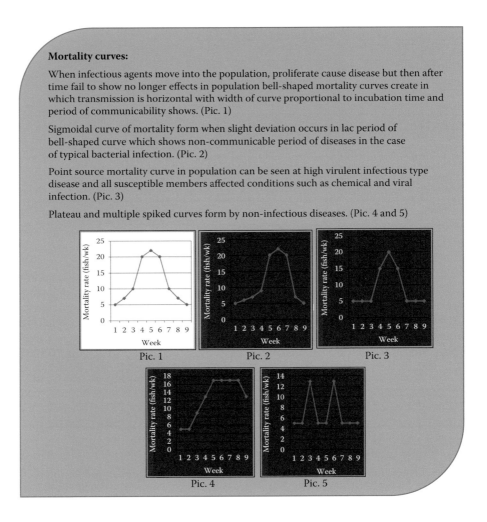

Pic. 1   Pic. 2   Pic. 3

Pic. 4   Pic. 5

(1) susceptible host, (2) pathogenic agents, and (3) environment unfavorable to host and favorable to agent(s). Disease agents always try to find a proper host → then a way for internal access → find a home → and then multiply in the present host until they can be transmitted to a new host. By the nature of agent, infection may be acute (high degree of mortality in short period of time, i.e., virus), chronic (gradual mortality, i.e., bacteria), or latent (little or no mortality).

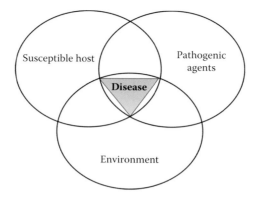

Drugs and chemicals are the easiest and most common ways to control diseases, and they have been used for centuries. In the past, people used only traditional chemicals like salt, potassium permanganate, formalin, and bleaching powder to control infection (especially in aquatic bodies), but today, several drugs and antibiotics are produced by pharmaceutical companies. The antibiotics used frequently in aquaculture are oxytetracycline, chlorotetracycline, amoxicillin, cotrimoxazole, and sulfamethoxazole [1]. They remain in aquatic environments for a long time, with detrimental side effects, including the emergence of antibiotic-resistant bacteria, the presence of antibiotic residue in the flesh, and variations in aquaculture environment microbiota [2,3]. The use of such chemotherapeutic medications as disease control measures has become questionable because of the development of resistant species of pathogens [4–6]. Drugs and chemicals have had a positive impact on aqua production and disease recovery, but they cause remarkable pathological changes in fish and create harmful resistant power in microbes. This in turn has led to a quest for alternative antibiotics and vaccinations to prevent the diseases [7,8].

Some alternative strategies, such as vaccination and immune-stimulants, have emerged. Vaccination cannot prevent disease outbreaks in immunologically immature individuals [9]. Live microbial feed supplements, such as probiotics, benefit the host by improving its intestinal balance and act as immunostimulant for the body. Probiotics are becoming the most beneficial and cost-effective disease prevention strategies.

Parker (1974) [10] defines probiotics as "[o]rganisms and substances which contribute to intestinal microbial balance." Probiotics are microorganisms (such as friendly bacteria) that provide healthful benefits. A healthy environment requires a balance between the beneficial bacteria and bad bacteria, a phenomenon known as eubiosis. Dysbiosis is the respective imbalance, when harmful bacteria proliferate and disease occurs, which can lead to heavy economic losses.

The term *probiotic* originates from the Greek words "pro" and "bios," and means "for life" [11]. Élie Metchnikoff, a Russian analyst, presented first described probiotics in the early 1900s when he observes the longevity of Bulgarian workers who drank fermented milk items [12]. Lilly and Stillwell (1965) originally used the concept of probiotics to mean a substance which stimulates growth of other microorganisms [13,14]. That's why the principle of probiotics refers both to a response to diseases but also the improvement of the ambient environment.

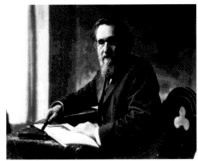
Élie Metchnikoff, 1845–1916

Microbial adjuncts are designed to do the following:

1. Prevent the proliferation of pathogens in the gut or elsewhere.
2. Improve digestibility.
3. Deliver improved nutrition to aquatics.
4. Enhance host response to acquired diseases.
5. Improve environmental quality.

CHARACTERISTICS OF PROBIOTIC BACTERIA

The main purpose of probiotics is to establish or maintain the association between useful and harmful bacteria that are usually present in the intestines or gut [15,16]. Many obstacles to be overcome in probiotic research are due to the selection of the wrong microorganisms, which need to be adjusted for different situations and host species. For the selection of probiotics, it is imperative to comprehend the mechanisms of probiotic activity [17].

The reliability of effective probiotics depend on certain qualities of each probiotic. To have a positive impact on the growth of beneficial microbiota or to protect the host against various pathogenic bacteria, the microbes form an association with the host's gut, resulting in the formation of essential substances analogous to vitamins [16]. The first criterion that probiotics must meet to be able to colonize the host is the ability to attach to the host. Viability factors also play an important role in the attachment of probiotics with the host [18,19]. When probiotics are given to the host, they must have no negative side effects on the host species [20,21]. Various tests, such as the challenge test, grip test, and test of enmity, can be performed to check the potential of probiotics in in vitro conditions [22].

For use as a probiotic, bacteria must meet the following criteria:

- Resistance to stomach acid.
- Ability to attach to the intestinal epithelia and colonize.
- Nonpathogenic and nontoxic properties.
- Ability to impart beneficial effects on the host.
- Stability of desired characteristics during processing, storage, and transportation
- Anti-inflammatory, antimutagenic, and immunostimulatory properties.

Techniques for *In Vitro* Evaluation of Desired Probiotic Bacteria for Pisciculture

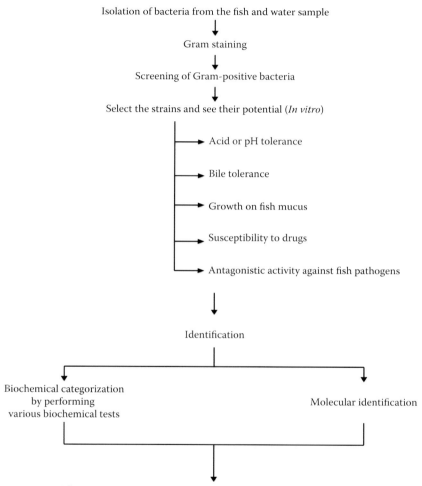

Isolation of bacteria from the fish and water sample

↓

Gram staining

↓

Screening of Gram-positive bacteria

↓

Select the strains and see their potential (*In vitro*)

→ Acid or pH tolerance

→ Bile tolerance

→ Growth on fish mucus

→ Susceptibility to drugs

→ Antagonistic activity against fish pathogens

↓

Identification

Biochemical categorization by performing various biochemical tests

Molecular identification

↓

After *In vitro, In vivo* evaluation as probiotic activity and optimization!

Acid and Bile Tolerance

Inoculate the culture bacteria in broth with pH levels of 2, 3, 4, 5, and 6 at 37°C for 24–48 hours. After this, observe the culture tubes for the presence of growth or count the number of viable cells by using the plate-counting method. Agar medium that contains 0.3% ox-gall is used to check the bile tolerance. Determine the viability by counting the value of colony-forming units per milliliter (CFU/mL).

Growth of Bacteria on Fish Mucus

Collect the mucus from the skin and intestines of fish immediately after killing them. Sterilized mucus that is not inoculated serves as the control. To determine viable bacterial cells in mucus, dilute (up to 10^{-5}) 24, 48, and 72 hours. Inoculate the cultures (0.1 mL) onto agar plates, and incubate at 30°C for 24 hours. Count the CFU/mL.

Salt Tolerance

Salt tolerance is estimated by observing the growth rate of bacteria in agar medium with different salt concentrations, that is, 2%, 3%, 4%, 5%, 6%, and 7%. In the salt-containing medium, 0.1 mL of culture bacteria is inoculated. Incubate at 37°C for 24–48 hours.

Gastric and Pancreatic Juice Tolerance

The gastric and pancreatic juices are prepared by adding 3 g/L of pepsin and 1 g/L of pancreatin in sterile saline and adjusting the pH to 2.0 and 8.0 by using HCl or NaOH, respectively. The viability of bacteria is determined by plating the gastric juice–treated bacteria onto De Man, Rogosa, and Sharpe (MRS) agar medium.

Susceptibility to Drugs

Susceptibility of bacteria to various antibiotics like ampicillin, amoxicillin, penicillin, cloxacillin, chloramphenicol, ciprofloxacin, tetracycline, kanamycin, vancomycin, methicillin, gentamycin, and erythromycin can be checked by the disc diffusion method on Mueller Hinton Agar (MHA) plates with octadiscs. The zone of inhibition determines that either a bacterium is resistant (no clear zone) or it is not resistant (clear zone) after an incubation period of 24 hours.

Antagonistic Activity against Common Fish Pathogens

The antagonistic activity of probiotic bacteria can be evaluated by the cross-streaking method, agar well-diffusion method, and pour plate method by using several pathogens: *Aeromonas hydrophila*, *Aeromonas salmonicida*, *Vibrio anguillarium*, *Flavobacterium* species, and so on. Spread the 100 µL of each the test organisms listed above onto Mueller-Hinton agar plates, make the wells 6 mm in diameter, fill with live culture of isolates, and incubate the petri plates for 24 hours. Then observe the zone of inhibition to determine the activity against the disease-causing fish pathogens.

POSSIBLE MODES OF ACTION

The modes of action for probiotics is an emerging field, so less is known about them currently. What is known about the modes of action are largely circumstantial and based on imperial arguments. Possible modes of actions include the following:

1. *Competition for space.* Pathogenic bacteria require attachment to the mucosal layer of the host gastrointestinal tract to initiate development of a disease. An important mechanism of action in probiotic bacteria is competition for adhesion sites, also known as "competitive exclusion."

2. *Production of inhibitory substances.* Probiotic bacteria produce substances with bactericidal or bacteriostatic effects on other microbial populations [23], such as bacteriocins, hydrogen peroxide, siderophores, lysozymes, proteases, among many others [24,25].
3. *Competition for nutrients.* The existence of any microbial population depends on its ability to compete for nutrients and available energy with other microbes in the same environment [26]. Probiotics can out-contend the pathogens by expending the supplements that would somehow be devoured by pathogenic microorganisms.
4. *Improving water quality.* Application of gram-positive bacteria, such as *Bacillus* spp., is beneficial in improving the quality of the water system. *Bacillus* spp. convert organic matter into carbon dioxide more efficiently compared to the gram-negative bacteria, which converts a greater proportion of organic matter into bacterial biomass or slime [6,27].
5. *Disruption of quorum sensing.* Quorum sensing (QS) is a bacterial regulatory mechanism that is responsible for controlling the expression of various biological macromolecules such as the virulence factors in a cell density–dependent manner. Biodegradation of N-Acyl homoserine lactones (AHLs) proves to be an efficient way to interrupt QS because AHLs are the main family of QS auto-inducers used in gram-negative bacteria [28].

TYPES OF PROBIOTIC BACTERIA USED IN AQUACULTURE

Two types of probiotics are (1) natural and (2) manufactured, or business, probiotics. Probiotic microbes can be segregated from the gastrointestinal tract (GIT) of a fish, that is, from the gut, stomach, gill, kidney, and gonads. They can likewise be obtained from the interior organs of different animals [29].

The business sources for probiotics include already synthesized probiotics and those commercially available. The probiotic microorganisms used most often are those from *Lactobacillus* or *Bifidobacterium* species. Portions of the financially accessible probiotics are shown in the table below [29]:

1. *Lactobacillus* Species	2. *Bifidobacterium* Species
Lactobacillus acidophilus	*Bifidobacterium bifidum*
Lactobacillus casei	*Bifidobacterium breve*
Lactobacillus fermentum	*Bifidobacterium lactis*
Lactobacillus gasseri	*Bifidobacterium longum*
Lactobacillus lactis	3. *Streptococcus* Species
Lactobacillus plantarum	*Streptococcus thermophiles*
Lactobacillus salivarius	*Streptococcus cremoris*
Lactobacillus rhamnosus	4. *Saccharomyces* Species
Lactobacillus johnsonii	*Saccharomyces boulardii*
Lactobacillus paracasei	5. *Bacillus* Species
Lactobacillus reuteri	*Bacillus subtilis*
Lactobacillus helveticus	*Bacillus cereus*
Lactobacillus bulgaricus	*Bacillus pumilus*

HOW TO SELECT PROBIOTIC STRAINS

The aim of probiotics is maintaining or reestablishing the balance between good and bad microbes that comprise the microbiota of the intestinal or skin mucus of a host. Beneficial probiotics are those that have certain qualities to address certain conditions for the host. With a specific end goal of advancing beneficial development or combating certain pathogens, the strains should also be able to colonize the host by attachment [16] and deliver critical substances such as vitamins. Attachment is the most critical criterion for probiotic microorganisms because it is essential for colonization [18]. The microorganisms must be viable for long stretches under capacity and in field conditions [19], although nonviable microbes have the capacity to hold fast to tissue culture cells, showing attachment without conferring any benefits to the host [20,21]. Probiotic microorganisms must be nonpathogenic and nontoxic to the host species to avoid any detrimental side effects. Enmity, grip, and challenge tests in in vitro conditions are necessary to choose among the probiotic species [22].

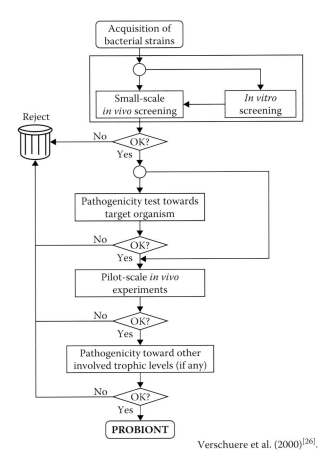

Verschuere et al. (2000)[26].

AQUACULTURE

Aquaculture is the most important and rapidly growing sector to meet the food demands of an increasing global human population. It has a large role in achieving global protein food availability. Different types of fish are dominant in aquaculture, with more than 200 species of fish produced for commercial sale. Because of the diversity and nutritional value of many types of fish, fisheries always attract attention from farmers and from researchers or fishery engineers to improve quality and productivity. But a high production of fish by intense aquaculture practices, high stocking densities of fish, the decay of biotic materials, and intense feeding and fertilization cause not only stress and health issues but also degrade water quality. The slurry water influences the proliferation of pathogenic microorganisms, which cause disease and reduce aquaculture productivity [30]. Fish are permanently exposed to different external hazards because of their intimate contact with the aquatic habitat. Microbial infection is an important and limiting factor in intensive fish production because it diverts energy toward immunity development and health maintenance. The body of a fish acts as a platform for bacterial growth, but due to immunity in adult fish, major problems are generally avoided. Pathogenic bacteria have the potential to proliferate or maintain themselves in the aquatic environment, and they are constantly taken up by the fish through feeding and osmoregulation processes [31]. Microorganisms emit extracellular enzymes or toxins that can harm the intestinal coating. Recently, the rate of contamination and cell harm (particularly the assault on tight junctions and desmosomes) has increased [32].

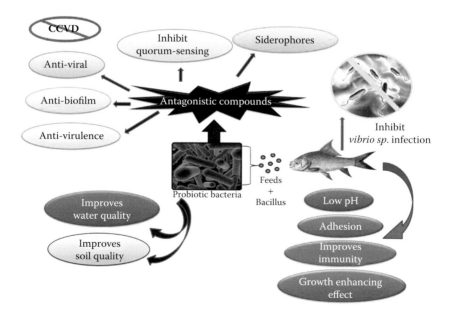

The physiological effects from using probiotic microorganisms are a decrease in the pH level of the gut; production of some digestive chemicals; creation of antimicrobial secretions, for example, organic acids, H_2O_2, bacteriocins, diacetyl, lactoperoxidase, acetaldehyde, lactones, and other unidentified substances; reproduction of ordinary gut microflora modifications brought on by diarrhea; antimicrobial treatment; reduced blood cholesterol levels; increased immune function; concealment of microbial diseases; reduction in the number of cancer-causing agents; changes in calcium ingestion; and a decrease in fecal enzyme activity [33–36].

Toward the beginning of the twentieth century, probiotics were thought to benefit the host by enhancing intestinal microbial parity, therefore hindering pathogens and toxin-releasing microorganisms [12]. Today, specific benefits are being researched and archived, including interminable intestinal incendiary maladies [37], treatment of pathogen-instigated looseness of the bowels and urogenital diseases [38], and atopic sicknesses [39].

Lactic acid bacteria (LABs) are gram-positive, anaerobic, and catalase negative, and they do not form spores and lack cytochromes. Most general microorganisms are used as starters for the modern preparation of fermented dairy, meat, vegetable, and grain items. Decrease in pH levels and transformation of sugars to natural acids are the essential protective activities that these microorganisms give to fermented foods [40]. The isolated microorganisms were distinguished as *Lactobacillus* species by watching their morphological qualities and by Gram staining, motility test, catalase test, endospore test, and milk coagulation experiments [41].

Lactobacilli are critical probiotic microbes that hinder undesirable microflora in the gut and maintain balance in the midst of intestinal pathogens. Their biochemical makeup is the essential part of recognizing the culture or the isolates obtained. The catalase test is the exclusive test for identifying *Lactobacilli* species.

Catalase is a typical enzyme found in nearly every single living creature that breathes. It catalyzes hydrogen peroxide to form water and oxygen [42]. Hydrogen peroxide is a destructive by-product of numerous ordinary metabolic procedures. To avoid harm, it must be immediately changed into other, less dangerous substances. Catalase is frequently used by cells to quickly catalyze H_2O_2 into oxygen and water particles. Probiotic isolates, according to Bergey's manual, are catalase negative, which is a desirable characteristic of probiotics [43].

Not enough satisfactory research has been done on probiotics in pond aquaculture. This is unfortunate because numerous organizations are marketing these items, and they maintain that probiotics can improve the environment and enhance production. The standard methodology is to use low concentrations of probiotics for remediation and higher focuses when a particular issue has been identified [44].

The healthful benefits of *Lactobacillus acidophillus* and *Bifidobacterium* spp. have led to their expanded use in dairy food, for example, yogurt. On the other hand, these probiotic microorganisms do not survive as long as the shelf life of yogurt [45].

High stocking density to raise profitability has been followed by biological effects, including the development of a broad variety of pathogens and bacterial resistance. These effects are caused to some extent by the indiscriminate use of chemotherapeutic drugs as an aftereffect of management practices in production series. The utility of antibacterial agents as preventive measures has been addressed, and the development of antibacterial resistance among pathogenic microbes has been well documented [46]. The use of probiotics or other beneficial microorganisms, which control pathogens via many factors, is progressively seen as a distinct option for antibiotic treatment. The use of probiotics in human and animal foods is well documented [47–49]; recently, probiotics have started to be used in aquaculture [22,26,46,50–52].

Starliper (2011) concluded that cold water disease (CWD) is a bacterial illness that influences a broad range of animal and fish groups that inhabit cold and freshwater. CWD occurs in cultured and free-range fish populations, but hatchery-reared young trout and salmon species are especially vulnerable. *Flavobacterium psychrophilum* is the etiological agent of CWD, and no vaccines are commercially available to protect fish against the disease [53].

Because of their habitat, fish are in ceaseless contact with complex and dynamic microbiota, some of which may have repercussions for the well-being of fish. The manipulation of the host microflora may signify a new avenue for the inhibition or management of pathological and physiological disorders [54].

In aquaculture, the use of *Bacillus* probiotics enhances water quality. The gram-positive microbes are better converters of natural matter back to CO_2 than are gram-negative microorganisms. Large numbers of gram-positive microbes can minimize the development of dissolved and particulate natural carbon. *Bacillus* sp. enhances water quality, improves the survival and development rates of aquatic living beings, and reduces diseases [55]. Among the *Bacillus* spp., some of the species that have been most widely analyzed are *B. subtilis, B. clausii, B. cereus, B. coagulans, and B. licheniformis*. Spores that are heat-stable have a number of advantages because products made from them can be dried and stored at room temperature without reducing viability, and the spore is capable of surviving in the low pH of the gastric barrier [56,57].

Vine and his colleagues isolated the microbes from the gut of clownfish (*Amphiprion percula*) under sterile conditions and investigated their *in vitro* potential against fish pathogens such as *Aeromonas salmonicida, Vibrio harveyi, Vibrio anguillarium*, and *Vibrio damsela*. All five candidate probiotics (AP1, AP2, AP3, AP4, and AP5) showed antagonism to various aquatic pathogens. Candidate probiotic AP3 showed the greatest antagonistic activity against aquatic pathogens. The researchers also investigated the potential of probiotics to grow in fish mucus by growing them in marine broth and fish intestinal mucus [58].

Balcazar et al. (2008) isolated the LAB strains from the intestinal microbiota of rainbow trout and investigated the in vitro adhesion assay, pH, and bile tolerance activity by growing the probiotics in a range of pH levels (1.0–6.5) by adding HCl and 2.5%–10% v/v fish bile and determined the viable bacteria by the plate count method using MRS agar. Antimicrobial activity against several fish pathogens (*Aeromonas hydrophila, Aeromonas salmonicida, Yersinia ruckeri*, and *Vibrio anguillarum*) was determined by the disc-diffusion method using Mueller-Hinton agar. The outcomes demonstrate that only *Lc. lactis* (CLFP 101) reduced the attachment of all fish pathogens, whereas *L. plantarum* (CLFP 238) reduced the attachment of *A. hydrophila* and *A. salmonicida*. With the exception of *V. anguillarum*, the adhesion of all fish pathogens to intestinal mucus was reduced by *L. fermentum* (CLFP 242) and by a mixture of the three LAB strains. In addition, only *Lc. lactis* (CLFP 101) showed antibacterial activities against all fish pathogens. All LAB strains had the capacity to survive in relatively low pH levels and in high fish bile concentrations. Based on the positive results of this study, *Lc. lactis* (CLFP 101), *L. plantarum* (CLFP 238), and *L. fermentum* (CLFP 242) should be further studied to investigate their probiotic effects [4].

Microbes (i.e., *Bacillus* spp. *Bacillus laterosporus, Bacillus subtilis, Lactobacillus* spp. *and Lactococcus lactis*) from the digestive tract of different healthy fish were investigated for their antagonistic capacity against pathogenic bacteria (*Citrobacter freundii, Enterobacter sakasakii, Klebsiella oxytoca, Proteus vulgaris*, and *Vibrio fluvialis*) at different dilutions (10^9, 10^8, 10^7, 10^6, 10^5, and 10^4). Probiotic strains of *B. subtilis* were better at inhibiting the growth of pathogenic bacteria *P. vulgaris*, *E. sakazakii, V. fluvialis, K. oxytoca*, and *C. freundii* in most of the tested dilutions. *E. sakazakii* does not show sensitivity to *B. laterosporus* (10^6, 10^5, and 10^4 dilutions), *Lactobacillus* sp. (10^9, 10^6, and 10^4 dilutions), and *Bacillus* sp. (10^6 and 10^4 dilutions). Other dilutions with the used probiotic gave a positive result in sensitivity against the employed pathogen. *K. oxytoca* pathogen does not show sensitivity to *B. subtilis* (10^6 dilution), *B. laterosporus* (10^8, 10^7, 10^6, 10^5, and 10^4 dilutions), and *Lactobacillus* sp. (10^9, 10^8, 10^7, and 10^6 dilutions). Only probiotic *L. lactis* gave a positive result against *K. oxytoca* [59,60].

Jamal and Faragi isolated the bacteria from the intestines of 50 common carp and grew them on nutrient agar supplemented with 1.5% NaCl (w/v). They investigated the inhibition activity of selected *B. subtilis* against *Aeromonas hydrophila*. The results showed that *Bacillus subtilis* could produce antibacterial substances at the highest levels in 2 days, and that amount was about 4.8 mm as measured by the size of the clear zone. Thus, it has been exhibited that *Bacillus subtilis* delivered some antimicrobial substances that could restrain or strongly exclude the development of the pathogenic microbes. *Bacillus* spp. could protect aquatic animals against the disease caused by pathogenic microbes and may be applied as a beneficial probiotic in aquaculture [61].

The bacterial isolated from the gut of *Labeo rohita* tolerated low pH levels (2.0–5.0) and high bile concentrations (2%–6% v/v) during the experiment by Giri et al. The probiotic strains were also capable of adhering to intestinal mucus but not to skin mucus. All the isolates were susceptible to amoxicillin, penicillin, gentamycin, ampicillin, and so on, and showed strong protective characteristics against *A. salmonicida*, *A. hydrophila, V. harveyi*, and *V. alginolyticus. Bacillus subtilis* (VSG1) failed to show antimicrobial effects against *V. alginolyticus* (MTCC4439), but it did show moderate activity against other pathogens. The researchers concluded that these selected strains should be further examined to address their probiotic impacts on fish in in vivo settings. These isolates should be further examined by via test analyses on fish to discover if these probiotics can work in real-life situations [62,63].

A probiotic blend may be more powerful than applying a solitary species because not all desirable probiotic attributes are present in a solitary isolated strain. The quick spread of multiresistant bacterial pathogens has made it necessary to create alternative techniques for fighting pathogens. New substances are needed for efficient antibacterial activity against drug-resistant strains [64]. Today, fish aquaculture is experiencing setbacks because of incurable diseases. The use of antimicrobial medications, pesticides, and disinfectants in aquaculture for infection prevention and growth advancement has prompted the development of resistant strains of microbes. Thus, there is increased interest in research into the use of eco-friendly probiotics for sustainable aquaculture. The advantages of such supplements would enhance feed value, enzymatic contribution to digestion, inhibition of pathogenic microbes, and increased immune response. These probiotics are safe microbes that are beneficial to the host animal and contribute, directly or indirectly, to protect the host animal against harmful bacterial pathogens. The researchers concluded that the use of probiotics in aquaculture needs additional significant further research to confirm the viability of probiotics for use in aquaculture [65].

Probiotics play a very important role in maintaining optimum water quality parameters like dissolved oxygen, ammonia, phosphates, nitrite, nitrate, bacterial loads, and zooplanktons throughout the culture period. Their use resulted in better growth and survival of fish species in aquaculture ponds [30].

The effectiveness of probiotic isolates from tropical freshwater species has not been studied extensively and requires detailed exploration [63]. Starting about two decades ago, probiotics are used more frequently in aquaculture. The use of commercial probiotics in fish is somewhat futile (incapable of producing any useful results), however, because most of the commercial formulations contain strains isolated from nonfish sources and might not remain viable at high cell density in the intestinal microenvironment of fish. Also screening and characterization of efficient probiotic isolates from tropical freshwater species has not been studied as much and thus merits require further exploration [66].

CONCLUSION

The use of probiotics in aquaculture is a safe and useful technique for mitigating the harmful effects of excessive use of antibiotics. Because of its uncertainty and slow action, it is not in regular practice. Education, awareness, and support are needed to bring the issue to the fore. A major problem with the use of probiotics in aquaculture is the lack of diversity of probiotics. Available effective strains act and maintain habitat (water and soil quality) of the host, and studies are needed to determine which strains benefit which species of fish. Uncertainty and ineffectiveness are the result of using strains isolated from different habitats (terrestrial and fermented food). For aquaculture, probiotic strains should be selected from aquatic fauna, flora, and their habitats. *In vivo* testing is necessary for all strains.

REFERENCES

1. Plumb, J. A., 1992. Disease control in aquaculture. Disease in Asian Aquaculture. Fish health Section of the Asian Fisheries Society, Manila, Philippines, 3–17.
2. Munoz-Atienzal, E., Gomez-Sala, B., Araujo, C., Campanerol, C., Del Campo, R., et al. 2013. Antibiotic susceptibility and virulence factors of Lactic Acid Bacteria of aquatic origin intended for use as probiotics in aquaculture. *BMC Microbiology*, *13*, 15.
3. Azevedo, R. V. D., Fosse Filho, J. C., Cardoso, L. D., Mattos, D. D. C., Junior, V., et al. 2015. Economic evaluation of prebiotics, probiotics and symbiotics in juvenile Nile tilapia. *Revista Ciencia Agronomica*, *46*(1), 72–79.

4. Balcazar, J. L., Vendrell, D., de Blas, I., Ruiz-Zarzuela, I., Muzquiz, J. L., and Girones, O., 2008. Characterization of probiotic properties of lactic acid bacteria isolated from intestinal microbiota of fish. *Aquaculture, 278*(1), 188–191.
5. Mancuso, M., Rappazzo, A. C., Genovese, M., El Hady, M., Ghonimy, A., et al. 2015. In vitro selection of bacteria and isolation of probionts from farmed Sparus aurata with potential for use as probiotics. *International Journal of Animal Biology, 1*(4), 93–98.
6. Luis Balcazar, J., Decamp, O., Vendrell, D., De Blas, I., and Ruiz-Zarzuela, I., 2006. Health and nutritional properties of probiotics in fish and shellfish. *Microbial Ecology in Health and Disease, 18*(2), 65–70.
7. Kwon, A. S., Kang, B. J., Jun, S. Y., Yoon, S. J., Lee, J. H., and Kang, S. H., 2017. Evaluating the effectiveness of Streptococcus parauberis bacteriophage Str-PAP-1 as an environmentally friendly alternative to antibiotics for aquaculture. *Aquaculture, 468,* 464–470.
8. McEwen, S. A., and Fedorka-Cray, P. J., 2002. Antimicrobial use and resistance in animals. *Clinical Infectious Diseases, 34*(Supplement 3), S93–S106.
9. Defoirdt, T., Boon, N., Sorgeloos, P., Verstraete, W., and Bossier, P., 2007. Alternatives to antibiotics to control bacterial infections: Luminescent vibriosis in aquaculture as an example. *Trends in Biotechnology, 25*(10), 472–479.
10. Paker, R. B., 1974. Probiotics, the other half of the antibiotics story. *Aimal Nutrition & Health, 29,* 4–8.
11. Gismondo, M. R., Drago, L., and Lombardi, A., 1999. Review of probiotics available to modify gastrointestinal flora. *International Journal of Antimicrobial Agents, 12*(4), 287–292.
12. Metchnikoff E., 1907. *The Prolongation of Life. Optimistic Studies.* London, UK: William Heinemann.
13. Lilly, D. M., and Stillwell, R. H., 1965. Probiotics: Growth-promoting factors produced by microorganisms. *Science, 147*(3659), 747–748.
14. Chukeatirote, E., 2003. Potential use of probiotics. *Songklanakarin Journal of Science Technology, 25,* 275–282.
15. Thirumurugan, R., and Vignesh, V., 2015. Probiotics: Live boon to aquaculture. In *Advances in Marine and Brackishwater Aquaculture* (pp. 51–61). New Delhi, India: Springer.
16. Olsson, J. C., Westerdahl, A., Conway, P. L., and Kjelleberg, S., 1992. Intestinal colonization potential of turbot (Scophthalmus maximus)-and dab (Limanda limanda)-associated bacteria with inhibitory effects against Vibrio anguillarum. *Applied and Environmental Microbiology, 58*(2), 551–556.
17. Havenaar, R., and Marteau, P. 1994., Establishing a scientific basis for probiotic R&D. *Trends in Biotechnology, 12,* 6–8.
18. Beachey, E. H., 1981. Bacterial adherence: Adhesin-receptor interactions mediating the attachment of bacteria to mucosal surfaces. *Journal of Infectious Diseases, 143*(3), 325–345.
19. Fuller, R. 1989. Probiotics in man and animals. *Journal of Applied Bacteriology, 66*(5), 365–378.
20. Hood, S. K., and Zoitola, E. A., 1988. Effect of low pH on the ability of Lactobacillus acidophilus to survive and adhere to human intestinal cells. *Journal of Food Science, 53*(5), 1514–1516.
21. Coconnier, M. H., Bernet, M. F., Chauvière, G., and Servin, A. L., 1993. Adhering heat-killed human Lactobacillus acidophilus, strain LB, inhibits the process of pathogenicity of diarrhoeagenic bacteria in cultured human intestinal cells. *Journal of Diarrhoeal Diseases Research,* 235–242.

22. Gatesoupe, F. J., 1999. The use of probiotics in aquaculture. *Aquaculture, 180*(1), 147–165.
23. Servin, A. L., 2004. Antagonistic activities of lactobacilli and bifidobacteria against microbial pathogens. *FEMS Microbiology Reviews, 28*(4), 405–440.
24. Panigrahi, A., and Azad, I. S., 2007. Microbial intervention for better fish health in aquaculture: The Indian scenario. *Fish Physiology and Biochemistry, 33*(4), 429–440.
25. Tinh, N. T. N., Dierckens, K., Sorgeloos, P., and Bossier, P., 2008. A review of the functionality of probiotics in the larviculture food chain. *Marine Biotechnology, 10*(1), 1–12.
26. Verschuere, L., Rombaut, G., Sorgeloos, P., and Verstraete, W., 2000. Probiotic bacteria as biological control agents in aquaculture. *Microbiology and Molecular Biology Reviews, 64*(4), 655–671.
27. Mohapatra, S., Chakraborty, T., Kumar, V., DeBoeck, G., and Mohanta, K. N., 2013. Aquaculture and stress management: A review of probiotic intervention. *Journal of Animal Physiology and Animal Nutrition, 97*(3), 405–430.
28. Chu, W., Zhou, S., Zhu, W., and Zhuang, X., 2014. Quorum quenching bacteria Bacillus sp. QSI-1 protect zebrafish (Danio rerio) from Aeromonas hydrophila infection. *Scientific Reports, 4*, 5446.
29. Nwanna, L. C., 2015. Use of probiotics in aquaculture. *Applied Tropical Agriculture, 15*(2), 76–83.
30. Sunitha, K., and Padmavathi, P., 2013. Influence of probiotics on water quality and fish yield in fish ponds. *International Journal of Pure and Applied Sciences and Technology, 19*(2), 48.
31. Hansen, G. H., and Olafsen, J. A., 1999. Bacterial interactions in early life stages of marine cold water fish. *Microbial Ecology, 38*(1), 1–26.
32. Ringø, E., Løvmo, L., Kristiansen, M., Bakken, Y., Salinas, I., et al. 2010. Lactic acid bacteria vs. pathogens in the gastrointestinal tract of fish: A review. *Aquaculture Research, 41*(4), 451–467.
33. Zubillaga, M., Weill, R., Postaire, E., Goldman, C., Caro, R., and Boccio, J., 2001. Effect of probiotics and functional foods and their use in different diseases. *Nutrition Research, 21*(3), 569–579.
34. Holzapfel, W. H., and Schillinger, U., 2002. Introduction to pre-and probiotics. *Food Research International, 35*(2), 109–116.
35. Ouwehand, A. C., Kirjavainen, P. V., Grönlund, M. M., Isolauri, E., and Salminen, S. J., 1999. Adhesion of probiotic micro-organisms to intestinal mucus. *International Dairy Journal, 9*(9), 623–630.
36. Ouwehand, A. C., Kirjavainen, P. V., Shortt, C., and Salminen, S., 1999. Probiotics: Mechanisms and established effects. *International Dairy Journal, 9*(1), 43–52.
37. Mach, T., 2006. Clinical usefulness of probiotics. *Journal of Physiology and Pharmacology, 57*(2333), 89.
38. Yan, F., and Polk, D. B., 2006. Probiotics as functional food in the treatment of diarrhea. *Current Opinion in Clinical Nutrition & Metabolic Care, 9*(6), 717–721.
39. Vanderhoof, J. A., 2008. Probiotics in allergy management. *Journal of Pediatric Gastroenterology and Nutrition, 47*, S38–S40.
40. Axelsson, L. T., Chung, T. C., Dobrogosz, W. J., and Lindgren, S. E., 1989. Production of a broad spectrum antimicrobial substance by Lactobacillus reuteri. *Microbial Ecology in Health and Disease, 2*(2), 131–136.
41. Hoque, M. Z., Akter, F., Hossain, K. M., Rahman, M. S. M., Billah, M. M., and Islam, K. M., D. 2010. Isolation, identification and analysis of probiotic properties of Lactobacillus spp. from selective regional yoghurts. *World Journal of Dairy & Food Sciences, 5*(1), 39–46.

42. Chelikani, P., Fita, I., and Loewen, P. C., 2004. Diversity of structures and properties among catalases. *Cellular and Molecular Life Sciences*, *61*(2), 192–208.

43. Gaetani, G. F., Ferraris, A. M., Rolfo, M., Mangerini, R., Arena, S., and Kirkman, H. N., 1996. Predominant role of catalase in the disposal of hydrogen peroxide within human erythrocytes. *Blood*, *87*(4), 1595–1599.

44. Boyd, C. E., and Gross, A., 1998. Use of probiotics for improving soil and water quality in aquaculture ponds. *Advances in Shrimp Biotechnology*, 101–105.

45. Talwalkar, A., and Kailasapathy, K., 2004. The role of oxygen in the viability of probiotic bacteria with reference to L. acidophilus and Bifidobacterium spp. *Current Issues in Intestinal Microbiology*, *5*(1), 1–8.

46. Balcázar, J. L., De Blas, I., Ruiz-Zarzuela, I., Cunningham, D., Vendrell, D., and Muzquiz, J. L., 2006. The role of probiotics in aquaculture. *Veterinary Microbiology*, *114*(3), 173–186.

47. Fuller, R., 1992. History and development of probiotics. In: Fuller, R. (Ed) *Probiotics: The Scientific Basis*. London, UK: Chapman and Hall, pp. 1–45.

48. Mulder, R. W. A. W., Havenaar, R., and Huis, J. H. J., 1997. Intervention strategies: The use of probiotics and competitive exclusion microfloras against contamination with pathogens in pigs and poultry. In *Probiotics 2* (pp. 187–207). Dordrecht, the Netherlands: Springer.

49. Rinkinen, M., Jalava, K., Westermarck, E., Salminen, S., and Ouwehand, A. C., 2003. Interaction between probiotic lactic acid bacteria and canine enteric pathogens: A risk factor for intestinal Enterococcus faecium colonization. *Veterinary Microbiology*, *92*(1), 111–119.

50. Gomez-Gil, B., Roque, A., and Turnbull, J. F., 2000. The use and selection of probiotic bacteria for use in the culture of larval aquatic organisms. *Aquaculture*, *191*(1), 259–270.

51. Irianto, A., and Austin, B., 2002. Use of probiotics to control furunculosis in rainbow trout, Oncorhynchus mykiss (Walbaum). *Journal of Fish Diseases*, *25*(6), 333–342.

52. Bachère, E., 2003. Anti-infectious immune effectors in marine invertebrates: Potential tools for disease control in larviculture. *Aquaculture*, *227*(1), 427–438.

53. Starliper, C. E., 2011. Bacterial coldwater disease of fishes caused by Flavobacterium psychrophilum. *Journal of Advanced Research*, *2*(2), 97–108.

54. Perez, T., Balcázar, J. L., Ruiz-Zarzuela, I., Halaihel, N., Vendrell, D., et al. 2010. Host–microbiota interactions within the fish intestinal ecosystem. *Mucosal Immunology*, 3(4), 355–360.

55. Dalmin, G., Kathiresan, K., and Purushothaman, A., 2001. Effect of probiotics on bacterial population and health status of shrimp in culture pond ecosystem. *Indian Journal of Experimental Biology*, 39, 939–942.

56. Barbosa, T. M., Serra, C. R., La Ragione, R. M., Woodward, M. J., and Henriques, A. O., 2005. Screening for Bacillus isolates in the broiler gastrointestinal tract. *Applied and Environmental Microbiology*, *71*(2), 968–978.

57. Spinosa, M. R., Braccini, T., Ricca, E., De Felice, M., Morelli, L., et al. 2000. On the fate of ingested Bacillus spores. *Research in Microbiology*, *151*(5), 361–368.

58. Vine, N. G., Leukes, W. D., and Kaiser, H., 2004. In vitro growth characteristics of five candidate aquaculture probiotics and two fish pathogens grown in fish intestinal mucus. *FEMS Microbiology Letters*, *231*(1), 145–152.

59. Monroy-Dosta, M. C., Castro-Barrera, T., Fernández-Perrino, F. J., and Mayorga-Reyes, L., 2010. Inhibition of Aeromonas hydrophila by probiotic strains isolated from the digestive tract of Pterophyllum scalare. *Revista Mexicana de Ingeniería Química*, *9*(1), 37–42.

60. Monroy-Dosta, M. C., Castro-Mejia, J., Castro-Mejia, G., De Lara-Andrade, R., Ocampo-Cervantes, J. A., and Cruz-Cruz, I., 2015. Use of five probiotic strains to determine sensitivity in vitro on pathogenic bacteria growth isolated from sick fishes. *Digital Journal of El Hombrey su Ambiente Department*, *1*(7), 23–28.

61. Al-Faragi, J. K., and Alsaphar, S. A., 2012. Isolation and identification of Bacillus subtilus as (probiotic) from intestinal microflora of common carp Cyprinus carpio L. In *Proceedings of the Eleventh Veterinary Scientific Conference*, Vol. 355, p. 361.

62. Giri, S. S., Sukumaran, V., and Dangi, N. K., 2012. Characteristics of bacterial isolates from the gut of freshwater fish, *Labeo rohita* that may be useful as potential probiotic bacteria. *Probiotics and Antimicrobial Proteins*, 4(4), 238–242.

63. Sahoo, T. K., Jena, P. K., Nagar, N., Patel, A. K., and Seshadri, S., 2015. In vitro evaluation of probiotic properties of lactic acid bacteria from the gut of Labeo rohita and Catla catla. *Probiotics and Antimicrobial Proteins*, 7(2), 126–136.

64. Balakrishna, A., and Keerthi, T. R., 2012. Screening of potential aquatic probiotics from the major microflora of guppies (Poecilia reticulata). *Frontiers of Chemical Science and Engineering*, 6(2), 163–173.

65. Pandiyan, P., Balaraman, D., Thirunavukkarasu, R., George, E. G. J., Subaramaniyan, K., et al. 2013. Probiotics in aquaculture. *Drug Invention Today*, 5(1), 55–59.

66. Dutta, D., and Ghosh, K., 2015. Screening of extracellular enzyme-producing and pathogen inhibitory gut bacteria as putative probiotics in mrigal, Cirrhinus mrigala (Hamilton, 1822). *International Journal of Fisheries and Aquatic Studies*, 2(4), 310–318.

17 Impact of Biogenic Silver Nanoparticles on Plant Pathogenic Fungi

Monika and Gaurav Kumar

CONTENTS

INTRODUCTION

The human diet consists mainly of carbohydrates, proteins, fats, fiber, minerals, and water as its major components, and humans obtain these from various animal and plants sources. Throughout history, plant crops have been used as a very significant source of food, and they form the backbone of life on earth. Humans depend either directly or indirectly on plants for their food and nutrition. Worldwide, humans use about 7,000 various species of plants for obtaining their food and nutrition. Among these, around 300 plants species are widely cultivated, and only 11 are responsible for 95% of human food production. Human nutrition significantly depends on 10 major crops: corn, rice, wheat, millet, sorghum, sugar cane, beans, banana, and coconut; other important staples are cassava and potato. Humans' food also embraces a variety of herbs, spices, flowers, nuts, fruits, and vegetables from plant sources. In recent years, food security has emerged as an important global issue; approximately 1 billion people do not have access to sufficient food supplies, and over 2 billion people are not getting the required daily nutrients and vitamins (Fang and Ramasamy, 2015). This could be largely attributed to the significant reduction in agricultural land and issues related to pre-harvesting, harvesting and post-harvesting of agriculture products. Among various issues, microorganisms are one of the leading problems associated with crop loss, and they can largely affect productivity during pre- and post-harvesting periods. It is estimated that the demand for food will continue to increase due to an increase in the global population, and by 2050 an additional 70% of the present food supply will be required (Godfray et al., 2010). Therefore, now is the right time to improve agricultural productivity in order to meet future demands for food.

MICROBIAL DISEASES OF PLANTS

Microbial diseases are turning into a global problem and generating a lot of concerns for agriculture professionals. Microbes such as fungi, oomycetes, bacteria, viruses, viroids, virus-like organisms, phytoplasmas, protozoa, and nematodes are responsible for causing serious diseases of important plants, leading to enormous crop losses and eventually to large economic losses. As explained earlier, crop loss can occur at different times, starting from the sowing of seeds in the field to the harvesting of crops, to storage of crops. It is estimated that plant pathogens can lead to significant reduction in plant yield, ranging between 20% and 40%, and leads to miserable economic loss (Savary et al., 2012). A plant disease is any abnormal condition that alters the appearance and functioning of a plant. According to the American Phytopathological Society, a disease is referred to as the change from the normal working conditions of physiological activities for some interval of time or the concentration that can cause imbalance in the activities of the plant that are necessary for its survival. The occurrence of plant disease normally requires the interaction of three components: susceptible plant host, suitable environment, and a virulent pathogen. Such interactions are commonly referred to as the disease triangle (Figure 17.1) (Singh, 2007). Unavailability of any of the factors involved in the disease triangle significantly affects the occurrence of plant

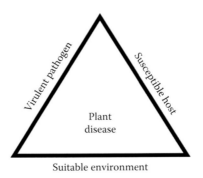

FIGURE 17.1 Plant diseases triangle.

diseases. Many factors that influence disease development in plants include hybrid/variety genetics, the age of the plant at the time of infection, soil type, climate, atmospheric temperature, rainfall, wind, hail, and so on.

PLANT PATHOGENIC FUNGI

Fungi are an important group of microorganisms responsible for causing infections in cultivated plants. They represent the largest group of plant pathogens, with an array of serious diseases in economically important crops, and cause considerable yield losses worldwide. The history of phytopathogenic fungal outbreaks represents an unforgettably devastating past and impact on human civilization. Some prominent instances include the Irish famine/late blight of the potato (*Phytophthora infestans*) in Ireland during 1845 and 1846, which resulted in widespread hunger and reduced the Irish population by half. Another prominent outbreak of brown spot of rice (*Bipolaris oryzae*) took place in Bengal, India (then British India), in 1942 and resulted in approximately 3.5 million deaths due to starvation and malnutrition. Another classic example that had an impact on the economy of a country includes the outbreak of coffee rust in Sri Lanka during 1967, which resulted in a 93% decline in the export of coffee from the country. These examples demonstrate the huge impact of fungal epidemics of plants on human life and national economies.

Among the 1.5 million fungal species (yeast, mold, and mushrooms), about 15,000 species of fungi are known to cause disease in plants. The majority of these fungi belong to the Ascomycetes and Basidiomycetes. It is estimated that phytopathogenic fungi are responsible for nearly 10%–35% of crop loss during pre- and post-harvesting processes, resulting in a loss of USD 200 billion every year (Dunlap, 2007). Fungi that can harm plants can be classified into two groups: necrotrophs, and biotrophs. Pathogens commonly interfere with the host defense mechanism to cause disease, necrotrophs produce harmful toxins to kill their host plants and feed on dead organic material, and biotrophs manipulate the host metabolism to grow and colonize the living tissue (Doehlemann et al., 2016). One more group of fungi are known as hemibiotrophs; they show some unique properties because they initially grow as biotrophs to colonize the plant tissue and, in the later stage of the disease, damage the plants as necrotrophs (Laluk and Mengiste, 2010). Fungal pathogens can infect a wide range of plant species, at other times, they might be restricted to one or a few host species. Some of the phytopathogenic fungi are obligate parasites requiring the presence of the living host to grow and reproduce, but most of them are saprophytic and can survive in the soil, water, and air without the presence of living plants. The widespread presence of fungal spores in nature and their ability to survive in harsh conditions help them to spread over large geographic areas to spread a disease rapidly and efficiently. Prevalent signs and symptoms produced by phytopathogenic fungi in their hosts include rust, rot, shot holes, spot, scabs, warts, wilt, blight, blast, canker, powdery mildew, Sclerotinia, Phytophthora, stunting growth, chlorosis, anthracnose, and so on. Specific phytopathogenic fungi can produce a specific set of symptoms while causing disease in their host. Some common phytopathogenic fungi, their target plants, diseases, and associated symptoms are summarized in Table 17.1.

TABLE 17.1
Common Phytopathogenic Fungi and Associated Symptoms

Organism	Target Plant	Disease	Symptoms
Alternaria solani	Tomato, potato, and pepper	Alternaria blight	Brown to black spots that can develop into concentric rings
Puccinia graminis, *P. sorghi*, *P. coronata*, *Uromyces phaseoli*	Wheat, apple, and asparagus	Rusts	Browning or reddening of the small twigs and needles; release of rusty, powdery spores
Colletotrichum lindemuthianum	Beans and other leguminous plants	Anthracnose	Small dead spots that have concentric rings of pink and brown
Macrophomina phaseoli, *Rhizoctonia solani*	*Zea mays*, *Pinus elliotti*	Damping off	Charcoal rot on many plant species
Phytophthora capsici	Potatoes, tomatoes, and peppers	Late blight	Dark blotches through the tuber and formation of sunken lesions
Ustilago nuda, *U. maydis*	Grains, grasses, barley, and corn	Smut	Smutted grain heads, which contain masses of black or brown spores
Peronospora belbahrii, *P. manshurica*	Grapes, basil, and soybean	Downy mildew	Large, angular, or blocky yellow areas visible on the upper surface; as lesions mature, they expand rapidly and turn brown
Venturia inaequalis	Apple	Apple scab	Scabby spots are sunken and tan and may have velvety spores in the center
Fusarium oxysporum	Banana, tomato, muskmelon, tobacco	Fusarium wilt	Stunting of the plant, yellowing of the lower leaves, defoliation, marginal necrosis, and plant death
Fusarium graminearum	Wheat, barley, oats, corn, and rye	Fusarium head blight	Masses of colored spores form on the base of glumes or over head
Cercospora personata	Groundnuts	Tikka disease	Leaflets of lower leaves have dark spots that, at a later stage, are surrounded by yellow rings
Phakopsora pachyrhizi	Soybean	Asian soybean rust	Brown or reddish lesions with globe-like orifices
Magnaporthe oryzae	Wheat, rice, rye, barley, and millet	Blast/blight disease	White-gray-green spots with shady margins on plant shoots; in later stage, may kill the whole leaf
Botrytis cinerea	Wine grapes	Botrytis bunch rot	Formation of dull green spots on grapes that later turn brownish and necrotic
Blumeria graminis	Wheat and barley	Powdery mildew	White powdery growth on leaves that turn gray to brown or black and are surrounded by chlorosis

NANOTECHNOLOGY

In the 1950s, before the world knew about nanomaterials, Richard Feynman, an American physicist, introduced the concept of nanotechnology in one of his popular lectures entitled "There's Plenty of Room at the Bottom" at an annual meeting of the American Physical Society at the California Institute of Technology. In the 1980s, Eric Drexler coined the term *nanotechnology* and did lots of pioneer work to popularize the field. Today, nanotechnology is one of the most important scientific fields and involves imaging, developing, measuring, modeling, and manipulating materials at the nano scale. The word prefix "nano" is derived from the Greek word "nanos," which means "dwarf." The size of nanomaterials ranges from 1 to 100 nm in at least one dimension. Nanoparticles are considered to be the fundamental building units in nanotechnology. The most important property of nanoparticles includes a large surface area–to–volume ratio, which compliments various unique properties in them (Alagumuthu and Kirubha, 2012). In recent years, a variety of metallic (gold, silver, titanium, copper, zinc, etc.) and nonmetallic (silica, carbon, etc.) nanoparticles are being synthesized because of their wide application in various industrial processes/products such as biosensors, composite fibers, cryogenic superconducting materials, electronic components, cosmetics, textiles, drug delivery, biolabeling, and water treatment.

SYNTHESIS AND CHARACTERIZATION OF NANOPARTICLES

Synthesis of nanoparticles is a relatively complex mechanism and relies on various factors, including the pH of the reaction, the presence of ions, temperature, viscosity, the concentration of the substrate material, and so on. These conditions are highly influential in determining the quantity and various physiochemical properties of the end product. Therefore, specific conditions must be present in order to obtain particles with unique physiochemical properties. Materials science has seen significant progress in methods for developing nanoparticles, and numerous methods are currently used for the effective production of nanoparticles. Current methods fall into three major categories: physical, chemical, and biological. Some of the popular physical methods involved in nanoparticles synthesis include arc-discharge and physical vapor condensation. Chemical reduction, electrochemical techniques, photochemical reduction, and pyrolysis are some of the popular chemical methods for nanoparticle synthesis. Biosynthesis of nanoparticles is relatively different and complex method of nanoparticle synthesis. Biosynthesis of nanoparticles includes the use of cell-free extract from plants, algae, and microbes and sometimes the whole organism. Figure 17.2 summarizes the popular physical, chemical, and biological methods with the target nanoparticles for which they are used.

The physical, chemical, and biological methods follow either a top–down or a bottom–up approach for the synthesis of nanoparticles. The top–down approach

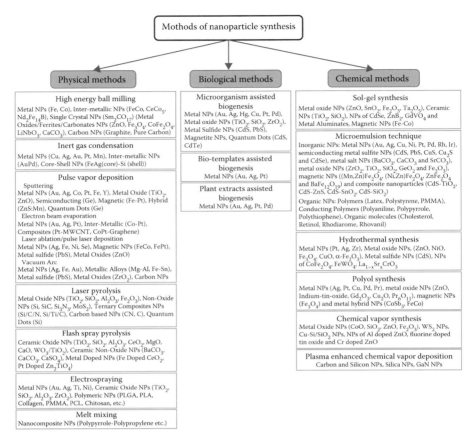

FIGURE 17.2 Methods of nanoparticles synthesis and target nanoparticles. (From Dhand, C. et al., *Rsc Adv.*, 5, 105003–105037, 2015.)

includes breaking of bulk materials into smaller structures by using any physical, chemical, or biological approach. The bottom–up approach includes building up nanoparticles by joining atoms. Figure 17.3a summarizes the top–down approach/ bottom–up approach. Figure 17.3b clarifies the approaches, followed by various methods of nanoparticle synthesis (Mittal et al., 2013).

Characterization of nanoparticles is relatively an analytical approach and includes the application of various advanced instruments for studying the physiochemical properties of nanoparticles. Major physiochemical properties studied for the characterizations of nanoparticles include particle size, particle size distribution, particle structure, molecular weight, surface charge, surface hydrophobicity, and surface chemical composition. Various analytical methods used for studying these properties are summarized in Table 17.2.

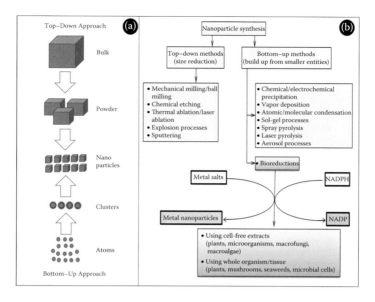

FIGURE 17.3 Top–down and bottom–up approach for the synthesis of nanoparticles: (a) diagrammatic presentation of nanoparticle synthesis; (b) methods followed for top–down and bottom–up approach. (From Mittal, A. K. et al., *Biotechnol. Adv.*, 31, 346–356, 2013.)

TABLE 17.2
Methods Studying the Physiochemical Properties of Nanoparticles

Physiochemical Properties	Methods Used
Particle shape, size, and size distribution	Atomic force microscopy (AFM)
	Dynamic light scattering (DLS)
	Scanning tunneling microscopy (SEM)
	Transmission electron microscopy (TEM)
Surface charge	Zeta potentiometer
	Laser Doppler anemometry
Molecular weight crystallinity	X-ray diffraction spectroscopy (XRD)
	Differential scanning calorimetry (DSC)
	Gel permeation chromatography
Surface hydrophobicity	Rose Bengal (dye) binding
	Water contact angle measurement
Surface chemical analysis	X-ray photoelectron spectroscopy
	Nuclear magnetic resonance (NMR)
	Secondary ion mass spectrometry
	Fourier transform infrared spectroscopy (FTIR)
	Sorptometer

Source: Bhatia, S., 2016, Nanoparticles types, classification, characterization, fabrication methods and drug delivery applications, In *Natural Polymer Drug Delivery Systems*, pp. 33–93, Cham, Switzerland: Springer International Publishing.

SILVER NANOPARTICLES

Silver nanoparticles (SNPs) are nanoparticles fabricated from silver. They come in various sizes ranging from 1 to 100 nm. Their shape can vary greatly, from spherical to octagonal, hexagonal, and diamond, based how they have been synthesized. SNPs are considered one of the most important nanomaterials used in consumer products because of its numerous unique optical, electrical, antioxidant, antimicrobial, and thermal properties (Lok et al., 2007; Sharma et al., 2009; Marambio-Jones and Hoek, 2010; Sotiriou and Pratsinis, 2010). These properties of SNPs enable them to be used in various products, such as the following:

- *Diagnostics*: Biosensors and numerous assays, where the SNPs are used as biological tags for quantitative detection.
- *Antibacterial*: Apparel, footwear, paints, wound dressings, appliances, cosmetics, and plastics.
- *Conductive*: Conductive inks and integration into composites to enhance thermal and electrical conductivity.
- *Optical*: SNPs harvest light efficiently, and they are used for enhanced optical spectroscopies including metal-enhanced fluorescence (MEF) and surface-enhanced Raman scattering (SERS).

The properties of SNPs applicable to humans are under investigation in laboratory and animal studies to assess their potential efficacy, toxicity, and costs. The exclusive physical and chemical properties of SNPs always intensify the efficacy of silver. Chemical and physical approaches of SNPs synthesis have been used in the past, but they are costly and slightly toxic too. A biological method would be an effective alternative.

BIOSYNTHESIS OF SILVER NANOPARTICLES

It is clear from Figure 17.2 that the biological synthesis of SNPs is a bottom–up approach of synthesis and represents a remarkable low-cost and environmentally friendly manufacturing alternative to various hazardous physical and chemical methods, which usually involve the application of various chemicals, use of lower ambient temperatures and lower pressures for the synthesis of nanoparticles (Mukherjee et al., 2008; Pearce et al., 2008; Dobias et al., 2011). Biological organisms such as fungi, bacteria, algae, mushrooms, yeast, lichens, and plants represent some of the very potent methods for the synthesis of SNPs. Their potential to synthesize SNPs can be attributed to their ability to synthesize antioxidant compounds and to reduce the number of enzymes, which are typically responsible for the reduction of the metal salt into nanoparticles. Biosynthesis of SNPs can take place either intracellularly or extracellularly based on the presence of cellular metabolites with reducing properties (Ahmad et al., 2003; Saifuddin et al., 2009).

ANTIFUNGAL ACTIVITY OF BIOLOGICALLY SILVER NANOPARTICLES AGAINST PLANT PATHOGENS

SNPs are widely used for controlling microbial population in numerous ways. Various recent reports have also emphasized the powerful, broad-spectrum, antimicrobial nature of SNPs in relation to a wide range of bacteria, fungi, and other microorganisms. The global focus has centered on studying the antimicrobial potential of SNPs toward human pathogens, while plant pathogens have not been explored as much. Strong and broad-spectrum antimicrobial properties of biologically synthesized SNPs are being explored for controlling plant fungal diseases. In numerous studies, biologically synthesized SNPs have been reported to display significant antifungal activity against a variety of plant pathogens, including *Fusarium gramineous*, *Colletotrichum* spp., *Phakopsora pachyrhizi*, *Magnaporthe oryzae*, *Fusarium oxysporum*, *Blumeria graminis*, *Botrytis cinerea*, *Puccinia* spp., *Mycosphaerella graminicola*, *Ustilago maydis*, *Melampsora lini*, and *Rhizoctonia solani*. Table 17.3 summarizes the antifungal activity of biologically synthesized SNPs against a variety of plant pathogenic fungi.

TABLE 17.3
Antagonistic Activity of Biogenic SNPs against Plant Pathogenic Fungi

SNPs Synthesized from …	Target Plant Fungi	References
Streptomyces spp.	*Fusarium oxysporium*	Krishnakumar and Bai (2015)
Proteus mirabilis	*Alternaria alternata, Sclerotinia sclerotiorum, Macrophomina phaseolina, Rhizoctonia solani, Curvularia lunata*	Krishnaraj et al. (2012)
Bacillus subtilis	*Alternaria alternata, Fusarium oxysporum, Aspergillus nidulans, Cladosporium herbarum, A. niger, Fusarium* spp., *Trichoderma harzianum*	Bholay et al. (2013)
Macrophomina phaseolina	*Fusarium semitectum, Aspergillus niger*	Chowdhury et al. (2014)
Trichoderma viridae	*Bipolaris oryzae*	Gomathinayagam et al. (2010)
Trichoderma longibrachiatum	*Fusarium oxysporium*	Elamawi and Al-Harbi (2014)
Trichoderma reesei	*Aspergillus fumigatus, Fusarium oxysporum*	Vahabi et al. (2011)
Macrophomina phaseolina	*Pythium aphanidermatum, Sclerotinia sclerotiorum*	Mahdizadeh et al. (2015)
Aspergillus versicolor	*Sclerotinia sclerotiorum, Fragaria × ananassa*	Elgorban et al. (2016)

(Continued)

TABLE 17.3 (*Continued*)
Antagonistic Activity of Biogenic SNPs against Plant Pathogenic Fungi

SNPs Synthesized from …	Target Plant Fungi	References
Alternaria alternata	*Phoma glomerata, P. herbarum, Fusarium semitectum, Trichoderma* sp.	Gajbhiye et al. (2009)
Trichoderma viride	*Alternaria solani*	Ismail et al. (2016)
Alternaria solani (endophyte)	*Alternaria solani*	Abdel-Hafez et al. (2016)
Citrus	*Alternaria alternata, A. citri, Penicillium digitatum*	Abdelmalek and Salaheldin (2016)
Oak wilt	*Raffaelea* sp.	Kim et al. (2009)
Svensonia hyderabadensis, Boswellia ovalifoliolata, Shorea tumbuggaia	*Aspergillus niger, Fusarium oxysporum, Curvularia lunata,* and *Rhizopus arrhizus*	Savithramma et al. (2011)
Raspberry extract	*Cladosporium cladosporoides, Aspergillus niger*	Pulit et al. (2013)
Garcinia kola	*Aspergillus niger, Rhizopus stolonifer*	Hassan et al. (2016)
Lagerstoemia spp.	*Aspergillus flavus, A. niger, Curvularia spp.*	Sundararajan and Kumari (2014)
Conyza ambigua	*Aspergillus niger, A. flavus, Sclerotium rolsfii*	Elumalai and Kumar (2013)
Raphanus sativus	*Aspergillus flavus, A. fumigatus, A. japonicus, Cochliobolus spicifer, Penicillium duclauxii, Rhizopus stolonifer, Trichoderma harzianum*	Ali et al. (2015)
Thalictrum foliolosum	*Trichophyton rubrum, Aspergillus versicolor*	Hazarika et al. (2016)
Calotropis procera	*Fusarium solani, F. oxysporum, Colletotrichum gloesporoides, Macrophomina phaseolina*	Mohamed et al. (2014)
Murraya koengii	*Trichoderma, Rhizopus, Aspergillus niger, A. flavus*	Indhumathi and Rajathi (2013)

ANTIFUNGAL MECHANISM OF SILVER NANOPARTICLES

SNPs exhibit a strong and broad-spectrum antifungal activity toward fungal isolates, although the exact molecular mechanism elucidating the antifungal activity is currently unknown. However, several scientists have reported the effect of SNPs on fungal growth, which is very helpful in understanding the antifungal effect of SNPs. In one study, Xia et al. (2016) used SEM and TEM to study the effect of SNPs on the surface and intracellular organelles of *Trichosporon asahii*. This study suggests that the treatment of fungi with SNPs leads to mycelium deformation, fracture, and

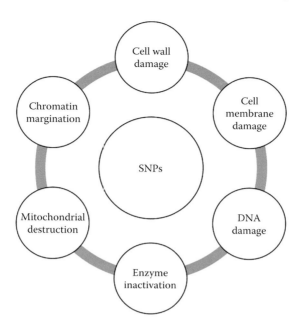

FIGURE 17.4   Antifungal activity of silver nanoparticles.

shrinking, which results in the outflow of intracellular materials and shrinkage of the mycelium. Further TEM imaging revealed the infiltration of SNPs inside the cell and severe damage in the fungal cell wall and cell membrane. In addition, severe degeneration was observed in other cellular organelles such as condensation and margination of chromatin, depolymerization of ribosomes, thinning of the matrix, and fragmentation of mitochondria. Ouda (2014) reported that the SNP treatment of *Alternaria alternata* and *Botrytis cinerea* resulted in damage to the fungal hyphae, which may result in the leakage of intracellular material from fungal hyphae. Common properties of SNPs that may be responsible for the death of fungal cells are summarized in Figure 17.4.

CONCLUSION

SNPs are some of the most widely studied metallic nanoparticles because of their promising antimicrobial properties against a wide range of microorganisms. This chapter briefly discussed the various methods for synthesizing and characterizing SNPs. Various laboratory studies cited in the chapter provide a clear overview that SNPs possess strong antifungal activity and suggest that they could perhaps be used for controlling plant pathogenic fungi. Additional research is needed to fully decode the antimicrobial mechanism of SNPs. In addition, systemic studies are required to learn of any possible toxic effects of SNPs on higher organisms, including humans.

REFERENCES

Abdel-Hafez, S. I., Nafady, N. A., Abdel-Rahim, I. R., et al., 2016. Assessment of protein silver nanoparticles toxicity against pathogenic *Alternaria solani*. *3 Biotech* 6(2): 1–12.

Abdelmalek, G. M. A., and Salaheldin, T. A., 2016. Silver nanoparticles as a potent fungicide for Citrus phytopathogenic fungi. *Journal of Nanomedicine Research* 3: 00065.

Ahmad, A., Mukherjee, P., Senapati, S., et al., 2003. Extracellular biosynthesis of silver nanoparticles using the fungus *Fusarium oxysporum*. *Colloids and Surfaces B: Biointerfaces* 28(4): 313–318.

Alagumuthu, G., and Kirubha, R., 2012. Synthesis and characterisation of silver nanoparticles in different medium. *Open Journal of Synthesis Theory and Applications* 1(2): 13–17.

Ali, S. M., Yousef, N. M., and Nafady, N. A., 2015. Application of biosynthesized silver nanoparticles for the control of land snail *Eobania vermiculata* and some plant pathogenic fungi. *Journal of Nanomaterials*. doi:10.1155/2015/218904.

Bhatia, S., 2016. Nanoparticles types, classification, characterization, fabrication methods and drug delivery applications. In *Natural Polymer Drug Delivery Systems*, S. Bhatia (Ed.), 33–93. Cham, Switzerland: Springer International Publishing.

Bholay, A. D., Nalawade, P. M., and Borkhataria, B. V., 2013. Fungicidal potential of biosynthesized silver nanoparticles against phytopathogens and potentiation of fluconazole. *World Research Journal of Pharmaceutical Research* 1: 12–15.

Chowdhury, S., Basu, A., and Kundu, S., 2014. Green synthesis of protein capped silver nanoparticles from phytopathogenic fungus *Macrophomina phaseolina* (Tassi) Goid with antimicrobial properties against multidrug-resistant bacteria. *Nanoscale Research Letters* 9(1): 365.

Dhand, C., Dwivedi, N., Loh, X. J., et al., 2015. Methods and strategies for the synthesis of diverse nanoparticles and their applications: A comprehensive overview. *Rsc Advances* 5(127): 105003–105037.

Dobias, J., Suvorova, E. I., and Bernier-Latmani, R., 2011. Role of proteins in controlling selenium nanoparticle size. *Nanotechnology*, 22(19): 195605.

Doehlemann, G., Ökmen, B., Zhu, W., et al., 2016. Plant Pathogenic Fungi. *Plant Pathogenic Fungi. Microbiol Spectrum* 5(1): FUNK-0023-2016.

Dunlap, J., 2007. *Fungal Genomics*. San Diego, CA: Academic Press.

Elamawi, R. M., and Al-Harbi R. E., 2014. Effect of biosynthesized silver nanoparticles on *Fusarium oxysporium* fungus the cause of seed rot disease of faba bean, tomato and barley. *Journal of Plant Protein and Pathology Mansoura University* 5(2): 225–237.

Elgorban, A. M., Aref, S. M., Seham, S. M., et al., 2016. Extracellular synthesis of silver nanoparticles using *Aspergillus versicolor* and evaluation of their activity on plant pathogenic fungi. *Mycosphere* 7(6): 844–852.

Elumalai, E. K., and Vinothkumar, P., 2013. Role of silver nanoparticle against plant pathogens. *Nano Biomedicine and Engineering* 5(2): 90–93.

Fang, Y., and Ramasamy, R. P., 2015. Current and prospective methods for plant disease detection. *Biosensors* 5(3): 537–561.

Gajbhiye, M., Kesharwani, J., Ingle, A., et al., 2009. Fungus-mediated synthesis of silver nanoparticles and their activity against pathogenic fungi in combination with fluconazole. *Nanomedicine: Nanotechnology, Biology and Medicine* 5(4): 382–386.

Godfray, H. C. J., Beddington, J. R., Crute, I. R., et al., 2010. Food security: The challenge of feeding 9 billion people. *Science* 327(5967): 812–818.

Gomathinayagam, S., Rekha, M., and Murugan, S. S., 2010. The biological control of paddy disease brown spot (*Bipolaris oryzae*) by using *Trichoderma viride in vitro* condition. *Journal of Biopesticides* 3(1): 93–95.

Hassan, L. A., Elijah, A. T., Ojiefoh, O. C., et al., 2016. Biosynthesis of silver nanoparticles using *Garcinia kola* and its antimicrobial potential. *African Journal of Pure and Applied Chemistry* 10(1): 1–7.

Hazarika, S. N., Gupta, K., Shamin, K. N. A. M., et al., 2016. One-pot facile green synthesis of biocidal silver nanoparticles. *Materials Research Express* 3(7): 075401.

Indhumathi, T., and Rajathi, K., 2013. A study on synthesis of silver nanoparticles from *Murraya koengii* leaf and its antifungal activity. *International Journal of Drug Delivery & Research* 5(3): 294–298.

Ismail, A. W. A., Sidkey, N. M., Arafa, R. A., et al., 2016. Evaluation of *in vitro* antifungal activity of silver and selenium nanoparticles against *Alternaria solani* caused early blight disease on potato. *British Biotechnology Journal* 12(3): 1–11.

Kim, S. W., Kim, K. S., Lamsal, K., et al., 2009. An *in vitro* study of the antifungal effect of silver nanoparticles on oak wilt pathogen *Raffaelea* sp. *Journal of Microbiology and Biotechnology* 19(8): 760–764.

Krishnakumar, S., and Bai, V., 2015. Extracellular biosynthesis of silver nanoparticles using-terrestrial *Streptomyces* sp-SBU3 and its antimicrobial efficiency against plant pathogens. *International Journal of Chem Tech Research* 1: 112–118.

Krishnaraj, C., Jagan, E. G., Ramachandran, R., et al., 2012. Effect of biologically synthesized silver nanoparticles on *Bacopa monnieri* (Linn.) Wettst. plant growth metabolism. *Process Biochemistry* 47(4): 651–658.

Laluk, K., and Mengiste, T., 2010. Necrotroph attacks on plants: Wanton destruction or covert extortion? *The Arabidopsis Book* 8: e0136.

Lok, C. N., Ho, C. M., Chen, R., et al., 2007. Silver nanoparticles: Partial oxidation and antibacterial activities. *JBIC Journal of Biological Inorganic Chemistry* 12(4): 527–534.

Mahdizadeh, V., Safaie, N., and Khelghatibana, F., 2015. Evaluation of antifungal activity of silver nanoparticles against some phytopathogenic fungi and *Trichoderma harzianum*. *Journal of Crop Protection* 4(3): 291–300.

Marambio-Jones, C., and Hoek, E. M., 2010. A review of the antibacterial effects of silver nanomaterials and potential implications for human health and the environment. *Journal of Nanoparticle Research* 12(5): 1531–1551.

Mittal, A. K., Chisti, Y., and Banerjee, U. C., 2013. Synthesis of metallic nanoparticles using plant extracts. *Biotechnology Advances* 31(2): 346–356.

Mohamed, N. H., Ismail, M. A., Abdel-Mageed, W. M., et al., 2014. Antimicrobial activity of latex silver nanoparticles using *Calotropis procera*. *Asian Pacific Journal of Tropical Biomedicine* 4(11): 876–883.

Mukherjee, P., Roy, M., Mandal, B. P., et al., 2008. Green synthesis of highly stabilized nanocrystalline silver particles by a non-pathogenic and agriculturally important fungus *T. asperellum. Nanotechnology* 19(7): 075103.

Ouda, S. M., 2014. Antifungal activity of silver and copper nanoparticles on two plant pathogens. *Alternaria alternata* and *Botrytis cinerea. Research Journal of Microbiology* 9(1): 34–42.

Pearce, C. I., Coker, V. S., and Charnock, J. M., 2008. Microbial manufacture of chalcogenide-based nanoparticles via the reduction of selenite using *Veillonella atypica*: An in situ EXAFS study. *Nanotechnology* 19(15): 155603.

Pulit, J., Banach, M., Szczygłowska, R., et al., 2013. Nanosilver against fungi. Silver nanoparticles as an effective biocidal factor. *Acta Biochimica Polonica* 60(4): 795–798.

Saifuddin, N., Wong, C. W., and Yasumira, A. A., 2009. Rapid biosynthesis of silver nanoparticles using culture supernatant of bacteria with microwave irradiation. *Journal of Chemistry* 6(1): 61–70.

Savary, S., Ficke, A., Aubertot, J. N., and Hollier, C., 2012. Crop losses due to diseases and their implications for global food production losses and food security. *Food Security* 4(4): 519–537.

Savithramma, N., Rao, M. L., Rukmini, K., et al., 2011. Antimicrobial activity of silver nanoparticles synthesized by using medicinal plants. *International Journal of ChemTech Research* 3(3): 1394–1402.

Sharma, V. K., Yngard, R. A., and Lin, Y., 2009. Silver nanoparticles: Green synthesis and their antimicrobial activities. *Advances in Colloid and Interface Science* 145(1): 83–96.

Singh, D. V., 2007. *Introductory Plant Pathology.* New Delhi, India: NISCAIR.

Sotiriou, G. A., and Pratsinis, S. E., 2010. Antibacterial activity of nanosilver ions and particles. *Environmental Science & Technology* 44(14): 5649–5654.

Sundararajan, B., and Kumari, B. R., 2014. Biosynthesis of silver nanoparticles in *Lagerstroemia* species (L.) pers and their antimicrobial activities. *International Journal of Pharmacy and Pharmaceutical Sciences* 6(3): 30–34.

Vahabi, K., Mansoori, G., and Karimi, S., 2011. Biosynthesis of silver nanoparticles by fungus *Trichoderma reesei* (A route for large-scale production of AgNPs). *Insciences Journal* 1(1): 65–79.

Xia, Z. K., Ma, Q. H., Li, S. Y., et al., 2016. The antifungal effect of silver nanoparticles on *Trichosporon asahii. Journal of Microbiology, Immunology and Infection* 49(2): 182–188.

18 Engineering Microbial Cell Factories for Improved Whey Fermentation to Produce Bioethanol

Deepansh Sharma, Arun Beniwal, Priyanka Saini, Shailly Kapil, and Shilpa Vij

CONTENTS

INTRODUCTION OF WHEY AS A SOURCE OF BIOFUEL

Ethanol is produced by anaerobic fermentation of different sugars by a variety of microorganisms, especially yeast. Various agro-industrial residues were used for the production of bioethanol on a pilot scale and on a commercial scale. One important substrate for bioethanol production today is lactose, which is the main sugar in milk and is an underutilized waste residue from all the different kinds of cheese produced worldwide by dairy-processing industries. Lactose can be either hydrolyzed or fermented, which leads to ethanol as an end product with traces of other organic acids (Mawson, 1994; Siso, 1996; Sansonetti et al., 2009). Rapidly depleting fossil fuels

353

and environmental pollution led to a global search for alternative fuels. Ethanol is considered a promising renewable fuel because of its distinct and well-documented advantages and applications (Galbe and Zacchi, 2002; Brethauer and Wyman, 2010). In developing countries such as India, which has a large population, diversion of food crops to ethanol production is neither viable nor sustainable. In India, ethanol is generally produced from molasses, but because molasses has limited availability and alternative uses, the government of India is strongly advocating research in developing second-generation fuel, that is, ethanol.

Global whey production is over 160 million tons per year, showing a 1%–2% annual growth rate (OECD-FAO, 2008; Smithers, 2008). In India, various indigenous and traditional fermented dairy foods are prepared and consumed. Chhana (a type of milk preparation) is in huge demand for the preparation of Rasogolla, Sandesh, and their variations. Whey is obtained as a by-product in the production of chhana. India at present produces 1.2 million tons of chhana every year (Saxena, 1997), which results in an annual production of 8.0 million tons of whey. Whey constitutes just about all nutrients present in the milk. Generally it contains about half the milk solids, most of the lactose, about one-fifth of the protein, and most of the vitamins and minerals. Whey, a by-product of the dairy industry, is comprised of about 85%–95% of the milk volume and retains 55% of milk nutrients. The whey composition changes with the components present in milk that is used for making cheese, the variety of cheese made, and the cheesemaking process employed. Whey contains approximately 0.3% butterfat, 0.8% whey proteins, 4.9% lactose, and 0.5% minerals. Whey also contains other components like lactic acid, vitamins, and nonprotein nitrogen compounds (Siso, 1996). Butterfat is considered to be of high value, and it is further used as an ingredient during processing. Whey may be separated into whey proteins, and the remaining whey is then disposed of. The high organic content of the whey leads to a high Biological Oxygen Demand (BOD) content of 30,000–50,000 ppm and COD content of 60,000–80,000 ppm (Marwaha and Kennedy, 1988; Gardner, 1989; Kemp and Quickenden, 1989; Mawson, 1994). Lactose moiety is mainly responsible for the high BOD and Chemical Oxygen Demand (COD) content because the protein recovery reduces the COD of the whey only by about 10,000 ppm (Mawson, 1994).

Cheese whey disposal became a major environmental problem because of the high volume generated during cheese processing. Methods of disposing of surplus whey include animal feeding, land spreading, or discharging it after treatment for BOD reduction. With increased demand for cheese, production simultaneously generated a huge amount of whey (Rajeshwari et al., 2000; De Wit, 2001), and cheese factories are usually built near rivers so that whey can be dumped easily into them (Kosikowski, 1979). Discharging of whey by spreading it on land results in another problem; that is, the soil becomes unfit for use. The issues in handling the large volume of surplus whey profitably still include a zero discharge policy and conversion of agro-industrial waste to beneficial products. The disposal of whey is expensive and is still an environmental problem for dairy-processing sectors. However, approximately half of the world's cheese whey production is not treated and is being discarded as effluent. Making cheese whey profitable has been a challenge for dairy industries around the globe.

Treating whey by fermentation of lactose to ethanol has received considerable attention recently, and various large-scale technologies have been developed for efficient utilization of whey and fuel production. Production of bioethanol by lactose-fermenting microorganisms may be a promising alternative. Several industries produce ethanol from whey in different parts of world, especially in countries with large milk production, such as Ireland, the United States, and mainly New Zealand, where nearly 50% of the cheese-whey production has been utilized to produce ethanol (Mawson, 1994; Pesta et al., 2007). In last 30 years, functional plants have been established to use cheese whey for bioethanol production from the whey. The fermentation of the whey into ethanol using yeast has been reported over last 50 years (Webb and Whittier, 1948). The first commercially functional whey-to-ethanol plant was built in April 1978 by Carbery Milk Products Ltd. of Ireland for the large-scale production of alcohol. Anchor Ethanol Ltd., a New Zealand dairy cooperative, is one of the main ethanol producers using whey. The ethanol produced has been utilized for food, beverage, and industrial applications.

The yeast cells that are able to assimilate lactose aerobically are widespread but only a few, such as *Kluyveromyces lactis*, *Kluyveromyces marxianus*, and a few strains of *Candida* spp., can ferment the lactose significantly. The commercial production of ethanol from various substrates such as sugar cane molasses and hydrolyzed starch from corn or other grains with yeast *Saccharomyces cerevisiae* is an established process on an industrial scale. Direct fermentation of whey to ethanol is not economical: It does not yield maximal ethanol because of the low lactose content, which ultimately yields a low ethanol titer at the end of fermentation. But a high concentration of lactose yields maximal bioethanol at the end of fermentation, and a higher lactose concentration could be achieved with ultrafiltration or reverse osmosis. Other methods that can be used involve the addition of high-sugar-containing substrates like molasses, sugar beets, and other high-sugar-content biomass.

KLUYVEROMYCES FOR PRODUCTION OF ETHANOL

A combination of high temperature, ethanol, and sugar is for the fermentation process. *Kluyveromyces marxianus* is a homothallic, hemiascomycetous yeast; is genetically related to *S. cerevisiae*; and is a sister species to the better-known *Kluyveromyces lactis* (Lachance, 1998; Llorente et al., 2000). *K. lactis* has been the major research species within Kluyveromyces, primarily for studies on lactose metabolism, but it has since been regarded as a model for nonconventional yeasts (Breunig, 2000). *Kluyveromyces marxianus* is a yeast species with several biotechnological applications because of its ability to be used in a variety of substrates; its high growth rate, with typical generation times of approximately 70 minutes; and its thermotolerance, or its ability to withstand temperatures up to 52°C (Fonseca et al., 2008). This strain has already been generally recognized as safe (GRAS). Kluyveromyces is a genus within the hemiascomycetous yeasts that has been classified to six species following the reclassification into monophyletic genera based on the 26S rDNA sequence (Kurtzman, 2003; Lachance, 2007). *K. marxianus* is having ability to ferment facultatively and regarded as Crabtree-negative (van Dijken et al., 1993). *K. marxianus* and *K. lactis* assimilate lactose (O-β-D-galactopyranosyl-(1–4)-β-D-glucose), use this disaccharide sugar as a carbon source, and are thus lactose positive. The lactose is the only fermentable carbohydrate in whey, and it is used in selective fermentations involving microorganisms that are capable of breaking down lactose with the enzyme β-galactosidase. *Kluyveromyces* β-galactosidase is a very advantageous tool for biotechnology and the food industry. It is useful in the elimination of lactose from certain foods and in the synthesis of galacto-oligosaccharides (GOSs); it has significant potential for human health and nutrition (Yang and Silva, 1995). The ability to utilize lactose is conferred by two genes, *LAC12*, which encodes a lactose permease required for lactose uptake into the cell, and *LAC4*, which encodes a beta-galactosidase that hydrolyzes lactose to the monomers glucose and galactose. Intracellular glucose follows glycolysis pathway, while galactose enters into the Leloir pathway. Cheese whey cultivation with *Kluyveromyces marxianus* have been proposed as a means of reducing pollution caused by this industrial waste stream (Harden, 1996; Aktas et al., 2005). The adaptation of new, genetically engineered systems is also increasing the use of Kluyveromyces yeasts in high-scale heterologous protein production (Schaffrath and Breunig, 2000).

In general, industrial yeast strains are able to grow and efficiently ferment ethanol at pH values of 3.5–6.0 and temperatures of 28°C–30°C, with efficiency reducing rapidly at higher temperatures. But thermotolerant yeasts have several possible benefits, particularly when used in the production of industrial alcohol. Ethanol production at elevated temperatures has received much attention because fermentation processes operating at high temperatures will appreciably diminish cooling costs. Other advantages of high temperatures include more efficient fermentation, a continuous change from fermentation to distillation, minimal risk of contamination, and suitability for use in tropical countries. The tolerance of all species decreased with increasing temperature, but in general, *Kluyveromyces* strains are more thermotolerant than *Saccharomyces*, which in turn can produce higher ethanol yields. *Kluyveromyces marxianus* species has been reported to grow at 47°C (Anderson et al., 1986), 49°C (Hughes et al., 1984), and even 52°C (Banat et al., 1992), and to produce ethanol at temperatures above 40°C (Fonseca et al., 2008). It is important to note that *K. marxianus* cannot grow under strictly anaerobic conditions, and the rate of ethanol formation is linked completely to oxygen limitation (Visser et al., 1990; van Dijken et al., 1993). Yeast *Kluyveromyces* sp. ZMS1 GU133329 and *Kluyveromyces* sp. ZMS3 GU1333331 show good growth up to 45°C and give maximum production of ethanol at 20%–25% sugar concentration (Hashem et al., 2013).

Kluyveromyces marxianus strain MTCC 1288 was able to metabolize lactose within 22 hours to give 2.10 g L^{-1} ethanol and 8.9 g L^{-1} biomass. The specific ethanol formation rate obtained the maximum value of 0.046 h^{-1} between 6 and 8 hours of batch fermentation. The link between ethanol concentration and specific growth rate suggested a strong inhibitory effect of ethanol on the specific culture growth rate (Zafar and Owais, 2005). Oda and Nakamura (2009) have recently identified a *K. marxianus* strain insensitive to catabolite repression using 2 deoxyglucose–resistant mutants able to produce the ethanol from a mixture of whey and molasses. Fonseca et al. (2013) reported that *K. marxianus* CBS 6556 does not require any special nutritional requirements; it grows well in the range of 30°C–37°C on different sugars; and it is capable of growing on sugar mixtures in a shorter period of time than *Saccharomyces cerevisiae*, which is interesting from an industrial point of view. There are many inhibitory effects and problems in the fermentation of concentrated lactose. Slow fermentation and high residual sugar was found when lactose concentration increases to 200 g L^{-1}. This high lactose concentration leads to osmotic sensitivity of yeast. Such problems like low ethanol tolerance and osmotic sensitivity seem to be strain dependent. There is a direct correlation between fermentation efficiency and stress resistance, which refers to the ability of a yeast strain to adapt efficiently to a changing environment and unfavorable growth conditions (Bauer and Pretorius, 2000). Yeast cells must compete with fluctuations in temperature, osmolarity and acidity of their environment, the presence of radiation and toxic chemicals, and long periods of nutrient starvation. Yeast cells use a general mechanism of cellular protection that is forced when cells are exposed to stressful stimuli. A reserve carbohydrate trehalose (α-D-glucopyranosyl α-D-glucopyranoside) acts as a potential stress protectant under harsh conditions and accumulates in cells shifted to higher temperatures; thus, the disaccharide represents a stress response product. Genes involved in heat shock proteins encode HSPs that are induced under ethanol and heat stress response (Piper et al., 1994).

Different strain development programs involve the selection of naturally stress tolerant isolates or the metabolic engineering of strains. During fermentation, yeast survival is also affected by oxygen availability. Fermentative metabolism has been favored by low oxygen levels, leading to higher ethanol production in hypoxic, followed by anoxic, and then aerobic conditions. The ethanol production ability of a *K. marxianus* strain was also improved by ultraviolet (UV) irradiation and N-methyl-N′-nitro-N-nitrosoguanidine (NTG) mutagenesis. *Kluyveromyces marxianus* GX-15 was mutated multiple times by alternate treatment with UV irradiation and NTG for two cycles. Four mutant strains were obtained with improved ethanol yield. The maximum ethanol concentration, ethanol yield coefficient, and theoretical ethanol yield of the best mutant strain, GX-UN120, was 69 g L^{-1}, 0.46 g g^{-1}, and 91%, respectively, when fermenting 150 g glucose l^{-1} at 40°C (Pang et al., 2010). *S. cerevisiae* is an ethanol overproducer that is unable to metabolize lactose (lactose-negative), while *K. marxianus* initiates the hydrolysis of lactose to fermentable sugars. These released sugars can then be utilized by *S. cerevisiae*. This coculture system might be able to generate an increase in ethanol production. In a study by Magalhatilde et al. (2013), the coculture of *S. cerevisiae* UFLA KFG33 (ethanol overproducer) and *K. marxianus* (UFLA KF22) showed the highest value of ethanol production (16.02 ± 0.11 g L^{-1}) and the highest yield of ethanol by fermentation time (0.22 ± 0.05 g L h^{-1}). These yeasts also showed the highest cell mass concentration in final fermentation (1.02 ± 0.01 g L^{-1}). This methodology is a promising technique for the production of ethanol using deproteinized cheese whey. *K. lactis* was chosen among non-Saccharomyces yeasts and was able to improve the survival of *S. cerevisiae* cells in mixed cultures. Thus, co-cultivation of *K. lactis* seems to cause *S. cerevisiae* to be ethanol tolerant by forming favorable metabolites such as glycerol and alanine and changing the intracellular amino acid pool. In mixed cultures, the glycerol contents increased and the alanine contents decreased when compared with the pure culture of *S. cerevisiae* (Yamaoka et al., 2014).

Another strategy is response surface methodology (RSM), which is a combination of mathematical and statistical equations for obtaining empirical models for the development, improvement, and optimization of processes using composite experimental designs (Myers and Montgomery, 1995). Diniz et al. (2014) optimize the conditions for the production of ethanol by *K. marxianus* UFV-3 from cheese whey permeate using RSM and central composite rotational design (CCRD) to evaluate the effects of pH (4.5–6.5), temperature (30°C–45°C), lactose concentration (50–250 g L^{-1}), and cell biomass concentration (A_{600} 2–4). It was found that the temperature was the most significant factor in optimizing ethanol production, followed by pH, cell biomass concentration, and lactose concentration. Several tools, namely, the genetic and metabolic engineering techniques, are available for the improvement of yeast strains (Nevoigt, 2008; Nielsen, 2001). In addition, the so-called conventional methodologies of mutagenesis with screening are still very useful in microbial improvement programs (Parekh et al., 2000). The combination of such tools with evolutionary engineering strategies (Çakar et al., 2009; Sauer, 2001) constitutes a powerful approach for the improvement of strains in specific harsh conditions typical of certain industrial fermentation processes. Evolutionary engineering follows nature's "engineering" principle by variation and selection, and this is a powerful strategy for improving industrially important characteristics of *S. cerevisiae*. Cell immobilization techniques can also improve continuous fermentation (CF) by enhancing ethanol productivity and protecting cells from inhibitory products and environmental variations, resulting in smaller bioreactor volumes and lower operational costs (Kourkoutas et al., 2004). Cell immobilization offers many advantages, such as enhanced fermentation productivity; utility of continuous processing; cell constancy; and lower costs of recovery, recycling, and downstream processing (Margaritis and Merchant, 1984; Stewart and Russel, 1986).

Because of their high lactose content, whey and scotta could be considered as media for biotechnological transformation into bioethanol. In a study conducted by Zoppellari and Bardi (2013), different fermentation managements were tested for best ethanol yields and process performance, considering the yeast physiology. They focused on oxygen availability, temperature, growth medium, and semicontinuous fermentation. The best performance was observed at low temperatures (28°C); high temperatures are also compatible with good ethanol yields in whey fermentations but not in scotta fermentations. Semicontinuous fermentation in the dispersed phase gave the best fermentation performance, particularly with scotta. Both effluents can thus be considered suitable for ethanol production.

ENGINEERING OF *SACCHAROMYCES CEREVISIAE* STRAINS

S. cerevisiae is generally regarded as model sugar-fermenting organisms and is a major bioethanol producer worldwide. Fermentation with *S. cerevisiae* has various advantages over other microorganism in relation to ethanol production:

- It is generally recognized as safe (GRAS).
- It has a high potential for alcoholic fermentation even under aerobic conditions (Crabtree effect), thereby making *S. cerevisiae* Crabtree positive (Pronk et al., 1996). The yeast, which is crab-positive, has the ability to transport a greater flux for the formation of fermentation products such as ethanol.
- The high degree of ethanol tolerance of *S. cerevisiae* strains is also a beneficial attribute of this microbial cell factory (Aguilera et al., 2006; Snowdon et al., 2009).

- *S. cerevisiae* cells are able to produce a high ethanol titer (Antoni et al., 2007).
- Its ability to grow promptly under anaerobic conditions is the key factor for the application of *S. cerevisiae* as a model fermentation catalyst.
- The metabolic and structural properties of the *S. cerevisiae* cell make it the appropriate organism of choice for bioethanol production, and biomass obtained after downstream processing may be used as a single-cell protein (SCP) for animal feed (Bai et al., 2008).

S. cerevisiae lacks the necessary cellular machinery to utilize lactose as a carbon source because it lacks the membrane protein lactose permease (*LAC12*), which is responsible for transporting the lactose across the cell membrane. *S. cerevisiae* also lacks the β galactosidase (*LAC4*) structural genes responsible for the breakdown of lactose into its monomers, that is, glucose and galactose. The problem can be solved by using the *S. cerevisiae* strains in whey fermentation, where the lactose is pre-hydrolyzed to yield glucose and galactose. But the main drawback of this strategy is the requirement of pre-hydrolyzed suspension of lactose, which is ultimately responsible for the high production cost. *S. cerevisiae* ferments glucose preferentially and forms galactose, which also increases the length of time for the fermentation process because of the diauxic lag phase after glucose is depleted from the production media. The possible solution is to select the catabolite repression–resistant mutants. The 2-deoxyglucose is the main agent generally used for selecting the mutants. A mutant strain of Saccharomyces cerevisiae ferments a rich medium containing a mixture of glucose and galactose simultaneously with an ethanol titer of 90 g L^{-1} (Bailey et al., 1982).

CONSTRUCTION OF LACTOSE-UTILIZING *S. CEREVISIAE* STRAINS

PROTOPLAST FUSION

The development of a *S. cerevisiae* strain with the ability to ferment lactose is an important technical aspect for successful and economical production of cheese whey. The main approach to constructing the Lac+ (lactose fermenting) *S. cerevisiae* is the protoplast fusion. Protoplast fusion is used for development of important industrial strains of yeast (Ferenczy and Maraz, 1977; Scheinbach, 1983). Protoplast fusion was used to transfer the nuclear genes interspecifically and intraspecifically into strains of yeast. Taya et al. (1984) constructed a protoplast fusion of *S. cerevisiae* kyokai 7 and *K. lactis* T396 and obtained a stable hybrid strain PN13 that produced ethanol at a higher rate than the parental *K. lactis* strain. In another study by Farahnak et al. (1986), a hybrid strain was constructed using auxotrophic strain of *S. cerevisiae* having high ethanol tolerance and an auxotrophic strain of *K. fragilis* having a natural ability to ferment lactose. The strain obtained was capable of fermenting lactose and yielded higher amounts of ethanol (13% v/v) compared to the parental strain. Ryu et al. (1991) constructed a strain showing high ethanol tolerance, β galactosidase production, and lactose fermentation by protoplast fusion of *S. cerevisiae* STV 89 and *K. fragilis* CBS397. The fusant obtained was found to be more ethanol tolerant because of its higher unsaturated fatty acid (linoleic acid) content and less accumulation of intracellular ethanol due to the increased diffusion rate of ethanol. The ethanol production rate was also increased with greater β galactosidase secretion. Tahoun et al. (2002) reported a fusant strain capable of fermenting both sweet and salted whey by protoplast fusion of *S. cerevisiae* and *K. lactis*.

CO-IMMOBILIZATION

Another vital strategy proposed by various researchers is to ferment the whey lactose by using the enzyme β-galactosidase co-immobilized with *S. cerevisiae* strain for successful ethanol production. Rosenberg et al. (1996) reported the use of permeabilized *K. marxianus* with *S. cerevisiae* for simultaneous hydrolysis of lactose from concentrated whey and achieved higher ethanol productivity compared to direct fermentation with the *K. marxianus* strain. Wild strains of *S. cerevisiae* cannot utilize the lactose; however, *S. cerevisiae* can metabolize the hydrolyzed product, galactose, by a membrane permease (*GAL2*) through the Leloir pathway (Nehlin et al., 1989). Thus, *S. cerevisiae* can be used in whey fermentation after the lactose is hydrolyzed into glucose and galactose.

DIRECT METABOLIC ENGINEERING

The various strain development programs that use the metabolic engineering of *S. cerevisiae* are important for lactose-to-ethanol fermentation with increased productivity. Some microorganisms are natural lactose fermenters, and their lactose-utilizing genes are a target for cloning in *S. cerevisiae* cells in a direct metabolic engineering approach. The main organisms containing essential lactose pathway genes are *E. coli*, *Kluyveromyces*, and *Aspergillus niger*. Two different approaches were used for the construction of recombinant *S. cerevisiae* *Lac+*: primarily cloning of both the lactose permease and β-galactosidase genes, and β-galactosidase production in the extracellular medium. A different methodology involves the secretion of the *E. coli* galactosidase in *S. cerevisiae* cells. In *E. coli*, the effort to direct β-galactosidase to the membrane by means of the signal sequence of a membrane protein was ineffective. In *S. cerevisiae*, various signal sequences, *SUC2*, *MF*, and *STA2*, genes were used, but these attempts were also unsuccessful. With the *STA2* signal sequence Vanoni et al. (1989) were able to detect 76% of β-galactosidase activity in the periplasmic space, but activity of the enzyme was not detected in the culture medium. Thus, the first engineered strain of *S. cerevisiae* that could produce the intracellular β-galactosidase did not utilize lactose. The problem was first solved by constructing a Lac+ strain using a plasmid that carries the β-galactosidase (*LAC4*) and lactose permease (*LAC12*) from *K. lactis*. The Lac+ transformed cell had integrated copies of the vector into the host chromosome (Sreekrishna and Dickson, 1985). But the strain was found to grow poorly on the lactose medium. In addition, the strain was found to be mitotically unstable. Later Porro et al. (1992) were able to grow *S. cerevisiae* on a medium with lactose by expressing the *S. cerevisiae Gal4* gene with the *E. coli* lac Z gene. Both genes were placed under the control of an inducible promoter. An increase in the expression of the β-galactosidase causes lysis of the cell, which in turn causes release of the β-galactosidase into the medium. β-Galactosidase causes the breakdown of lactose into glucose and galactose, which in turn are assimilated by yeast.

Kumar et al. (1992) constructed Lac+ *S. cerevisiae* with the β-galactosidase of *A. niger* (Lac A). The filamentous fungi *A. niger* is an efficient producer of various extracellular enzymes that are important for different reasons from an industrial point of view. Among these enzymes is β-galactosidase, which is used mainly to hydrolyze lactose in acid whey. The cloning of the *LACA* gene (coding for *A. niger* β-galactosidase) with its own signal sequence resulted in recombinant *S. cerevisiae* cells secreting β-galactosidase. Cells expressing the *LACA* gene on a multicopy plasmid secrete up to 40% of total β-galactosidase into the growth medium, and the *S. cerevisiae* was found to grow on whey permeate (4% w/v lactose). But the Lac+ phenotype was unstable, and the assimilation of the lactose was subject to diauxic growth. Rapid and complete lactose hydrolysis and higher ethanol (0.31 g g^{-1} of sugar) and biomass (0.24 g g^{-1} of sugar) production were observed with distiller's yeast grown under aerobic conditions. However, plasmid stability was low.

LACTOSE UTILIZATION BY FLOCCULANT *S. CEREVISIAE*

Domingues et al. (1999) constructed a flocculent *S. cerevisiae* strain secreting β-galactosidase using the vector developed by Kumar et al. (1992). Optimization of the culture condition, such as lactose concentration, with bioreactor operation together led to a 21-fold increase in the extracellular β-galactosidase produced compared to preliminary shake-flask fermentations. For improving the genetic stability of the strains, the *LACA* gene expression cassette was targeted to the δ-sequences in the genome. It was found that these strains produced ethanol from lactose/whey with close-to-theoretical yields in batch and in high-cell-density CFs with a complete utilization of lactose. Domingues et al. (1999) constructed a flocculant Lac+ strain expressing the *LAC4* and *LAC12* gene of *K. lactis* using the 13-kb genome sequence that included the two genes and the intergenic region between them. The original recombinant strain (T1) reported a slow growth on lactose with a doubling time of 5 hours and with a low ethanol yield. After the adaption of the strain on lactose, however, the result was an increase in ethanol production. The rheology of the flocculated strain determined in a reactor was studied by Klien et al. (2005). But the adapted strain lost its features after storage at −80°C. Evolutionary engineering was used to improve the stability of the strain. The evolved strain formed from the original T1 was named T1E, and this strain was found to have a higher ethanol yield and greater flocculation than the original recombinant strain. Transcriptome analysis and molecular differences were investigated, and the molecular events responsible were found to be 1,593 bp gene deletion in the intergenic region. It was also found that the plasmid copy number is decreased in the evolved strain. Therefore, it was projected that the expression of the *LAC* genes in the evolved recombinant was due to both the decreased copy number of *LAC4* and *LAC12* genes and different levels of transcriptional induction for both genes due to changed promoter structure. The stable, lactose-fermenting, evolved strain T1E conferred highly flocculent phenotype with efficient fermentation of lactose to ethanol. The ethanol production was found to be 8% ethanol from media containing 150 g L^{-1} lactose, and showed an ethanol productivity of 1.5–2.0 g L^{-1}h^{-1} (Guimarães et al., 2008a).

Systemwide analysis of the cell using the DNA microarrays is an important tool for strain development (Bro et al., 2005). These techniques can be used to study the strains undergoing improvement programs. The difference between the strains can be measured by checking the desired phenotype and by measuring the genes and other factors responsible for that phenotype. This is an important part of inverse metabolic engineering approaches (Bailey et al., 1996; Nielsen and Olsson, 2002; Bro and Nielsen, 2004). Once a strain with a desired feature is obtained, for example, by an evolutionary engineering method, systemwide tools can be used to elucidate main metabolic pathways and targets for future engineering of cell factories. The identified genes and factors contributing to the desired phenotype can also be incorporated into other cells for getting the desired phenotype (Çakar et al., 2006; Guimarães et al., 2008b).

Gene Deletion of *GAL* Regulatory Genes

Metabolic engineering, that is, the intentional redirection of metabolic fluxes, has played a unique role in improving yeast strains. In contrast to classical methods of genetic strain improvement such as selection, mutagenesis, mating, and hybridization, metabolic engineering has major advantages, one of them being that the directed modification of strains takes place without the accumulation of unfavorable mutations. The way to modify the level of gene expression is by regulating the copy number and regulatory sequence (promoter) upstream of a gene. Most metabolic engineering has involved modification of only a single gene, for example, disruption of a pathway or expression of a particular gene for protein production (Ostergaard et al., 2000).

CELLULAR CONTROL FOR GALACTOSE METABOLISM

The expression and regulation of genes are essentially important for maintaining the metabolic functions and growth in all types of cells. As mentioned, the prehydrolyzed lactose containing both glucose and galactose is treated as a substrate for *S. cerevisiae*. There remains the glucose repression phenomenon, and the utilization of galactose is not optimal because the sugars are consumed sequentially. First, the glucose is utilized; then the utilization of the galactose sugar takes place. The alleviation of glucose repression results in a more simultaneous ingestion of both glucose and galactose present in the medium and is therefore of significant industrial interest because it results in short cultivation time.

Therefore, the focus is on engineering the *GAL* system of *S. cerevisiae*, which contains the genes encoding the proteins responsible for galactose utilization, and the system is under dual control. The system is induced by galactose and repressed by the glucose present in the cultivation media. *GAL* system induction requires the presence of intracellular galactose, which acts as a signal molecule by the ATP-dependent mechanism. The genetics of the *GAL* system has served as a eukaryotic model system for transcriptional control. Galactose metabolism occurs with the help of the Leloir pathway.

The Leloir pathway requires five enzymes to convert galactose into glucose-6-phosphate. Mutation in some of the enzymes of this pathway in mammals is responsible for genetic diseases, for example, galactosemia (Timson, 2006). In *S. cerevisiae*, the enzyme activities are controlled mainly by these five proteins: Gal1p, Gal7p, Gal10p, PGM1p, and PGM2p. Gal1p is a galactokinase responsible for conversion of galactose to galactose-1-phosphate (Schell and Wilson, 1977; Timson, 2007). It also combines with UDP glucose to form D-glucose-1-phosphate and UDP galactose by the Gal 7p. UDP-glucose is regenerated from UDP Gal by Gal10p enzyme. The final step of the pathway is catalyzed with the help of phosphoglucomutase by isomerization of glucose-1-phosphate to glucose-6-phosphate. In *S. cerevisiae*, two phosphoglucomutase forms are present: *PGM1* and *PGM2*. *PGM2* is responsible for 80% of the total enzyme activity (Tsoi and Douglas, 1964).

In *S. cerevisiae*, three genetically defined regulatory genes—*GAL4* (a transcriptional activator), *GAL80* (a repressor), and *GAL3* (a ligand sensor)—control the expression of genes of the Leloir pathway, which codes for enzymes required for galactose utilization. Considerable genetic evidence indicates that the *GAL4* and *GAL80* regulatory genes function via diffusible proteins to activate or inactivate the transcription of the structural genes (Gill, 1988; Leuther, 1992).

Regulation of transcription requires coupling of gene-specific transcription activators to regulatory signals. Galactose-inducible genes (*GAL* genes) in yeast *S. cerevisiae* are efficiently transcribed only when the sequence-specific transcription activator Gal4p is activated. Activation of Gal4p requires interaction between the Gal4p inhibitory protein Gal80p and the galactokinase paralog, Gal3p. Gal3p binds to a Gal80p-Gal4p complex in the nucleus to activate Gal4p. Gal3p-Gal80p interaction occurs in the cytoplasm, and concurrently, Gal80p is removed from Gal4p at the *GAL* gene promoter. The results indicate that galactose-triggered Gal3p-Gal80p association in the cytoplasm activates Gal4p in the nucleus (Suzuki-Fujimoto et al., 1996; Yano and Fukasawa, 1997; Peng and Hopper, 2002). The Gal4 protein acts as a positive regulator for the Gal regulon. The *GAL3* function is necessary for normal rapid induction, and the *GAL3* mutants exhibit slower induction. The Gal80 protein is thought to be necessary to prevent structural gene expression in the absence of galactose, as proposed by the constitutive phenotype of cells with recessive *GAL80* mutations and the noninducible phenotype of cells with dominant *GAL80S* mutations.

Another strategy for increasing ethanol yield is increasing the overall flux of galactose in the Leloir pathway (Niederberger et al., 1992). This can be achieved by reducing the level of the negative regulator or by increasing the level of the positive activator of the gene expression. Three main negative regulators control the expression of *GAL* genes found in the case of *S. cerevisiae*: Gal80, Mig1, and Gal6 proteins. First, the Gal 80 p is the transcription factor (repressor) of the *GAL* genetic switch, which, as mentioned, is responsible for preventing the *GAL* gene expression in the presence of glucose. The Mig1p is another protein that, in the presence of glucose, is responsible for repressing the expression of *GAL* genes. The two other proteins—Mig2p and Nrg1p—are also found to substitute partially for the Mig1p (Lutfiyya et al., 1998; Zhou and Winston, 2001). But the main role belongs to the Mig1p protein only. Mig1p is a Zinc-finger DNA binding protein that senses the glucose but does not bind directly to glucose. It has a binding site upstream of the *GAL* genes, and this site is found close to or overlapping with Gal4p (activator) binding sites (Frolova et al., 1999). Papamichos-Chronakis et al. (2004), has reported that even during active transcription, Mig 1p can remain bound to the upstream sequences of *GAL* genes. Mig 1p is also found to be responsible for forming a complex with general transcription co-repressor complex Ssn6p-tup1p (Keleher et al., 1992; Treitel and Carlson, 1995), which represses the transcription of the *GAL* genes. This complex maintains the chromatin in inert form by recruiting the histone deacetylase complex (Wu et al., 2001; Malave and Dent, 2006).

The third negative regulator, Gal 6p, is a bleomycin hydrolase that is a highly conserved and ubiquitous protein whose cellular function is other than hydrolyzing. Bleomycin is part of an autoregulatory circuit that downregulates the *GAL* system by changing the production, stabilization, and degradation of the *GAL1*, *GAL2*, and *GAL7* mRNA, but the mechanism responsible for this is still not known (Zheng et al., 1997). Cells with *GAL6* deletion, when transferred from glucose to galactose medium, show a faster induction of *GAL1* and a higher level at stationary phase. This indicates that deletion of *GAL6* allows relief of glucose repression faster, with a higher total output of *GAL1* (Zheng et al., 1997). The *GAL* genes are tightly regulated, being repressed by glucose and induced by galactose up to 1,000 times (Johnston and Carlson, 1992). *GAL* gene expression requires the well-studied transcriptional activator protein Gal4, which binds to the *GAL* gene promoters. Gal4 function is inhibited by Gal80, which binds directly to Gal4, and by Mig1, which represses expression of *GAL1* and *GAL4* in the presence of glucose. Three known negative regulators of the *GAL* system—Gal6, Gal80, and Mig1—were the main targeted regulatory genes. Deletion of the genes encoding the transcriptional repressor Mig1 and the Gal80 increased the flux through the galactose utilization pathway 15% compared to the wild-type strain. Deletion of *GAL6*, which encodes a protein that negatively regulates *GAL* gene expression by an unknown mechanism, increased the flux through the pathway by 24%. The maximum increase in flux (41%) was achieved by eliminating all three proteins that impose downregulation of the *GAL* gene regulatory network. The improved galactose consumption of the gal mutants did not favor biomass formation; instead, it caused excessive respire fermentative metabolism, with the ethanol production rate increasing linearly with glycolytic flux (Ostergaard et al., 2000). The increase in the flux of galactose has a positive impact on ethanol formation. The ethanol yield is increased from 5 mmol EtOH/g gal, in the case of the wild-type strain, to 8.48 mmol EtOH/g gal, in the case of the triple mutant strain (Δgal6 Δgal80Δmig 1) (Ostergaard et al., 2000).

Further increasing the expression of *GAL4* by using a high-copy-number plasmid containing *GAL4* gene caused a 26% higher maximum specific galactose consumption rate compared with the wild-type strain, which is less when compared with the increase in flux obtained by eliminating Gal6, Gal80, and Mig1. This may perhaps be due to expression of both *GAL6* and *GAL80* when the level of Gal4 is increased, and they have an indirect negative impact on expression of GAL enzyme (Igarashi et al., 1987; Ostergaard, 2000).

IMPROVING GALACTOSE UPTAKE BY USING THE *PGM2* GENE

Inverse metabolic engineering is used for determining another target gene responsible for increasing the galactose uptake rate in *S. cerevisiae* under increasingly aerobic conditions in expression of *PGM2*, which leads to a 70% increase in the maximum specific galactose uptake rate and a threefold increase in the maximum specific ethanol production rate compared to the rates of the reference strain. The maximum specific growth rate on galactose of the *PGM2* strain was 0.23 ± 0.02 h^{-1} compared to 0.17 ± 0.01 h^{-1} for the reference strain. Bro et al. (2005) report that phosphoglucomutase plays a key role in controlling the flux through the Leloir pathway, possibly due to the increased conversion of glucose-1-phosphate to glucose-6-phosphate. This makes a more efficient shunting of galactose from the Leloir pathway into glycolysis. The increased intracellular levels of glucose-6-phosphate and fructose-6-phosphate in the *PGM2* overexpressing strain may ensure that the flux through glycolysis can be increased. Sanchez et al. (2010) found that, under anaerobic conditions, the overexpression of *PGM2* using an integrative plasmid increased the *PGM* activity five to six times, which considerably lessens the lag phase of glucose pregrown cells in an anaerobic galactose culture. PGM2 overexpression also increased the anaerobic-specific growth rate, but ethanol production was not significantly changed.

FURTHER DEVELOPMENTS NEEDED FOR BIOFUEL DEVELOPMENT

The requirements still needed to develop a process for increasing whey utilization for large-scale production of the ethanol are as follows:

- Simultaneous fermentation of both glucose and the galactose.
- New strains for biofuel fermentation from whey.
- Strains of yeast with higher fermentation temperature and better ethanol tolerance.
- Improvement in various factors such as the substrate concentration, growth, and product separation.
- Improved methods of whey disposal and its proper management.

CONCLUSION

With blending, biofuels produced from renewable resources can be used as supplements to fossil fuels. In this chapter, we discussed whey, which is considered a waste product, as a value-added product similar to bioethanol. Fermentation of the lactose in whey by yeast to produce ethanol is an area that needs to be studied. As a model cell factory in classical and modern biotechnological processes, the yeast *S. cerevisiae* is of great importance in the production of ethanol. Various strategies were employed for creating a lactose-utilizing strain. The genetic engineering of yeast using recombinant strains of *S. cerevisiae* for lactose fermentation resulted in an increase in ethanol production and thereby holds promising results, but it needs to be scaled up for industrial production of ethanol. Another target organism is the dairy yeast *Kluyveromyces marxianus*, which can ferment lactose and carry the lactose permease and β-galactosidase gene pair, which are responsible for the uptake and subsequent cleavage of lactose into glucose and galactose and are thus the targets for ethanol production. For industrial production of ethanol from whey, there is still the need of good fermentation technology to enhance ethanol production. Therefore, the development of appropriate strains using genetic engineering will help in generating the robust strain that can increase ethanol production efficiently. Promising results were obtained for the recombinant *S. cerevisiae* strains, but the procedure needs to be scaled up for larger-scale production of ethanol. Whole genome transcript analysis will also help in discovering newer target genes that will be essential in improving particular traits of particular cell factories.

REFERENCES

Anderson, P. J., McNeil, K., Watson, K., 1986. High-efficiency carbohydrate fermentation to ethanol at temperatures above 40°C by *Kluyveromyces marxianus var. marxianus* isolated from sugar mills. *Appl. Environ. Microbiol.* 51(6), 1314–1320.

Aguilera, F., Peinado, R. A., Millan, C., Ortega, J. M., Mauricio, J. C., 2006. Relationship between ethanol tolerance, H+-ATPase activity and the lipid composition of the plasma membrane in different wine yeast strains. *Intern. J. Food Microbiol.* 110(1), 34–42.

Antoni, D., Zverlov, V. V., Schwarz, W. H., 2007. Biofuels from microbes. *Appl. Microbiol. Biotechnol.* 77, 23–35.

Bai, F. W., Anderson, W. A., Moo-Young, M., 2008. Ethanol fermentation technologies from sugar and starch feedstocks. *Biotechnol. Adv.* 26(1), 89–105.

Bailey, R. B., Benitez, T., Woodward, A., 1982. *Saccharomyces cerevisiae* mutants resistant to catabolite repression: Use in cheese whey hydrolysate fermentation. *Appl. Environ. Microbial.* 44(3), 631–639.

Bailey, J. E., Sburlati, A., Hatzimanikatis, V., Lee, K., Renner, W. A., Tsai, P. S., 1996. Inverse metabolic engineering: A strategy for directed genetic engineering of useful phenotypes. *Biotechnol. Bioeng.* 52(1), 109–121.

Banat, I. M., Nigam, P., Marchant, R., 1992. Isolation of thermotolerant, fermentative yeasts growing at 52°C and producing ethanol at 45°C and 50°C. *World. J. Microbiol. Biotechnol.* 8, 259–263.

Bauer, F. F., Pretorius, I. S., 2000. Yeast stress response and fermentation efficiency: How to survive them making of wine-a review. *South African J. Enol. Viticulture* 21, 27–51.

Brethauer, S., Wyman, C. E., 2010. Review: Continuous hydrolysis and fermentation for cellulosic ethanol production. *Bioresource Technol.* 101(13), 4862–4874.

Breunig, K. D., Bolotin–Fukuhara, M., Bianchi, M. M., Bourgarel, D., Falcone, C., et al., 2000. Regulation of primary carbon metabolism in *Kluyveromyces lactis. Enz. Microbiol. Technol.* 26(9), 771–780.

Bro, C., Knudsen, S., Regenberg, B., Olsson, L., Nielsen, J., 2005. Improvement of galactose uptake in *Saccharomyces cerevisiae* through overexpression of phosphoglucomutase: Example of transcript analysis as a tool in inverse metabolic engineering. *Appl. Environ. Microbial.* 71(11), 6465–6472.

Bro, C., Nielsen, J., 2004. Impact of "ome" analyses on inverse metabolic engineering. *Metabolic Eng.* 6(3), 204–211.

Çakar, Z. P., Alkım, C., Turanlı, B., Tokman, N., Akman, S., et al., 2009. Isolation of cobalt hyper-resistant mutants of *Saccharomyces cerevisiae* by in vivo evolutionary engineering approach. *J. Biotechnol.* 143(2), 130–138.

Çakar, Z. P., Seker, U. O. S., Tamerler, C., Sonderegger, M., Sauer, U., 2005. Evolutionary engineering of multi-stress resistant *Saccharomyces cerevisiae*. *FEMS Yeast* 5, 569–578.

De Wit, J. N., 2001. *Lecturer's Handbook on Whey and Whey Products.* Brussels, Belgium: European Whey Products Association.

Diniz, R. H., Rodrigues, M. Q., Fietto, L. G., Passos, F. M., Silveira, W. B., 2014. Optimizing and validating the production of ethanol from cheese whey permeate by *Kluyveromyces marxianus* UFV-3. *Biocat. Agri. Biotechnol.* 3(2), 111–117.

Domingues, L., Dantas, M. M., Lima, N., Teixeira, J. A., 1999. Continuous ethanol fermentation of lactose by a recombinant flocculating *Saccharomyces cerevisiae* strain. *Biotechnol. Bioeng.* 64, 692–697.

Farahnak, F., Seki, T., Ryu, D. D., Ogrydziak, D., 1986. Construction of lactose-assimilating and high ethanol producing yeasts by protoplast fusion. *Appl. Environ. Microbiol.* 51, 362–367.

Ferenczy, L., Maráz, A., 1977. Transfer of mitochondria by protoplast fusion in Saccharomyces cerevisiae. *Nature* 268, 524–525.

Fonseca, G. G., Heinzle, E., Wittmann, C., Gombert, A. K., 2013. The yeast *Kluyveromyces marxianus* and its biotechnological potential. *Appl. Microbio. Biotechnol.* 79(3), 339–354.

Frolova, E., Johnston, M., Majors, J., 1999. Binding of the glucose-dependent Mig1p repressor to the GAL1 and GAL4 promoters *in vivo*: Regulation by glucose and chromatin structure. *Nucleic Acids* 27: 1350–1358.

Galbe, M., Zacchi, G., 2002. A review of the production of ethanol from softwood. *Appl. Microbial. Biotechnol.* 59(6), 618–628.

Gardner, D., 1989. New technologies in the conversion of whey to high protein products. *Modern Dairy* 68, 15–17.

Gill, G., Ptashne, M., 1988. Negative effect of the transcriptional activator GAL 4. *Nature* 334(6184), 721–724.

Guimaraes, P. M. R., Francois, J., Parrou, J. L., Teixeira, J. A., Domingues, L., 2008a. Adaptive evolution of a lactose-consuming *Saccharomyces cerevisiae* recombinant. *Appl. Environ. Microbiol.* 74: 1748–1756.

Guimarães, P. M., Teixeira, J. A., Domingues, L., 2008b. Fermentation of high concentrations of lactose to ethanol by engineered flocculent *Saccharomyces cerevisiae*. *Biotechnol. Lett.* 30(11), 1953–1958.

Harden, T. J., 1996. The reduction of BOD and production of biomass from acid whey by *Kluyveromyces marxianus. Food Australia* 48(10), 456–457.

Hashem, M., Zohri, A. N. A., Ali, M. M., 2013. Optimization of the fermentation conditions for ethanol production by new thermotolerant yeast strains of Kluyveromyces sp. *Afr. J. Microbiol. Res.* 7(37), 4550–4561.

Hughes, D. B., Tudroszen, N. J., Moye, C. J., 1984. The effect of temperature on the kinetics of ethanol production by a thermotolerant strain of *Kluveromyces marxianus. Biotechnol. Lett.* 6, 1–6.

Igarashi, M., Segawa, T., Nogi, Y., Suzuki, Y., Fukasawa, T., 1987. Autogenous regulation on the *Saccharomyces cerevisiae* regulatory gene GAL80. *Mol. General Gen.* 207(2–3), 273–279.

Johnston, M., Carlson, M., 1992. In *The Molecular and Cellular Biology of the Yeast Saccharomyces: Gene Expression.* Cold Spring Harbor, NY: Cold Spring Harbor Laboratory Press, pp. 193–281.

Keleher, C. A., Redd, M. J., Schultz, J., Carlson, M., Johnson, A. D., 1992. Ssn6-Tup1 is a general repressor of transcription in yeast. *Cell* 68(4), 709–719.

Kemp, D. L., Quickenden, J., 1989. Whey processing for profit-a worthy alternative. In *Resources and Applications of Biotechnology,* London, UK: The New Wave, pp. 323–331.

Kosikowski, F. V., 1979. Whey utilization and whey products. *J. Dairy Sci.* 62, 1149–1160.

Kourkoutas, Y., Bekatorou, A., Banat, I. M., Marchant, R., Koutinas, A. A., 2004. Immobilization technologies and support materials suitable in alcohol beverages production: A review. *Food Microbiol.* 21(4), 377–397.

Kumar, V., Ramakrishnan, S., Teeri, T. T., Knowles, J. K., Hartley, B. S., 1992. *Saccharomyces cerevisiae* cells secreting an *Aspergillus niger* β-galactosidase grow on whey permeate. *Nature Biotechnol.* 10(1), 82–85.

Kurtzman, C. P., 2003. Phylogenetic circumscription of *Saccharomyces, Kluyveromyces* and other members of the Saccharomycetaceae, and the proposal of the new genera *Lachancea, Nakaseomyces, Naumovia, Vanderwaltozyma* and *Zygotorulaspora*. *FEMS Yeast Res.* 4(3), 233–245.

Lachance, M. A., 2007. Current status of Kluyveromyces systematics. *FEMS Yeast Res.* 7(5), 642–645.

Lachance, M. A. 1998. Kluyveroixyces., In *The Yeasts, A Taxonomic Study*, 4th ed., Amsterdam, the Netherlands: Elsevier Science, pp. 227–247.

Leuther, K. K., Johnston, S. A., 1992. Nondissociation of GAL4 and GAL80 in vivo after galactose induction. *Science* 256(5061), 1333–1335.

Llorente, B., Malpertuy, A., Blandin, G., Artiguenave, F., Wincker, P., Dujon, B., 2000. Genomic Exploration of the Hemiascomycetous Yeasts: 12. *Kluyveromyces marxianus* var. *marxianus*. *FEBS Lett.* 487(1), 71–75.

Lutfiyya, L. L., Iyer, V. R., DeRisi, J., DeVit, M. J., Brown, P. O., Johnston, M., 1998. Characterization of three related glucose repressors and genes they regulate in *Saccharomyces cerevisiae*. *Genetics* 150(4), 1377–1391.

Magalhatilde, K. T., Rodrigues, A. K., Gervasio, I. M., Gervasio, I., Schwan, R. F., 2013. Ethanol production from deproteinized cheese whey fermentations by co-cultures of *Kluyveromyces marxianus* and *Saccharomyces cerevisiae*. *Afr. J. Microbiol. Res.* 7(13), 1121–1127.

Malave, T. M., Dent, S. Y., 2006. Transcriptional repression by Tup1-Ssn6. *Biochem. Cell Bio.* 84(4), 437–443.

Margaritis, A., Merchant, F. J. A., 1984. Advances in ethanol production using immobilized cell systems. *Crit. Rev. Biotechnol.* 1, 339–393.

Marwaha, S. S., Kennedy, J. F., 1998. Whey—pollution problem and potential utilization. *Int. J. Food Sci. Technol.* 23(4), 323–336.

Mawson, A. J., 1994. Bioconversions for whey utilization and waste abatement. *Biores. Technol.* 47, 195–203.

Myers, R. H., Montgomery, D. C., 1995. *Response Surface Methodology: Process and Product Optimization Using Designed Experiments*, New York, NY: Wiley.

Nehlin, J. O., Carlberg, M., Ronne, H., 1989. Yeast galactose permease is related to yeast and mammalian glucose transporters. *Gene* 85, 313–319.

Niederberger, P., Prasad, R., Miozzari, G., Kacser, H., 1992. A strategy for increasing an in vivo flux by genetic manipulations. *Biochem. J.* 287, 473–479.

Nielsen, J., Olsson, L., 2002. An expanded role for microbial physiology in metabolic engineering and functional genomics: Moving towards systems biology. *FEMS Yeast Res.* 2(2), 175–181.

Nevoigt, E., 2008. Progress in metabolic engineering of *Saccharomyces cerevisiae*. *Microbiol. Mol. Biol.* 72, 379–412.

Nielsen, J., 2001. Metabolic engineering. *Appl. Microbiol. Biotechnol.* 55(3), 263–283.

Oda, Y., Nakamura, K., 2009. Production of ethanol from the mixture of beet molasses and cheese whey by a 2-deoxyglucose-resistant mutant of *Kluyveromyces marxianus*. *FEMS Yeast Res.* 9(5), 742–748.

OECD, 2008. Agricultural Outlook 2008–2017. Ostergaard, S., Olsson, L., Johnston, M., Nielsen, J., 2000. Increasing galactose consumption by *Saccharomyces cerevisiae* through metabolic engineering of the GAL gene regulatory network. *Nature Biotechnol.* 18(12), 1283–1286.

Pang, Z. W., Liang, J. J., Qin, X. J., Wang, J. R., Feng, J. O., Huang, R. B., 2010. Multiple induced mutagenesis for improvement of ethanol production by *Kluyveromyces marxianus. Biotechnol. Lett.* 32(12), 1847–1851.

Papamichos-Chronakis, M., Gligoris, T., Tzamarias, D., 2004. The Snf1 kinase controls glucose repression in yeast by modulating interactions between the Mig1 repressor and the Cyc8–Tup1 co-repressor. *EMBO Rep.* 5, 368–372.

Parekh, S., Vinci, V. A., Strobel, R. J., 2000. Improvement of microbial strains and fermentation processes. *Appl. Microbiol. Biotechnol.* 54(3), 287–301.

Peng, G., Hopper, J. E., 2002. Gene activation by interaction of an inhibitor with a cytoplasmic signaling protein. *Proceedings of the National Academy of Sciences* 99(13), 8548–8553.

Pesta, G., Meyer-Pittroff, R., Russ, W., 2007. Utilization of whey. In *Utilization of By-Products and Treatment of Waste in the Food Industry*, New York: Springer, pp. 193–207.

Piper, P. W., Talreja, K., Panaretou, B., Moradas-Ferreira, P., Byrne, K., et al., 1994. Induction of major heat-shock proteins of Saccharomyces cerevisiae, including plasma membrane Hsp30, by ethanol levels above a critical threshold. *Microbiology* 140(11), 3031–3038.

Porro, D., Martegani, E., Ranzi, B. M., Alberghina, L., 1992. Lactose/whey utilization and ethanol production by transformed Saccharomyces cerevisiae cells. *Biotechnol. Bioeng.* 39(8), 799–805.

Pronk, J. T., Steensma, H. Y., Van Dijken, J. P., 1996. Pyruvate metabolism in *Saccharomyces cerevisiae. Yeast* 12(16), 1607–1633.

Rajeshwari, K. V., Balakrishnan, M., Kansal, A., Lata, K., Kishore, V. V. N., 2000. State-of-the-art of anaerobic digestion technology for industrial wastewater treatment. *Renew. Sust. Energ. Rev.* 4(2), 135–156.

Rosenberg, M., Tomáška, M., Kanuch, J., Surdík, E., 1996. Improved ethanol production from whey with *Saccharomyces cerevisiae* using permeabilized cells of *Kluyveromyces marxianus. Acta Biotechnologica* 15(4), 387–390.

Ryu, Y. W., Jang, H. W., Lee, H. S., 1991. Enhancement of ethanol tolerance of lactose assimilating yeast strain by protoplast fusion. *J. Microbiol. Biotechnol.* 1(3), 151–156.

Sanchez, R. G., Hahn-Hägerdal, B., Gorwa-Grauslund, M. F., 2010. Research PGM2 overexpression improves anaerobic galactose fermentation in *Saccharomyces cerevisiae. Microb. Cell Fact.* 9, 40.

Sansonetti, S., Curcio, S., Calabrò, V., Iorio, G., 2009. Bio-ethanol production by fermentation of ricotta cheese whey as an effective alternative non-vegetable source. *Biomass. Bioeng.* 33(12), 1687–1692.

Sauer, U., 2001. Evolutionary engineering of industrially important microbial phenotypes. *Adv. Biochem. Eng. Biotechnol.* 129–169.

Saxena, R., 1997. Demand for milk and milk products. Dairy India.

Schaffrath, R., Breunig, K. D., 2000. Genetics and Molecular Physiology of the Yeast *Kluyveromyces lactis. Fungal Genet. Biol.* 30(3), 173–190.

Scheinbach, S., 1983. Protoplast fusion as a means of producing new industrial yeast strains. *Biotechnol. Adv.* 1(2), 289–300.

Schell, M. A., Wilson, D. B., 1977. Purification and properties of galactokinase from *Saccharomyces cerevisiae. J. Bio. Chem.* 252(4), 1162–1166.

Siso, M. I., 1996. The biotechnological utilization of cheese whey: A review. *Bioresour. Technol.* 57(1), 1–11.

Smithers, G. S., 2008. Whey and whey proteins—from 'gutter-to-gold'. *International Dairy Journal* 18(7), 695–704.

Snowdon, C., Schierholtz, R., Poliszczuk, P., Hughes, S., Van Der Merwe, G., 2009. ETP1/ YHL010c is a novel gene needed for the adaptation of *Saccharomyces cerevisiae* to ethanol. *FEMS Yeast Res.* 9(3), 372–380.

Sreekrishna, K., Dickson, R. C., 1985. Construction of strains of Saccharomyces cerevisiae that grow on lactose. *Proceedings of the National Academy of Sciences* 82(23), 7909–7913.

Stewart, G. G., Russel, I., 1986. One hundred years of yeast research and development in the brewing industry. *J. Inst. Brew.* 92, 537–558.

Suzuki-Fujimoto, T., Fukuma, M., Yano, K. I., Sakurai, H., Vonika, A., et al., 1996. Analysis of the galactose signal transduction pathway in Saccharomyces cerevisiae: Interaction between Gal3p and Gal80p. *Mol. Cell. Bio.* 16(5), 2504–2508.

Tahoun, M. K., El-Nemr, T. M., Shata, O. H., 2002. A recombinant *Saccharomyces cerevisiae* strain for efficient conversion of lactose in salted and unsalted cheese whey into ethanol. *Mol. Nutr. Food Res.* 46, 321–326.

Taya, M., Honda, H., Kobayashi, T., 1984. Lactose-utilizing hybrid strain derived from *Saccharomyces cerevisiae* and *Kluyveromyces lactis* by protoplast fusion. *Agri. Biol. Chem.* 48, 2239–2243.

Timson, D. J., 2006. The structural and molecular biology of type III galactosemia. *IUBMB Life* 58(2), 83–89.

Timson, D. J., 2007. Galactose metabolism in *Saccharomyces cerevisiae*. *Dyn. Biochem. Process Biotechnol. Mol. Biol.* 1(1), 63–73.

Treitel, M. A., Carlson, M., 1995. Repression by SSN6-TUP1 is directed by MIG1, a repressor/ activator protein. *Proceedings of the National Academy of Sciences* 92(8), 3132–3136.

Tsoi, A., Douglas, H. C., 1964. The effect of mutation on two forms of phosphoglucomutase in Saccharomyces. *Biochim. Biophys. Acta* 92(3), 513–520.

van Dijken, J. P., Weusthuis, R. A., Pronk, J. T., 1993. Kinetics of growth and sugar consumption in yeasts. *Antonie Van Leeuwenhoek* 63(3–4), 343–352.

Vanoni, M., Lotti, M., Alberghina, L., 1989. Expression of cloned *Saccharomyces diastaticus* glucoamylase under natural and inducible promoters. *Biochim. Biophys. Acta* 1008(2), 168–176.

Visser, W., Scheffers, W. A., Batenburg-van der Vegte, W. H., van Dijken, J. P., 1990. Oxygen requirements of yeasts. *Appl. Environ. Microbiol.* 56, 3785–3792.

Webb, B. H., Whittier, E. O., 1948. The utilization of whey: A review. *J. Dairy Sci.* 31(2), 139–164.

Wu, A. M., 2001. Expression of binding properties of Gal/GalNAc reactive lectins by mammalian glycotopes. *The Mol. Immunol. Complex Carbohydrates* 2, 55–64.

Yamaoka, C., Kurita, O., Kubo, T., 2014. Improved ethanol tolerance of *Saccharomyces cerevisiae* in mixed cultures with *Kluyveromyces lactis* on high-sugar fermentation. *Microbiol. Res.* 169, 907–914.

Yang, S. T., Silva, E. M., 1995. Novel products and new technologies for use of a familiar carbohydrate, milk lactose. *J. Dairy. Sci.* 78(11), 2541–2562.

Yano, K. I., Fukasawa, T., 1997. Galactose-dependent reversible interaction of Gal3p with Gal80p in the induction pathway of Gal4p-activated genes of *Saccharomyces cerevisiae*. *Proceedings of the National Academy of Sciences* 94(5), 1721–1726.

Zafar, S., Owais, M., 2006. Ethanol production from crude whey by *Kluyveromyces marxianus*. *Biochem. Eng. J.* 27(3), 295–298.

Zheng, W., Xu, H. E., Johnston, S. A., 1997. The cysteine-peptidase bleomycin hydrolase is a member of the galactose regulon in yeast. *J. Bio. Chem.* 272(48), 30350–30355.

Zhou, H., Winston, F., 2001. NRG1 is required for glucose repression of the SUC2 and GAL genes of *Saccharomyces cerevisiae*. *BMC Genet.* 2, 5.

Zoppellari, F., Bardi, L., 2013. Production of bioethanol from effluents of the dairy industry by *Kluyveromyces marxianus*. *New Biotechnol.* 30(6), 607–613.

19 Analytical Potential of Bacterial Spores for Assessment of Milk Quality

Nimisha Tehri, Naresh Kumar, Rajesh Gopaul,
Pradip Kumar Sharma, and H. V. Raghu

CONTENTS

INTRODUCTION

Surveillance data obtained from different sources reveal the presence of various microbial and nonmicrobial contaminants in milk and its products. The presence of these contaminants has been attributed mainly to unhygienic environmental conditions during production, processing, transport, and storage, which is cause for serious concern (Thakur et al., 2014). In recent years, widespread outbreaks from various contaminated food products, including milk, have been reported. This contamination is linked to melamine in China, pesticides in India, and *Listeria monocytogenes* and *Salmonella typhimurium* in the United States. As a result, standards that include Colony forming Units (CFUs) and Maximum Residue Limits (MRLs) of potential contaminants, of both microbial and nonmicrobial origin, for different types of food matrices have been laid down by various regulatory bodies, for example, Codex Alimentarius, the European Union, Food Safety and Standards Authority of India, and so on (Kumar et al., 2013). This indicates the need for effective monitoring tools for targeting potential contaminants in various types of food matrices in order to comply with regulatory standards. Today, several conventional methods are available for detection of these contaminants. These methods are sensitive, efficient, and reliable, but they have inherent drawbacks: They have a limited scope of application under field conditions, are time-consuming, and require complex pretreatment steps during estimation. Therefore, faster screening methods are in demand. Biosensors represent an interesting approach for detecting various contaminants in food. They are analytical devices composed of two types of components, including a biological recognition element and a suitable transducer. Biosensors as reported in previous studies have been developed using enzymes, antibodies, aptamers, whole cells, and so on. This chapter explores the analytical potential of bacterial spores for their use as biorecognition molecules for targeting various types of contaminants in order to provide safe and wholesome consumer food products.

BACTERIAL SPORES

Spores are dormant structures produced by a process of sporulation in a few species of both gram-positive and gram-negative bacteria such as *Bacillus*, *Clostridium*, *Sporomusa*, and so on. They are meant to survive unfavorable environmental conditions. Endospores have a very hardy and robust structure comprised of many layers: a core, inner membrane, germ cell wall, cortex, outer membrane, coat, and sometimes exosporium, as depicted in Figure 19.1. These structural properties of spores allow them to preserve genetic material and to resist a wide temperature range, pressure, radiation, toxic chemicals, and many other extreme environmental conditions (Tehri, 2016).

SPORULATION AND GERMINATION

The process of spore formation is known as sporulation. Cells undergoing this process first divide into two unequal-sized progenies by the formation of a polar septum.

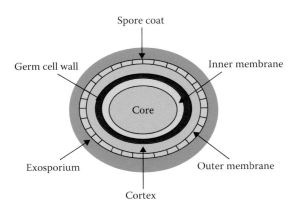

FIGURE 19.1 Structure of bacterial spore.

The septum leads to the development of a smaller forespore compartment and a larger mother cell. This step is followed by engulfment of the forespore by the mother cell. Its cytoplasm chiefly forms the core region of developing spore (Piggot and Hilbert, 2004). Thick cell wall material called the cortex is synthesized around the core, followed by a dense multilayered proteinaceous coat, which in turn is assembled by the mother cell onto the surface of forespore. An additional outermost layer of the spore, the crust, has also been identified. These outer layers of cortex, coat, and crust provide the spore with mechanical protection by excluding undesirable molecules. Eventually, when sporulation is complete, the mature spore is liberated by lysis of the mother cell (Piggot and Hilbert, 2004).

Even though spores are resting bodies and are formed under conditions of starvation and stress, they persistently search their external environment for various types of germinants, which are molecules that trigger spore germination. Germinants are normally divided into two types: nutrient and nonnutrient. Nutrient types include mainly sugars, amino acids, and so on and nonnutrient types include other driving forces like temperature, pressure, and so on, that allow spores to germinate and thus convert them into metabolically active vegetative cells. Spores possess the unique ability to recognize stereoisomerically distinct forms of nutrient germinants (Tehri et al., 2017).

PARAMETERS FOR DETECTING SPORE GERMINATION

Germination is an irreversible event; therefore, germination can be detected by the use of different markers known as physiobiochemical, or signature markers of the germination process. These markers can directly correlate changes in properties, occurring during germination, to the process of germination (Foster and Johnstone, 1990; Ferencko et al., 2004). Such various markers have been used successfully as unique tools for assessing germination in bacterial spores either qualitatively or quantitatively. These markers mainly include measurement of absorbance, Adenosine triphosphate (ATP), di-pic-o-lin-ic acid, enzymes, heat resistance, refractility, and nucleic acids.

DIFFERENT APPROACHES USED FOR DEVELOPMENT OF ASSAYS EMPLOYING BACTERIAL SPORES

Four different types of approaches have mainly been used for the development of spor-based biosensors for detection of different contaminants. Spores have been used to target different analytes, like antibiotics and aflatoxin M1 in milk (Singh et al., 2013; Khan, 2014), on the basis of inhibition of the germination process. A germinogenic substrate based concept has also been used to detect various pathogens such as *E. coli*, *L. monocytogenes*, *Enterococci*, and so on (Thakur, 2014). This principle of sugar uptake has been used to detect pathogens. Target bacteria present in the sample are incubated with selected sugars and substrates. Subsequently, germination in spores is measured with these same sugars and substrates alone and in combination with pathogen. The reduced rate of germination in the spores can be detected by the significant uptake of sugars by target pathogen. However, spores are germinated fully when they are allowed to incubate in the presence of sugars only, without pathogen. This principle has been used successfully to detect and differentiate *E. coli* and *E. coli* O157:H7 on the basis of sorbitol and gentiobiose percentage uptake in milk system. The developed spore based assay was highly specific because uptake signals for these pathogens for combination with different sugars/ or substrates were exclusive and did not coincide with any of the gram-positive and gram-negative bacterial strains when evaluated in buffer systems (Yadav, 2014).

SPORE BASED ASSAYS FOR DETECTION OF DIFFERENT CONTAMINANTS IN MILK

Spores of different species of bacilli have been used as biosensing elements to detect various contaminants of microbial and nonmicrobial origin (Table 19.1). The potential of developed spore-based biosensors has been evaluated by determining the sensors' suitability in terms of their application in the analysis of contaminants in real food samples, that is, milk and milk products. The design and analytical performance of developed sensors employing spores as biorecognition molecule for different types of contaminants are explained below.

DETECTION OF NONMICROBIAL CONTAMINANTS

Pesticides

Illness outbreaks caused by pesticides in contaminated food products, including milk and milk products, are well documented in the literature. This has led to regulations setting MRL levels for pesticides in different food matrices. To meet stringent regulations, the dairy industry needs sensitive alternatives for the standard conventional chromatographic methods for detecting pesticides because these methods include lengthy protocols and a large infrastructure. Attempts have been made to develop spore germination and enzyme inhibition based sensors to detect pesticide residues (toxic xenobiotics) in milk. The working principle of this spore based sensor is based on the inhibition of enzymes released during germination of spores by the presence of pesticides in milk and its products. The signal produced due to inhibition in enzyme activity by the target pesticide was captured by the addition of a chromogenic substrate in tube, and fluorogenic substrate in 96 micro well plate/micro well chip. This work explored the analytical potential of bacterial spores in terms of their use as a source of marker enzymes for pesticide analysis, and the detection of pesticides in contaminated milk samples within 2.0–2.5 h at ≥MRL values (Thakur et al., 2014; Gopaul, 2015; Kumar et al., 2015; Tehri, 2016).

Antibiotics

Antibiotics are widely used for the treatment of diseases in livestock. They are used specifically to treat mastitis in dairy animals which is known to cause reduction in milk production (Mesele et al., 2012). Currently, approximately 80% of all food-producing animals receive medication for part or most of their lives (Lee et al., 2001). The improper use of antibiotics may result in its occurrence in milk, which has several harmful effects, including interference with starter activity leading to improper acid production and off-flavors in fermented milk products and ripened

TABLE 19.1

Spore-Based Biosensors for Detection of Different Contaminants in Milk System

Type of Contaminant	Principle	Biorecognition Molecule	Transducer	Parameter for Detection	Detection Limit	Time of Analysis	References
Antibiotics	Spore germination inhibition	*B. stearothermophilus* Spores	Colorimetric, (Naked eyes)	DPA	≥MRL	3.0–3.15 h	Kumar et al. (2006)
Pesticides	Inhibition of enzyme released on germination	*B. megaterium* Spores	Colorimetric, (Naked eyes) and Fluorescence	Esterase	≥MRL	2.0–2.15 h	Kumar et al. (2015); Tehri (2016)
Listeria monocytogenes	Germinogenic substrate concept	*B. megaterium* Spores	Fluorescence reader and EMCCD	GS-methyl β-D-gluco-pyranoside; PE-β-D-glucosidase; SE-esterase	5.0 log (96 well plate) 3.0 log (Biochip)	4 h (+12 h enrichment); 2 h (+8 h enrichment)	Balhara et al. (2013)
***E. coli/E. coli* O157:H7**	% Sugar uptake	*B. megaterium* Spores	Fluorescence reader and EMCCD	Sorbitol and gentiobiose	5.0 log (96 well plate) 3.5 log (Biochip)	2.30 h (+6 h enrichment); 1.30 h (+4 h enrichment)	Kumar et al. (2014)
Enterococci	Germinogenic substrate concept	*B. megaterium* Spores	Fluorescence reader and EMCCD	GS-; esculin PE-β-D-glucosidase; SE-esterase	5.6 log (96 well plate) 5.0 log (Biochip)	2.30 h (+10 h enrichment); 45 min (+8 h enrichment)	Kumar et al. (2012)

Note: GS—germinogenic substrate; PE—enzyme from pathogen; SE—enzyme from spores.

cheeses. Allergic reactions can occur in highly sensitive consumers, which can lead to potential carcinogenicity, mutagenicity, and long-term toxic effects (Epstein et al., 2000). The presence of antibiotic residues in milk can be attributed to a number of reasons, including indiscriminate use of antibiotics, lack of medication records for livestock, use of unapproved drugs, contaminated milking equipment, purchase of treated cows, and failure to observe the proper withdrawal period in lactating cows. The presence of antibiotics in milk has created alarm in the dairy sector. Hence, there is increasing need to detect antibiotics in milk and as early as possible, before the contaminated milk reaches consumers.

A number of test kits are presently available in the market for the detection of antibiotics, and microbial inhibitor tests have gained global popularity for the detection of antibiotic residues in milk (Mitchell et al., 1998). Commercial test kits based on the microbial inhibition principle include Delvo SP, BR, Copan, Charm Farm, and Charm Aim 96, as well as the multiple-drug-resistant (MDR) test kit developed by NDRI, Karnal (Kumar et al., 2006). These tests have a number of advantages, including cost effectiveness and ease of use. However, long incubation periods are hindering their performance for farms and manufacturing units. Various rapid methods have also been developed to test for antibiotic residues, for example, the microbial receptor assay (Charm II assay), enzyme colorimetric assay (Penzym test), receptor binding assay (SNAP test), immunoassay (Fluorophos beta screen test), and immunochromatographic assay (ROSA test).

Spores based detection systems are inexpensive, rapid, and easy to perform, and they require almost negligible infrastructure, have a long shelf life, and are easy to produce in the laboratory. An analytical system using dormant spores as biosensors for broad spectrum detection of antibiotic residues in milk has been developed and patented (Kumar et al., 2006).

A cost-effective and rapid test kit, one that can be used at both farm and manufacturing level, has been developed. A novel rapid enzyme spore based assay can detect antibiotics in milk within 2 hours and 15 minutes. The assay is based on the specific enzyme substrate reaction, which can be observed visually using a chromogenic substrate. Different *B. stearothermophilus* strains were screened for marker enzymes, and strain 69 was found to have the highest α-D-glucosidase activity. This strain and substrate were selected for the assay. Five different media were evaluated for spore germination, and AK medium was found to be the most suitable. With some modifications, it also became cost effective. The optimum spore concentration was found to be 100 ± 10 µL, volume of germination medium 200 ± 10 µL, chromogen concentration 100 ± 10 µL, quantity of milk 100 ± 10 µL, and temperature/time combination of spore heating $100 \pm 1°C/15 \pm 1$ min. The limit of detection of different antibiotics (namely, gentamycin, neomycin, streptomycin, kanamycin, amoxicillin, penicillin, ampicillin, cephazolin, cephalexin, oxacillin, tetracycline, erythromycin, sulfadimidine, and chloramphenicol) was set after spiking milk at MRL levels set by Codex. The assay was also checked for the inhibitory effects of detergents, aflatoxin M1, and pesticides and was found to be insensitive to the assay. The assay was also evaluated with milk samples and the assay was similar to Charm and ROSA. The novel assay has been patented and can now be part of routine monitoring of antibiotics in milk for the dairy industry.

A rapid method was also developed in our lab for the specific detection of β-lactam antibiotics. The β-lactam is one of the major groups of antibiotics found in milk that induces β-lactamase enzyme production in some of the spore forming bacteria (i.e., *B. cereus* and *B. licheniformis*). Enzyme production is proportional to the concentration of inducer present in milk, and this hypothesis was the approach used to detect the presence of β-lactam antibiotics in milk and milk products. Three strains of *B. cereus* and one strain of *B. licheniformis* were screened for β-lactamase production using an iodometric method. Enzyme induction was greater in *B. cereus* NCDC 66 and less in *B. licheniformis* NCDC 266 by MRL doses of six antibiotic residues belonging to β-lactam group (amoxicillin, penicillin, ampicillin, cephazolin, cephalexin, cloxacillin). In addition, enzyme induction was greater in spores compared to vegetative cells. The analytical system was validated using milk samples spiked with the six different β-lactam antibiotics and compared with Association of Official Analytical Chemists (AOAC) approved Charm 6602 system; consistent results were obtained.

DETECTION OF MICROBIAL CONTAMINANTS

Enterococci

Enterococci are important indicator organisms for monitoring the microbiological quality of milk. They are gram-positive bacteria of intestinal origin and hence are good indicator organisms for fecal contamination and the hygiene status of the milk supply. The enumeration of *Enterococci*, because of its association with food, feed, and the environment, has become an important issue in dried products, especially infant formula. Earlier *Enterococci* were thought to be harmless commensals, but they are now recognized as serious nosocomial pathogens. They also cause infections of nonhospitalized populations because of growing antibiotic resistance (Murray, 1990). The control of *Enterococci* constitutes a special challenge because of their robust nature, wide distribution, and stability in the external environment. In the dairy environment, their sources include the dairy water supply, working personnel, and dairy equipment (Batish et al., 1986).

Conventional detection methods rely on specific media such as citrate azide agar for enterococcal isolation in dairy products. These methods involve multiple steps like selective enrichment on liquid and solid media, followed by biochemical screening and serological confirmation. These tests are reference standard methods, but they are time consuming. Hence, rapid and low-cost techniques with bioanalytical sensors utilizing enzymes are needed. Enzyme-based detection methods are rapid, sensitive, and less time consuming compared to traditional culture-based methods. It is useful to assay directly the activity of enzymes for the detection of microorganisms (Manafi, 1998). These methods can detect viable but nonculturable cells (VNCs) and can be used for real-time monitoring. The majority of *Enterococci* spp. produce β-D-glucosidase enzyme (β-GLU), and substrates such as 4-methylumbelliferyl-β-D-glucosidase and indolyl-β-D-glucosidase have been used consistently in the detection of *Enterococci* using chromogenic or fluorogenic substrate. Based on this approach, partial development of medium for selective enrichment of *Enterococci* and its enumeration in milk by employing an enzyme-based biosensing system was carried out in our lab (Thakur, 2010; Kaur, 2011).

Spores can be used effectively as biosensors for tracking the presence of *Enterococci* in milk because of their ability to sense environmental changes by using molecular mechanisms that transform into rapidly growing cells. A spore germination based bioassay was developed for the rapid detection of *Enterococci* using β-D-glucosidase as a marker enzyme and its specific action on the marker enzyme substrate. The system consisted of target bacteria, microbial spores suspended in buffer containing a marker enzyme substrate and diacetate fluorescein (DAF), a fluorogenic compound that produces fluorogenic signal when hydrolyzed by acetyl esterase enzyme released as a result of spore germination. The quantification of fluorescent signals produced indicated the presence of *Enterococci* in milk. Eight *B. megaterium* strains were screened for acetyl esterase activity. MTCC-3 was the most prominent and was selected for spore production. The optimal working conditions for the assay were incubation time (2 h), concentration of esculin (5 mM), and volume of spore suspension. The limit of detection (LOD) was determined with pure cells. The sensitivity of the bioassay was determined by immobilizing spores on a sensor disc by air drying in an incubator at 37°C/3.30 h. The lowest detection limit was 5.66 log counts in 2.30 h. The bioassay was also carried out by immobilizing spores (4.71 log counts) on a gold chip for its miniaturization based on integrated optical density. The sensitivity of the assay on the gold chip was improved to 5.43 log counts, and the assay time was also reduced to 45 min. The optimized spore based assay on the sensor disc was also carried out with milk spiked with *Enterococci*, following the protocol already developed in our lab. The developed bioassay offered better sensitivity, that is, 5.66 log counts compared to 7.52 log counts with Esculin Based Sodium Azide Medium (EBSAM) medium and reduction in time up to 2–3 h.

Listeria

Members of *Listeria* spp. are gram-positive, facultative anaerobic, catalase positive, and oxidase negative bacteria. Currently, the genus contains the species *L.monocytogenes*, *L. ivanovii*, *L. innocua*, *L. seeligeri*, *L. welshimeri*, *L. murrayi*, and *L. grayi*. Two species have been identified more recently, namely, *L. marthii*, from the natural environment of the Finger Lakes National Forest, United States, by Graves et al. (2010), and *L. rocourtiae* from precut lettuce by Leclercq et al. (2010). Out of the nine species, only two, *L. monocytogenes* and *L. ivanovii*, are pathogenic. *L. monocytogenes* is known to be a food-borne human pathogen causing listeriosis, whereas *L. ivanovii* is an animal pathogen found mainly in sheep and cattle. *Listeria monocytogenes* has gained a lot of attention due to numerous multinational outbreaks in dairy products that have resulted in a high mortality rate and thus has become a major public health concern (Jamali et al., 2013). *L. monocytogenes* is a serious pathogen associated with milk and milk products; it causes a high incidence of listeriosis due to increased consumption of raw milk and dairy products prepared from unpasteurized milk such as cheese and ice cream. Dairy products have been linked to both invasive and noninvasive listeriosis outbreaks. Invasive listeriosis causes meningoencephalitis, encephalitis, sepsis, and abortion and has a high mortality rate (20%–30%). Invasive listeriosis occurs mainly in people belonging to specific risk groups, including newborn infants, the elderly, pregnant women, and immune-compromised persons. Noninvasive listerosis causes fever, diarrhea, muscle pain, headache, nausea, vomiting, and abdominal pain in healthy adults (Parisi et al., 2013). Early detection is a very good way to counter this harmful pathogen and to prevent outbreaks. Sensitive and specific methods are needed to detect this pathogen. The existing methods for detection of *L. monocytogenes* in dairy products still rely on conventional ISO: 11290-1:1996 method, which requires at least a 5- to 7-day protocol for its identification (Curtis and Lee, 1995). An assay based on germinant–germinogenic substrate, where specific marker enzymes act on germinogenic substrates and release germinants, was developed. These germinants trigger spores to germinate, and the enzymatic signal resulting from target bacteria after their selective enrichment is captured using fluorogen on micro well biochip/96 microwell plate. Marker enzymes were screened in *Bacillus megaterium* 2949 spores used as biosensing agents based on a germination signal. A number of germinants and germinogenic substrates specific for targeted marker enzymes were screened. These germinogenic substrates were optimized for different parameters for assay development, and the optimized conditions included the following: 20 µL of *L. monocytogenes* (5.0 ± 0.5 log cells), 10 µL of spore suspension (6.0 ± 0.5 log spores), and 4.0 ± 0.30 h of incubation for assay at 37°C. The optimized protocol was transformed into 96 well plate spore germination based assay giving a germination signal. The LOD of the developed assay in buffer was found to be 5.0 ± 0.5 log cells/mL in 4.0 ± 0.3 h with each germinogenic substrate. The sensitivity of the assay was also established in milk after selective enrichment of target bacteria at 1.0 ± 0.14 log cells/mL in Listeria Selective Enrichment Medium (LSEM) for 16.0 ± 1.0 h. The assay was further miniaturized on micro well biochip to develop spore-based biosensor by adding 0.5 µL of reaction mixture. The measurements were done based on Integrated Optical Density (IOD) signals captured using the Electron Multiplying Charged Couple Device (EMCCD) as a transducer. The spore-based biosensor was specific for *L. monocytogenes* and was sensitive enough to detect 1.0 ± 0.14 log cells/mL within 14.0 ± 1.0 h. The developed assay was validated via conventional method ISO11290-1:1996, lab-developed method two-stage enzyme assay, and AOAC approved VIDAS® bioMérieux system by screening 25 milk samples each of raw and pasteurized milk samples procured from different sources.

E. coli

E. coli are gram-negative short rods commonly found in the lower intestine of warm-blooded organisms. They are considered part of the normal flora of the intestinal tract of humans and other warm-blooded animals (Drasar and Hill, 1974). Pathogenic *E. coli*, especially *E. coli* 0157:H7, is a serious and high-risk food-borne pathogen. *E. coli* serotype O157:H7 is a rare strain of *E. coli* that produces large quantities of one or more related and potent toxins that cause severe damage to the lining of the intestine. The consumption of unpasteurized and raw milk is a recognized risk factor for diarrheal illnesses due to bacteria such as *Campylobacter*, *Salmonella*, and Shiga toxin-producing *E. coli* (STEC) including *E. coli* O157:H7. Human infection is associated with the consumption of a number of contaminated milk products such as raw milk, yogurt, and cheese. Its detection is essential to prevent disease outbreaks. Earlier conventional methods, considered the gold standard for food-borne pathogen detection, were used; they rely on specific media to enumerate and isolate viable bacterial cells in food (Gracias and McKillip, 2004). These methods are very sensitive and inexpensive, and they can give qualitative information; they involve the basic steps of pre-enrichment, selective enrichment, selective plating, biochemical screening, and serological confirmation (Bhunia, 2008). These methods are very reliable but they are lengthy, cumbersome, and often ineffective because they are not compatible with the speed at which the products are manufactured and the short shelf life of products. To overcome the challenges of time and sensitivity, rapid methods are needed to give instant or real-time results. Conventional culture-based techniques require 3–4 days for confirmation. The developed spore germination assay involved the use of selected marker sugars that trigger spore germination and release of marker enzymes that produce fluorescence signals. Different strains of *B. megaterium* (spores/cells), and *E. coli* were screened. Different sugars and nitrogenous compounds were screened as germinant. The assay conditions were optimized with different concentrations of sugars as germinant (100–300 mM), volumes of spore suspension (20 µL/6.65 $\pm$ 0.25 log CFU), incubation time (3.00 h at 37°C), and inoculum level of target bacteria (20 µL/7.02 $\pm$ 0.21 log CFU). The sensitivity of the assay was found to be 5.24 $\pm$ 0.25 log count with detection time of 3.00 h after pre-enrichment (5.00 $\pm$ 0.30 h) of pure cells/spiked milk in *E. coli* selective medium (EC-SM) at 37°C. The selectivity of the bioassay was checked with different gram-negative and gram-positive contaminants. The assay was also evaluated with milk samples under field conditions, and positive signals were achieved. The assay was further miniaturized on a biochip by adding 0.5 µL of reaction mixture, and measurement was based on IOD values using the EMCCD system.

CONCLUSION

Using spore-based biosensors for detection of a varying range of contaminants offers many advantages over existing methods. These biosensors have been reported to be highly sensitive, reliable, user friendly, and cost effective. They have a long shelf life and are suitable for their on-site application for detection of contaminants. This chapter highlighted the importance of bacterial spores for their use as biorecognition molecules. Apart from contaminants discussed herein, spores hold great promises for targeting a broad range of other contaminants. These contaminants may include different groups of pesticides, heavy metals, detergents, sanitizers, spoilage types, pathogenic microorganisms and several others that may be important for public health. Spore-based sensing technologies can be developed to target many emerging contaminants in different types of food matrices, including milk and milk products, in order to ensure food safety and high quality.

REFERENCES

Balhara, M., Kumar, N., Thakur, G., Raghu, H. V., Singh, N., et al., 2013. A Novel enzyme substrate based bioassay for real time detection of *Listeria monocytogenes* in milk. Indian Patent Reg. No. 1357/DEL/2013.

Batish, V. K., Chander, H., and Ranganathan, B., 1986. Enterocin typing of enterococci isolated from dried infant foods. *J Dairy Sci* 69:983–989.

Bhunia, A. K., 2008. Biosensors and bio-based methods for the separation and detection of food borne pathogens. *Adv Food Nutr Res* 54:1–44.

Curtis, G., and Lee, W., 1995. Culture media and methods for the isolation of *Listeria monocytogenes*. *Int J Food Microbiol* 26:1–13.

Drasar, B. S., and Hill, M. J., 1974. The distribution of bacterial in the intestine. In *Human Intestinal Flora*, London, UK: Academic Press, pp. 36–43.

Epstein, J. B., Chong, S., and Lee, N. D., 2000. A survey of antibiotics used in dentistry. *J Am Dent Assoc* 131:1600–1609.

Ferencko, L., Cote, M. A., and Rotman, B., 2004. Esterase activity as a novel parameter of spore germination in *Bacillus anthracis*. *Biochem Biophys Res Commun* 319:854–858.

Foster, S. J., and Johnstone, K., 1990. Pulling the trigger: The mechanism of bacterial spore germination. *Mol Microbiol* 4:137–141.

Gopaul, R., 2015. Paper-strip based spore sensor for pesticide residues in milk. Doctoral Thesis Submitted to NDRI, Karnal.

Graves, L. M., Helsel, L. O., Steigerwalt, A. G., Morey, R. E., Daneshvar, M. I., et al., 2010. *Listeria marthii* sp. nov., isolated from the natural environment, Finger Lakes National Forest. *Int J Syst Evol Microbiol* 60:1280–1288.

Gracias, K. S., and McKillip, J. L., 2004. A review of conventional detection and enumeration methods for pathogenic bacteria in food. *Can J Microbiol* 50:883–890.

Jamali, H., Radmehr, B., and Thong, K. L., 2013. Prevalence, characterisation and antimicrobial resistance of *Listeria* species and *Listeria monocytogenes* isolates from raw milk in farm bulk tanks. *Food Control* 34:121–125.

Kaur, G., 2011. Spore germination: An innovative approach for detecting Enterococci in milk. MSc. Thesis. Submitted to NDRI, Karnal.

Khan, A., 2014. Development of enzyme-spore sensor for monitoring antibiotic residues in milk. Doctoral Thesis. Submitted to NDRI, Karnal.

Kumar, N., Kaur, G., Thakur, G., Raghu, H. V., Singh, N., et al., 2012. Real time detection of Enterococci in dairy foods using spore germination based bioassay. Indian Patent Reg. No. 119/DEL/2012.

Kumar, N., Lawaniya, R., Yadav, A., Arora, B., Vishweswaraiah, H. R., et al., 2014. Marker enzymes and spore germination based assay for detection of E. coli in milk and milk products. Indian Patent Reg. No. 2214/DEL/2014.

Kumar, N., Sawant, S., Malik, R. K., and Patil, G. R., 2006. Development of analytical process for detection of antibiotic residues in milk using bacterial spores as biosensor. Indian Patent Reg. No. 1479/DEL/2006.

Kumar, N., Thakur, G., Raghu, H. V., Singh, N., Sharma, P. K., et al., 2013. Bacterial spore based biosensor for detection of contaminants in milk. *J Food Process Technol* 4:277.

Kumar, N., Tehri, N., Gopaul, R., Sharma, P. K., Kumar, B., et al., 2015. Rapid spores-enzyme based miniaturised assay (s) for detection of pesticide residues. Indian Patent Reg. No. 3819/DEL/2015.

Leclercq, A., Clermont, D., Bizet, C., Grimont, P. A. D., Le Fleche Mateos, A., et al., 2010. *Listeria rocourtiae* sp. nov. *Int J Sys Evol Microbiol* 60:2210–2214.

Lee, H. J., Lee, M. H., and Ruy, P. D., 2001. Public health risks: Chemical and antibiotic residues. *Asian-Aust J Anim Sci* 14:402–413.

Manafi, M., 1998. Culture media containing fluorogenic and chromogenic substrates. De ware (n) Chemicus. *Int J Food Microbiol* 28:12–17.

Mesele, A., Belay, E., Kassaye, A., Yifat, D., Kebede, A., and Desie, S., 2012. Major causes of mastitis and associated risk factors in small holder dairy cows in Shashemene, Southern Ethiopia. *Afr J Agri Res* 7:3513–3518.

Mitchell, J. M., Griffiths, M. W., McEwen, S. A., McNab, W. B., and Yee, A. J., 1998. Antimicrobial drug residues in milk and meat: Cause, concerns, prevalence, regulation, tests and test performance. *J Food Prot* 61:742–756.

Murray, B. E., 1990. The life and times of Enterococcus. *Clin Microbiol Rev* 3:45–45.

Parisi, A., Latorre, L., Fraccalvieri, R., Miccolupo, A., Normanno, G., et al., 2013. Occurrence of *Listeria* spp. in dairy plants in Southern Italy and molecular sub typing of isolates using AFLP. *Food Control* 29:91–97.

Piggot, P. J., and Hilbert, D. W., 2004. Sporulation of *Bacillus subtilis. Curr Opin Microbiol* 7:579–586.

Singh, N. A., Kumar, N., Raghu, H. V., Sharma, P. K., Singh, V. K., et al., 2013. Spore inhibition-based enzyme substrate assay for monitoring of aflatoxin M1 in milk. *Toxicol Environ Chem* 95:765–777.

Tehri, N., 2016. Spore based sensor for pesticide residues in milk. Doctoral Thesis Submitted to NDRI, Karnal.

Tehri, N., Kumar, N., Raghu, H. V., Thakur, G., and Sharma, P. K., 2017. Role of stereo-specific nature of germinants in *Bacillus megaterium* spores germination. *3 Biotech* 7:259.

Thakur, G., 2010. Development of off-line enzyme substrate based assay for monitoring Enterococci in milk. M.Sc Thesis. Submitted to NDRI, Karnal.

Thakur, G., 2014. Development of spore based biosensor for detection of *Listeria monocytogenes* in milk. Doctoral Thesis. Submitted to NDRI, Karnal.

Thakur, G., Raghu, H. V., Tehri, N., Kumar, N., Yadav, A., and Malik, R. K., 2014. Biochip based detection-An emerging tool for ensuring safe milk: A review. *J Innov Biol* 1:147–154.

Yadav, A., 2014. Development of spore germination based bioassay for detection of *E. coli* 0157:H7 in milk and milk products. Doctoral Thesis. Submitted to NDRI, Karnal.

Index

Note: Page numbers followed by f and t refer to figures and tables respectively.